S0-DPD-559

Electron Microscope Laboratory
Department of Pathology
MCV Hospitals

Ultrastructural Pathology
of the Cell and Matrix

By the same author:

Fine Structure of Synovial Joints
Diagnostic Ultrastructural Pathology
Diagnostic Electron Microscopy of Tumours, 2nd edn

To Edna
My wife and grand companion
With unabated love and esteem

Ultrastructural Pathology of the Cell and Matrix

A Text and Atlas of Physiological and Pathological Alterations in the Fine Structure of Cellular and Extracellular Components

Third Edition

Volume I

Feroze N. Ghadially

MB BS (Bom.), MB BS (Lond.), MD, PhD, DSc (Lond.), Hon. DSc (Guelph), FRCPath., FRCP(C), FRSA
Isaak Walton Killam Laureate of the Canada Council, W.S. Lindsay Professor of the College of Medicine and Professor of Pathology, University of Saskatchewan, Saskatoon, Canada

Formerly Reader in Neoplastic Diseases and Senior Lecturer in Experimental Pathology, University of Sheffield, England

Butterworths
London Boston Singapore Sydney Toronto Wellington

All rights reserved. No part of this publication may be
reproduced or transmitted in any form or by any means,
including photocopying and recording, without the written
permission of the copyright holder, application for which
should be addressed to the Publishers, or in accordance with
the provisions of the Copyright Act 1956 (as amended), or
under the terms of any licence permitting limited copying
issued by the Copyright Licensing Agency, 7 Ridgmount
Street, London WC1E 7AE, England. Such written permission
must also be obtained before any part of this publication is
stored in a retrieval system of any nature.

Any person who does any unauthorized act in relation to this
publication may be liable to criminal prosecution and civil
claims for damages.

This book is sold subject to the Standard Conditions of Sale of
Net Books and may not be re-sold in the UK below the net
price given by the Publishers in their current price list.

First published 1975
Reprinted 1977, 1978
Second edition 1982
Third edition, in two volumes, 1988

© F. N. Ghadially, 1988

British Library Cataloguing in Publication Data

Ghadially, Feroze N. (Feroze Novroji), *1920–*
    Ultrastructural pathology of the cell and
    matrix.—3rd ed.
    1. Animals. Cells. Ultrastructure.
    Pathology
    I. Title II. Killam, Isaac Walton
    III. Lindsay, W.S.
    591.87′65

    ISBN 0–407–01571–X Vol. 1

    ISBN 0–407–01572–8 Vol. 2

Library of Congress Cataloging-in-Publication Data

Ghadially, Feroze N. (Feroze Novroji), 1920–
    Ultrastructural pathology of the cell and matrix : a text and
atlas of physiological and pathological alterations in the fine
structure of cellular and extracellular components / Feroze N.
Ghadially. — 3rd ed.
        p.   cm.
    Includes bibliographies and index.
    ISBN 0–407–01570–1 (set) :
    ISBN 0–407–01571–X (v. 1). ISBN 0–407–01572–8 (v. 2)
    1. Pathology, Cellular. 2. Ultrastructure (Biology)—Atlases.
3. Diagnosis, Electron microscopic—Atlases. I. Title.
    [DNLM: 1. Cells—pathology. 2. Cells—pathology—atlases.
3. Cells—ultrastructure. 4. Cells—ultrastructure—atlases. QZ 4
G411u]
    RB25.G4   1988
    616.07′582—dc19
    DNLM/DLC
    for Library of Congress   88–22192
                                                                      CIP

Typeset by Scribe Design, Gillingham, Kent
Printed and bound in Great Britain by Butler and Tanner, Frome, Somerset

Preface to the third edition

The laudatory reviews and warm reception accorded to the second edition of this book have encouraged me to produce a larger third edition which deals with many more ultrastructural changes and lesions. The task of cataloguing and classifying them is endless as David Lagunoff surmises in his review (*Journal of the American Medical Association* 1982, **248**, 1246). He states: 'For his inhospitality to Perseus, Atlas was forced to bear the burden of the heavens through eternity. Sisyphus, for his greater transgression, became responsible for repeatedly pushing a large stone up a hill and on nearing the summit having it escape his grasp and roll down. I don't know if Ghadially's task in producing his book was freely assumed or thrust upon him, but his labors seem closer to those of Sisyphus than Atlas. He has (in his own words) directed his efforts to "cataloguing, classifying, describing and illustrating virtually every intracellular lesion." Each time he must think he is about to roll the last abnormality up his mountainous catalog, a new group of changes comes rolling out of the journals.'

The task of producing this work was self-imposed in the mistaken belief that it would be quick and easy: by the time I discovered otherwise it was too late to turn back. I have, however, learnt that there is no better way of learning a subject than writing a book about it!

A substantial number of new ultrastructural changes and lesions have come 'rolling out of the journals'. Incorporation of this new knowledge has been accomplished by adding 43 new sections and enlarging and rewriting several old ones. The remaining sections have been revised and updated. The number of: (1) pages has increased from about 950 to over 1300; (2) sections from 186 to 229; (3) electron micrographs from 885 to 1227; (4) line drawings from one to 26; and (5) references from about 3500 to a little over 5800. I trust these additions and changes will enhance the value of this book to those who examine pathological tissues with the electron microscope.

F. N. Ghadially

Preface to the second edition

Ultrastructural Pathology of the Cell and Matrix is a revised and expanded second edition of *Ultrastructural Pathology of the Cell*. The change in title is necessitated by the addition of a chapter on the extracellular matrix (extracellular components). This was done on the advice of colleagues who felt that the usefulness of the book was marred by the omission of such common structures as collagen and elastic fibres.

I wrote the first edition of this book with the aim of cataloguing, classifying, describing and illustrating virtually every intracellular lesion within the covers of a modest-sized volume. It seemed to me that although this goal was clearly impossible to attain, striving to attain it might produce a useful book. The net result was that the first edition was never 'finished', it had to go to press when it had grown to a size and price apparently incompatible with economic viability.

The unexpected demand for the book, leading to two reprintings of the first edition have allayed our (publisher's and author's) fears, and encouraged the production of a larger work that comes closer to the original goal or, to be more accurate, the expanded goal which now includes various extracellular components.

Altogether 56 completely new sections have been added. Many old sections have been enlarged and others rewritten or revised, and the book has grown from 560 pages to nearly 1000 pages. The number of illustrations has increased from 520 to 885 and the references from about 1800 to a little over 3500. I trust that this has enhanced the value and utility of this book to those who use the electron microscope to examine pathological tissues.

F. N. Ghadially

Preface to the first edition

There can hardly be a disease or pathological process where electron microscopy has not added new details and dimensions to existing knowledge. The innumerable published papers and books on the ultrastructure of tissues altered by disease or experimental procedures bear eloquent testimony to the many major contributions made by this technique.

Although the student interested in the pathology of certain systems, organs and tissues such as liver (David, 1964), muscle (Mair and Tomé, 1972), synovial joints (Ghadially and Roy, 1969), kidney (Dalton and Haguenau, 1967) and peripheral nervous system (Babel *et al.*, 1970) is now catered for and excellent books dealing with the ultrastructure of normal cells and tissues are available (e.g. Fawcett, 1966; Porter and Bonneville, 1973); Lentz, 1971; Rhodin, 1974), there is as yet no book from which one may learn in a systematic fashion about the numerous changes that occur in cellular organelles and inclusions as a result of disease or experimental procedures. On confronting an unfamiliar or unknown morphological alteration in some particular cellular structure the questions that arise are: (1) has this been seen before? (2) if so, in what situations has such a change been seen? (3) what is the significance of the change? and (4) how can one retrieve information on this point from the formidable, scattered literature on the ultrastructure of normal and pathological tissues?

It is my hope that this book will help to answer such questions and serve as a brief textbook and atlas of cellular pathology at the ultrastructural level. Within its covers I have collected, classified, described and illustrated various alterations that are known to occur in cellular organelles and inclusions as a result of changing physiological states, diseases and experimental situations.

In keeping with the traditional practice adopted in many past pathology texts, each chapter commences with a discourse on normal structure and function. This is followed by essays devoted to various morphological alterations that have hitherto been witnessed. The introduction and preliminary essays on well known normal structures (e.g. nucleus and mitochondria) are, of necessity, brief. They do little more than set the scene and outline the classification and nomenclature employed. The advanced electron microscopist may find that some of the passages in these essays are of a rather elementary nature, but this material is included on the assumption that some readers may not be too familiar with current electron microscopic concepts and topics. Less well known normal structures (e.g. rod-shaped tubular bodies and nuclear bodies) are dealt with more fully, for information on such structures is often not easy to find and unfamiliarity with such structures is likely to lead to errors of interpretation.

The sections dealing with morphological alterations and lesions follow a fairly standard pattern in most instances. A brief introduction dealing with matters such as definition, nomenclature, correlations with light microscopy, and historical aspects of the subject is followed by a morphological description supported by accompanying illustrations. After this comes a section where I have listed the sites and situations in which the particular morphological alteration has been seen and the authors who have reported its occurrence. This section often contains numerous references. (Some readers may find these lists irksome, but they are essential for the research worker and student seeking further information.) Then follows a discussion and interpretation of the morphological change under survey. The principle I have followed here is to present as many known theories and ideas as possible even though I may not be in sympathy with some of them. I have also often indicated what I have come to think about the matter as a result of my own studies and reading of the literature. However, I do not feel that an author should judge every issue, and I have, at times, done little more than report as faithfully as I can the views propounded by others. Not all essays follow the above-mentioned pattern for there are instances where the story is told more profitably within a different format. For example, instead of devoting a section to every change in mitochondrial morphology which has been suspected as representing an involuting or degenerating mitochondrion, I have collected these changes into a section entitled 'mitochondrial involution and elimination'.

One of the functions I would like this book to serve is as a gateway to the relevant literature. Since this is not a book primarily devoted to normal structure and function (even though a substantial number of pages are devoted to such matters), the references in sections dealing with well known normal structures are somewhat sparse. When dealing with little known normal structures or with alterations and lesions, I have tried to include virtually every reference on the subject that I am aware of. When such citations are few they are all presented in the text; when too many, I have included review articles and also tried to include the earliest and latest paper on the topic.

Although the format is designed primarily for those who examine pathological tissues with the electron microscope, I hope that this book will also be of interest to the teacher of pathology and the practising pathologist. This book is not for the individual who has no knowledge of cell fine structure at all (there can be few who fall into this category today!) nor is it for the expert ultrastructural pathologist. It is addressed to the much larger intermediate group of workers who may wish to acquire a basic knowledge of general ultrastructural pathology on which they may pursue their own special interests with greater confidence and a wider understanding.

The teacher of pathology attempting to relate classic pathology with the now familiar concepts of cell ultrastructure has had to search through a wide variety of books and journals and at best may only find patchy information. The hospital pathologist, similarly, has up to now had little reason to embark on the exhausting pursuit through the published literature, often in journals which are not on his usual reading list, in search of clues which might lead to a better understanding, or an earlier or more precise diagnosis of human disease. However, in some fields such as the interpretation of the liver, renal and muscle biopsy and the diagnosis of viral and storage diseases and certain tumours the electron microscope is already proving its worth. The scope of electron microscopy will undoubtedly extend into wider areas of diagnostic histopathology. Further, more and more papers in journals of pathology now incorporate the results of ultrastructural studies, and the reader unfamiliar with the range and limitations of electron microscope technology may well be at a loss in attempting to interpret published work.

Today it is not possible to present to the student an up-to-date account of many pathological processes and disease states without discussing ultrastructural changes. Cell injury, cloudy swelling, necrosis, fatty degeneration of the liver, the detoxification of many drugs by the liver, brown atrophy of the heart and lipofuscin, pigmentary disorders of the skin and melanomas, haemorrhage, haemosiderin, erythrophagocytosis and siderosomes, glycogen storage diseases, lipoidoses, Wilson's disease, silicosis, rheumatoid arthritis and melanosis coli are all better understood by virtue of a knowledge of the underlying fine structural changes.

Correlations between light and electron microscopic findings are singularly interesting and satisfying and I have lost no opportunity of dwelling upon such matters. However, the function of electron microscopy is not simply the resolving of old controversies bequeathed by light microscopists. Electron microscopy is a science in its own right with its practitioners, problems and preoccupations. Many structures such as the endoplasmic reticulum and polyribosomes were unheard of in the light microscopic era, while the structural details of others such as the nucleolus, centrioles and cilia were but poorly resolved. The presence of the nuclear envelope and the cell membrane were suspected and the existence of the Golgi complex doubted. Clearly, alterations in such structures belong to the realms of ultrastructual pathology, and correlations with light microscopy are often tenuous and at times non-existent. Such findings may not have a direct appeal to the light microscopist but such matters cannot be ignored for they have materially altered our thinking about cellular physiology and pathology. Indeed, the main preoccupation of this book is with such matters, but I hope that I have presented this material in a manner which will make interesting reading for both light and electron microscopists.

F.N.G.

References

Babel, J., Bischoff, A. and Spoendlin, H. (1970). *Ultrastructure of the Peripheral Nervous System and Sense Organs*. Stuttgart: Georg Thieme

Dalton, A.J. and Haguenau, F. (1967). *Ultrastructure of the Kidney*. New York and London: Academic Press

David, H. (1964). *Submicroscopic Ortho- and Patho-Morphology of the Liver*. Oxford: Pergamon Press

Fawcett, D.W. (1966). *The Cell: Its Organelles and Inclusions*. Philadelphia and London: Saunders

Ghadially, F.N. and Roy, S. (1969). *Ultrastructure of Synovial Joints in Health and Disease*. London: Butterworths

Lentz, T.L. (1971). *Cell Fine Structure*. Philadelphia and London: Saunders

Mair, W.G.P. and Tomé, F.M.S. (1972). *Atlas of the Ultrastructure of Diseased Human Muscle*. Edinburgh and London: Churchill Livingstone

Porter, K.R. and Bonneville, M.A. (1973). *Fine Structure of Cells and Tissues*, 4th Edn. Philadelphia: Lea and Febiger

Rhodin, J.A.G. (1974). *Histology*. New York and London: Oxford University Press

Acknowledgements

It is my pleasant duty to acknowledge the help given by my friends and colleagues and also the skill and dedication of my co-workers and technicians.

Dr O.G. Dodge, Dr T.E. Larsen and Dr J.D. Newstead read through the typescript and offered many useful criticisms and suggestions. Most of their suggestions have been incorporated; any errors are my responsibility entirely.

My thanks are due to Mrs M. Boyle, Mrs C.E. Dick, Mr J-M.A. Lalonde and Mr N.K. Yong for collecting and processing tissues, cutting ultrathin sections and preparing innumerable prints from which a few were selected for publication in this book. In the latter task, Mr J. Junor and Mr R. Van den Beuken also assisted, particularly when special techniques were required to obtain prints from a less than perfect negative. The line drawings in this book were also executed by Mr J. Junor and Mr R. Van den Beuken.

Several colleagues have been most helpful in supplying me with specimens or blocks of tissues from which some of the illustrations in this book were derived. They include: Dr R.J. Adams, Dr R. Baumal, Dr D. Beju, Dr S. Bhuta, Dr A.H. Cameron, Dr S. Cinti, Dr I. Dardick, Dr W.E. DeCoteau, Dr H.P. Dienes, Dr M. Djaldetti, Dr G. Finkel, Dr R. Ghadially, Dr V.E. Gould, Dr E.I. Grodums, Dr G.A. Herrera, Dr K.O. Hewan-Lowe, Dr S. Holt, Dr E. Horvath, Dr M. Imamura, Dr J.V. Johannessen, Dr K. Kovacs, Dr B. Lane, Dr Y.S. Lee, Dr A. Levene, Dr E. Liepa, Dr B. Mackay, Dr P.B. Marcus, Dr G. Mariuzzi, Dr J.H. Martin, Dr G. Mierau, Dr K.W. Min, Dr T.M. Mukherjee, Dr L.W. Oliphant, Dr E.W. Parry, Dr B.E.F. Reimann, Dr B. Rozdilsky, Dr T.A. Seemayer, Dr T. Stanley, Dr T.K. Shnitka, Dr J.G. Swift, Dr M. Takeya, Dr J.H. Wedge and Dr I. Wilkie. Their contributions are also acknowledged in the legends.

The task of searching the massive literature on the ultrastructure of normal and pathological tissues, classifying and filing reprints and xeroxed copies of papers (in well over a thousand files), preparing reference lists and correcting and organizing the text into publishable format was executed by my wife, Mrs E.M. Ghadially. The expert assistance of our library staff, Dr Wilma P. Sweaney and Mrs Eva Wong in running Medline and Medlar searches on innumerable subjects is gratefully acknowledged. The text was typed by Mrs E.M. Ghadially. Her skill at promptly converting an almost illegible manuscript into well-laid out error-free sheets was a major factor in accelerating the production of this work.

The task of producing this work has been greatly facilitated by the skill and knowledge of the editorial staff of Butterworths.

The electron micrographs published in this work spring mainly from work carried out with various colleagues and co-workers. These include Dr R.L. Ailsby, Mr R. Bhatnager, Dr T. Cunningham, Mrs C.E. Dick, Dr J.A. Fuller, Mr J-M.A. Lalonde, Dr T.E. Larsen, Dr Emma Lew, Dr P.N. Mehta, Dr A.F. Oryschak, Dr E.W. Parry, Dr S. Roy, Dr L.F. Skinnider, Dr S-E. Yang-Steppuhn and Mr N.K. Yong. In the text and/or legends to the illustrations their contributions are duly identified.

Of the 1227 electron micrographs (on 546 plates) published in this work, 187 come from external sources. For these illustrations I am indebted to the following authors and journals.

Afzelius, B.A. (unpublished): *Plate 509, Fig. 1*

Barland, P., Novikoff, A.B. and Hamerman, D. (1964) *Am. J. Path.* **44**, 853: *Plate 253, Fig. 1*

Bockus, D., Remington, F., Friedman, S. and Hammar, S. (1985) *Ultrastruct. Path.* **9**, 1: *Plate 391, Fig. 1; Plate 522*

Cain, H. and Kraus, B. (1977) *Virchows Arch. B Cell Path.* **26**, 119: *Plate 395, Figs. 1 and 2*

Carstens, P.H.B. (1984) *Ultrastruct. Path*, **6**, 99: *Plate 212, Figs. 1 and 2*

Chalvardjan, A., Picard, L., Shaw, R., Davey, R. and Cairns, J.D. (1980) *Am. J. Obstet. Gynecol.* **138**, 391: *Plate 298*

Chandra, S. (unpublished): *Plate 220, Fig. 1; Plate 227, Fig. 1.* (1968) *Lab. Invest.* **18**, 422: *Plate 220, Fig. 2*

Cinti, S., Osculati, F. and Parravicini, C. (1982) *Ultrastruct. Path.* **3**, 263: *Plate 242, Fig. 2*

Coimbra, A. and Lopez-Vaz, A. (1967) *Arthritis Rheum.* **10**, 337: *Plate 253, Figs. 2–5*

Cook, M.L. and Stevens, J.G. (1970) *J. Ultrastruct. Res.* **32**, 334: *Plate 428, Figs. 1–3*

Dahl, H.A. (1963) *Z. Zellforsch. mikrosk. Anat.* **60**, 369: *Plate 502, Fig. 5*

Davis, W.C., Spicer, S.S., Greene, W.B. and Padgett, G.A. (1971) *Lab. Invest.* **24**, 303: *Plate 284, Figs. 1 and 2*

Dienes, H.P. (unpublished): *Plate 400*

Dingemans, K.P. (unpublished): *Plate 309, Fig. 1*

Djaldetti, M. (1976) In *Case Histories in Human Medicine* No. 9. Philips Monographs: *Plate 195, Fig. 2*

Djaldetti, M., Landau, M., Mandel, E.M., Har-Zaav, L. and Lewinski, U. (1974) *Blut* **29**, 210: *Plate 195, Figs. 1 and 3*

Djaldetti, M., Bessler, H., Fishman, P. and Machtey, I. (1975) *Nouv. Rev. Franc. d'Hemat.* **15**, 567: *Plate 5, Fig. 2*

Duncan, J.R. and Ramsey, F.K. (1965) *Am. J. Path.* **47**, 601: *Plate 505, Figs. 1–3*

Dustin, P. (unpublished): *Plate 311, Fig. 2; Plate 313, Fig. 2*

Dustin, P. and Libert, J. (unpublished): *Plate 311, Fig. 1*

Erlandson, R.A. (unpublished): *Plate 3, Fig. 3; Plate 154, Fig. 1*

Erlandson, R.A. and Tandler, B. (1972) *Arch. Path.* **93**, 130: *Plate 154, Fig. 2*

Feremans, W.W., Neve, P. and Caudron, M. (1978) *J. Clin. Path.* **31**, 250: *Plate 416, Figs, 1–3*

Flaks, B. and Flaks, A. (1970) *Cancer Res.* **30**, 1437: *Plate 40, Figs. 1–3; Plate 45, Fig. 2*

Frasca, J.M., Auerbach, O., Parks, V. and Stoeckenius, W. (1965). *Expl. Molec. Path.* **4**, 340: *Plate 24;* (1967) **6**, 261: *Plate 247, Figs. 1–4*

Ganote, C.E. and Otis, J.B. (unpublished): *Plate 230*

Godman, G.C. and Lane, N. (1964) *J. Cell Biol.* **21**, 353: *Plate 146, Figs. 1 and 2*

Gonatas, N.K., Margolis, G. and Kilham, L. (1971) *Lab. Invest.* **24**, 101: *Plate 401, Figs. 1 and 2*

Gouranton, J. and Thomas, D. (1974) *J. Ultrastruct. Res.* **48**, 227: *Plate 59, Figs. 1 and 2*

Grodums, E.I. (unpublished): *Plate 56, Figs. 1 and 2; Plate 134, Figs. 1 and 2; Plate 227, Fig. 2; Plate 438, Figs. 1–3*

Grunnet, M.L. and Spilsbury, P.R. (1973) *Archs Neurol.* **28**, 231: *Plate 267*

Hammar, S. (unpublished): *Plate 461, Figs. 1 and 2*

Harris, M., Vasudev, K.S., Anfield, C. and Wells, S. (1978) *Histopathology* **2**, 177: *Plate 434, Figs. 1–4*

Helyer, B.J. and Petrelli, M. (1978) *J. Natl. Cancer Inst.* **60**, 861: *Plate 238, Fig. 1*

Ho, K.L. (1985) *Acta Neuropathol. (Berl.).* **66**, 117: *Plate 417, Figs. 1–3*

Ishikawa, T. and Pei, Y.F. (1965) *J. Cell Biol.* **25**, 402: *Plate 132, Figs. 1–5*

Mahley, R.W., Gray, M.E., Hamilton, R.L. and Lequire, V.S. (1968) *Lab. Invest.* **19**, 358, *Plate 150, Fig. 2*

Martinez-Palomo, A. (unpublished): *Plate 463, Figs. 1 and 2;* (1970) *Lab. Invest.* **22**, 605: *Plate 467, Figs. 1 and 2*

Matsuda, H. and Sugiura, S. (1970) *Invest. Ophthal.* **9**, 919: *Plate 352, Figs. 1–5*

Maynard, J.A., Cooper, R.R. and Ponseti, I.V. (1972) *Lab. Invest*, **26**, 40: *Plate 243, Figs. 1 and 2*

Michaels, J.E., Albright, J.T. and Pati, D.I. (1971) *Am. J. Anat.* **132**, 301: *Plate 257, Figs. 1–3*
Mukherjee, T.M. and Swift, J.G. (unpublished): *Plate 442, Fig. 2; Plate 451, Fig. 1; Plate 464; Plate 465*
Murdock, L.L., Cahill, M.A. and Reith, A. (1977) *J. Cell Biol.* **74**, 326: *Plate 92, Figs. 1–3*
Nagano, T. and Ohtsuki, I. (1971) *J. Cell Biol.* **51**, 148: *Plate 415*
Nakai, T., Shand, F.L. and Howatson, A.F. (1969) *Virology* **38**, 50: *Plate 68, Figs. 1–3*
Newstead, J.D. (unpublished): *Plate 183, Fig. 2; Plate 368, Fig. 1; Plate 440, Fig. 2; Plate 501, Figs. 1 and 2*
Otkjaer-Nielsen, A., Johnson, E., Hentzer, B., Danielsen, L. and Carlsen, F. (1977) *J. Invest. Derm.* **69**, 376: *Plate 532, Figs. 1 and 2*
Otkjaer-Nielsen, A., Christensen, O.B., Hentzer, B., Johnson, E. and Kobayasi, T. (1978) *Acta Dermatovener. (Stockholm)* **58**, 323: *Plate 526, Figs. 3 and 4*
Oteruelo, F.T. (unpublished): *Plate 358*
Parry, E.W. (unpublished): *Plate 135, Fig. 2; Plate 466, Fig. 3*; (1969) *J. Path.* **97**, 155: *Plate 304, Fig. 1*; (1970) *J. Anat.* **107**, 505: *Plate 368, Fig. 2*
Petrelli, M. (unpublished): *Plate 238, Fig. 2*
Porte, A., Stoeckel, M.-E., Sacrez, A. and Batzenschlager, A. (1980) *Virchows Arch. A. Path. Anat. Histol.* **386**, 43: *Plate 380, Figs. 1 and 2*
Pfeifer, U. and Altmann, H.-W. (unpublished): *Plate 386, Figs. 1–3*
Roberts, D.K., Horbelt, D.V. and Powell, L.C. (1975) *Am. J. Obstet. Gynecol.* **123**, 811: *Plate 57*
Roberts, D.K., Horbelt, D.V., Powell, L.C. and Walker, N. (unpublished): *Plate 49, Figs. 1–3*
Roy, S. (1967) *Ann. rheum. Dis.* **26**, 517: *Plate 149, Fig. 1*
Rutsaert, J., Menu, R. and Resibois, A. (1973) *Lab. Invest.* **29**, 527: *Plate 312*
Sanel, F.T. and Lepore, M.J. (1968) *Expl. Molec. Path.* **9**, 110: *Plate 240, Fig. 2*
Schneeberger, E.E. (1972) *J. Histochem. Cytochem.* **20**, 180: *Plate 327*
Schneeberger-Keeley, E.E. and Burger, E.J. (1970) *Lab. Invest.* **22**, 361: *Plate 479, Figs. 1 and 2*
Seïte, R., Escraig, J. and Couineau, S. (1971) *J. Ultrastruct. Res.* **37**, 449: *Plate 55, Fig. 4*
Seïte, R., Mei, N. and Vuillet-Luciani, J. (1973) *Brain Research* **50**, 419: *Plate 55, Fig. 1*
Seïte, R., Escraig, J., Luciani-Vuillet, J. and Zerbib, R. (1975) *J. Microscopie Biol. Cell* **24**, 387: *Plate 55, Fig. 3*
Seïte, R., Leonetti, J., Luciani-Vuillet, J. and Vio, M. (1977) *Brain Research* **124**, 41: *Plate 55, Fig. 2*
Senoo, A. (unpublished): *Plate 10*
Shipkey, F.H. (unpublished): *Plate 414, Fig. 1*
Shipkey, F.H., Lieberman, P.H., Foote, F.W.Jr. and Stewart, F.W. (1964) *Cancer* **17**, 821: *Plate 414, Fig. 2*
Shipkey, F.H., Erlandson, R.A., Bailey, R.B., Babcock, V.I. and Southam, C.V. (1967) *Expl. Molec. Path.* **6**, 39: *Plate 21, Figs. 1–4*
Sondergaard, K., Henschel, A. and Hou-Jensen, K. (unpublished): *Plate 343, Fig. 1*; (1980) *Ultrastruct. Path.* **1**, 357: *Plate 343, Fig. 2*
Stanley, T. (unpublished): *Plate 226, Figs. 1 and 2; Plate 433, Fig. 2*
Stass, S.A., Perlin, E., Jaffe, E.S., Simon, D.R., Creegan, W.J., Robinson, J.J., Holloway, M.L. and Schumacher, H.R. (unpublished): *Plate 495, Fig. 1*; (1978) *Am. J. Hemat.* **4**, 67: *Plate 495, Fig. 2*
Stubblefield, E. and Brinkley, B.R. (1967) In *Formation and Fate of Cell Organelles* Vol. 6, 175. Ed. K.B. Warren, Academic Press: *Plate 80; Plate 81, Figs. 1 and 2; Plate 82, Figs. 1 and 2*
Takahashi, K., Terashima, K., Kojima, M., Yoshida, H. and Kimura, H. (1977) *Acta Path. Jap.* **27**, 775: *Plate 269, Fig. 2*
Tandler, B. (unpublished): *Plate 118; Plate 300; Plate 301, Fig. 4; Plate 507, Fig. 1*
Tandler, B. and Rossi, E.P. (1977) *J. Oral Path.* **6**, 401: *Plate 301, Figs. 2 and 3*
Tandler, B., Hutter, R.V.P. and Erlandson, R.A. (1970) *Lab. Invest.* **23**, 567: *Plate 133, Figs. 1–3*
Threadgold, L.T. and Lasker, R. (unpublished): *Plate 94, Fig. 4*; (1967) *J. Ultrastruct. Res.* **19**, 238: *Plate 94, Figs. 1–3*
Tillack, T.W. and Marchesi, V.T. (1970) *J. Cell Biol.* **45**, 649: *Plate 441, Figs. 1 and 2*
Wheatley, D.N. (unpublished): *Plate 500, Fig. 1; Plate 502, Figs. 1, 2 and 4*
Willett, G.D. and Clayton, F. (1985) *Ultrastruct. Path.* **8**, 115: *Plate 437, Figs. 1 and 2*
Wong, Y.C. and Buck, R.C. (1971) *Lab. Invest.* **24**, 55: *Plate 504, Fig. 4*
Yamamoto, T. (unpublished): *Plate 66, Fig. 2*; (1969) *Microbiology* **1**, 371: *Plate 66, Fig. 1*
Zucker-Franklin, D. (1969) *J. Clin. Invest.* **48**, 165: *Plate 398, Figs. 1–4*

I am also grateful to the following journals and publishers for permission to use illustrations from past publications of which I am author or co-author.

Ann. Pathol. Paris: Masson
Ghadially, F.N., Fergus Murphy and Lalonde, J-M.A. (1982) **2**, 57: *Plate 310, Fig. 2*

Ann. rheum. Dis. London: British Medical Association
Ghadially, F.N. and Mehta, P.N. (1971) **30**, 31: *Plate 371, Fig. 1; Plate 372, Figs. 1–3*
Ghadially, F.N. and Roy, S. (1967) **26**, 426: *Plate 302, Figs. 1–3; Plate 303*
Ghadially, F.N., Meachim, G. and Collins, D.H. (1965) **24**, 136: *Plate 264, Figs. 4 and 5*
Ghadially, F.N., Oryschak, A.F. and Mitchell, D.M. (1976) **35**, 67: *Plate 323, Fig. 2*
Mehta, P.N. and Ghadially, F.N. (1973) **32**, 75: *Plate 151, Fig. 1; Plate 412, Figs. 1 and 2*
Roy, S. and Ghadially, F.N. (1966) **25**, 402: *Plate 268, Fig. 1;* (1967) **26**, 26: *Plate 145, Fig. 2; Plate 473,*
   Fig. 1

Archs Path. Chicago: American Medical Association
Ghadially, F.N., Fuller, J.A. and Kirkaldy-Willis, W.H. (1971) **92**, 356: *Plate 26*
Skinnider, L.F. and Ghadially, F.N. (1973) **95**, 139: *Plate 318, Fig. 3; Plate 406, Fig. 2;* (1974) **98**, 58: *Plate*
   286

Br. J. Cancer. London: H.K. Lewis
Skinnider, L.F. and Ghadially, F.N. (1977) **35**, 657: *Plate 486, Figs. 1 and 2; Plate 488, Fig. 4; Plate 491,*
   Fig. 1

Cancer. Philadelphia, J.B. Lippincott
Ghadially, F.N. and Mehta, P.N. (1970) **25**, 1457: *Plate 2, Fig. 1; Plate 237, Fig. 2*
Ghadially, F.N. and Parry, E.W. (1966) **19**, 1989: *Plate 120, Fig. 1; Plate 148, Fig. 1; Plate 244, Fig. 1; Plate*
   263, Fig. 1; (1965) **18**, 485: *Plate 304, Fig. 2*
Ghadially, F.N. and Skinnider, L.F. (1972) **29**, 444: *Plate 492, Figs. 2 and 3; Plate 494, Fig. 3*
Parry, E.W. and Ghadially, F.N. (1965) **18**, 1026: *Plate 255, Figs. 2 and 3; Plate 304, Fig. 2;* (1966) **19**, 821:
   Plate 101; Plate 102

Experientia. Basel: Birkhauser Verlag
Ghadially, F.N. and Lalonde, J-M.A. (1977) **33**, 1600: *Plate 272, Fig. 2;* (1980) **36**, 59: *Plate 41, Figs. 1–4;*
   Plate 42, Figs. 2 and 3
Ghadially, F.N., Lalonde, J-M.A. and Dick, C.E. (1978) **34**, 1212: *Plate 473, Fig. 3*
Ghadially, F.N., Oryschak, A.F. and Mitchell, D.M. (1974) **30**, 649: *Plate 477, Figs. 1 and 4*
Ghadially, F.N. and Skinnider, L.F. (1971) **27**, 1217: *Plate 493, Fig. 4;* (1976) **32**, 1061: *Plate 491, Fig. 2*

J. Anat. London: Cambridge University Press
Ghadially, F.N. and Lalonde, J-M.A. (1981) **132**, 481: *Plate 542, Fig. 2; Plate 543, Figs. 1, 2 and 5*
Ghadially, F.N., Thomas, I., Yong, N. and Lalonde, J-M.A. (1978) **125**, 499: *Plate 423, Figs. 1 and 2; Plate*
   424, Plate 530, Figs. 2 and 3

J. Bone & Joint Surg. London: Royal College of Surgeons
Ghadially, F.N., Mehta, P.N. and Kirkaldy-Willis, W.H. (1970) **52A**, 1147: *Plate 151*
Roy, S. and Ghadially, F.N. (1967) **49A**, 1636: *Plate 268, Fig. 3*

J. Path. Bact. Edinburgh: Longman
Ghadially, F.N. and Parry, E.W. (1966) **92**, 313: *Plate 293, Figs. 1 and 2; Plate 294, Figs. 1 and 2*
Roy, S. and Ghadially, F.N. (1967) **93**, 555: *Plate 147, Figs. 1 and 2*

J. Path. Edinburgh: Longman
Ailsby, R.L. and Ghadially, F.N. (1973) **109**, 75: *Plate 503; Plate 504, Fig. 3*
Ghadially, F.N., Ailsby, R.L. and Yong, N.K. (1976) **120**, 201: *Plate 275; Plate 277, Fig. 1*
Ghadially, F.N., Lowes, N.R. and Mesfin, G.M. (1977) **122**, 157: *Plate 234, Figs. 1–3*
Ghadially, F.N., Thomas, I. and Lalonde, J-M.A. (1977) **123**, 181: *Plate 322, Figs. 3 and 4; Plate 324, Figs.*
   3 and 4
Ghadially, F.N., De Coteau, W.E., Huang, S. and Thomas, I. (1978) **124**, 77: *Plate 308, Figs. 1–3*
Ghadially, F.N., Lalonde, J-M.A., Thomas, I. and Massey, K.L. (1978) **125**, 219: *Plate 324, Figs. 1 and 2*
Ghadially, F.N., Lalonde, J-M.A. and Dick, C.E. (1979) **127**, 19: *Plate 274, Figs. 1 and 2*
Ghadially, F.N., Lalonde, J-M.A. and Yong, N.K. (1980) **130**, 147: *Plate 525, Figs. 2 and 3*
Lalonde, J-M.A., Ghadially, F.N. and Massey, K.L. (1978) **125**, 17: *Plate 273, Fig. 1*
Larsen, T.E. and Ghadially, F.N. (1974) **114**, 69: *Plate 500, Fig. 2; Plate 506*
Skinnider, L.F. and Ghadially, F.N. (1973) **109**, 1: *Plate 493, Figs. 1 and 2; Plate 494, Figs. 1 and 2*
Ghadially, F.N. and Skinnider, L.F. (1974) **114**, 113: *Plate 125*

J. Rheum. Toronto: Journal of Rheumatology
Ghadially, F.N. (1979) (Suppl. No. 5), 45: *Plate 323, Figs. 1 and 3*

J. Submicr. Cytol. Basle: S. Karger
Ghadially, F.N. (1979) **11**, 271: *Plate 268, Fig. 2; Plate 276*
Ghadially, F.N. and Lalonde, J-M.A. (1979) **11**, 413: *Plate 39, Figs. 1, 2 and 4; Plate 42, Fig. 1*
Ghadially, F.N., Lalonde, J-M.A. and Yong, N.K. (1980) **12**, 447: *Plate 373, Fig. 1; Plate 425, Figs. 1 and 2*
Ghadially, F.N., Lock, C.J.L., Yang-Steppuhn, S-E. and Lalonde, J-M.A. (1981) **13**, 223: *Plate 325, Fig. 1*
Ghadially, F.N., Stinson, J.C., Payne, C.M. and Leibovitz, A. (1985) **17**, 469: *Plate 43, Figs. 1–4; Plate 44, Figs. 1–4*
Ghadially, F.N., Harawi, S. and Khan, W. (1985) **17**, 269: *Plate 46, Figs. 2 and 3; Plate 157, Fig. 2; Plate 158, Fig. 3; Plate 159, Fig. 1–3*
Senoo, A., Fuse, Y. and Ghadially, F.N. (1984) **16**, 379: *Plate 73, Figs. 1–4; Plate 75, Figs. 1–6*
Ghadially, F.N., Senoo, A. and Fuse, Y. (1985) **17**, 687: *Plate 73, Figs. 6–7; Plate 75, Figs. 7–12*
Ghadially, F.N. and Block, H.J. (1985) **17**, 435: *Plate 119, Fig. 2; Plate 139, Figs. 1–3; Plate 546, Figs. 1 and 2*
Ghadially, F.N., Chisholm, I.A. and Lalonde, J-M.A. (1986) **18**, 189: *Plate 156, Figs. 1–3*
Pounder, D.J., Ghadially, F.N., Mukherjee, T.M., Hecker, R., Rowland, R., Dixon, B. and Lalonde, J-M.A. (1982) **14**, 389: *Plate 296, Figs. 1–3*
Ghadially, F.N., McNaughton, J.D. and Lalonde, J-M.A. (1983) **15**, 1055: *Plate 375, Fig. 1*
Ghadially, F.N. and Mierau, G.W. (1985) **17**, 645: *Plate 521, Figs. 1 and 2*
Ghadially, F.N., Ghadially, R. and Lalonde, J-M.A. (1986) **18**, 417: *Plate 309, Fig. 3; Plate 349, Figs. 1 and 2; Plate 350, Figs. 1 and 2*
Ghadially, F.N., Senoo, A., Fuse, Y. and Chan, K.W. (1987) **19**, 175: *Plate 206, Figs. 1 and 2; Plate 207, Figs. 1–5; Plate 208, Figs. 1–8; Plate 209, Figs. 1 and 2*
Nimmo Wilkie, J.S. and Ghadially, F.N. (1987) **19**, 433: *Plate 210, Figs. 1 and 2*
Kostianovsky, M. and Ghadially, F.N. (1987) **19**, 509: *Plate 213, Figs. 1 and 2; Plate 214, Figs. 1–3*

Ultrastructural Pathology. Washington, DC: Hemisphere Publishing Corp.
Robertson, D.M. and Ghadially, F.N. (1983) **5**, 369: *Plate 346; Plate 347, Figs. 1–4*

Virchows Arch. B. Cell Path. New York: Springer Verlag
Ghadially, F.N. and Parry, E.W. (1974) **15**, 131: *Plate 251, Figs. 1 and 2*
Ghadially, F.N. and Yong, N.K. (1976) **21**, 45: *Plate 63; Plate 64, Figs. 1–4*
Ghadially, F.N., Lalonde, J-M.A. and Yong, N.K. (1979) **31**, 81: *Plate 523, Figs. 1 and 2; Plate 524*
Ghadially, F.N., Lock, C.J.L., Lalonde, J-M.A. and Ghadially, R. (1981) **35**, 123: *Plate 325, Fig. 2*
Lalonde, J-M.A. and Ghadially, F.N. (1977) **25**, 221: *Plate 271, Fig. 2; Plate 273, Fig. 2; Plate 278, Figs. 1 and 2*
Oryschak, A.F. and Ghadially, F.N. (1976) **20**, 29: *Plate 322, Fig. 2*

Diagnostic Electron Microscopy of Tumours. London: Butterworths.
First Edition. Ghadially, F.N. (1980)
Plate 134, Fig. 5; Plate 182, Figs. 1 and 2; Plate 290, Figs. 1 and 2; Plate 291, Figs. 1 and 2; Plate 299; Plate 362, Fig. 2; Plate 363, Fig. 1; Plate 367, Figs. 1 and 2; Plate 373, Fig. 2; Plate 399; Plate 429, Figs. 1 and 2; Plate 432, Figs. 1–3; Plate 447, Figs. 2 and 3; Plate 471, Figs. 1 and 2; Plate 472, Figs. 1–3; Plate 519, Fig. 1
Second Edition. Ghadially, F.N. (1985)
Plate 4, Figs. 1, 2 and 4; Plate 15, Figs. 1 and 2; Plate 47, Fig. 2; Plate 128, Fig. 1; Plate 129; Plate 152; Plate 160, Figs. 1 and 2; Plate 164; Plate 165, Fig. 1 and 2; Plate 166, Figs. 1 and 2; Plate 168; Plate 169, Figs. 1 and 2; Plate 171, Figs. 1 and 2; Plate 198, Figs. 1 and 2; Plate 336, Fig. 1; Plate 366, Fig. 2; Plate 431, Figs. 1–3; Plate 455

Fine Structure of Joints in **The Joints and Synovial Fluid.** London: Academic Press. Volume 1, Chapter 3, p. 105. Ed. by L. Sokoloff
Ghadially, F.N. (1978) *Plate 520, Fig. 2; Plate 541, Fig. 2*

Fine Structure of Synovial Joints. London: Butterworths.
Ghadially, F.N. (1983) *Plate 473, Fig. 2*

Ultrastructure of Synovial Joints in Health and Disease. London: Butterworths
Ghadially, F.N. and Roy, S. (1969) *Plate 13, Fig. 1 and 2; Plate 37, Fig. 1; Plate 144; Plate 145, Fig. 1; Plate 149, Fig. 2; Plate 180, Figs. 1–3; Plate 181, Fig. 2; Plate 186; Plate 200; Plate 263, Fig. 3; Plate 272, Fig. 1; Plate 273, Fig., 3; Plate 351, Fig. 1; Plate 446, Fig. 2; Plate 499, Fig. 1; Plate 544, Fig. 2*

Contents, Volume 1

xviii

5 Endoplasmic reticulum

6 Annulate lamellae

Contents, Volume 2

14   Cell membrane and coat

15   Cell junctions

16   Endocytotic structures and cell processes

17   Extracellular matrix (extracellular components)

Nucleus

Introduction

Early ultrastructural studies were concentrated mainly on the new and intriguing structures revealed by the electron microscope in the cytoplasm and not the nucleus, which revealed only an assortment of granules intermingled with some filamentous and amorphous material. The sentiments of that era are recorded by Moses (1956), who stated 'Most electron microscopists acknowledge that the nucleus appears to be as remarkable for its lack of obvious ordered detail as the cytoplasm is for the richness in it'. Dissatisfaction with the state of affairs was expressed by many workers and is epitomized by Bernhard and Granboulan (1963), who stated 'In electron microscopical cytology the interphase nucleus of the normal somatic cell has been the neglected orphan compared with cytoplasmic organelles'. Such sentiments have been reiterated by others, for example by Kaye (1969), who states 'Research on the nucleus seems remarkably unfruitful compared with that on cytoplasmic organelles when results achieved by similar efforts are considered'.

However, disenchantment with electron microscopic studies on the nucleus is no longer warranted, because later studies have revealed much that is new and interesting, as evidenced by the fact that this chapter on the nucleus is the largest in this book.

Outstanding among these achievements are the studies on the nuclear envelope, and the nucleolus. There is much here of interest for both the student of normal structure and the pathologist. Similarly, our knowledge of viral and non-viral inclusions has been enhanced, and many an old controversy regarding the nature of these inclusions has been settled. This subject, of course, is of great interest to pathologists; hence I have dealt with it in some detail in this chapter. It is amazing how much more one can discern in these inclusions with the light microscope once their ultrastructural features are recognized.

On the other hand, light microscopic studies of the mitotic nucleus have proved more rewarding than studies of ultrathin sections through these structures. Hence, only the interphase nucleus is dealt with in this chapter; the mitotic nucleus receives only passing mention in this and later chapters.

Nuclear shape

In ultrathin sections examined with the electron microscope, many nuclei show a degree of irregularity of form quite beyond that expected from their light microscopic appearance. It need hardly be pointed out that this is no shrinkage artefact, since other organelles such as mitochondria are not crenated or shrunken. This phenomenon, although at first perplexing, can be readily explained when one considers that the thinness of the sections employed in electron microscopy gives a virtually two-dimensional view of the state of affairs at the plane of section, while the much thicker sections employed for light microscopy may be regarded as several superimposed thin sections where projections and indentations which overlie each other cancel out and give a smooth appearance to the nuclear margin. No doubt the higher magnification employed in electron microscopy also contributes to this phenomenon by revealing small irregularities which would appear insignificant or be beyond the resolving power of the light microscope.

Thus the electron microscope shows that many nuclei which one had come to regard as smooth and round or oval, can in fact be quite irregular and at times beset by an unsuspected slender deep invagination*. The significance of such irregularity of nuclear shape is obscure and the operative mechanisms poorly understood. However, a few interesting studies and speculations regarding this point are worth recording.

Perhaps the best known example here is the nucleus of smooth and striated muscle which in ultrathin sections often shows a markedly folded or convoluted appearance. This has now been correlated with the state of the cell, the nucleus being unfolded and elongated in the relaxed phase and ovoid and invaginated after contraction of the muscle cell (Lane, 1965; Panner and Honig, 1967; Franke and Schinko, 1969; Bloom and Cancilla, 1969; Crissman et al., 1978). Similar changes also occur in the nuclei of endothelial cells of blood vessels (Plate 1), and it is reasonable to assume that this, too, may be correlated with the state of the vessel wall (Majno et al., 1970). Several hypotheses have been proposed to explain the folding of the nucleus in muscle cells. These include: (1) changes in the ionic concentration (Franke and Schinko, 1969); (2) mechanical compression (Bloom and Cancilla, 1969) and structural connections extending between myofibrils and the nuclear envelope (Franke, 1970a; Crissman et al., 1978).

Instances may be cited where complexity of nuclear form is related to maturation and ageing of the cell. The classic example here is the neutrophil leucocyte where the nucleus becomes segmented and lobed as the cell increases in age. In mature normal articular cartilage there is a population of cells which very rarely divide, but suffer in situ necrosis with the passage of time. Barnett et al. (1963) have observed an increased complexity of nuclear form in this population of cells as animals (rabbits) grow older. There is also evidence that human hepatic and adrenal cell nuclei (Kleinfeld and Koulish, 1957; Sobel et al., 1969a) show invaginations of the nuclear envelope and complexity of nuclear form more frequently in older age groups.

*Invaginations of the nuclear envelope lead to the formation of pseudoinclusions. These and discussion on the mode of formation of such invaginations are dealt with on page 74.

*Invaginations of the nuclear envelope lead to the formation of pseudoinclusions. These and discussion on the mode of formation of such invaginations are dealt with on page 74.

Plate 1
Folded and invaginated nuclei (E) are seen in the endothelial cells of this collapsed blood vessel from the subsynovial tissue of man. × 14 000 (Ghadially and Roy, unpublished electron micrograph)

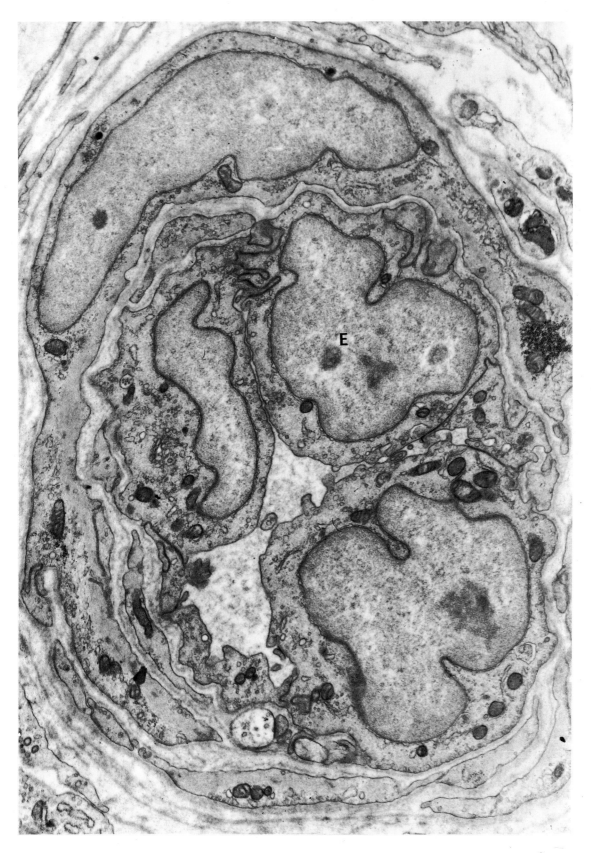

3

Other examples of age-associated irregularity or lobation of nuclear form have been noted in: (1) the dog myocardium (Munnell and Getty, 1968); (2) anterior pituitary cells (Weiss and Lansing, 1953); (3) astrocytes of chinchillas (Cammermeyer, 1963); (4) Purkinje cells and hepatic cells of mice (Andrew, 1955, 1962); (5) the macronucleus of the unicellular protozoan *Tokophyra infusionum* (Rudzinska, 1961a, b); (6) cultured chick fibroblasts (Brock and Hay, 1971); and (7) cultured fibroblasts from Werner's syndrome (one of the premature ageing syndromes) (Basler *et al.*, 1979).

Irregularity of nuclear form provides an increased area of contact between the nucleus and the cytoplasm, and in some cases at least this seems to denote increased nucleocytoplasmic exchanges and heightened metabolic activity. In this connection it is interesting to note that some of the most irregular and branched nuclei occur in the cells of silk-spinning glands of certain insects, and that such nuclei evolve by a series of steps from unremarkable oval nuclei of the cells of the Malpighian tubule (Lozinski, 1911). Here increasing metabolic activity is clearly associated with an increasing complexity of nuclear form.

After ultrasonic radiation of the rabbit knee joint, Zichner and Engel (1971) found that the nuclei of the synovial intimal cells, especially the type A cells became markedly irregular and segmented. This, taken in conjunction with other changes, led them to conclude that this was a sign of increased metabolic activity.

Support for this hypothesis may also be found in the case of tumours where complex nuclear form is associated with a high metabolic activity. The marked irregularities of shape assumed by neoplastic nuclei are well known to the light microscopist and this feature is of some value in the diagnosis of malignant tumours. The electron microscope reveals even more dramatically the extremes of complex and bizarre forms the nuclei of tumour cells can assume (*Plate 2, Fig. 1*). At times the nucleus is so extensively segmented or invaded by numerous invaginations (*Plate 2, Fig. 2*) that it assumes a sponge-like character.

Plate 2

Fig. 1. Giant cell from a well differentiated osteogenic sarcoma showing two irregular nuclear profiles with small pedunculated masses of nuclear substance connected by complex slender stalks. × 7000 (*From Ghadially and Mehta, 1970*)

Fig. 2. A nucleus from a metastatic malignant melanoma. Invaginations of the nuclear envelope (arrows) have produced numerous pseudoinclusions (P) which give the nucleus a sieve-like or sponge-like appearance. × 15 000

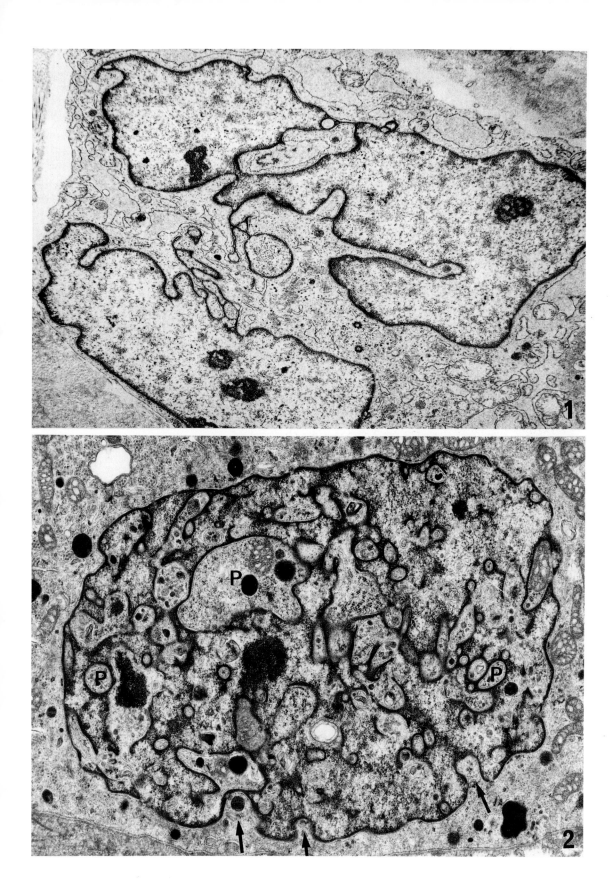

However, as is well known the nuclei of some malignant tumours can be quite small and may show little or no irregularity of form even with the electron microscope and conversely one may sometimes find a few irregular nuclei even in normal tissue or a benign tumour. An example of this is the fibroadenoma of the breast where a rare tumour contains a few fibroblasts with surprisingly bizarre lobulated nuclei (*Plate 3, Figs. 1 and 2*). Irregular nuclei somewhat similar to this have also been seen (Hashimoto *et al.*, 1974; Alguacil-Garcia *et al.*, 1978; Zina and Bundino, 1979; Erlandson, 1981) in some but not all specimens of dermatofibrosarcoma, a tumour with a strong tendency to recur after removal but one which very rarely metastasizes (*Plate 3, Fig. 3*). Thus, it is obvious that in rare instances markedly irregular nuclei are seen in benign or not too aggressive tumours. However, such exceptions are so rare that they do not detract materially from the generalization that nuclei of malignant tumours are markedly irregular in form compared with those found in corresponding benign tumours or corresponding normal cells, and that this is a feature of diagnostic value when viewed in conjunction with other criteria of malignancy.

The neoplastic nucleus, although irregular and altered often continues to bear some resemblance to its normal counterpart. This is best demonstrated by the fact that crenated, folded or concertina-like nuclei of contractile cells, like smooth muscle cells, striated muscle

Plate 3

Fig. 1. Fibroadenoma of breast. A neoplastic fibroblast from the fibrous component of the tumour showing a lobulated nucleus. Such atypical nuclei are rare exceptions, usually the nuclei of this benign tumour are only moderately enlarged and relatively speaking quite smooth. × 15 500

Fig. 2. Fibroadenoma of breast. Same tumour as *Fig. 1*. The nucleus of this cell is beset by meandering invaginations (arrows). When such invaginations are transected they present as pseudoinclusions (P) in the nucleus. × 10 500

Fig. 3. Dermatofibrosarcoma protuberans. The nuclei of the fibroblastic cells are lobulated. × 8700 (*Electron micrograph supplied by Dr R. A. Erlandson*)

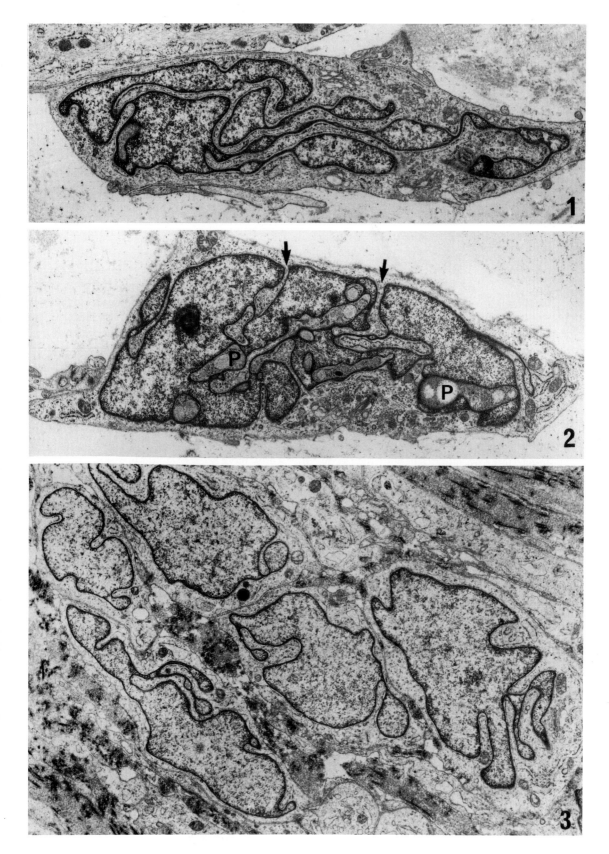

cells and myofibroblasts, are also often seen in tumours of these cells (*Plate 4*) and this is a point of some diagnostic value★.

The nuclei of some but not all leukaemic cells tend to be somewhat more irregular in form than their normal counterparts and at times cells may be found where the nucleus may be segmented, lobulated or beset by numerous invaginations so that the nuclear form is quite irregular. However, the nuclei of leucocytes in the Sézary syndrome† are so bizarre that they are almost in a class by themselves (*Plate 5*). This is a point of value in diagnosing this condition. In smears of blood and in replicas from freeze-etched preparations of unfixed cells, these nuclei usually show a cerebriform appearance, but they appear serpentine or drawn out into a mass of overlapping narrow ribbons in ultrathin sections examined with the electron microscope (Lutzner and Jordan, 1968; Tan *et al.*, 1974; Djaldetti *et al.*, 1975).

An hypothesis often offered in the literature is that intracytoplasmic filaments may be responsible for producing irregularity of nuclear form in some instances. Abundant intracytoplasmic filaments were clearly demonstrated in Sézary cells by Zucker-Franklin *et al.* (1974) and they state: 'the abundance of such fibrils in Sézary cells raises the question of their relationship to the deformity of the nucleus'. Frequent nuclear lobulation and abundant intracytoplasmic filaments were found in circulating plasma cells in a case of plasma cell leukaemia by Beltran and Stuckey (1972) who suggest that these filaments 'may have played a role in the production of nuclear lobulation'. A similar view was also expressed by Bessis (1961) who found lobulation of nuclei and abundant intracytoplasmic filaments in mononuclear cells from normal blood that had been incubated with an oxalate solution. He speculated that the filaments were probably contractile and induced nuclear lobulation. These were, in fact, radial segmented nuclei and it is now clear (*see* page 12) that microtubules rather than filaments are involved in the production of radial segmented nuclei. What is more, the filaments illustrated in mononuclear cells by Bessis (1961) and in plasma cells by Beltran and Stuckey (1972) are clearly intermediate filaments (presumably vimentin) not actin filaments. Similarly from the many published electron micrographs of Sézary cells it is clear that the intracytoplasmic filaments are in fact intermediate filaments which as we now know have no contractile function. Thus there is little reason to believe that 'filaments' are responsible for producing nuclear lobulation or irregularity of nuclear form. An increase in intracytoplasmic filaments (not always clear whether actin or intermediate filaments) has been seen in diverse cell types and pathological states (*see* Chapter 12) without nuclear lobulation. Conversely, one can think of examples of cells with lobulated or irregular nuclei (e.g. *Plates 2* and *3*) where intracytoplasmic filaments would be hard to find.

★Nuclear morphology is one of the features which at times assists the histopathologist in distinguishing myomas (e.g. leiomyosarcoma, rhabdomyosarcoma) from other neoplasms, particularly fibroblastic neoplasms. At the light microscopic level neoplastic myocytes tend to have wrinkled nuclei (equivalent to the folded nucleus seen with the electron microscope) with blunt poles, while neoplastic fibroblasts usually contain smoother nuclei with pointed poles.
†The Sézary cell nucleus and current views about the diagnosis of Sézary syndrome are discussed on page 10.

Plate 4

Fig. 1. Leiomyoma of uterus. Neoplastic smooth muscle cell showing the folded nucleus characteristic of this cell type. × 17 000 (*From Ghadially, 1985*)

Fig. 2. Leiomyosarcoma. The nucleus presents the corrugated profile reminiscent of that seen in muscle cells. The detached profile (arrow) would most likely be continuous with the main nuclear mass in another plane of sectioning. × 13 500 (*From Ghadially, 1985*)

Fig. 3. Rhabdomyosarcoma. The nuclear profiles are not so deeply indented as in *Figs. 1* and *2*, but shallower indentations are present. This gives the nuclear profiles a crenated appearance. × 4600

Fig. 4. Myofibroblastoma. The nucleus presents the crenated or corrugated profile one expects to find in contractile cells (For details about this not-too-well-known tumour or tumour-like lesion *see* Chapter 38 in Ghadially, 1985). × 5400

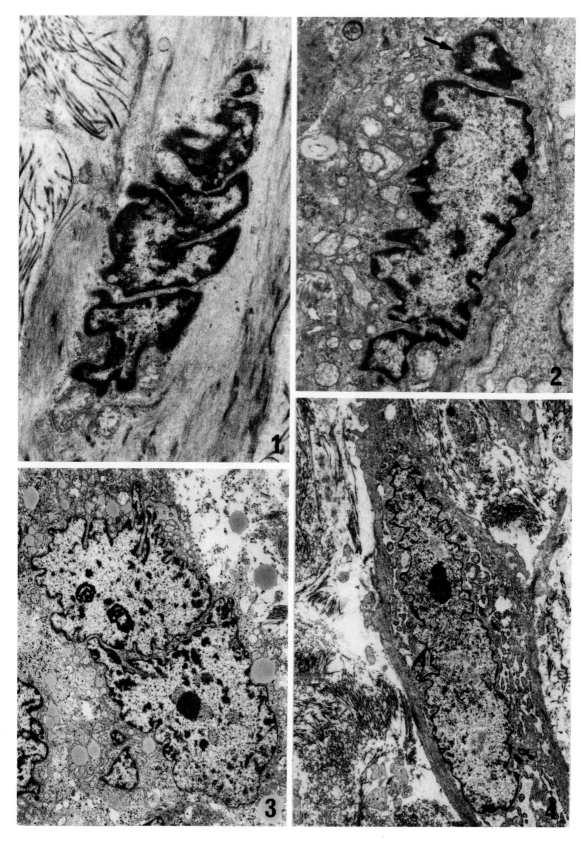

9

Cerebriform nucleus

In 1949 Sézary described a syndrome manifested by oedematous and pigmented erythroderma, leonine facies, lymphadenopathy and large abnormal cells with strikingly irregular nuclei in circulating blood. The apt term 'cerebriform nucleus' was used by Lutzner and Jordan (1968) to describe the nucleus of the Sézary cell. Sézary considered these cells to be giant histiocytes[*] which proliferated in the skin and then invaded the blood stream creating a leukaemic state. The condition was at first regarded as a rare fatal reticulosis and hence called 'Sézary's reticulosis'. It is now called 'Sézary syndrome' which is the leukaemic manifestation or phase of mycosis fungoides, a disease which is considered to be a malignant dermotrophic lymphoma of T cells.

In smears of blood and in freeze-etched preparations, the typical Sézary cell nucleus presents a cerebriform appearance. In ultrathin sections (*Plate 5*), it appears serpentine or drawn out into a mass of narrow, overlapping ribbons (Lutzner and Jordan, 1968; Tan et al., 1974; Djaldetti et al., 1975; Johannessen, 1977). At one stage it was thought that this nuclear morphology (*Plate 5*) was diagnostic of Sézary syndrome (if in the skin, mycosis fungoides), but since then cells with similar nuclei have also been found in patients with several benign dermatoses and at times in the blood of apparently normal individuals (Flaxman et al., 1971; Lutzner et al., 1971; Schwartz and Bangert, 1979; Cinti et al., 1985).

Litovitz and Lutzner (1974) studied the nuclear contour index[†] of normal and leukaemic lymphocytes (including Sézary cells) using the technique of Schrek (1972). They found that the mean nuclear contour index for: (1) cells of chronic lymphocytic leukaemia was 3.9; (2) cells of chronic lymphosarcoma cell leukaemia was 4.4; (3) normal lymphocytes was 4.4; and (4) Sézary cell was 6.8. They state: 'Rarely except in Sézary syndrome were circulating lymphocytes found with a contour index > 8.6'.

Fletcher et al. (1984) calculated the number of cells (in blood of patients with Sézary syndrome and control cases) bearing nuclear indentations (light microscopic study) whose total length exceeded one and a half times the greatest nuclear diameter. Such cells they called Sézary cells and they conclude that: '(1) 0% to 9% Sézary cells negative for Sézary syndrome; (2) 10% to 29% Sézary cells suggestive of Sézary syndrome; and (3) 30% or more Sézary cells consistent with Sézary syndrome'. The consensus of opinion now is that only when more than 25 per cent of the cells have markedly irregular nuclei can one support the diagnosis of Sézary syndrome. Payne et al. (1984) have developed an ultrastructural method for diagnosing mycosis fungoides (said to be 100 per cent accurate) on skin biopsy specimens, by scoring the number of sharply angulated nuclear invaginations in lymphocytes.

Investigators wishing to emphasize the non-specificity of the Sézary cell often quote the work of Yeckley et al. (1975) which purports to show that in vitro stimulation of lymphocytes with pokeweed mitogen or phytohaemagglutinin produces Sézary-like cells. However, the studies of Payne et al. (1985) show that: (1) various mitogens and antigens do not produce Sézary-like cells[‡]; and that (2) nuclear contour indices determined on electron micrographs published by Yeckley et al. (1975) are within normal limits[§]. Thus it would appear that objective quantitative methods are better suited for confidently identifying the Sézary cell than subjective assessment of cells in electron micrographs.

[*]In smears of peripheral blood Sézary cells range in size from 7–19 μm, while normal lymphocytes range from 6–13 μm. (Litovitz and Lutzner, 1974)
[†]The nuclear contour index is the ratio of the nuclear circumference (length of perimeter) to the square root of the nuclear cross-sectional area. This is a size-independent, quantitative indicator of irregularity of nuclear form. The higher the nuclear contour index the more irregular the nucleus. A perfectly circular sectional profile has the theoretical minimum index of 3.54.
[‡]Various other reports make no mention of Sézary cells developing from stimulated lymphocytes (for references see Dardick et al., 1981).
[§]This is also the case for so-called 'Sézary-like' cells found in various benign dermatoses (Payne et al., 1984).

Plate 5
Sézary cell with characteristic nucleus. (*From Djaldetti, Bessler, Fishman and Machtey, 1975*). × 23 000

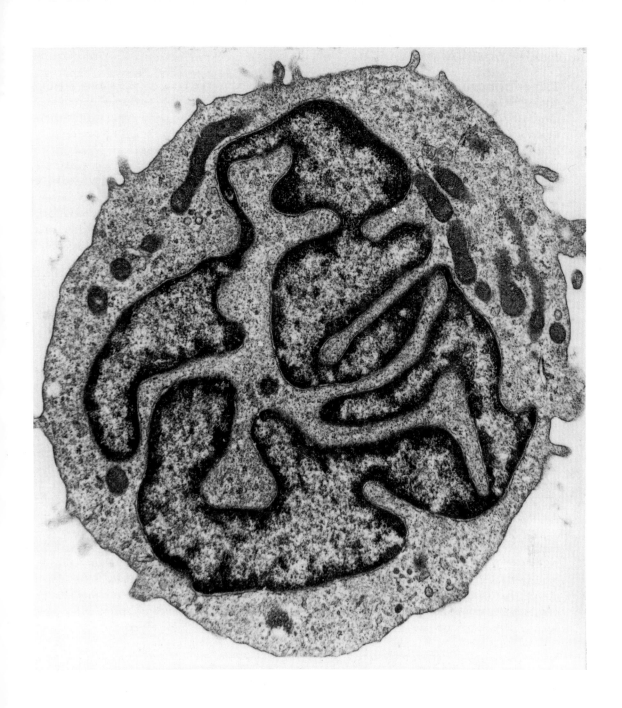

11

Radially segmented nucleus

This peculiar but quite characteristic aberration of nuclear shape is distinguished by a radial arrangement of nuclear segments (lobes) around a central zone thought to correspond to the cell centre (i.e. the centrosomal region). The appearance created by this arrangement of nuclear lobes is akin to the petals of a flower or a clover leaf. Hence such a nucleus is at times referred to as a 'clover leaf nucleus' (*noyau en trèfle*).

Radial segmentation of the nucleus was first noted by Reider (1893) in leukaemic cells. Hence cells bearing such nuclei are referred to as 'Reider cells' (*Plate 6*). Radial segmented nuclei have been found in[*] (1) leukaemic cells from the peripheral blood in various acute leukaemias[†], particularly acute lymphoblastic leukaemia (Hayhoe *et al.*, 1964; Ito, 1974; Ito and Hattori, 1974); (2) leukaemic cells from the peripheral blood in chronic lymphocytic leukaemia (Undritz, 1952; Cawley, 1972); (3) leukaemic cells from the bone marrow in cases of acute myeloid leukaemia (Stenstam *et al.*, 1975); (4) leukaemic cells in the peripheral blood in chronic myelomonocytic leukaemia (Skinnider *et al.*, 1977); (5) cells of malignant B-cell lymphomas in lymph nodes (van der Putte *et al.*, 1984); (6) virus-infected cells (Nii and Kamahora, 1963; Engel *et al.*, 1969; Levinson, 1967, 1970); (7) irradiated cells (Roy-Taranger *et al.*, 1965); and (8) monocytes and lymphocytes from normal oxalated blood (Bessis and Breton-Gorius, 1965; Norberg, 1969, 1970, 1971).

Ultrastructural studies show microtubules in the clefts between the lobes and a study of various profiles shows that microtubules from the centriolar region loop around each bridge between the lobes. It is thought that these microtubules are the interphase remnants of the mitotic spindle and shortening[‡] of these microtubules folds the nucleus in, from the cytoplasmic aspect of the nuclear envelope towards the cell centre (Norberg, 1971).

Bessis and Breton-Gorius (1965) found filaments instead of microtubules in the clefts between the lobes of radial segmented nuclei in oxalate-treated blood. However, this may be explained by the fact that in quite a few situations when microtubules disintegrate filaments are seen in their place (*see* Chapter 12). Further, it may be noted that primary fixation in glutaraldehyde at room temperature is desirable if not absolutely essential for adequate demonstration of microtubules of the spindle apparatus.

That microtubules rather than filaments are involved in radial segmentation is attested by the fact that physicochemical agents (e.g. low temperatures, colchicine, demecolcine and vinblastine) which depolymerize microtubules inhibit the formation of Reider cells in oxalate-treated blood (Norberg and Söderström, 1967; Norberg, 1969). Finally, it is worth noting that oxalate salts are not absolutely essential for radial segmentation for this change occurs in heparinized blood and to a much lesser extent in blood to which no anticoagulant has been added.

[*]In some of the references quoted Reider cells are evident in the illustrations but the authors do not mention them in the text, or describe them in other ways (e.g. 'fragmented nuclei' and 'severely deformed atypical nuclei').
[†]In some cases up to 80 per cent of the leukaemic cells may be Reider cells (Bessis, 1973).
[‡]Microtubules do not contract; they shorten. When a structure contracts its mass is unchanged so that a reduction in length is accompanied by an increase in girth or thickness. Microtubules shorten by losing tubulin units (depolymerization); there is no increase in the diameter of the shortened microtubule. (*See* Chapters 2 and 12 for more details.)

Plate 6

Figs. 1–6. Leukaemic cells with radial segmented nuclei from a case of myelomonocytic leukaemia. Various patterns and degrees of segmentation are depicted, leading ultimately (*Fig. 6*) to images suggesting fragmentation of the nucleus. × 11 000; × 11 500; × 17 000; × 12 000; × 11 000; × 11 500

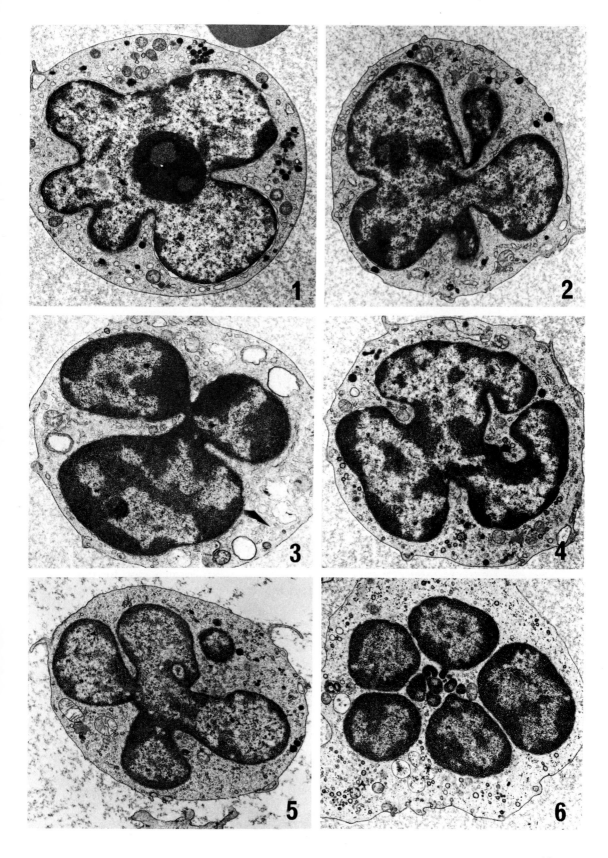

Chromatin in normal, neoplastic and necrotic cells

DNA occurs in the nucleus combined with histones and other proteins. This combination constitutes chromatin. Two forms of chromatin are known to occur in the interphase nucleus: (1) a condensed, presumably inactive, form called 'heterochromatin', which is basophilic with the light microscope and presents as collections of rounded or irregular-shaped electron-dense granules in ultrathin sections (*Plate 7*); and (2) an active form called 'euchromatin', which is dispersed in the nuclear matrix and stains feebly or not at all with basic dyes. This form cannot be confidently identified in electron micrographs either.

In the mitotic nucleus (*Plate 8*) the chromosomes present as elongated bodies constricted at one or more places, and are seen to be composed of heterochromatin which has a structure similar to the heterochromatin areas of the interphase nucleus, except that it is somewhat more densely packed (particularly at metaphase). Thus the heterochromatin of the interphase nucleus is generally looked upon as the unexpanded segments of chromosomal chromatin, while the euchromatin is regarded as the functional expanded portion of the chromosome engaged in synthetic activity within the interphase nucleus. In the mature spermatozoa the chromatin is highly compacted so that it appears as a homogeneous electron-dense mass in the sperm head (*Plate 9*). Even so it can be shown by treatment with alkaline thioglycolate that the chromatin is still strikingly fibrous (Lung, 1972), while treatment with sarkosyl followed with dithiothreitol further decondenses the heterochromatin to reveal the characteristic beads-on-a-string structure (*see below*) of the chromatin fibre (Sobhon *et al.*, 1982).

For some time now the term chromatin, coined on the basis of the tinctorial reaction of this nuclear material to basic dyes, has been restricted to indicate only the DNA-containing Feulgen-positive areas in the nucleus and not the basophilic, but Feulgen-negative, nucleolus. In suitably prepared tissues viewed with the electron microscope, aggregates of electron-dense granules having the characteristic intranuclear chromatin distribution (chromatin pattern) are visualized. Hence, the term chromatin has been retained by electron microscopists even though no tinctorial reaction is involved and the ultrastructural techniques used are not specific for the demonstration of DNA.

In ultrathin sections through interphase nuclei, aggregates of chromatin have a granular appearance. However, it is well established that the structural units of chromatin are fibrous and at high magnifications images that can be interpreted as fibres★ cut in various planes can be discerned. It would appear that ultrathin sections are singularly unsuitable for studying the structure of chromatin and other techniques, such as negative staining, whole mounts of chromosomes and scanning electron microscopy, have been employed to elucidate the structure of chromatin. Even so, despite numerous studies the size and arrangement of chromatin fibres in the interphase and mitotic nucleus has not been unequivocally established.

★One does not as a rule (*see* pages 1215–1221) call a 25 nm thick thread-like structure a 'fibre', but as explained on the next page three levels of organization are evident in chromatin and it is convenient to refer to these as fibres, fibrils and filaments, even though the classic concepts of a fibre being composed of fibrils which, in turn, are composed of a collection of filaments are not met.

Plate 7
Plasma cell from human bronchial mucosa showing the characteristic cartwheel or clockface distribution of heterochromatin aggregates. Centrally placed nucleolus (N), marginated chromatin (A), chromatin centres (B), and nucleolus-associated chromatin (C) can be readily identified in this material, which was fixed in cacodylate-buffered osmium and stained with uranium and lead. × 34 000

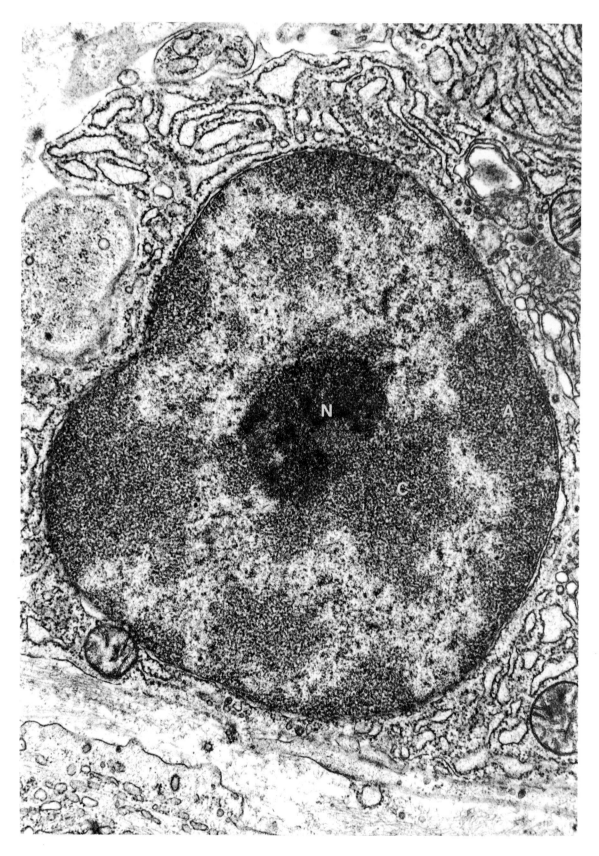

15

Early studies on tissues of higher plants, insects and various vertebrates have given figures for the diameter of chromatin fibres, fibrils or filaments which range from 3–50 nm (4–15 nm in ultrathin sections) (De Robertis, 1956; Ris, 1956, 1962; Moses, 1960; Porter, 1960; Miyai and Steiner, 1965; Abuelo and Moore, 1969; Kaye, 1969; Golomb and Bahr, 1971; Golomb et al., 1971). In suitably treated whole mounts of chromosomes the chromatin fibres were found to have a diameter of about 24 ± 5 nm. Most of the material, however, is protein which can be removed by treatment with trypsin, leaving behind a trypsin-resistant DNA core 2.5–5 nm in diameter.

It is generally believed that the granular appearance of chromatin seen in ultrathin sections results from sections through a tightly coiled structure, but some believe that the chromatin fibres form an interlacing, branching network (Yasuzumi, 1960; Hay and Revel, 1963). Yet others (Hozier et al., 1977; Beçak and Fukuda, 1979) believe that native chromatin may be composed of globules or beads (20–30 nm in diameter) because chromatin presents a 'beads-on-a-string' appearance when subjected to a condition of low salinity. Each bead★ is thought to be an agglomerate of eight to ten nucleosomes about 8 nm in diameter†. Each nucleosome is said to contain 200 base pairs of DNA. The interbead filament (3 nm thick) presumably contains DNA but is looked upon as an artefact resulting from stresses produced during specimen preparation. This is supported by the fact that in some types of preparations nucleosomes are present but the interbead filament is absent (Rattner and Hamkalo, 1979).

There are other studies (Finch and Klug, 1976; Haggis and Bond, 1978; Ris 1978; Cameron et al., 1979; Thoma et al., 1979; Woodcock et al., 1984) which suggest three levels of organization in chromatin. Based on this one can present a tentative plan for the structure of chromatin as follows. There is virtually unanimous agreement that the double stranded DNA occurs as a filament which measures 2 nm in diameter (one to several metres in length). This probably has a thin protein coat of its own (which brings the diameter of the filament up to about 3.2–5.2 nm) and it seems likely that it is wrapped around a core of histone to form a fibril about 10 nm in diameter. The 10 nm fibril is packaged by either folding or spiralling (i.e. a solenoid-like structure) to form a chromatin fibre 20–30 nm in diameter.

In tissues fixed in osmium (collidine- or veronal-acetate-buffered) and stained with lead, nuclei have a somewhat homogeneous appearance and condensations of chromatin with the pattern familiar to light microscopists are either absent or barely discernible (see for example Plate 1). The closest approach to the familiar chromatin pattern is seen when tissues are fixed in glutaraldehyde, post-fixed in osmium and stained with uranium and lead.

This difference is attributable to the staining techniques employed (see Plates 50, 51 and 407 and also to the fixative and buffer used. It is clear that lead is a poor stain for chromatin, while uranium, particularly alcoholic uranium, stains chromatin intensely. (Uranium can combine with DNA in amounts sufficient to increase the dry weight by a factor of almost two (Huxley and Zubay, 1961).) In my experience, tissues fixed in cacodylate-buffered osmium, and stained with uranium and lead, give a good visualization of the familiar chromatin pattern (Plate 7) only a little less compact and dense than that obtained from glutaraldehyde fixation and double staining with uranium and lead.

★There is also another system of nomenclature where the nucleosomes are referred to as 'beads' and the structures composed of eight to ten nucleosomes are called 'superbeads'.
†Current view is that the nucleosome is not spherical but discoid (diameter 11 nm, thickness 5.5 nm) in shape.

Plate 8
Ultrathin section through chromosomes of a mitotic nucleus. From monkey kidney cells in culture. × 25 000

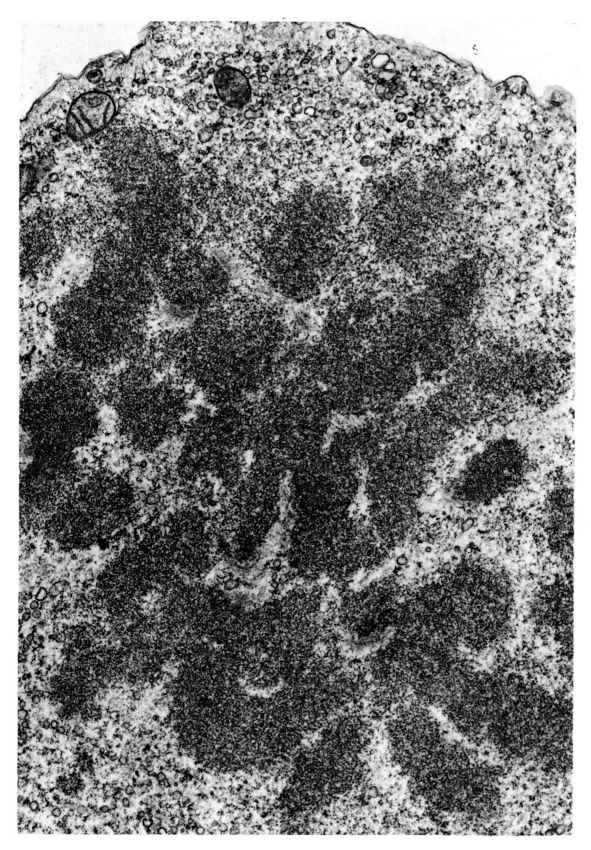

17

It has been argued in the past that osmium may be a poor fixative for chromatin and that the difference observed is due to loss of DNA. This idea has to be discarded, for ultraviolet spectrometry has shown that little, if any, DNA is lost by this process, and the work of Moses (1956) has shown that the characteristic chromatin pattern can be demonstrated with the Feulgen technique in osmium-fixed nuclei that do not show this pattern with the electron microscope.

Chromatin aggregates occur in certain preferred sites in the nucleus and it is this phenomenon which produces the familiar chromatin pattern. Such aggregates of chromatin may be designated as follows (*Plate 7*).

(1) *Peripheral or marginal chromatin:* irregular-shaped masses of chromatin adjacent to the nuclear envelope, between the nuclear pores. There is a clear area devoid of heterochromatin immediately behind the nuclear pores.
(2) *Chromatin centres:* randomly distributed chromatin aggregates within the nuclear matrix.
(3) *Nucleolus-associated chromatin:* focal aggregates of chromatin granules along the periphery of the nucleolus.
(4) *Intranucleolar chromatin:* although the nucleolus contains mainly protein and RNA and is Feulgen negative, numerous studies have shown that it contains a small amount of DNA also (*see* review by Miller and Beatty, 1969).

It is now clear that not only the distribution but also the proportion of heterochromatin to euchromatin varies from one cell type to another. Since it is well established that the average amount of DNA in the somatic cell nuclei from various tissues of a given species is constant, one can argue that in nuclei poorly endowed with heterochromatin there will be more of the metabolically active euchromatin (Fawcett, 1981). Thus one may expect that metabolically active cells will have a paler-staining nucleus with fewer and smaller heterochromatin masses. This thesis is borne out by the fact that stem cells or blast cells have paler nuclei, and that in a maturing series of cells such as the red blood cells an increasing concentration of heterochromatin masses becomes evident as the cell matures, and becomes metabolically less active.

An apparent exception to the rule is the plasma cell with its familiar chromatin pattern (clockface or cartwheel) of large heterochromatin masses. This cell, with its abundant rough endoplasmic reticulum, is known to be actively engaged in the synthesis of antibodies. Fawcett (1981) has put forward two interesting suggestions to explain this anomaly. He states 'It is conceivable that in a cell so highly specialized in its function only a small proportion of its DNA may be needed in an active form to direct the narrow range of synthetic activities in its cytoplasm. Alternatively one may speculate that all the transcription of information necessary for continuing synthesis of antibody took place at an earlier stage in the differentiation of the plasma cell before its nucleus acquired its definitive coarse chromatin pattern'.

One of the most striking transformations of heterochromatin to euchromatin occurs during the *in vitro* activation of peripheral blood lymphocytes by phytohaemagglutinin. During this blastic transformation the nucleus enlarges two- to fourfold, most of the heterochromatin is converted to euchromatin, the nucleolus enlarges in size and instead of monoribosomes polyribosomes are seen in the cytoplasm. These changes correlate well with the heightened RNA and protein synthesis occurring in these cells.

Plate 9
Mouse spermatozoon, showing extreme condensation of chromatin. In this form the chromatin is metabolically inert and serves only an archival function, transmitting genetic information to the next generation. × 23 000

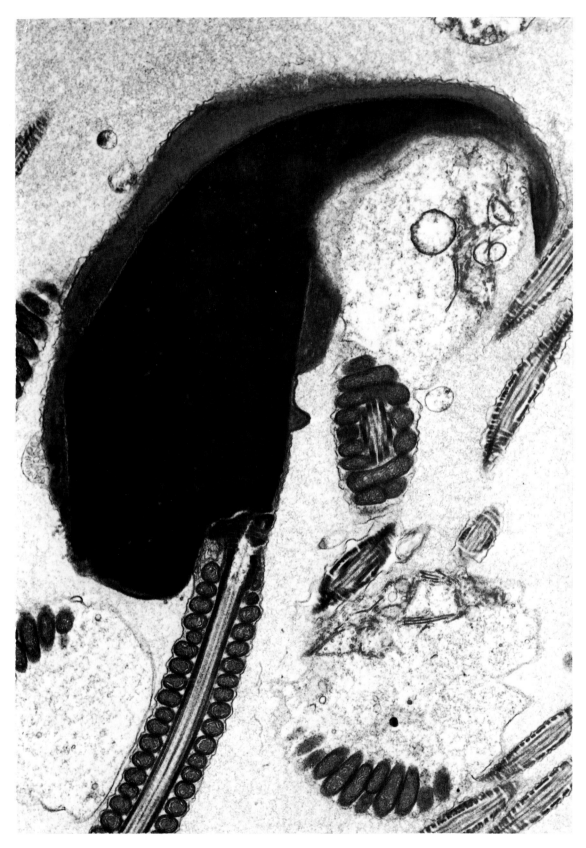

19

There is now a substantial body of evidence supporting the idea that euchromatin is active in RNA and DNA synthesis but heterochromatin shows little or no activity as a template for replication and transcription (*see* review by Frenster, 1974). In keeping with this is the observation that in regenerating rat liver 24 hours after partial hepatectomy when the synthesis of DNA and RNA reaches quite high levels almost all the chromatin in most nuclei is in the decondensed form (i.e. euchromatin) and only small and sparse heterochromatin aggregates are seen (Derenzini and Bonetti, 1975; Derenzini *et al.*, 1976). Conversely, various substances (e.g. ethionine, actinomycin D and α-amanitine) which inhibit RNA synthesis induce a condensation of chromatin (Shinozuka *et al.*, 1968; Goldblatt *et al.*, 1969a, b; Marinozzi and Fiume, 1971; Recher *et al.*, 1971; Magalhães and Magalhães, 1985).

However, when attempting to correlate the metabolic activity of a cell with its degree of nuclear staining by basophilic dyes, or with the degree of chromatin aggregation seen with the electron microscope, one must take another factor into consideration. Thus, although the total amount of DNA per nucleus is remarkably constant in a given species, the concentration of DNA is very variable, as evidenced by variations in nuclear size, and there is also a striking difference in the nature and amount of total protein of various nuclei. According to Mirsky and Osawa (1961) it is this factor which is largely responsible for the difference in staining characteristics of nuclei, and they point out that there is a significant correlation between the amount of residual protein (non-histone protein) and metabolic activity of the cell. Thus liver and kidney cells with high metabolic activity have relatively large amounts of nuclear residual protein compared with the nuclei of metabolically sluggish cells such as lymphocytes and nucleated erythrocytes.

Light microscopists have long been familiar with the nuclear changes seen in malignant tumour cells and also with the fact that none of these changes taken singly is specific for the neoplastic state. It had been hoped that the electron microscope would reveal specific morphological alterations which could be regarded as the hallmark of malignancy, but such a hope has not fructified. The chromatin pattern of tumour nuclei is very variable but not characteristic or distinctive (Bernhard and Granboulan, 1963; Ghadially, 1985). The electron microscope does little more than tell us what we already know, namely that tumour cell nuclei are highly pleomorphic. The well-known hyperchromasia of the neoplastic nucleus is now attributed to polyploidy. With the electron microscope, these hyperchromatic nuclei are seen to contain larger and/or more numerous heterochromatin masses. However, in tumours one also finds quite pale nuclei with a paucity of heterochromatin and, hence, presumably an excess of

---

Plate 10

Multiple myeloma. Clinically this was not a very aggressive condition. In keeping with this, the nucleus of this plasma cell is not quite as 'homogeneous-looking' as that found in highly aggressive versions of multiple myeloma (compare with *Plate 199* in Chapter 5), but on the other hand, the chromatin aggregates are much smaller than those seen in normal and reactive plasma cells (compare with *Plate 7*). Magnification is not known. (*Electron micrograph supplied by Dr A. Senoo*)

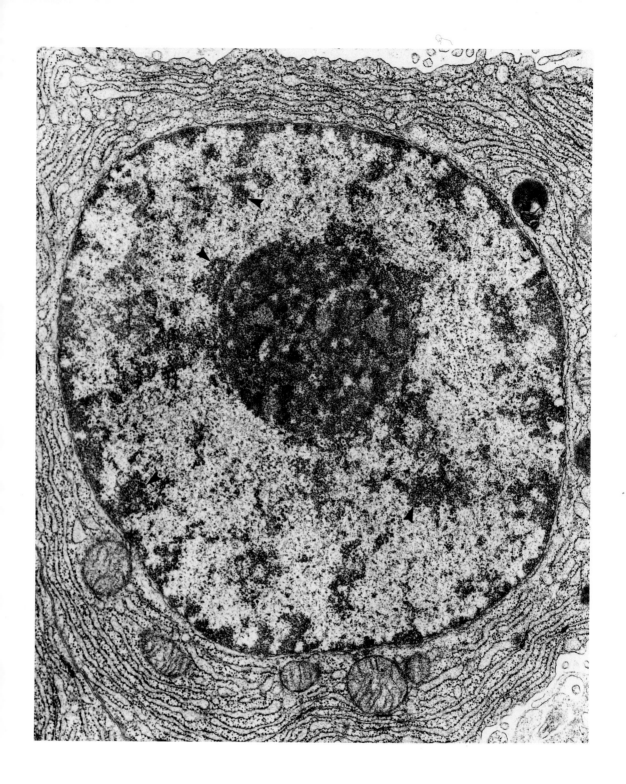

21

the more active euchromatin (*see* for example, *Plate 33*). This point* has perhaps not been sufficiently stressed despite early recognition of this phenomenon by light microscopists (Caspersson and Santesson, 1942; Montella, 1954), who referred to tumour cells with hyperchromatic nuclei and a not particularly enlarged nucleolus as type A cells and to cells with a pale nucleus and enlarged nucleolus as type B cells.

The significance of type A and B cells has not been probed, but applying the ideas discussed earlier, one is tempted to speculate that, while the hyperchromatic nucleus may be of diagnostic importance (as an indicator of polyploidy), it is the cell with the pale nucleus (an indicator of an increased amount of functionally active euchromatin) and an enlarged nucleolus (an indicator of active synthesis of ribosomal RNA and, hence, ribosomes and protein) which is more important from the point of view of active cell proliferation and, hence, growth of the tumour.

Neoplasms of plasma cells afford further support for such a thesis, for in benign plasmacytomas the characteristic heterochromatin pattern of the plasma cell nucleus is more or less retained, but in malignant versions such as multiple myeloma and plasma cell leukaemia this pattern is more or less lost and, indeed, in many cases the nucleus is large and pale, for it contains only scant small aggregates of heterochromatin (compare *Plates 7, 10* and *199*).

Students of pathology are well aware of the nuclear changes in necrosis, designated as pyknosis, karyorrhexis and karyolysis (*Plates 11* and *12*). The terms 'necrosis'† and 'cell death' are often used interchangeably, but I shall here use the term necrosis, in a stricter sense to imply morphological changes occurring after a lethal injury which leads to cell death. One need hardly point out that cells examined in fixed tissues, though dead, do not show the morphological features of necrosis, and that some time (at least eight hours for rat liver (Majno *et al.*, 1960)) must elapse between lethal injury (e.g. cutting off of blood supply) before the classic changes we call 'necrosis' are detectable in the nucleus by light microscopy. Viewed this way, necrosis may also be looked upon as an early stage prior to frank autolysis.

---

*One can find reports in the literature where it is claimed that the amount of heterochromatin in neoplastic nuclei is increased, and others which say it is decreased. However, the morphometric study (ultrastructural) of Nagl and Hiersche (1983) on the epithelial cells of the uterine cervix and adenocarcinomas again shows that 'carcinoma cell nuclei fall into two groups, some with less condensed chromatin than normal ones, and some with twice as much as normal ones'.

†At one time the term 'necrosis' was restricted to mean 'death of cells in the living animal' but this is not a useful point of distinction because the changes that occur in the cells of an excised piece of tissue maintained at body temperature and humidity are similar to those occurring after cutting off the blood supply to the tissue in the living animal or after death of the animal.

Plate 11
Cells harvested from a pleural effusion in a case of lymphocytic leukaemia.
Fig. 1. Pyknosis. × 20 000
Fig. 2. Karyorrhexis. × 20 000

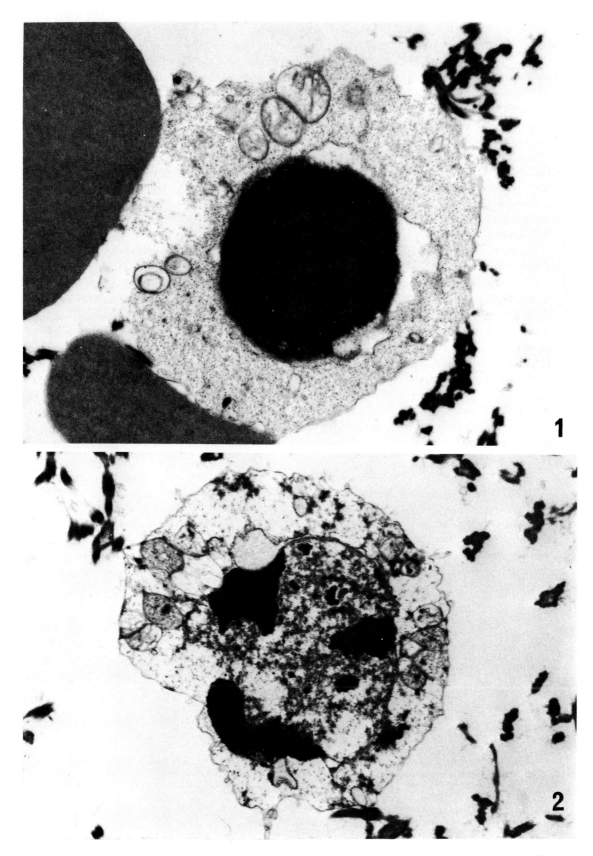

The large literature on cell injury, cell death, necrosis and autolysis can hardly be discussed here. My main purpose is to illustrate the electron microscopic equivalents of the nuclear changes associated with necrosis. Since these changes involve the distribution of chromatin they are considered in this section of the text, but changes also occur in the other nuclear components such as the nucleolus and nuclear envelope.

Pyknosis involves a shrinkage of the nucleus and condensation of the chromatin (*Plate 11, Fig. 1*). In karyorrhexis the nuclear chromatin is aggregated or clumped into numerous masses, and later released by rupture of the nuclear envelope (*Plate 11, Fig. 2*). In karyolysis the nuclear envelope remains reasonably intact but the contents are partially or completely lost (*Plate 12, Fig. 2*). Such ultrastructural appearances amply vindicate what has long been taught about these nuclear changes to students of pathology. But although one can find electron microscopic images that correlate well with our light microscopic concepts of pyknosis, karyorrhexis and karyolysis, there are also other images which cannot confidently be fitted into one of these three well known categories.

Electron microscopic studies have in fact focused attention on a much more common and consistent pattern of nuclear change in the necrotic cell, which is spoken of as chromatin margination. Here a condensation of the chromatin occurs along or adjacent to the inner membrane of the nuclear envelope, while chromatin disappears from other parts of the nucleus. Such a condensation may present in ultrathin sections as a complete ring, a crescent-shaped mass or irregular clumps of condensed chromatin (*Plate 12*) set at the periphery of the nucleus. Such changes are seen in necrosis resulting from the action of various noxious agents, such as viral infection, x-rays or ischaemia.

Margination of chromatin appears to be a fairly early change that occurs in the nucleus after irreversible injury leading to cell death. Trump *et al.* (1963, 1965a, b) studied this phenomenon in slices of mouse liver incubated in aseptic conditions for various periods of time prior to fixation. They noted various changes such as loss of mitochondrial dense granules, swelling of mitochondria, dilatation and vesiculation of the rough endoplasmic reticulum and margination of the chromatin which was detectable after 30 minutes but was not well developed until two hours after excision of liver tissue. On the other hand, Kalimo *et al.* (1977) report that ten minutes after permanent global cerebral ischaemia the nuclei of various cells in the brain showed chromatin clumping and margination. This was followed by the familiar cytoplasmic changes such as dilatation of endoplasmic reticulum and swollen mitochondria. In *Plate 12, Fig. 1*, we see a necrotic hepatocyte obtained from rabbit liver collected one hour after death of the animal. The rough endoplasmic reticulum is not dilated and most of the mitochondria are not obviously swollen but the nucleus shows a severe degree of chromatin margination. Thus it

---

Plate 12

Fig. 1. Rabbit liver fixed one hour after death of the animal. Chromatin margination is evident in this necrotic hepatocyte nucleus, as also are woolly focal densities in the mitochondria (arrow) which are considered to be evidence of irreversible cell injury. Endoplasmic reticulum and mitochondria are, however, not swollen in this instance. × 19 000

Fig. 2. Two nuclei from an ovarian carcinoma are seen in this electron micrograph. The one on the left shows karyolysis, while the one on the right may be interpreted as an intermediate stage between margination and lysis. × 10 500

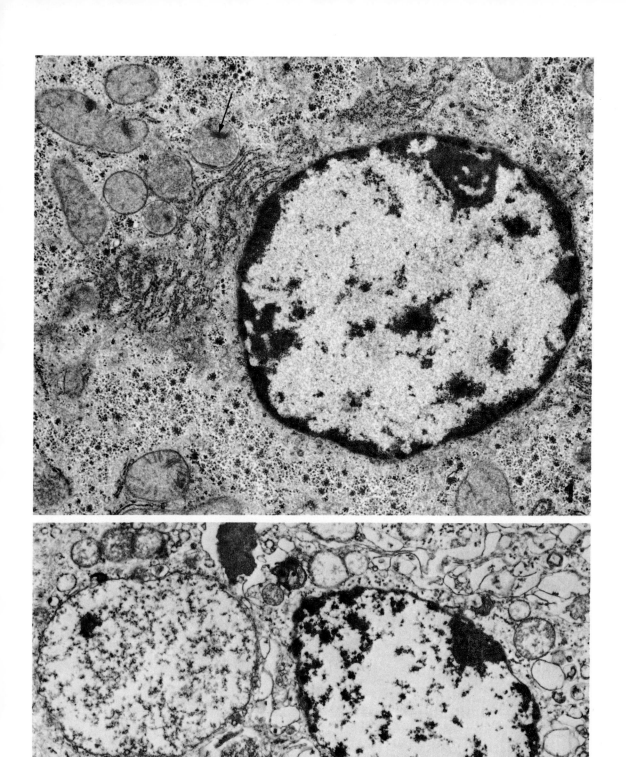

would appear that the familiar cytoplasmic changes, such as dilatation and vesiculation of the endoplasmic reticulum and mitochondrial swelling which are the equivalent of cloudy swelling seen with the light microscope (*see* page 248) do not always precede chromatin margination. One may therefore speculate that whether such cytoplasmic changes occur or not and the degree to which they occur probably depends on the amount of fluid available to swell various cell compartments.

Chromatin margination is also seen in so-called physiological necrosis (necrobiosis); that is to say, in cells that die normally in the body. An excellent site for studying this phenomenon is articular cartilage where *in situ* necrosis of chondrocytes normally occurs. We have occasionally noted chromatin margination in such cells. Another interesting alteration of nuclear morphology seen in a chondrocyte which has suffered *in situ* necrosis is illustrated in *Plate 13, Fig. 1*. Here the nucleus is crenated and the nuclear contents have a homogeneous appearance. No chromatin masses or nucleoli are discernible. Such a change may be designated 'homogenization' of the nucleus, and it is worth noting that this type of change is at times seen also in other cells besides chondrocytes. Necrosis of chondrocytes is followed by disintegration and dispersal of cell fragments (*Plate 13, Fig. 2*) and lipidic debris derived from them into the matrix (Ghadially *et al.*, 1965; Ghadially and Roy, 1969a).

This section began by noting that necrosis follows lethal injury producing cell death. However, the precise point at which a cell may be pronounced dead is debatable. In analogy with somatic death, one may argue that just as all the tissues do not die or cease functioning simultaneously, neither do the organelles. Electron microscopic studies tend to support such an idea, for sequential changes occur in cell organelles over a period of time after lethal cell injury. Further it should be noted that changes such as dilatation of the rough endoplasmic reticulum and mitochondrial swelling are reversible and so also are mild degrees of chromatin margination. Hence such changes do not necessarily indicate lethal injury or cell death. Trump *et al.* (1965a, b) from their study of necrosis in isolated liver slices concluded that when (one hour after excision of liver tissue) the mitochondria came to contain flocculent densities (*Plate 12, Fig. 1*) the point of no return had been reached. Since then numerous observations have attested to the validity of this observation and such flocculent densities in mitochondria have come to be recognized as the electron microscopic hallmark of lethally injured dead or dying cells. However, later studies (Myagkaya *et al.*, 1985) suggest that the point of no return for liver tissue incubated at 37°C is probably 1.5 hours when about 37 per cent of the mitochondria show flocculent densities (also called 'woolly' densities), and not at one hour when only 8 per cent of the mitochondria contain these densities (*see* pages 250–253 and page 296).

Plate 13

Necrotic chondrocytes from the articular cartilage of a six-month-old rabbit. (*From Ghadially and Roy, 1969a*)

Fig. 1. The nucleus (N) is crenated and its contents are homogeneous. The distended cisternae (C) of the rough endoplasmic reticulum and disintegrating mitochondria (M) can be easily recognized. × 23 000

Fig. 2. Another pattern of chondrocyte necrosis and disintegration is seen in this electron micrograph. In this shrunken cell lying in a lacuna (L) organelles can no longer be identified. The dark masses (M) probably represent fragmented nuclear remnants. Cell processes (P) and lipidic debris (D) derived from them are seen among the collagen fibrils (C) in the matrix. × 21 000

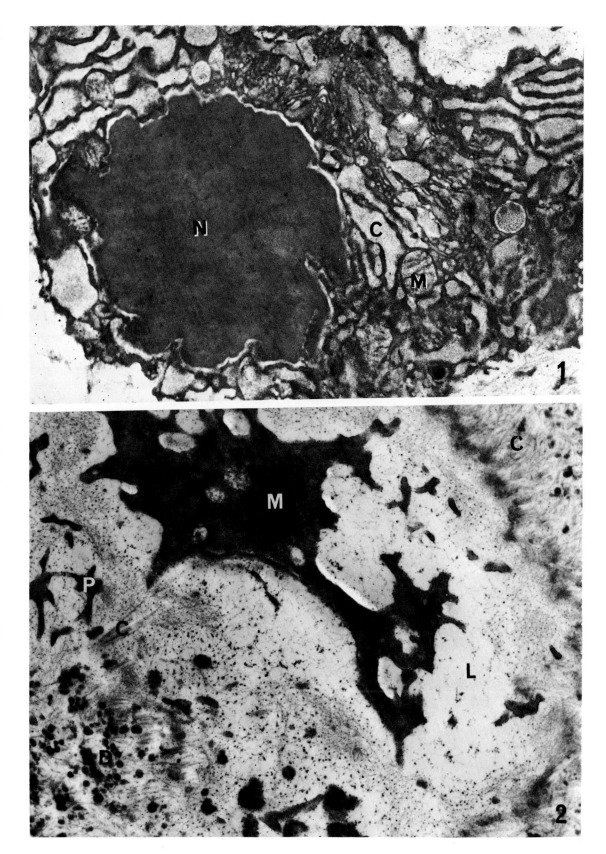

27

The nuclear matrix and interchromatin and perichromatin granules

The nuclear matrix★ (karyoplasm, nucleoplasm or nuclear sap) of living cells has a clear limpid appearance, but much filamentous and granular material can be discerned in this region by electron microscopy. Hence this region of the nucleus is sometimes referred to by electron microscopists as the interchromatin area or substance (that is to say, the material lying between the chromatin) and the two types of granules seen in this region as the interchromatin and perichromatin granules (*Plates 14* and *15*). Besides these granules the nuclear matrix also contains euchromatin and filamentous material of low density, believed to be protein.

Perichromatin granules, as their name implies, usually lie on the borders of chromatin areas. These electron-dense, solitary, spherical granules are separated from the adjacent chromatin by an electron-lucent halo. The granule itself measures 30–35 nm in diameter; the overall diameter including the halo is about 75 nm (Watson, 1962; Bernhard and Granboulan, 1963). It has been estimated that the hepatocyte nucleus contains 500–2000 such granules. Morphological and cytochemical studies (Vasquez-Nin and Bernhard, 1971; Bouteille, 1972) suggest that they are made up of coiled, packed 3–5 nm thick filaments of messenger RNA (mRNA) set in a proteinaceous matrix.

Interchromatin granules are highly electron-dense. They vary in diameter from 15–50 nm (Granboulan and Bernhard, 1961; Bernhard and Granboulan, 1963; Jézéquel and Marinozzi, 1963; Swift, 1963) and frequently have an angular shape. They often occur as clusters in the nuclear matrix, but single granules or short linear arrays of granules are also quite common.

At one time it was suggested (Watson, 1962; Bernhard and Granboulan, 1963) that both RNA and DNA were present in the perichromatin granules and both types of granules were nuclear ribosomes involved in the synthesis of nuclear proteins†. However, it has now been shown (Vasquez-Nin and Bernhard, 1971) that perichromatin granules are morphologically and cytochemically identical to Balbiani granules (found in Dipteran giant chromosomes) which are believed to contain mRNA. It has hence been suggested that perichromatin granules also contain mRNA and that the coiled, packed 3–5 nm thick filaments of mRNA probably unravel in the neighbourhood of the nuclear pores through which they migrate into the cytoplasm (Bouteille, 1972).

It is postulated that at least some of the perichromatin granules come from the nucleolus, because an accumulation of perichromatin granules is seen in the juxtanucleolar region after administration of various drugs such as: (1) corydycepin (Puvion *et al.*, 1976); (2) camptothecin (Gajkowska *et al.*, 1977); and (3) aflatoxin B_1 and α-amanitin (Derenzini and Moyne, 1978). It should be noted that such drugs also produce nucleolar segregation and fragmentation (page 70) and depressed protein synthesis.

★The term 'nuclear matrix' has long been used to designate the protein-rich fluid in which lie the chromatin and the nucleolus. However, in recent years a nuclear framework structure loosely referred to as the 'nuclear matrix' by some, but more properly referred to as the 'nuclear protein matrix' (or by some of the other proposed terms such as the 'nuclear skeleton', 'reversibly contractile nuclear matrix' and 'reversibly contractile nucleoskeleton'), has now been isolated and characterized. It comprises largely proteins (about 96 per cent) and traces of DNA, RNA, phospholipids and carbohydrates. Besides being responsible for the contraction of nuclei the nuclear protein matrix is thought to play a fundamental role in DNA replication, and synthesis and transport of RNA. (For references supporting these statements *see* Berezney and Coffey, 1977; Wunderlich and Herlan, 1977; Agutter and Richardson, 1980.)
†The collective evidence (Wassef, 1979) now shows that interchromatin granules contain mainly phosphorylated proteins. They may contain a small amount of stable RNA but there is no real proof of this.

Plate 14
Fig. 1. Human osteogenic sarcoma. The tumour cell nucleus contains clusters of markedly electron-dense interchromatin granules (IC), and a few perichromatin granules (arrows) separated from the adjacent chromatin by a halo. × 27 000
Fig. 2. High-power view of perichromatin granules (about 33 nm in diameter) from the nucleus of a rat hepatocyte (arrows). × 120 000

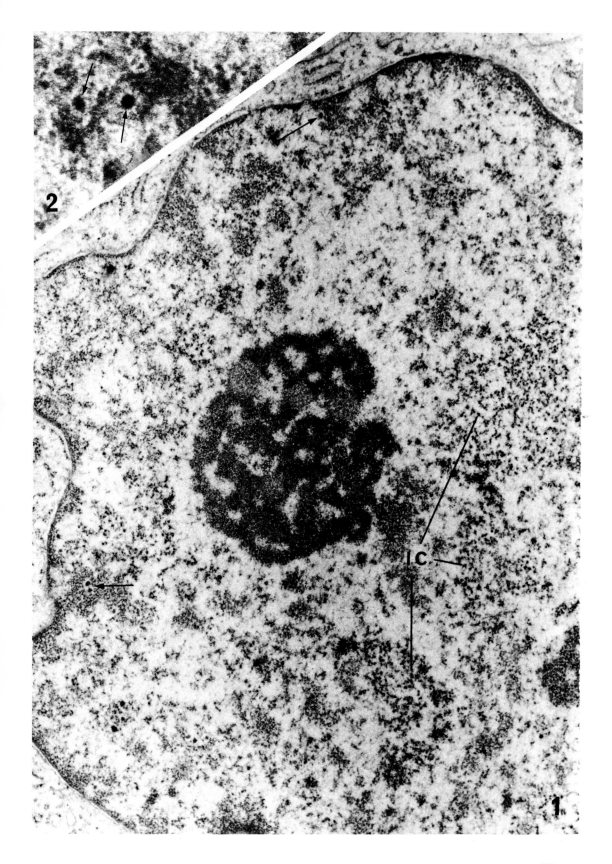

Little is known about the frequency and distribution of these granules in various cell types, but they can be easily demonstrated in hepatocytes and pancreatic acinar cells; many perichromatin granules are also said to occur in neurons and glial cells (Bouteille, 1972).

An abundance of interchromatin granules is seen in various tumours (*Plates 14* and *15, Fig. 1*). According to Bernhard and Granboulan (1963), interchromatin granules are seen more frequently in tumour cells, and Reddy and Svoboda (1968) have observed that, 'In chronic studies of carcinogenesis in rat liver the most consistent ultrastructural alteration is an apparent increase in interchromatinic granules'.

An abundance of perichromatin granules has also been noted in some tumours; for example, scirrhous carcinoma of the breast (Murad and Scarpelli, 1967). I, too, have at times been impressed by the abundance of either interchromatin or perichromatin granules in tumour cell nuclei. My experience is that in a given tumour one or the other type of granule is prominent, but not both.

Various studies indicate that an increase in the number of perichromatin granules (and often also some increase in size) may be an indicator of aberrations in protein synthetic activity for this change is noted after: (1) administration of drugs like the ones mentioned on page 28; (2) cycloheximide (an inhibitor of protein synthesis) (Daskal *et al.*, 1975); (3) galactoflavin (induces riboflavin deficiency) (Norton *et al.*, 1977); (4) hypo- or hyperthermic shock (depresses protein synthesis) to cells in culture (Heine *et al.*, 1971; Cervera, 1979); (5) neurons in Alzheimer's disease (deranged protein synthesis) (Mann *et al.*, 1981); (6) dichlorobenzimidazole riboside (impairs HnRNA and rRNA synthesis) (Puvion *et al.*, 1979); and (7) cadmium chloride and 8-methoxy psoralen (both inhibit protein synthesis) (Puvion-Dutilleul and Puvion, 1981; Ree *et al.*, 1982).

Plate 15

Fig. 1. Squamous cell carcinoma of the lip. Nucleus showing collections (demarcated by arrowheads) of interchromatin granules and a few perichromatin granules (arrows). × 34 000 (*From Ghadially, 1985*)

Fig. 2. Adenocarcinoma of lung. Nucleus showing prominent (about 45–50 nm in diameter) perichromatin granules (arrows). × 32 000 (*From Ghadially, 1985*)

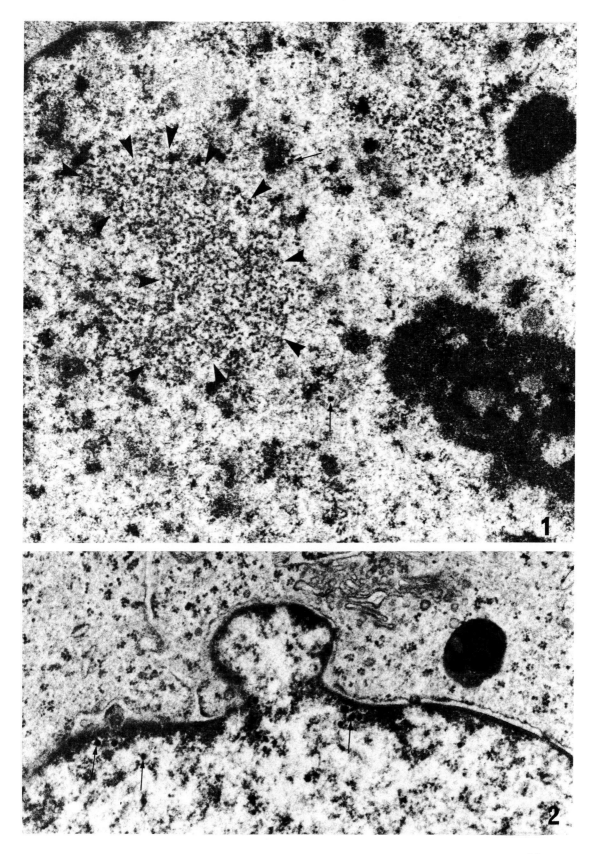

31

As noted before (page 28), the normal perichromatin granule is said to measure about 30–35 nm in diameter (Watson, 1962; Bernhard and Granboulan, 1963). However, somewhat more prominent, larger granules are at times seen in various pathological tissues, particularly tumours (*Plate 15, Fig. 2*) and on rare occasions they can attain almost twice the accepted normal size (i.e. up to about 60 nm in diameter) (*Plate 16*). Much larger granules (up to about 400 nm in diameter which I (Ghadially, 1985) have called 'giant perichromatin granules') have been recorded to occur only in the fibroblastic cells of nasopharyngeal angiofibroma. These giant perichromatin granules (*Plate 17*) are described in the next section of the text (page 34).

An increase in the number and size (up to about 50 nm) of perichromatin granules has also been seen during maturation and differentiation of keratinocytes of normal human skin (Karásek *et al.*, 1972). As is well known keratinocytes proliferate in the basal and suprabasal layers of the stratum germinativum; while in the more superficial layers the keratinocytes mature and finally transform into cornified cells. It is in the upper layers of the stratum granulosum that regressive changes heralding disintegration and final disappearance of the nuclei are prominent. Such changes include nucleolar segregation, formation of ring-shaped nucleoli★, together with an increase in perichromatin granules. Karásek *et al.* (1972) state that this 'might suggest that the RNA synthesis in these cells is inhibited first in the nucleoli before the cessation of extranucleolar synthesis and nuclear disintegration'.

Thus the collective evidence lends considerable support to the idea that accumulations and/or enlargement of perichromatin granules in the nucleus reflects a state of suppressed protein synthesis. One therefore wonders whether the prominence of perichromatin granules in some tumour cells is an indicator of naturally occurring aberrations of protein synthesis or whether it reflects the effectiveness of some therapeutic measure in inhibiting protein synthesis. I have at times seen quite prominent perichromatin granules in residual tumours after therapy. However, studies on animal and human tumours before and after various types of therapy are needed before one can evaluate such sporadic observations. At the moment we do not have precise information about the size and distribution of these granules in various normal and neoplastic cells. It would appear that most workers on tumour ultrastructure have ignored these granules, while a few have mistaken them for virus particles.

★The significance of these nucleolar changes are discussed on pages 70 and 62 respectively.

Plate 16

Fig. 1. Benign fibrous histiocytoma. Several enlarged perichromatin granules are associated with the marginal heterochromatin. The granule indicated by an arrow measures about 53 nm in diameter. Note also the prominent nuclear fibrous lamina (arrowheads). × 61 000

Fig. 2. From the same specimen as *Fig. 1*. Within and adjacent to the nucleolus-associated heterochromatin lie several enlarged perichromatin granules. A group of perichromatin granules surrounded by a ring of filamentous material (arrowheads) is also present. Filamentous material is at times also seen around solitary giant perichromatin granules (*Plate 17*), intranuclear glycogen inclusions (*Plate 51*), and nuclear bodies (*Plates 77 and 78*). The perichromatin granule indicated by an arrow measures about 64 nm in diameter. × 64 000

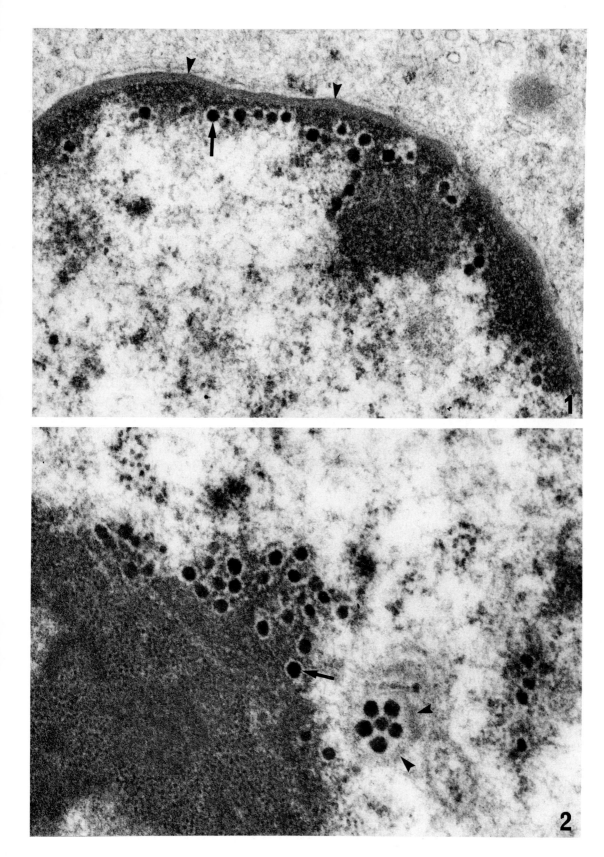

Giant perichromatin granules

I coined the term 'giant perichromatin granules' (Ghadially, 1985) to describe the large, round, electron-dense granules (up to about ten times bigger than normal perichromatin granules) which are found in the nuclei of the fibroblastic cells in nasopharyngeal angiofibroma, because there is now much evidence which shows that they are in fact grossly enlarged perichromatin granules (*Plate 17*). Several studies show that these granules, which can measure up to about 400 nm in diameter★ are pathognomonic of nasopharyngeal angiofibroma and that nothing quite like it is seen in any other site or situation (Svoboda and Kirchner, 1966; Albrecht and Küttner, 1970; Dorn *et al.*, 1971; Siefert, 1971; Stiller *et al.*, 1976; Topilko *et al.*, 1981; Hill, 1985). Like normal perichromatin granules, giant perichromatin granules lying adjacent to the heterochromatin are separated from it by a halo. Sometimes a giant granule is surrounded by a large filamentous ring or halo (*Plate 17, inset; see also Plate 16, Fig. 2*).

Until recently the nature of these granules remained obscure. Some suggested that they were virus particles†, but the morphology of these granules and the occurrence of granules of sizes ranging from normal perichromatin granules to the very large dense granules, clearly suggested that they were unusually large or giant perichromatin granules, but chemical proof that this was indeed the case was lacking. The elegant studies of Topilko *et al.* (1984) have now dispelled doubts about the nature of these granules. Their enzymatic digestion studies and cytochemical studies demonstrate that just like normal perichromatin granules, the giant granules also contain RNA and protein but no DNA.

However, the reason why the perichromatin granules in nasopharyngeal angiofibroma attain so large a size as to deserve to be called 'giant perichromatin granules' is not at all clear. Since an increase in number and size of perichromatin granules is now thought to be an indicator of a state of depressed protein synthesis (page 32), one may speculate that these are metabolically depressed cells and that tumour growth is probably achieved by cells that do not contain giant perichromatin granules. Such an idea is also in keeping with the fact that in the cells containing giant perichromatin granules there is a relative paucity of organelles and abundance of intermediate filaments in the cell cytoplasm; and this too is thought to be a regressive or degenerative change (pages 892–896).

The nuclei of cells containing giant perichromatin granules constantly show also a fairly prominent nuclear fibrous lamina (Topilko *et al.*, 1984; Ghadially, 1985; Hill, 1985). This is not too surprising since the nasopharyngeal angiofibroma is essentially a benign tumour (locally aggressive but very rarely metastasizes), and it is in such tumours (and tumour-like lesions and repair tissues) and not in malignant tumours that one finds a prominent nuclear fibrous lamina (page 54 and Ghadially, 1985). Such considerations also add weight to the idea that the giant perichromatin granule-containing cells are probably metabolically depressed cells.

★It is difficult to say at what point a perichromatin granule qualifies to be called a 'giant perichromatin granule'. However, one may tentatively fix this point at 100 nm (i.e. about three times normal size). It would appear that, until now, granules of this size and larger have been found only in nasopharyngeal angiofibroma.
†The idea that they are virus particles is quite untenable; the large differences in size strongly argue against such an idea. However, just about any electron-dense particles or granules including normal-sized perichromatin granules have at one time or other been mistaken for viral particles. *See* for example, illustrations and legends in Boyle *et al.* (1971) and Ahmed and Mukherjee (1974). *See also* page 138.

Plate 17

Figs. 1, 2 and inset. Nasopharyngeal angiofibroma. *Figs. 1* and *2* show nuclei of fibroblastic cells containing perichromatin granules which range in size from normal to giant. The thin arrow (*Fig. 1*) points to a granule which measures about 33 nm in diameter (i.e. normal size), the thick arrow (*Fig. 2*) to a giant granule which measures about 270 nm in diameter. The inset shows a giant granule (diameter about 397 nm) with a large filamentous halo. The cytoplasm of the cells shown in *Figs. 1* and *2* contains intermediate filaments (presumably vimentin) but few organelles. The nuclei show a nuclear fibrous lamina (arrowheads). × 32 000, × 37 000, Inset × 34 000

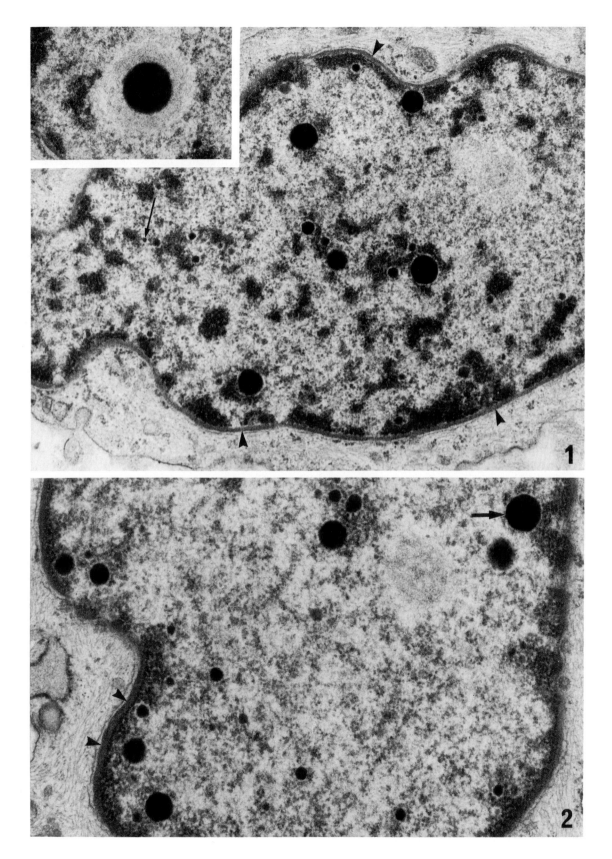

Nuclear envelope and pores

In electron micrographs the nuclear envelope is seen to consist of two membranes separated by a perinuclear cistern, generally about 20–30 nm wide (Watson, 1955, 1959). The outer membrane of the nuclear envelope is often studded with some ribosomes, and in favourable sections continuity between it and the rough endoplasmic reticulum are demonstrable, as is also a continuity between the cisternae of the rough endoplasmic reticulum and the perinuclear cistern (*Plate 18, Fig. 1*).

At intervals along the nuclear envelope the two membranes fuse (*Plate 18, Figs. 1-4*) producing 'fenestrations' called the nuclear pores (Watson, 1959; Oberling and Bernhard, 1961). In tangential sections each pore is seen (i.e. *en face* view) to be surrounded by, or delimited by, an annulus (*Plate 19*) and at times a granule or 'knob' is seen in the centre of the pore (Rhodin, 1963). Annuli demarcating pores are also seen in freeze-etched preparations (*Plate 20*) and preparations of isolated nuclear envelopes. Futher, annuli can be visualized on both the outer and inner aspects of the nuclear envelope where they are referred to as the 'outer ring' and 'inner ring' respectively. Although some quite wide variations in pore sizes have been reported, the diameter of the pore proper is usually about 55–70 nm while that of the outer rim of the annulus is about 100–120 nm.

The nuclear pores in certain cells may display a regular pattern of distribution on the nuclear envelope, but more often than not they appear to be randomly distributed. Various patterns have been described such as an 'orthogonal square pattern', 'hexagonal arrays' and 'clumped patterns' (for references and details *see* Wunderlich and Franke, 1968; Markovics *et al.*, 1974; Severs *et al.*, 1976; Pedro *et al.*, 1984). Since heterochromatin aggregates are absent behind nuclear pores, the pattern of pore distribution reflects the pattern of marginal heterochromatin aggregates abutting the nuclear envelope.

Often a diaphragm is seen guarding the pore but at times no such structure is visualized. Sometimes a thin lamina is seen extending across the pore, but as Barnes and Davis (1959) point out, such an image can be produced by non-equatorial sections through an annular opening. Whether a true diaphragm exists or whether such images are the product of sectioning geometry and thickness of section employed, have been extensively debated (*see* critique by Stevens and Andre, 1969). It would appear that pores both with and without diaphragms occur in nuclei of various cell types. In any case, the pores cannot be regarded as simple holes or fenestrations in the nuclear envelope through which material small enough can pass unimpeded. This is attested by many experimental studies (*see below*), including studies on the electrical properties of the nuclear envelope (Loewenstein and Kanno, 1963). The pores in fact delimit channels extending from the nucleoplasm to the cytoplasm, and at high magnifications are seen to contain oriented filamentous material (Watson, 1959). The channel material and pores are referred to as the 'pore complexes' by Watson (1959) and as the 'annular complexes' by Wischnitzer (1958).

Numerous studies on the passage of substances across the nuclear envelope show that small molecules such as sugars, amino acids and polypeptides readily pass from the cytoplasm into

---

Plate 18

Fig. 1. Nuclear envelope of rat hepatocyte, showing transversely cut nuclear pores (P) and continuity of the outer membrane of the nuclear envelope with the rough endoplasmic reticulum (arrows). × 58 000

Fig. 2. Tangentially sectioned rat hepatocyte nucleus showing an *en face* view of nuclear pores which present as annuli. × 34 000

Fig. 3. Profile of a pore with a diaphragm. From repair tissue in articular cartilage. Same nucleus as in *Plate 26*. × 82 000

Fig. 4. Nucleus of a polymorphonuclear neutrophil leucocyte showing profiles of two pores without diaphragms and one (arrow) where a thin lamina is seen across the pore opening. × 52 000

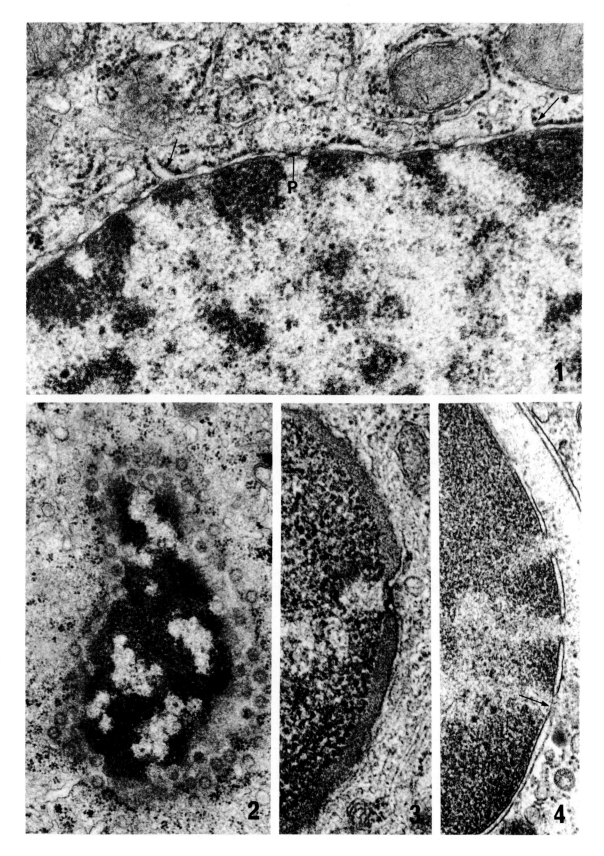

37

the nucleus but various proteins such as ovalbumin, serum albumin and globulin do not behave in this fashion even though the molecular size of these proteins is smaller than the diameter of nuclear pores (Mirsky and Osawa, 1961; Feldherr, 1962; Baud, 1963).

Several studies (Franke, 1970b; Feldherr, 1972; Wischnitzer, 1973) reveal that embedded in the diffuse or amorphous material comprising the annulus lie regularly spaced granules (called the 'annular granules'; eight granules on the so-called 'outer ring' and eight granules on the 'inner ring'). The central granule, knob or rod is attached to the pore wall and/or annular granules by filaments. It seems likely that the granules themselves may be made up of folded filaments. The dynamic variability of the morphology of the central granule has led to the suggestion that it represents ribonucleoproteins migrating from the nucleus to the cytoplasm. The material filling the pores comprises fine filaments which are resistant to digestion with nucleases but sensitive to digestion by pepsin and are hence considered to be protein in nature (Koshiba et al., 1970).

Since nuclear pores are potential pathways of nucleocytoplasmic exchanges, one may speculate that there might be a correlation between the metabolic activity of the cell and the number and size* of nuclear pores. Many studies support the former concept. A reduction in the number of pores with diminished metabolic activity is indicated by the studies of: (1) Yasuzumi et al. (1967), who found fewer nuclear pores in the testicular Leydig cells of old men (over 70 years) compared with young men (20–25 years); (2) Blackburn and Vinijchaikul (1969), who found, that in kwashiorkor where there is a severe amino-acid deficiency, there is a reduction in the number of nuclear pores/nuclear section (11/nuclear section compared with the normal 18.7/nuclear section), in the nuclei of pancreatic acinar cells; (3) Zucker-Franklin (1968), who found fewer nuclear pores in circulating polymorphonuclear neutrophil leucocytes than in their marrow precursors; (4) Liu and Davies (1972), who found 11.4 pores/μm^2† in microsporidian-infected fat-body cells of *Simulium vittatum* and 17.8 pores/μm^2 in non-infected cells (RNA and protein synthesis is depressed in these infected cells); and (5) Merriam (1962), who found a 28 per cent reduction in pores/unit area (also smaller annuli and fewer pores with a central knob) as the immature metabolically active frog oocyte turned into a mature resting oocyte. Conversely, an increase in the number of pores with increased metabolic activity is demonstrated by the studies of: (1) Jordan and Chapman (1973), who found a threefold increase in pore numbers as a result of activation of dormant carrot root cells; and (2) Maul et al. (1971), who found a doubling of the average number of pores/nucleus when lymphocytes were stimulated with phytohaemagglutinin‡.

Studies comparing the morphology and pore density of normal and neoplastic nuclei are remarkably few. An increase in pore density of various neoplastic nuclei was noted by Rejthar and Blumajer (1974) and Svejda et al. (1975), but a comparison (Banner et al., 1978) of nuclear pores of canine adenocarcinoma with normal pancreatic acinar cells showed a decrease in pore density. However, because of the increased nuclear surface area, the absolute nuclear pore density/nuclear volume was not significantly different in neoplastic as compared with normal

---

*Conflicting opinions have been expressed as to whether nuclear pores can expand and contract in diameter and thus regulate nucleocytoplasmic exchanges. Certainly at the moment there is no overwhelming evidence supporting this hypothesis (*see* Willison and Rajaraman, 1976; Severs and Jordan, 1978).
†The number of pores/μm^2 of nuclear surface is referred to as the 'pore density' or 'pore frequency'.
‡This occurs before the cells begin to divide, hence one may conclude that new pores can form in the interphase nucleus and that pores are not 'fixed' or 'permanent' structures which are laid down only in conjunction with reformation of the nuclear envelope after mitosis.

Plate 19
Hepatocyte nucleus (N) from the liver of a rat bearing a transplanted tumour in its flank. Numerous prominent pore annuli, some with a central dot (arrow), are seen in this section which cuts the nucleus at a little distance from the pole. Numerous polyribosomes (P) are abundant in the cytoplasm. × 48 000 (*Parry and Ghadially, unpublished electron micrograph*)

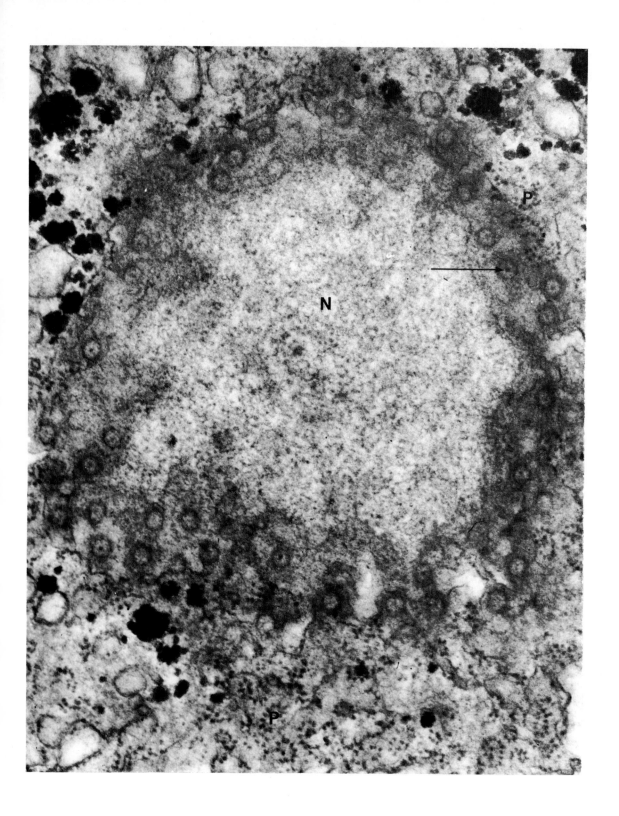

cells. Such variations in results are only to be expected when one realizes that not every tumour cell is in a state of heightened metabolic activity.

Remarkable differences in pore density (*Plate 20*) have been reported for various normal cell types in a large number of species. A few examples of these include: (1) log phase nuclear envelope of *Tetrahymena pyriformis*, 180 pores/μm^2 (Wunderlich and Franke, 1968); (2) yeast, 10–15 pores/μm^2 (Moor and Mühlethaler, 1963); (3) salivary gland of *Drosophila*, 65 pores/μm^2 (Wiener *et al.*, 1965); (4) salivary gland of larvae of *Simulium niditifrons*, 80–100 pores/μm^2 (MacGregor and Mackie, 1967); (5) frog oocyte, 25–35 pores/μm^2 (Merriam, 1962); (6) sea urchin oocytes, 40–80 pores/μm^2 (Afzelius, 1955); (7) hepatocytes of mouse, 35–55 pores/μm^2 (Franke, 1967); (8) canine pancreatic acinar cells, 12 pores/μm^2 (Banner *et al.*, 1978); (9) embryonal hamster fibroblasts, 12.5 pores/μm^2 (Rejthar and Blumajer, 1974); (10) human lymphocytes, 4.3 pores/μm^2 (Svejda *et al.*, 1975); and (11) HeLa cells, 11.24 pores/μm^2 (Maul and Deaven, 1977), 13 pores/μm^2 (Fisher and Cooper, 1967).

To what extent such differences in pore density are due to species differences, differences in cell type and differences in metabolic activity is difficult to evaluate. To obviate such differences a large variety of proliferating cells in culture were studied by Maul and Deaven (1977). Pore frequency, nuclear surface area and nuclear volume were determined and it was found that values for pore frequency were relatively constant in the species studied. They also state that 'when the pore to DNA ratio was plotted against the DNA content, there was a remarkable correlation which decreased exponentially for the cells of vertebrate origin'. Exceptions to this were the heteroploid mammalian cells which despite their higher DNA content showed the same ratio as the diploid mammalian cells. The results of this elegant study show that neither the nuclear surface, the nuclear volume nor the DNA content alone determines the number of pores, but rather an as yet undetermined combination of different factors.

Besides the numerical variations in pores already discussed, an interesting situation regarding nuclear pores in the liver of ethionine intoxicated rats (Miyai and Steiner, 1965) is worth mentioning. In this example, *en face* projections or pores with surrounding annuli were frequently seen, often in sections well away from the nuclear pole or even near the equator, a site where one would normally expect to see pore profiles and not annuli. These authors suggest that this phenomenon may be due to the stretching of the nuclear envelope and a consequent rotation of the pore complexes. However, as these authors themselves point out, it is difficult to see why, if this were the case, the pores retain their circular form and do not suffer distortion from stretching.

In non-neoplastic liver tissue adjacent to a human hepatoma (Ghadially and Parry, 1966) and in the livers of rats bearing subcutaneous carcinogen-induced or transplanted tumours (Parry and Ghadially, 1967), we found a high incidence of sections of nuclei showing numerous prominent pore annuli (near the nuclear pole, not near the equator as in the ethionine intoxicated rats) (*Plate 19*), but in normal rat liver such sections were rare and the pores appeared fewer and less distinct. The mechanism of production of this phenomenon is obscure. There is no evidence supporting the idea that a change in size or shape of the nucleus occurs in this condition.

It is, however, worth noting that while in ethionine intoxication there is a suppression of protein synthesis, the liver of the tumour-bearing host is markedly enlarged and there is evidence of increased protein synthesis in all but the terminal stages of life of the tumour-bearing host (Greenstein, 1954; Wiseman and Ghadially, 1958).

Plate 20

The remarkable variations in nuclear pore density that are encountered in freeze-fractured specimens is illustrated here. *Fig. 1.* shows a nucleus with sparse nuclear pores while *Fig. 2* depicts a nucleus with a large number of nuclear pores. Both these nuclei were found in a freeze-fractured preparation of normal mouse small intestine. The cell types could not be confidently identified. × 32 000; × 31 000 (*From a specimen supplied by Dr T. M. Mukherjee*)

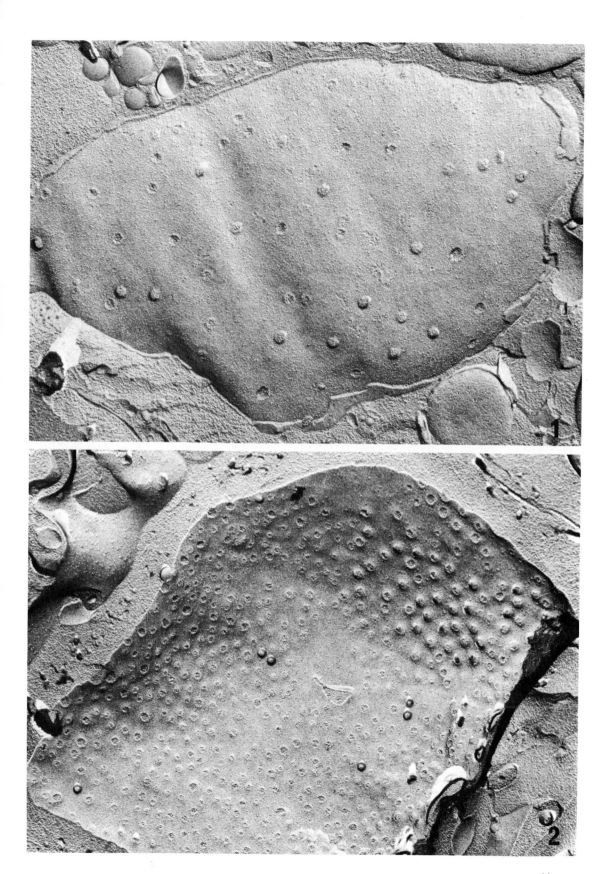

Thickening, proliferation and reduplication of nuclear envelope

The term 'proliferation of the nuclear envelope' describes a situation where there is an apparent excess of membranes of the nuclear envelope. The term 'reduplication' implies the folding and stacking of the redundant envelope to produce a multilayered structure. The 'thickening of the envelope' is due to the deposition of proteinaceous material in, and/or, on a membrane of the nuclear envelope. We will first deal with thickening, proliferation and reduplication of the nuclear envelope which is frequently seen in some virus-infected cells, and then we will look at proliferation of the nuclear envelope which is at times found in tumour cells.

Complex morphological changes occur in the nuclear envelope in cells infected with the herpes group of viruses (for references, *see* fourth paragraph), certain types of adenoviruses (Gregg and Morgan, 1959) and cytomegalovirus (Patrizi *et al.*, 1967). Details of the morphological picture vary, apparently depending upon the type of virus and variety of infected cell. These changes have been found in infected tissues of man, experimentally produced disease in laboratory animals and numerous infected tissue culture cell lines grown *in vitro*. We shall illustrate and discuss the changes that occur in the nuclear envelope using herpesvirus as an example.

A sequence of events that occurs in the nuclear envelope is clearly related to the passage of nucleocapsids from the nucleus to the cytoplasm (*Plate 21, Figs. 1-4*). The viral core and the surrounding shell, called the capsid (made of units called capsomeres), are assembled in the nucleus. The viral particle (core and capsid) then migrates to the nuclear envelope and, with the approach of the virus, the inner membrane of the nuclear envelope develops a focal thickening and becomes evaginated and encloses the virus. It is now clear from many studies (Shipkey *et al.*, 1967; Darlington and Moss, 1968; Leestma *et al.*, 1969) that, as the viral particle escapes from the nucleus, it acquires one or two membranous coats from the nuclear envelope. It may also derive further membranous coats from other membranous structures in the cell, and thus single virions or groups of virions may come to lie in vacuoles within the cytoplasm. Most workers believe that the primary membranous coat arises from the nuclear envelope but some contend that it can also be derived from cytoplasmic membranes and the Golgi (Epstein, 1962; Siminoff and Menefee, 1966; Leestma *et al.*, 1969).

Besides the changes in the nuclear envelope noted above, there also occur a variety of complex alterations which defy detailed description in the limited space available. These multitudinous morphological alterations stem from a combination of various changes designated as thickening, proliferation, reduplication and fusion of the membranes of the nuclear envelope. These patterns of change have been extensively studied and described in the

---

Plate 21

Figs. 1–4. Electron micrographs arranged in a sequence to depict the probable manner in which a virus particle migrates from the nucleus (N) to the cytoplasm. Thickening of the inner membrane of the nuclear envelope in proximity to the virus is clearly seen in *Figs. 1–3*, as is also an increasing evagination of the nuclear envelope. *Fig. 4* depicts the virus about to be detached from the nuclear envelope. From centre outwards one can discern the dense viral core, the capsid and two ensheathing membranous coats continuous with the inner and outer membranes of the nuclear envelope. All figs. × 100 000 (*From Shipkey, Erlandson, Bailey, Babcock and Southam, 1967*)

Figs 5. and 6. Nuclei of herpesvirus-infected monkey kidney cells in culture. These two electron micrographs show that the vesicular profiles (arrow) seen in *Fig. 5* could be sections through shelf-like elongations (arrow) of the inner membrane of the nuclear envelope as seen in *Fig. 6*. × 42 000; × 40 000

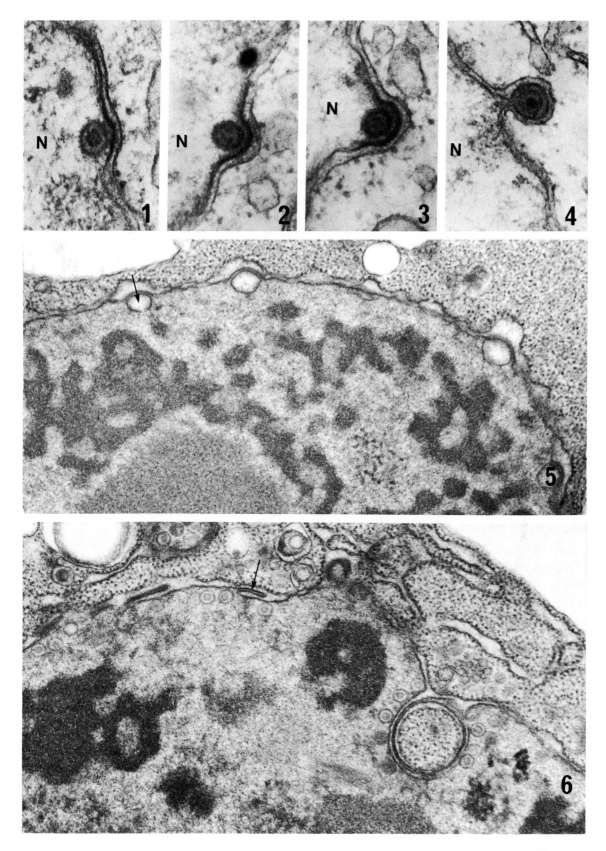

literature. They may be briefly catalogued as follows: (1) electron-opaque macular thickening of the inner membrane of the nuclear envelope and the associated portion of a round or flattened vesicle which is believed to develop by a process of reduplication of the inner membrane of the nuclear envelope (Swanson *et al.*, 1966; Moore and Pickren, 1967; Roy and Wolman, 1969); (2) proliferation of inner membrane of the nuclear envelope, forming vesicles within the nucleus containing virus particles (Darlington and Moss, 1968); (3) extensive proliferation of the membranes of the nuclear envelope, producing pod-like or finger-like extensions into the nucleus and/or cytoplasm (Shipkey *et al.*, 1967; Nii *et al.*, 1966, 1968); (4) thickening of long lengths of inner membrane of the nuclear envelope, even in areas where no contact with virus particles is observed (Swanson *et al.*, 1966; Shipkey *et al.*, 1967); (5) reduplication of inner membrane of the nuclear envelope (Epstein, 1962); (6) extensive proliferation and reduplication of the inner membrane of the nuclear envelope, with complex folds and macular densities along its length (Leestma *et al.*, 1969); and (7) proliferation, thickening and fusion, leading to the formation of concentric lamellar membranous arrays within and outside the nucleus (Nii *et al.*, 1968).

Some of these morphological alterations are shown in the accompanying illustrations (*Plates 21 and 22*). In *Plate 21, Fig. 5*, are depicted the 'vesicles' that have frequently been described in the literature and are believed to arise by a process of reduplication of the inner membrane of the nuclear envelope. However, as demonstrated in *Plate 21, Fig. 6*, at least some of these so-called vesicles may be sections through shelf-like extensions of the inner membrane of the nuclear envelope extending along the perinuclear cistern. *Plate 22, Fig. 1*, is a good example of how elaborate and extensive the membranous proliferations can be in herpesvirus-infected cells. Here the proliferated nuclear membranes have grown mainly outwards into the cytoplasm but in *Plate 22, Fig. 2*, the membranes have grown inwards into the nucleus to form membranous whorls. The dense 'lines' within these whorls have been interpreted as evidence of membrane thickening and/or fusion of adjacent membranes★.

The precise significance of the many alterations seen in the nuclear envelope has not been elucidated. Leestma *et al.* (1969) have proposed that 'the redundant foldings of the nuclear membranes may represent a proliferative reaction, to proteins or lipid-protein components of the nearby virus'. Watson and Wildy (1963) have shown that the capsid contains virus-specific antigens while the membranous coat contains host cell antigens. Fluorescent antibody studies by Shipkey *et al.* (1967) have shown that the thickened inner membrane of the nuclear envelope and the coat associated with it contain viral antigens also. Thus it would appear that thickening of the inner membrane of the nuclear envelope denotes the accumulation of viral antigens at this site.

As mentioned at the beginning of this section of the text, proliferation of the nuclear envelope is also at times seen in tumours. This change in its mildest form is seen in the lobulated nucleus (*Plate 3*). One can here regard the stalks (composed of apposed nuclear envelope) connecting the nuclear lobes as an example of excess or redundant membrane formation. Similarly, the

★Such formations referred to as confronting cisternae are dealt with on page 462.

Plate 22

Herpesvirus-infected monkey kidney cells in culture.

Fig. 1. The proliferated nuclear envelope is seen extending as complex folds into the cytoplasm. Note the marginated clumps of chromatin (C) and numerous viral particles in the nucleus and cytoplasm and also a few on the cell membrane (arrow). × 22 000

Fig. 2. Proliferation of the nuclear envelope extending into the nucleus, giving rise to whorled membranous structures (confronting cisternae). Note also the collection of virus particles in the nucleus (arrow). × 27 000

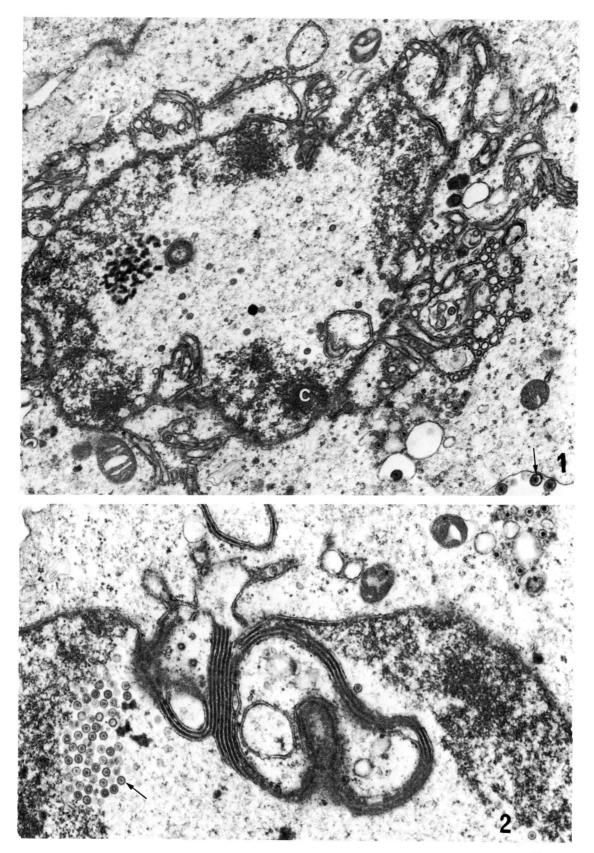

45

formation of a type 1 nuclear pocket (*Plate 72*) involves a focal proliferation of both membranes of the nuclear envelope to form a lamellar or cowl-like structure which entraps cytoplasmic material while the proliferation of the inner membrane (*Plate 73, Fig. 1*) of the nuclear envelope entrapping nuclear material to form a type 2 nuclear pocket is another example of proliferation of the nuclear envelope. In intranuclear annulate lamellae and some examples of intracytoplasmic annulate lamellae, we have further examples of proliferation of the inner or outer membrane of the nuclear envelope respectively (*see* Chapter 6). And finally, one may note that proliferation of the inner membrane of the nuclear envelope is involved in the production of intranuclear and intranucleolar tubular inclusions (*Plates 46–49*).

All the above-mentioned structures or abnormalities have a characteristic morphology which permits their identification and classification as distinct entities, and hence one refers to them by their proper names and not just as 'proliferations of the nuclear envelope' even though they do derive by a proliferation of one or both membranes of the nuclear envelope. If the term 'proliferation of the nuclear envelope' is to be of any use, it must be reserved and restricted for excess membrane formation which does not produce any of the above-mentioned specific structures. An example of this abnormality which deserves to be labelled as 'proliferation of the nuclear envelope' is shown in *Plate 23*. It comes from a benign or not too aggressive fibrous histiocytoma. In keeping with this is the easily visualized fibrous lamina (*see* pages 34 and 54 and Ghadially, 1985) in this nucleus.

In the literature, the term 'proliferation of the nuclear envelope' has not been used in the restricted manner as suggested above, and in fact this term and others such as nuclear projections, blebs, blisters and pockets have been used in a most indiscriminate manner. The occurrence of nuclear pockets or pocket-like structures* (*Plate 23*) in company with the change we here call 'proliferation of the nuclear envelope' compounds this difficulty.

A review of illustrations in the literature and my own experience leads me to conclude that florid proliferation of the nuclear envelope (as defined here) is a rather rare phenomenon and one that is more likely to be seen in mesenchymal rather than epithelial tumours, be they benign or malignant.

---

*In damaged cells or 'maltreated cells' the contents of the nucleus may escape or shrink so that a relative excess of nuclear envelope is present. Since such an envelope is thrown into folds and the chromatin has receded from the nuclear envelope, an illusion that nuclear pockets are present may be created. An excellent example of this phenomenon is demonstrated in *Fig. la* in Cinti *et al.* (1983) in a cell from human adipose tissue after digestion in collagenase and centrifugation. A true chromatin band (with a closely applied membrane on both sides) does not demarcate such pocket-like structures, but some chromatin adherent to the inner membrane of the nuclear envelope may create the illusion of a band.

Plate 23
From a benign or low-grade fibrous histiocytoma. Redundant folds of proliferated nuclear envelope and accompanying nuclear fibrous lamina (arrows) are depicted here. True nuclear pockets are bounded by a chromatin band or bands, but the pocket-like structures (arrowheads) clearly are not. What we are witnessing here is probably an early phase of excess membrane and lamina production which raises these structures above the main nuclear mass. × 35 000

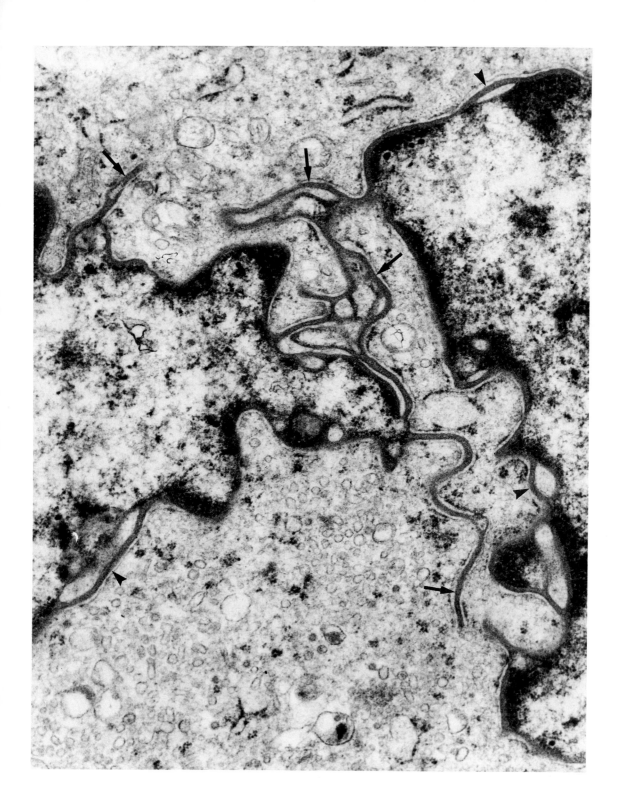

47

Evaginations or blebs of nuclear envelope

Many reports suggest that extrusion of nuclear or nucleolar material into the cytoplasm can occur via the formation of blebs, evaginations or pouches from the surface of the nucleus. Particularly interesting is the time-lapse cinematographic study by Hsu and Lou (1959) with Cloudman melanoma cells in culture where, upon adding fresh culture medium, a burst of nuclear activity and bleb formation was precipitated.

Bleb formation as a mechanism for nucleocytoplasmic exchanges has also been claimed to occur in: (1) oocytes and adenocarcinoma of frog kidney in culture (Duryee and Doherty, 1954; Duryee, 1956); (2) cultures of human tonsillar epithelium (Pomerat *et al.*, 1954); (3) salivary gland cells of third larval instar of *Drosophila melanogaster* (Gay, 1956); (4) dissociated cells of rat myocardium (Kyte, 1964); (5) ultraviolet irradiated cells of *Tetrahymena pyriformis* (Shepard, 1964); and (6) rat eggs approximately four and a half hours after sperm penetration (Szollosi, 1965).

In most of the above-mentioned examples one can be reasonably certain that both membranes of the nuclear envelope were involved in the formation of the bleb and that material was probably being conveyed from the nucleus, but in many other reports this is doubtful. Conversely there are other examples where presumably only the outer membrane of the nuclear envelope suffered evagination (Watson, 1955; Moses, 1956; Wischnitzer, 1958; Swift, 1959; Hadek and Swift, 1962; Baud, 1963; Wischnitzer, 1974; Birge and Doolin, 1974; Risueño *et al.*, 1975; Emura, 1978) producing cytoplasmic vesicles which then sometimes transform into annulate lamellae and/or rough endoplasmic reticulum.

Convincing electron microscopic evidence of bleb formation involving both layers of the nuclear envelope comes from the work of Clark (1960), on the exocrine cells of the rat pancreas, and Frasca *et al.* (1965), who have elegantly demonstrated this phenomenon in the ciliated columnar cells from the bronchial epithelium of four patients (*Plate 24*). Often a series of double-membrane-bound vacuoles derived from the nucleus were seen lying in the cytoplasm. Disintegration of the more distally placed vacuoles was noted, and it is suggested that this may provide a means of transfer of nuclear material to the cytoplasm.

The question raised by these studies on nuclear bleb formation is whether this is a normal phenomenon, or the sign of a damaged or a sick cell. Arguments supporting both these contentions can be given, but on the available data one cannot reach any definite conclusion. Certainly there is nothing overtly abnormal that one can detect from electron micrographs of cells showing this phenomenon. It is worth recalling that Clark (1960) found nuclear evagination in the pancreas of normal rats, and, although the patients studied by Frasca *et al.* (1965) had grave pathological changes in their lungs, the mucosa used for study was collected well away from the site of disease.

If, for the sake of argument, one concedes that nuclear bleb formation is a normal phenomenon, then it becomes difficult to explain why it has not been reported more frequently in the electron microscopy literature. Tissue culture studies indicate that this is an intermittent phenomenon which proceeds with some rapidity. It is conceivable, therefore, that the failure to visualize nuclear blebs more frequently may be related to the transient nature of this phenomenon and the ever-annoying problem of the smallness of the sample that can be examined with the electron microscope.

Plate 24

Multiple double-membrane-bound vacuoles, derived by a process of evagination of the nuclear envelope, are seen in this cell from the bronchial mucosa of man. The bleb (B) nearest to the nucleus (N) is seen to be an evagination with the limiting membranes of the bleb continuous with the two membranes of the nuclear envelope. Besides amorphous and electron-lucent material, this bleb also contains electron-dense granules resembling the chromatin in the nucleus. × 23 000 *(From Frasca, Auerbach, Parks and Stoeckenius, 1965)*

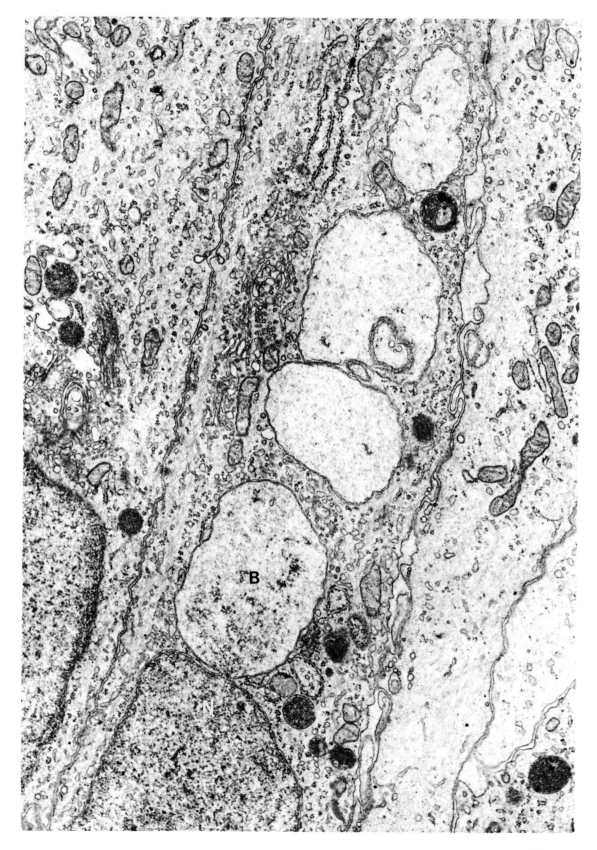

49

Nuclear fibrous lamina

In electron micrographs the nuclear fibrous lamina presents as a band of fine-textured material lying adjacent to the inner membrane of the nuclear envelope. In *Amoeba proteus* (Pappas, 1956; Mercer, 1959), *Gregarina melanopli* (Beams *et al.*, 1957) and neurons of the ventral nerve cord of *Hirudo medicinalis* (Gray and Guillery, 1963; Coggeshall and Fawcett, 1964), the fibrous lamina is a complex structure measuring 90–200 nm thick. Filaments 3–5 nm thick have been demonstrated in the fibrous lamina of *Hirudo* (Coggeshall and Fawcett, 1964). In sections perpendicular to the nuclear envelope, the fibrous lamina of *Amoeba proteus* (*Plate 25, Fig. 1*) is seen to delineate a system of cylindrical compartments. In tangential cuts through this region the lamina has a honeycombed appearance (*Plate 25, Figs. 2 and 3*). In the region of the nuclear pores this layer is either very thin or absent.

A nuclear fibrous lamina has now been demonstrated in some normal vertebrate cells also. However, the lamina in these instances is thinner (usually less than 30 nm) and presents as a band of medium to moderately high density lying between the inner surface of the nuclear envelope and the marginal condensates of heterochromatin. Fawcett (1966) has found that, in contrast to the situation in the leech where the fibrous lamina is absent over the pores, in the vertebrate cells studied by him the fibrous lamina continues either unaltered or as an attentuated band across the pores. Patrizi and Poger (1967), however, have failed to find such continuity in their material. Further they found that the lamina was thicker and more marked in glutaraldehyde-fixed material, but we (Ghadially *et al.*, 1974) found no statistically significant difference in thickness between the lamina of tissues fixed in cacodylate-buffered osmium or glutaraldehyde, but the lamina did appear somewhat denser and hence more prominent in material fixed in glutaraldehyde. In agreement with this are the results of a study on the nuclear fibrous lamina of a variety of normal and pathological cells from 1000 specimens of human biopsy material by Cohen and Sundeen (1976), who also found no evidence that variations in thickness depended on the type of fixation.

Filaments have been convincingly demonstrated in the lamina of *Hirudo* but not in the lamina of vertebrate cell nuclei. However, the texture of the lamina is in keeping with the idea that it contains filaments and in analogy with the lamina in invertebrates it is best to retain the term fibrous lamina★. The situation here is analogous to that of the chromatin where the fibrous nature is also difficult to demonstrate in ultrathin sections. Because of the fibrous nature of the lamina it has long been assumed that the lamina is proteinaceous in nature and cytochemical

---

★Various other terms such as 'zonula nucleum limitans', 'dense lamina', 'internal dense lamina' and 'nuclear limiting zone' have been proposed, but such terms have not been adopted by a majority of workers.

Plate 25

Nucleus of *Amoeba proteus*.
Fig. 1. Section through the nucleus, showing fibrous lamina delineating cylindrical compartments. × 42 000
Fig. 2. Tangential section, showing the honeycomb pattern of fibrous lamina. × 40 000
Fig. 3. Tangential cut through tip of nucleus, showing nuclear pores lying over the cylindrical openings in the lamina (arrow). × 44 000

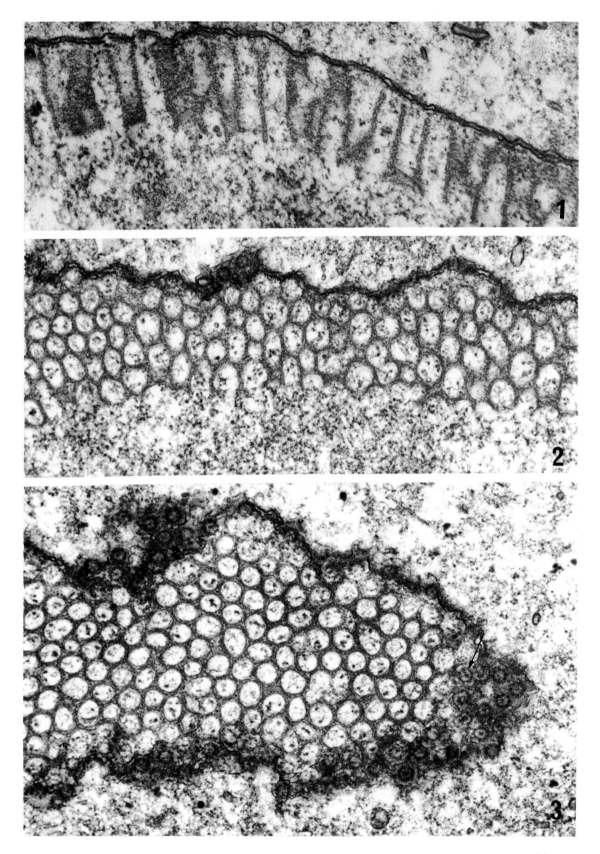

51

studies (Stelly *et al.*, 1970) on the neuronal nuclei of the leech (*Hirudo medicinalis*) indicate that this structure consists almost exclusively of acidic proteins and little or no DNA or RNA. Several workers have now isolated a fraction designated as a 'pore-complex-lamina-complex' or a 'non-membranous nuclear component' (said to be the equivalent of the nuclear fibrous lamina) (Dwyer and Blobel, 1976; Kirschner *et al.*, 1977; Gerace *et al.*, 1978) the major components of which appear to be three acidic proteins (molecular weight 60 000–70 000). These studies have been carried out on normal hepatocyte nuclei where a nuclear fibrous lamina is rarely if ever detectable in ultrathin sectioned material. This is explained away by Gerace *et al.* (1978) who stated that 'Although many eukaryotic cell types show no visible nuclear lamina, we feel that the functional counterpart may be ubiquitous, but often too thin to be recognized by conventional electron microscopy on whole cells'. It is unfortunate that so inappropriate a cell type was selected for such elaborate studies; whether their results have much bearing on the composition of the nuclear fibrous lamina is debatable.

The fibrous lamina is now known to occur in various normal vertebrate cells such as Schwann cells, endothelial cells, fibroblasts, smooth muscle cells, interstitial cells of the testis, intestinal epithelial cells, cells of Brunner's glands, osteoblasts and cultured amniotic cells (Fawcett, 1966b; Patrizi and Poger, 1967; Kalifat *et al.*, 1967; Leeson and Leeson, 1968; Rifkin and Heijl, 1979). In human biopsy material which included normal and pathological cells, Cohen and Sundeen (1976) found the nuclear fibrous lamina to be more prominent in mesenchymal cells, but a difficult-to-detect lamina also occurred in a large variety of epithelial cells. These authors therefore conclude that 'it is at least a transient structure in most human cell types'.

We (Oryschak *et al.*, 1974) have noted a fibrous lamina in chondrocytes of normal articular cartilage of man, rabbit, cow, horse and dog. However in two-month-old rabbits the lamina was undetectable or under 4.5 nm thick but in older rabbits and other animals mentioned, the mean thickness of the lamina lay between 20 and 30 nm. In a study of lumbosacral ventral root unmyelinated axon of the cat, Coggeshall *et al.* (1974) noted a prominent nuclear fibrous lamina in small Schwann cells, but in large Schwann cells the lamina was very thin or absent.

Nuclei with prominent fibrous lamina have also been found in experimental and pathological states such as: (1) cells of a mixed tumour of salivary gland (Kumegawa *et al.*, 1969); (2) chondroblastoma and chondromyxoid fibroma (Steiner, 1979; Ghadially 1985); (3) reticular cells and immature plasma cells from a case of Hodgkin's disease (Sanel and Lepore, 1968); (4) elastofibroma (Akhtar and Miller, 1977; Ramos *et al.*, 1978); (5) nasopharyngeal angiofibroma (*Plate 17*); (6) benign fibrous histiocytoma (*Plate 23*); (7) repair tissue filling surgically produced deep defects in articular cartilage (Ghadially *et al.*, 1971, 1972) (*Plate 26*); (8) injured human semilunar cartilages (Ghadially *et al.*, 1980a, b); (9) myofibroblasts in repair tissue (Ghadially, 1985) and avascular fibrous tissue (Ryan *et al.*, 1973); (10) synovial intimal cells, subsynovial fibroblasts and endothelial cells from a patient with multiple sclerosis, psoriasis and arthritis (Ghadially *et al.*, 1974); and (11) synovial intimal cells from cases of rheumatoid arthritis but not

Plate 26

From repair tissue filling a surgically produced deep defect (punched out hole) in articular cartilage. Nucleus of a cell showing a prominent fibrous lamina (F). Also seen is a nuclear pore with a well developed diaphragm (arrow), and others where no such diaphragm is evident in the plane of sectioning. Fixed in cacodylate-buffered osmium and stained with uranium and lead. × 58 000 (*From Ghadially, Fuller and Kirkaldy-Willis, 1971*)

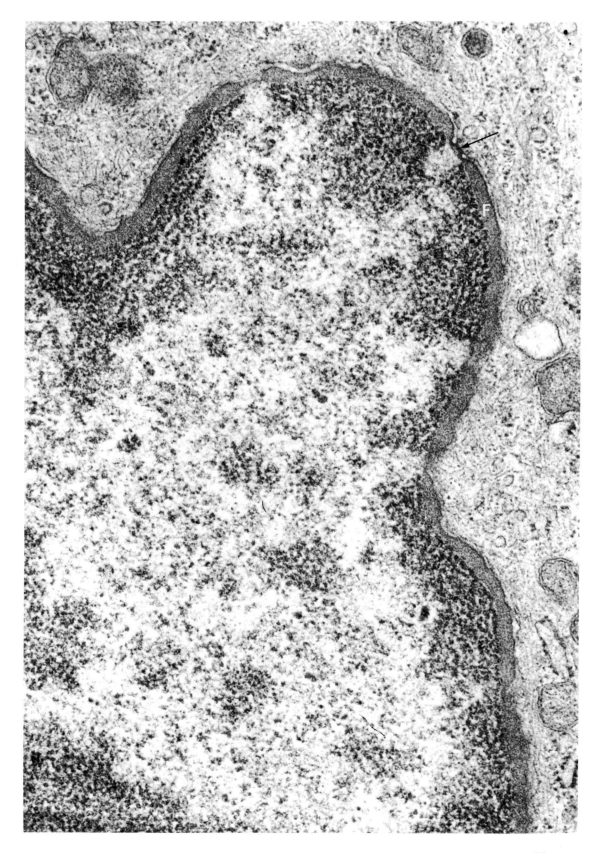

53

from non-rheumatoid cases (*Plate 27*) (Oryschak *et al.*, 1976). Personal observations lead me to conclude that a prominent nuclear fibrous lamina is rarely if ever seen in malignant tumours; (for a discussion on this *see* Ghadially, 1985) but in benign tumours or tumour-like lesions it has been seen in a few instances as attested by the list presented above.

During studies on the healing of surgically produced deep defects in articular cartilage of the knee joint of rabbits we found fibrous laminae up to 95 nm in thickness (Ghadially *et al.*, 1972). A hole passing through the articular cartilage and violating subchondral bone soon becomes filled with repair tissue arising from the marrow spaces. Later, metaplastic transformation to cartilage occurs. During the early stages (two weeks) the nuclei in the repair tissue show only a thin (35.5 ± 0.9 nm) fibrous lamina, but at three months the lamina is remarkably well developed (72.5 ± 1.5 nm). At six months the lamina is reduced in size (37 ± 1 nm).

Little is known about the function of the fibrous lamina. Its occurrence in large nuclei, such as those of the leech neurons, suggested that it might have a skeletal or supportive function, acting as a fibrous reinforcement to the nuclear envelope. However, the discovery that cells with not particularly large nuclei also have a fibrous lamina has now cast doubt on this theory. The waxing and waning of the lamina in repair tissue in articular cartilage (Ghadially *et al.*, 1972) shows that this is not a static structure of fixed dimensions for a given cell type, but that it is a dynamic component of the nucleus, capable of undergoing hypertrophy and involution in physiologically or pathologically altered states. Lending credence to this concept are the observations of Cohen and Sundeen (1976) who noted 'considerable variations in the prominence of the lamina in similar cells in the same tissue preparation'. Fawcett (1966b) has suggested that, since in vertebrates the fibrous lamina extends across the pores, it may function as a selective barrier in nucleocytoplasmic exchanges, while Kirschner *et al.* (1977) suggest that the major role of the nuclear fibrous lamina may be associated with the distribution, stability and perhaps also genesis of nuclear pore complexes.

Variations in thickness of lamina were also noted by Rifkin and Heijl (1979) in osteoblasts. They claim to have found laminae up to 80 nm thick in apparently quiescent osteoblasts and they suggest that the general metabolic state of the cell is not a factor in governing the size of the lamina. However, the so-called '80 nm thick lamina' shown in their *Fig. 2* is about 40 nm thick (the thickest part of the lamina measures 1.1 nm in their illustration at an alleged magnification of × 27 500) a figure not much in excess of that found in a variety of not particularly 'active' or 'inactive' normal cells. The literature is plagued not only with such palpable errors★ but also with measurements taken without monitoring the magnification of the microscope and enlarger.

★Some of the measurements of the lamina reported by Patrizi and Poger (1967) are also erroneous. (For a critique *see* Oryschak *et al.*, 1976.)

Plate 27

Fig. 1. Nucleus of a synovial intimal cell showing a thickened fibrous lamina. From the knee joint of a patient with rheumatoid arthritis. × 48 000

Fig. 2. Nucleus of a synovial intimal cell showing a very thin barely discernible fibrous lamina. From the knee joint of a patient with a torn meniscus. × 48 000

54

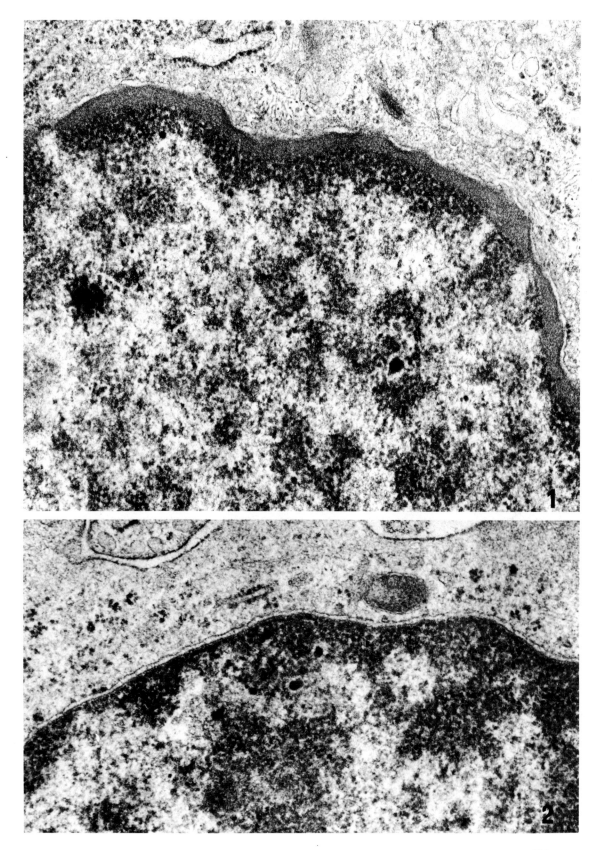

55

Nucleolus, structure and variations in size, shape and numbers

Nucleoli are readily visualized by a variety of light microscope techniques. The study of living cells shows them as refractile bodies that can move about in the nucleus and also fuse and divide. In fixed material the RNA-rich nucleolus stains intensely with a variety of basic dyes but is Feulgen negative, except for the rim of Feulgen-reactive nucleolus-associated chromatin. In suitable specimens, after silver impregnation the nucleolus shows two components: a branching anastomosing coarse thread-like structure called the 'nucleolonema', in the meshes of which are entrapped one or more rounded structures often called the 'pars amorpha' or 'fibrous centres' (best called 'filamentous centres', *see below*). Both the light microscope and the electron microscope show that not all nucleoli have an open or reticular nucleolonema, and in fact two main types of nucleoli are recognized (in normal and neoplastic tissues): 'open nucleoli' where the nucleolonema is thin and thread-like and spread out so that it is easily visualized and 'compact nucleoli' where the nucleolonema is not seen and it is thought that this is because the nucleolonema is absent or very closely packed (*Plates 28* and *29*). Between these two extremes (*Plate 30*) one finds not so compact nucleoli with 'holes' (rounded areas containing nuclear matrix) to somewhat more open nucleoli where the nucleolonema is quite plump rather than thread-like. In most open nucleoli, the nucleolonema is deployed in a reticular pattern but at times profiles of nucleolonema show a concentric or parallel stack pattern (*Plate 30*).

The significance of such variations in nucleolar pattern and structure are obscure. Often it is assumed that the open nucleolus reflects a metabolically active (RNA synthesizing and hence protein synthesizing) cell while the compact nucleolus indicates the converse, but there is as yet little evidence to support or refute such a hypothesis. The type of nucleolus (i.e. 'open' or 'compact') seems to be associated with cell-type rather than metabolic activity, but it is possible that both factors are involved in determining the form of the nucleolus. Be that as it may, tumours may contain open nucleoli or compact nucleoli and often both types and intermediate forms are seen in a given tumour.

With the electron microscope (in sectioned material) the nucleolus is seen to contain granules (15–20 nm in diameter) and filaments (about 5 nm in diameter and 30–40 nm long) but these are not dispersed homogeneously throughout the nucleolus (Swift, 1963; Granboulan and Granboulan, 1964; Marinozzi, 1964; Smetana and Busch, 1964; Brinkley, 1965; Hyde *et al.*, 1965; Terzakis, 1965; Bernhard, 1966; Bernhard and Granboulan, 1968; Hay, 1968). Besides these granules and filaments, which are susceptible to ribonuclease digestion and are hence believed to contain RNA, there is also some pepsin-digestible protein and some DNA in the nucleolus (Hay and Revel, 1962; Granboulan and Granboulan, 1964; Marinozzi and Bernhard, 1964; Schoefl, 1964; Lord and Lafontaine, 1969; Recher *et al.*, 1970).

Plate 28

Fig. 1. Nucleolus from dog myocardium with a reticular nucleolonema. Light granular (G) and dense filamentous (F) components can be discerned, as can rounded areas which might be called 'pars amorpha' or 'filamentous centres' (C). Note how the nuclear matrix extends into the interstices of the nucleolus (arrows). × 46 000

Fig. 2. Nucleolus from hypertrophic myocardium of man obtained at open heart surgery. A compact nucleolus is seen in which no obvious nucleolonema can be discerned. Dense filamentous zones (F), light granular zones (G) and filamentous centres (C) are easily discerned. × 35 000

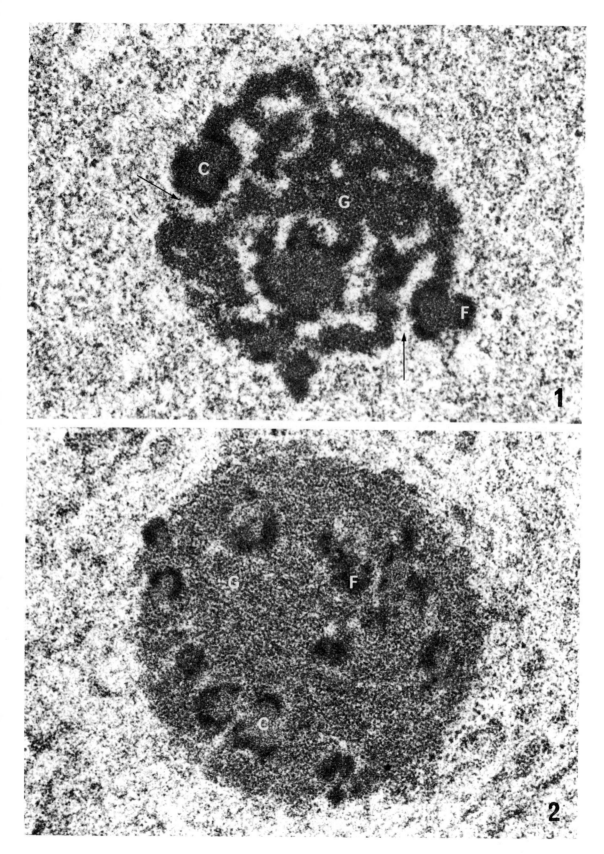

57

With the electron microscope the nucleolonema is seen to be composed of granules set in a filamentous matrix, but the proportion of granules and filaments varies in different zones in the nucleolonema. This produces light and dark areas at times referred to as the 'light' and 'dense' components of the nucleolus (*Plates 28* and *29*). The dense component (also called the 'filamentous component') contains compacted filaments (this is difficult to demonstrate except at high magnifications in suitable preparations) in which granules are scanty or absent. The light component (also called 'the granular component') is rich in granules set in a sparse filamentous matrix. Such zones are also discernible in compact nucleoli where a thread-like nucleolonema is not seen. It is now generally accepted that the filamentous component is the site of precursor ribosomal RNA synthesis while the granular component of the nucleolus represents a pool of accumulating partially completed ribosomal precursor particles (Busch and Smetana, 1970; Daskal *et al.*, 1974).

Much confusion exists regarding the electron microscopic equivalent of the light microscopist's pars amorpha. This is largely a continuation of the confusion which has reigned in the light microscopic literature where at times the pars amorpha is described as lying within the nucleolus and in other instances the nucleolus is described as embedded in a structureless mass called the 'pars amorpha'. The interstices of the nucleolonema are permeated by the nuclear matrix (*Plate 28, Fig. 1*) and at times such regions have erroneously been called 'pars amorpha' by electron microscopists.

If this term is to be retained at all by electron microscopists, it should be used, as by Fawcett (1981) and others, to describe the rounded zones of light density and texture that are encountered in nucleoli. However, such regions also contain 5 nm diameter filaments, similar to those in the rest of the nucleolus except that they are not compacted as in the dense zones of the nucleolonema. These rounded structures have now been described by various names besides 'pars amorpha' such as 'pars fibrosa', 'fibrous centres', 'fibrillar centres' and 'nucleolini'. Because of confusion over what exactly is the pars amorpha of the light microscopist and because this structure is not amorphous with the electron microscope, it is best to drop the term 'pars amorpha'. On the other hand it would be inaccurate or erroneous to call a structure composed of filaments as 'fibrous'. I shall therefore call it what it in fact is – a 'filamentous centre'.

It has long been known that the nucleolus usually breaks up at the onset of mitosis (prophase) and that it is not generally recognizable by the time metaphase is reached. Reconstitution of the nucleolus occurs in the daughter cells during late anaphase and telophase (*see* reviews by Bernhard and Granboulan, 1968; Busch and Smetana, 1970). This is almost universally true for somatic cells of animals, but in many plant species the nucleolus persists during mitosis. (For references *see* Goessens and LePoint, 1974; Chaly *et al.*, 1977). However, persistence of recognizable nucleolar material during mitosis has been seen in a number of cultured mammalian cells; (1) after treatment with cobalt salts (Heath, 1954); (2) after treatment with 5-fluorodeoxyuridine and thymidine (Hsu *et al.*, 1964); and (3) without any such treatment (Brinkley, 1965; Hsu *et al.*, 1965; Goessens and LePoint, 1974).

Plate 29

Figs. 1 and 2. Nucleolar pleomorphism in malignant tumours. *Fig. 1* shows a compact but enlarged nucleolus from an adenocarcinoma (primary site probably the stomach or colon). *Fig. 2* shows an enlarged irregular open nucleolus with a reticular nucleolonema (N), from an anaplastic bronchial carcinoma. Nucleolus-associated heterochromatin (H) is well demonstrated in *Fig. 1* while numerous small filamentous centres (F) are seen in *Fig. 2*. Nuclear matrix (M) extending into the nucleolus is also seen. × 32 000; × 28 000

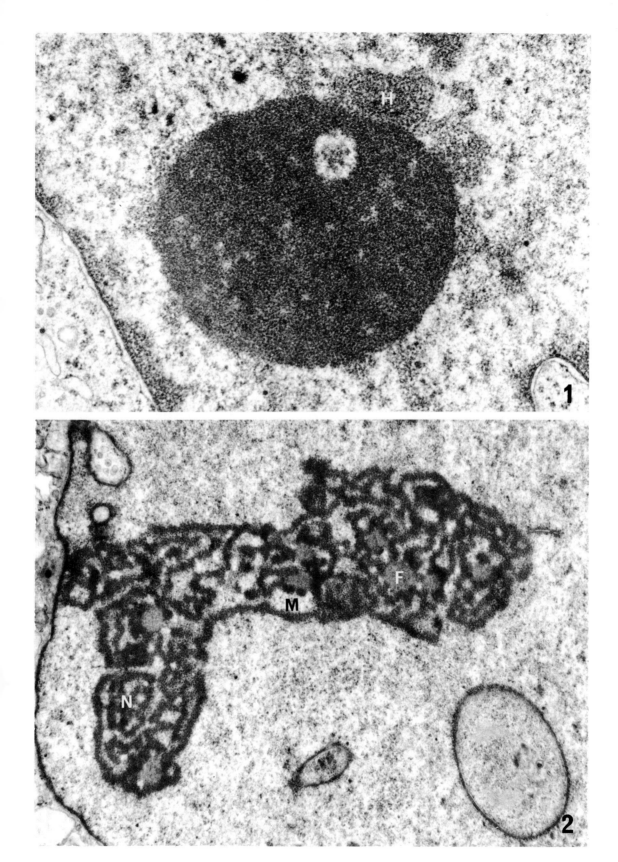

The prominence of the nucleolus in proliferating cells such as embryonic cells, stem cells, cells in tissue culture, tumour cells and cells producing a protein-rich secretory product such as pancreatic acinar cells has long suggested that the nucleolus plays a key role in protein synthesis (Caspersson and Schultz, 1940; Caspersson and Santesson, 1942; Caspersson, 1950). Since then evidence has accumulated which shows that this is because the nucleolus is involved in the production and distribution of RNA and is the site of synthesis of the precursors of ribosomal RNA (Perry, 1964, 1966, 1969). Such evidence includes the demonstration of a similarity of base composition between nucleolar and ribosomal RNA (Edstrom et al., 1961), the inhibition of ribosomal RNA synthesis after destruction of the nucleolus by ultraviolet microbeam irradiation (Perry, 1964) and work on the anucleolate mutant of Xenopus laevis which is unable to produce ribosomal RNA (Brown and Gurdon, 1964). The steps involved in the synthesis and maturation of ribosomal RNA and its combination with protein to form ribosomal subunits and ultimately ribosomes and polyribosomes in the cytoplasm have also been described (see review by Perry, 1969).

Enlargement of the nucleolus is a well known feature of tumour cells (Plate 29). This phenomenon, first observed by Pianese (1896), has been demonstrated by MacCarty (1937) and by many others* since to be true for a large number and variety of tumours. Although this enlargement can be quite impressive, and is a fairly constant feature of the neoplastic state, it is by no means the hallmark of malignancy. Thus Stowell (1949) showed the nucleoli larger than those occurring in malignant hepatoma can be found in regenerating rat liver after partial hepatectomy†. Early nucleolar enlargement has been observed in the skin of mice painted with carcinogens, but here also it is largely related to the hyperplastic rather than the neoplastic state engendered by such treatment (Cowdry and Paletta, 1941; Cooper, 1956). Other similar non-specific nucleolar changes in malignancy include margination of nucleolus (page 66), irregularity of shape, and an increase in numbers of nucleoli. The latter is said to be related to the aneuploidy of cancer cells, but splitting of pre-existing nucleoli also seems to be involved‡.

*An example of this is the study by Long and Sommers (1969) on papillary serous neoplasms of the ovary. They found that: (1) in both benign and borderline groups of tumours the nuclei contained up to four nucleoli, but nuclei with four nucleoli were four times more frequent in the borderline group; (2) increasing grade of malignancy was associated with five and sometimes 50 nucleoli in a nucleus; (3) the diameter of the nucleoli in the borderline group was significantly greater than in the benign group; and (4) with loss of differentiation the nucleoli became irregular in shape and markedly larger. A comparison of these nucleoli with those found in the less aggressive endometrioid tumours revealed that the latter had overall smaller nucleoli and fewer multiple nucleoli.
†Not surprising since the rate of growth of regenerating rat liver is about three to four times greater than carcinogen-induced (dimethylaminoazobenzene) rat hepatoma (personal experience based on several past studies).
‡Developmentally, several nucleoli appear on different organizer regions on certain chromosomes. These then fuse to produce usually one or two nucleoli. Failure of such a fusion process can also lead to an increase in the number of nucleoli.

Plate 30

Fig. 1. Rhabdomyosarcoma. A much enlarged nucleolus is seen here. This is a fairly compact nucleolus where only a few small areas ('holes') containing nuclear matrix (M) are evident. Compare with the much more compact nucleolus in *Plate 29, Fig. 1.* × 25 000

Fig. 2. Same case as *Fig. 1.* Two nucleolar profiles are seen here. In the one indicated by an arrow the strands of nucleolonema present as a stack of arcades, while in the one indicated by an arrowhead the nucleolus is fairly compact, only a few clear areas containing nuclear matrix are evident. × 17 000

Fig. 3. Mediastinal seminoma. In this nucleolar profile the strands of nucleolonema are concentrically arranged. × 31 000

Fig. 4. Rhabdomyosarcoma. Different case from *Figs. 1* and *2.* Multiple nucleolar profiles are evident. The nucleolonema is deployed in a reticular pattern. × 12 000

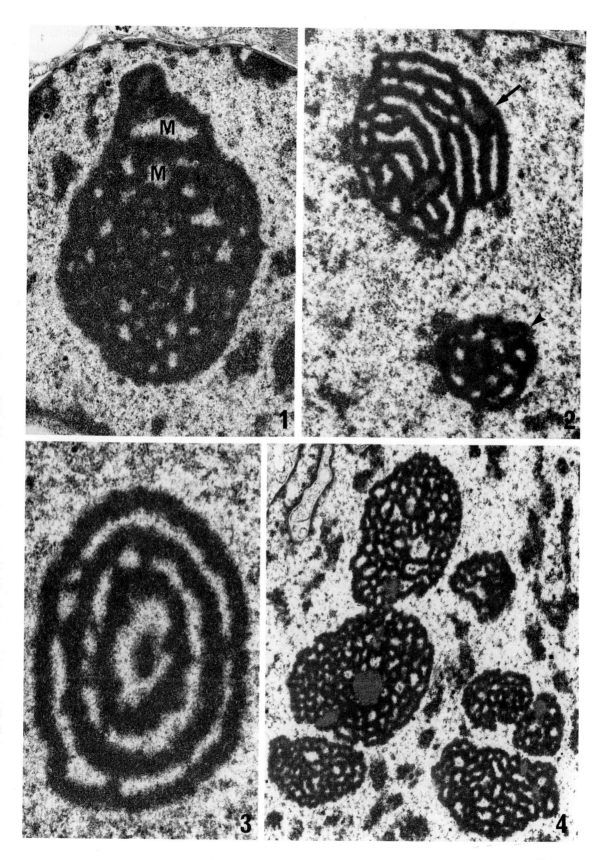

We have noted that nucleolar hypertrophy is associated with heightened protein synthesis. It is therefore conceivable that regressive changes might be evident in the nucleolus when cells, once engaged in such active synthesis, have ceased to be active.

It is interesting to note that light microscopists have for long described 'vacuoles' in nucleoli and noted that the number of vacuoles increase with the age of the cell, after irradiation, after treatment with acridine derivatives, or when growing cell cultures at low temperatures (for references, *see* Busch *et al.*, 1963) – situations where one would suspect that protein synthesis had been depressed. A pattern seen in ultrathin sections which probably reflects regressive changes is called the ring-shaped nucleolus. Here the nucleolonema forms a thin shell surrounding one or two pale filamentous centres (*Plate 31, Fig. 1*).

In a series of papers, Smetana and his colleagues (for references, *see* Smetana *et al.*, 1970a,b) have described ring-shaped nucleoli in various cells such as human lymphocytes, plasmacytes, monocytes, differentiated lymphosarcoma cells, myeloblasts and promyelocytes of acute myeloblastic leukaemia, and in mature (but not in immature) smooth muscle cells. They conclude from these studies that 'The finding of ring-shaped nucleoli in these different cell types apparently indicates that the presence and formation of such nucleoli represents a general phenomenon that reflects a reduced but continuing synthesis of ribosome precursors in the nucleolus'. Similarly, tissue culture studies (for references, *see* Love and Soriano, 1971) also show that when nucleolar RNA synthesis is inhibited by thymidine, or when the cells are in a quiescent state, the filamentous centres are few, large and prominent, while during active growth the nucleolonema is prominent and the filamentous centres form numerous small discrete spherules. My observations are in keeping with these findings, and in *Plate 31, Figs. 2 and 3*, are illustrated some extreme examples of nucleolar atrophy which I have encountered. One of these was found in a smooth muscle cell of the involuting rat uterus, two days after delivery. Here the nucleolus is reduced to a very thin shell-like structure and shows large spaces occupied by some filamentous material and nuclear matrix.

Plate 31

Fig. 1. Ring-shaped nucleolus from a plasmacytoid cell found in human bronchial mucosa. The nucleus of this cell showed the characteristic cartwheel pattern but little rough endoplasmic reticulum was evident in the cytoplasm. × 45 000

Fig. 2. Nucleolus from a rat kidney tubule cell. This animal had been on an Atromid S-containing diet for a long period. The cytoplasm of this cell appeared oedematous and contained few organelles. × 50 000

Fig. 3. Nucleolus from involuting rat uterus. The nucleolonema (N) is reduced to a thin shell-like structure, surrounding pools of nuclear matrix (M) and filamentous material (F). × 56 000

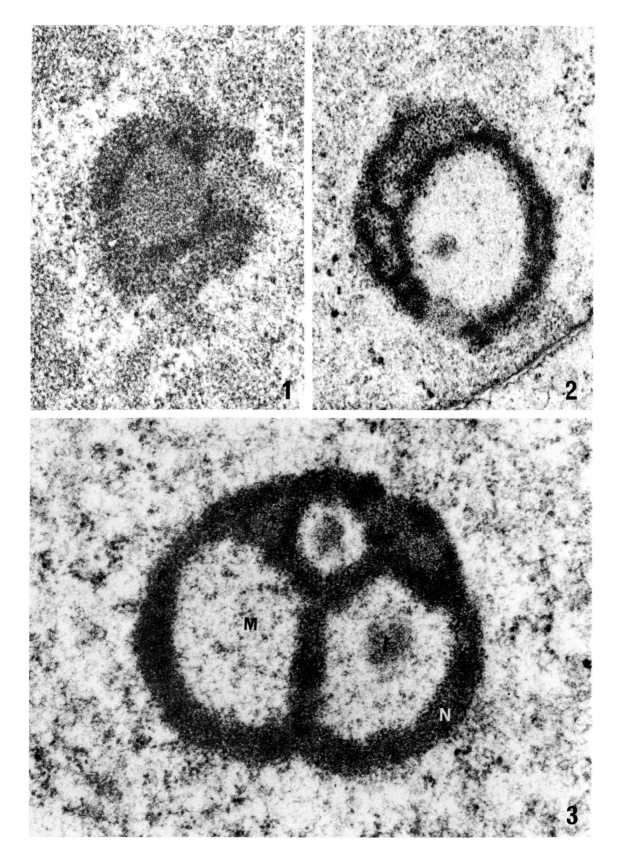

Meandering nucleolus

For some time now it has been apparent that some of the nucleoli in germinomas (seminomas and dysgerminomas) are sufficiently distinctive to be of diagnostic value (Ramsey, 1965; Pierce, 1966; Levine, 1973; Markesbery *et al.*, 1976; Ferenczy, 1976; Janssen and Johnston, 1978). Such nucleoli have been described as 'open nucleoli' and 'skein-like nucleoli', but terms such as these neither adequately describe these nucleoli nor distinguish them from other nucleoli, which are referred to by the same or similar terms.

The terms 'open' and 'compact' nucleoli or to be more precise nucleoli with an open or compact nucleolonema have been used to describe nucleoli found in various sites and situations both normal and neoplastic (page·56). In the open nucleolus, the nucleolonema is spread out and easily visualized as a thread-like structure (Gk *nēma* thread) forming a net or a skein, while in the compact nucleolus a nucleolonema is not seen, and it is assumed that this is because the nucleolonema is absent or closely packed. Since it is difficult to talk sensibly about an object without a name, I (Ghadially, 1985) coined the term 'meandering nucleolus' to describe certain nucleoli of characteristic morphology seen principally but not exclusively in germinomas.

In germinomas most nucleoli are of the open or very open variety, and as expected in malignant tumours they are enlarged, to a greater or lesser degree. These nucleoli present roughly rounded, oval or elongated profiles and occupy a fairly well circumscribed area in the nucleus. Such large open nucleoli are constantly seen in germinomas but they occur also in many other tumours (e.g *Plate 29, Fig. 2*).

The meandering nucleolus seems to result from a further 'opening up' of the nucleolonema which then 'wanders' or 'meanders' over quite a distance in the nucleus. The strands of nucleolonema may be interconnected to form a coherent structure, with a branching arboreal pattern or a stag-horn pattern, or fragments may break off and disperse in the nucleus, to form small ragged-looking daughter nucleoli.

In virtually all enlarged open nucleoli (in seminomas and other tumours) the peripheral nucleolonema presents as a more or less continuous strand and one does not find several finger-like or stag-horn-like projections emanating from the nucleolus but the converse is often the case with the meandering nucleolus.

As mentioned before, the meandering nucleolus is found in seminomas and dysgerminomas. In my experience, this aberration of nucleolar morphology is seen most constantly in seminomas (gonadal and extragonadal) but not so constantly (or frequently in a given case) in dysgerminomas. However, meandering nucleoli are not absolutely diagnostic or specific for germinomas, because such nucleoli are occasionally seen in other tumours (e.g. embryonal rhabdomyosarcoma and metastatic melanoma)*. Nevertheless, meandering nucleoli constitute an important feature which at times helps in distinguishing, for example, a mediastinal seminoma from a thymoma, lymphoma or Ewing's tumour (Erlandson, 1981 and personal experience), and primary or secondary intracranial dysgerminoma from many other primary and secondary intracranial neoplasms.

*Only when the differential diagnosis is narrowed down by history and histology does the presence of very open and meandering nucleoli become diagnostic of germinoma.

Plate 32

Meandering nucleoli from a mediastinal seminoma (*Figs. 1, 2 and 4*) which was difficult to diagnose with the light microscope (several pathologists thought that it was a lymphoma). *Fig. 3* is from a testicular seminoma. As much of the nuclear periphery as possible has been included in the illustrations to show how these nucleoli meander or sprawl out in the nucleus.

Figs. 1 and 2. May be regarded as irregularly open nucleoli where the peripheral strand of nucleolonema is not continuous, but broken, forming small projections (arrows). × 18 000; × 15 500

Fig. 3. This nucleolus has an arborescent or stag-horn-like appearance. The discontinuities in the nucleolar periphery are quite marked. × 15 000

Fig. 4. The nucleolonema is fragmented and scattered in the nucleus. × 11 500

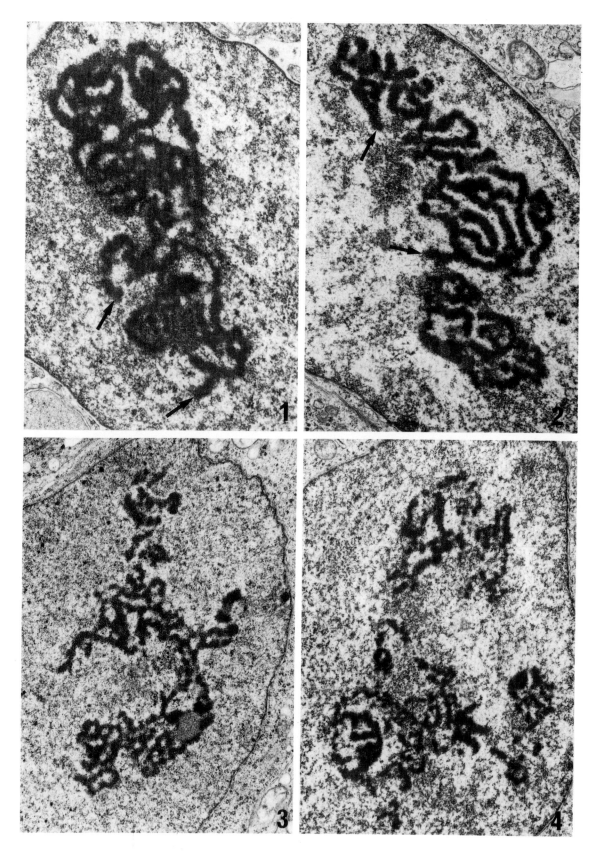

Nucleolar margination

The nucleolus can move within the nucleus and examples may be cited to show that, in states of active protein synthesis, it may come to lie against the inner membrane of the nuclear envelope. This phenomenon is referred to as nucleolar margination.

Thus in the growing oocyte of amphibia most of the numerous nucleoli that occur in this cell type are located at the inner membrane of the nuclear envelope. When the oocytes mature they shrink and lie in the central region of the nucleus, and after fertilization and during early cleavage, when protein synthetic activity is very low, the nucleoli are not visible (Mirsky and Osawa, 1961). Particularly interesting is the situation seen in the neurons of the fish, *Lophius*, for the direction of movement of the nucleolus which occurs with change in synthetic activity is towards the segment of nuclear envelope proximal to the axon base, and it is in the cytoplasm in this region where most of the synthetic activity is carried on (Hyden, 1943). Intense protein synthetic activity occurs in the regenerating liver of the rat after partial hepatectomy, and Swift (1959) has noted some 50 per cent of the nucleoli move to the nuclear margin.

Evidence of the type presented above indicates that nucleolar margination is a sign of increased protein synthesis. It is therefore not surprising to find that nucleolar margination is frequently seen in a variety of tumours, and that in some instances, such as the adenocarcinoma illustrated in *Plate 33*, several marginated nucleoli can be seen in a single field of view.

Although as a general rule there is a positive correlation between the degree of malignancy and the rate of growth of a tumour, this is not invariably so, and even some benign tumours are known to have a rapid growth phase. An example of this is the keratoacanthoma, a benign usually self-regressing tumour which mimics a carcinoma both in its histological appearance and in its rapid growth rate (Ghadially, 1961, 1971; Ghadially *et al.*, 1963). Such tumours can be produced experimentally (Ghadially, 1958) and we (Ghadially and Parry, unpublished observation) have observed frequent nucleolar margination during the growth phase of this benign tumour (*Plate 34, Fig. 1*).

Plate 33

A fragment of human adenocarcinoma (same case as *Plate 29, Fig. 1*) found in ascitic fluid. Most of the nucleoli seen in this electron micrograph are marginated (arrows). Note also the irregularity of nuclear shape and the variability of heterochromatin content. The two nuclei at the top corner of the electron micrograph contain abundant heterochromatin aggregates, and would thus appear hyperchromatic at light microscopy, while the remainder are poor in heterochromatin content and would present a paler appearance. × 7000

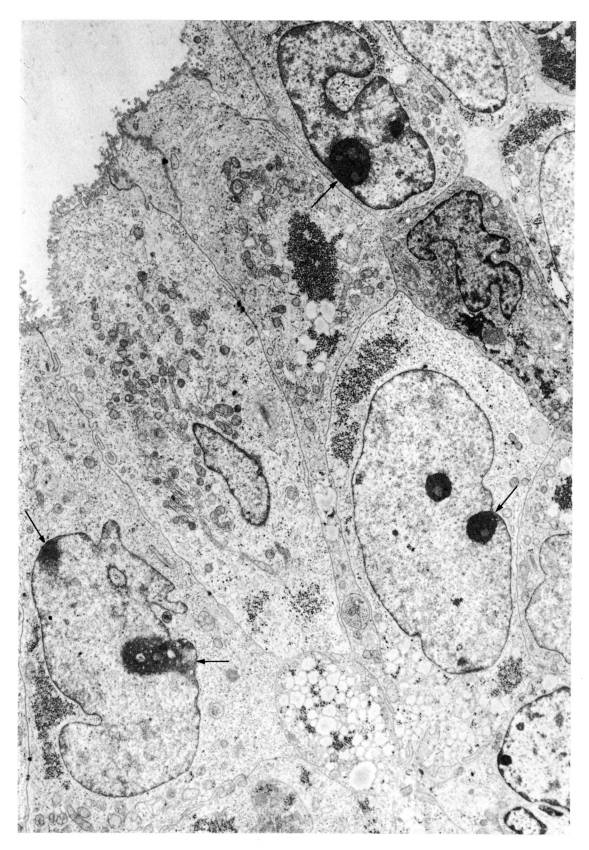

Irregularities of shape (page 4), invaginations of the nuclear envelope and pseudoinclusions (page 76) are common features of the neoplastic nucleus, and in some tumours such deep invaginations are seen to make contact with or penetrate the nucleolus (*Plate 34, Figs. 2 and 3*). This phenomenon has been observed in: (1) Ehrlich's ascites tumour (Oberling and Bernhard, 1961); (2) primary cultures of human hepatocytes, and established cell lines from human tumours and rabbit kidney (Bourgeois *et al.*, 1979); and (3) several human tumours (Ghadially, 1985), particularly bronchial carcinoma cells found in a pleural effusion (*Plate 34*). In this example innumerable tumour cells showed this close association between nucleolus and invaginations of the nuclear envelope. Examples were seen where multiple invaginations were present, in a single nucleus, each contacting one or more nucleoli.

The phenomenon of nucleolar margination has led many observers to speculate that such an arrangement facilitates nucleocytoplasmic exchanges. For although an occasional marginated nucleolus may be found in the cells of any tissue, it is seen much more frequently in rapidly growing cells and in cells engaged in the production of a protein-rich secretory product (e.g. pancreatic acinar cells). Thus regarding nucleolar margination, Oberling and Bernhard (1961) state, 'One can assume that transportation of nucleolar products towards the cytoplasm is highly facilitated by this arrangement'. Clear morphological evidence on this point is, however, lacking. If exchanges do occur at such sites of contact, they are probably at a molecular level undetectable by current techniques. One may at times find ribosomes in the cytoplasm adjacent to a marginated nucleolus, and even a nuclear pore may be detected in the area, but this cannot be accepted as proof of transfer from nucleolus to cytoplasm, as has sometimes been suggested.

Plate 34

Fig. 1. Cells from keratoacanthoma of rabbit skin, produced by repeated application of 7,12-dimethylbenz-α-anthracine. Enlarged and marginated nucleoli are seen in the nuclei of this tumour. × 5500

Fig. 2. Carcinoma of the bronchus. A deep invagination of the nuclear envelope (E) containing cytoplasmic material (C) is seen in contact with the nucleolus (NU). Nucleus (N), intracytoplasmic lipid droplet (L). × 17 500

Fig. 3. From the same specimen as *Fig. 2*. A pseudoinclusion containing cytoplasmic structures (C) is seen in close association with a nucleolus (NU). × 15 000

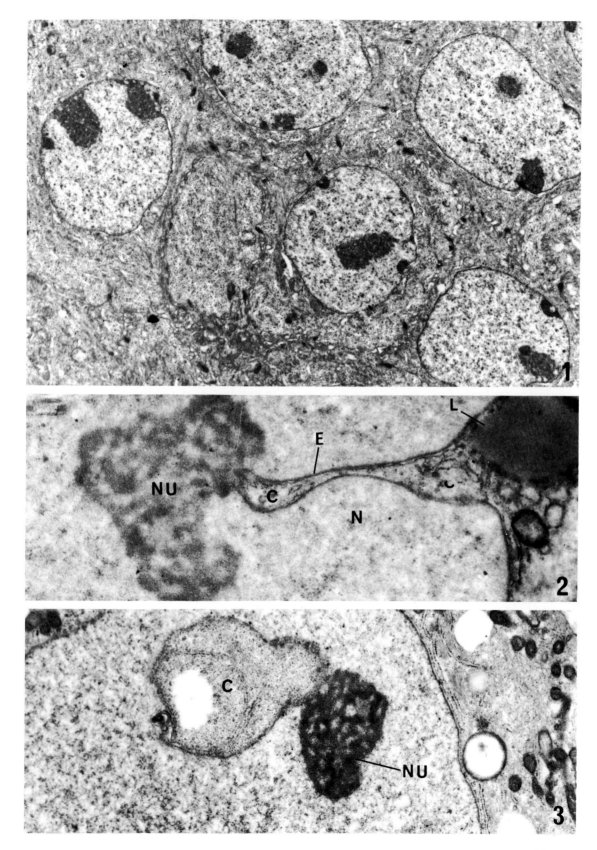

Segregation of nucleolar components

It has already been noted (page 58) that the nucleolus is largely made up of granules and filaments and that focal variations in the proportion of filaments and granules produce the light (granular component) and dark (filamentous component) zones of the nucleolus. In the phenomenon referred to as nucleolar segregation there is separation and migration of the filamentous from the granular component (*Plates 35* and *36*). This change is to some extent reversible but the process may lead to wide separation and dispersal of the components, and ultimately to a total disintegration of the nucleolus.

In assessing nucleolar segregation, two main points must be borne in mind: one is the degree of separation, that is to say how far the segregated components have moved apart, and the second is the purity of segregation. Thus in some instances the segregation may be quite pure and one can distinguish the dense filamentous component quite clearly from the much lighter granular component, but in other instances (impure segregation) there is only a marginal difference in densities, for both granules and filaments are present in each component, there being only a relative difference in the amount of granules and filaments in the segregated parts. Yet another not too common factor which may affect the final image seen in electron micrographs is the density of the filamentous component due to close packing of filaments. If these are not well packed, this component may also present as a light area.

It is worth recalling that the filaments of the nucleolus are extremely fine and, in the dense areas, form a closely packed meshwork. Thus, the filamentous nature of the dense component is difficult to demonstrate in sectioned material where only short lengths of the cut filaments are present. Examination of the margins of the dense areas at high magnifications usually demonstrates the filaments for here they are not so tightly packed.

Various patterns of nucleolar segregation are recognized, perhaps the best known being the nucleolar cap. Here, the dense filamentous component forms a crescentic, hemispherical, cone-shaped or cap-like mass over the granular component of the nucleolus (*Plate 35*). Sometimes two caps are formed and wider separation of segregated components may also occur.

In other instances the filamentous component departs from the granular component as numerous small dense masses, from one pole of the nucleolus or in a radial fashion (*Plate 36, Figs. 1, 2 and 4*). The significance and mechanisms involved in the production of these different patterns is not known. A correlation between aetiological agent and pattern of nucleolar segregation does not seem to exist. Thus nucleolar cap formation, which is the characteristic form of segregation seen after actinomycin D administration, has also been seen in herpesvirus infected cells (Sirtori and Bosisio, 1966).

Plate 35

Nucleolar segregation produced in rat hepatocyte nucleoli by actinomycin D (*Ghadially and Ailsby, unpublished electron micrographs*).

Figs 1–3. Nucleolar caps are shown here. The denser filamentous component forming the cap is indicated by arrows. Note also the nucleolus associated heterochromatin (H). × 29 000; × 35 000; × 56 000

Fig. 4. Further separation of segregated components is illustrated here. The segregation is quite impure; the component richer in filaments (arrow) can barely be identified as such. × 56 000

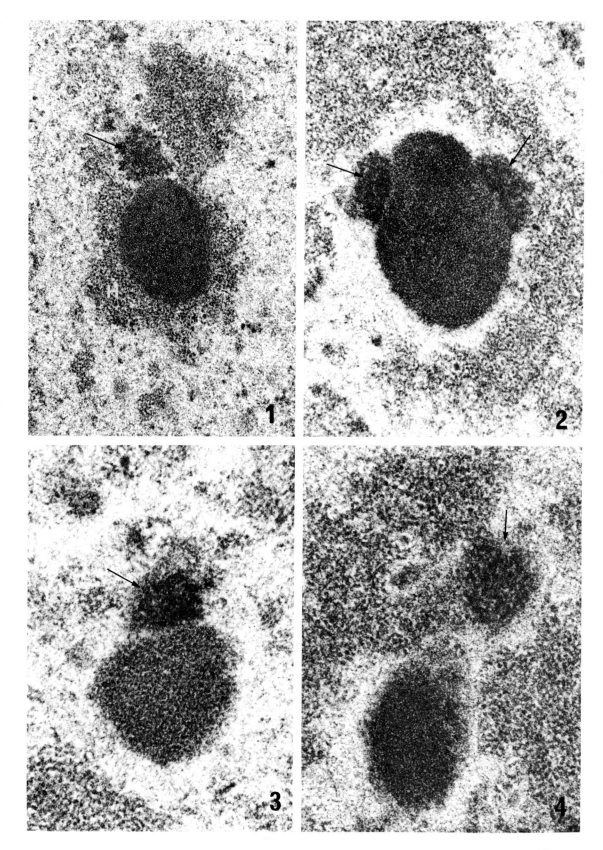

71

Nucleolar segregation has been produced in a variety of cells* by numerous agents† such as: (1) actinomycin D (Schoefl, 1964; Oda and Chiga, 1965; Chiga et al., 1966; De Man and Noorduyn, 1967; Goldblatt et al., 1969b; Magalhães and Magalhães, 1980); (2) mitomycin C (Lapis and Bernhard, 1965); (3) mithramycin (Kume et al., 1967); (4) adriamycin, carminomycin and marcellomycin (Merski et al., 1976; Daskal et al., 1978); (5) N-ethyl-N-nitrosourea (Lantos, 1971); (6) 4-nitroquinoline-N-oxide (Reynolds et al., , 1963; Lazarus et al., 1966); (7) proflavine, acridine orange (Simard, 1966; Reynolds and Montgomery, 1967); (8) ethionine (Miyai and Steiner, 1967; Shinozuka et al., 1968); (9) dimethylnitrosamine, 3′methyl-4-dimethyl-aminoazobenzene, aflatoxin B, lasiocarpine, tannic acid (Svoboda et al., 1966, 1967; Reddy and Svoboda, 1968); (10) cycloheximide (Harris et al., 1968); (11) herpesvirus (Sirtori and Bosisio, 1966; Swanson et al., 1966; Leestma et al., 1969); (12) Coxsackie virus (Weiss and Meyer, 1972); (13) mycoplasma (Jézéquel et al., 1967); and (14) flying spot ultraviolet nucleolar irradiation (Montgomery et al., 1966). It will be observed that the list of agents which produce nucleolar segregation contains many carcinogens and antimetabolites.

Simard and Bernhard (1966) postulated that nucleolar segregation probably reflects DNA binding and inhibition of DNA-dependent RNA synthesis because of the loss of template activity of DNA, and this view has found favour with many students of this subject. Reddy and Svoboda (1968) have pointed out that many hepatocarcinogens and also some other agents which produce nucleolar segregation produce a decrease in the activity of RNA polymerase, an enzyme known to catalyse the synthesis of RNA, and that two carcinogens, 3-methylcholanthrene and thioacetamide, which do not produce nucleolar segregation show an increase in RNA polymerase activity and RNA synthesis. Further, it can be observed that the list of agents which produce nucleolar segregation also contains many compounds not known to be carcinogenic. Hence one may conclude that this phenomenon is not a prerequisite for the production of a tumour.

*Most studies are on rat hepatocytes, a few deal with other cells such as cells in culture, cardiac myocytes, neurons, and adrenal fasciculata cells.
†Nucleolar segregation is not always produced by extrinsic agents. Examples of this are the partial nucleolar mutants of Xenopus laevis (Miller and Gonzales, 1976). These mutations are due to a partial deletion of the nucleolar organizer which results in a reduction of the rate of ribosomal RNA synthesis to about 50 per cent or 25 per cent of the normal. Segregated nucleoli are seen throughout the limited life-span of these mutants.

Plate 36

Fig. 1. Small dense masses comprising the filamentous component (F) are seen sequestrated from the main nucleolar mass containing numerous granules (G). From herpesvirus-infected monkey kidney cells in culture. × 41 000

Fig. 2. A more advanced form of segregation is seen in this electron micrograph. The filamentous component (F) is represented by small dense bodies radiating from the centrally placed granular component (G). Virus particles (V). From the same material as *Fig. 1.* × 33 000

Fig. 3. Another pattern of nucleolar segregation, where the granular (G) and filamentous components (F) have each formed a hemispherical mass. From the same material as *Fig. 1.* × 49 000

Fig. 4. An unusual pattern of nucleolar segregation is depicted here. In the centre of the nucleolus is an enlarged filamentous centre (C). Adjacent to this is the granular component (G) and, surrounding this, the dense filamentous component (F) which is broken up into discrete small masses. From an early tumour nodule (fibrosarcoma) produced in the subcutaneous tissue of the rat by an injection of 7,12-dimethylbenz-α-anthracine. × 40 000 (*Ghadially and Bhatnager, unpublished electron micrograph*)

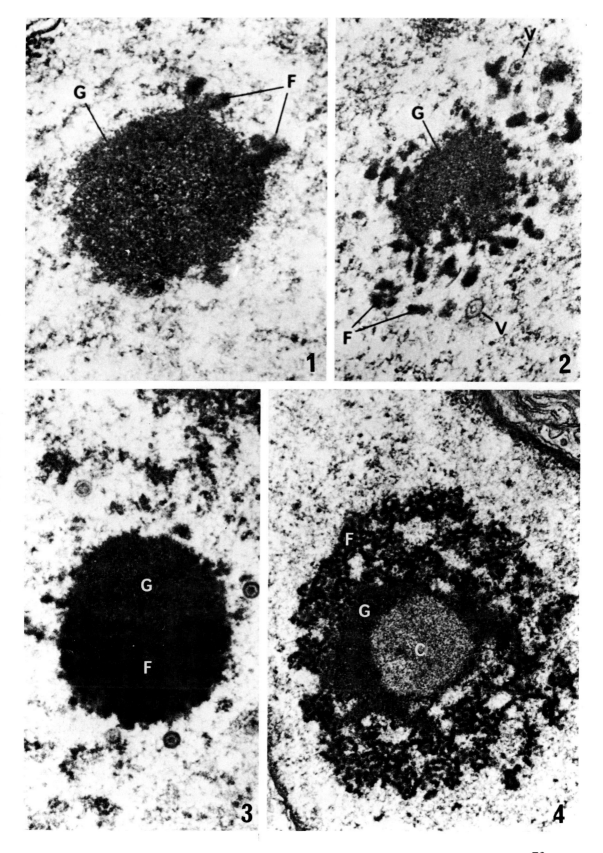

73

Pseudoinclusions and true inclusions

Nuclear inclusions occurring in a variety of tissues of man and other animals have been studied extensively by light microscopy for over 70 years (for references *see* Sobel *et al.*, 1969a). Distinction between viral and non-viral inclusions could not be made with confidence and many non-viral inclusions were assumed to be viral ones.

Electron microscopic studies have now made it amply clear that most nuclear inclusions contain cytoplasmic structures and are non-viral. It is also evident that a large majority of these inclusions are, in fact, pseudoinclusions (*Plate 37*), for the apparently included material does not lie free in the nuclear matrix but is separated from it by the two membranes derived from an invagination of the nuclear envelope. Virtually every cytoplasmic organelle or inclusion has, at one time or another, been found within such inclusions. There also occurs a somewhat rare variety of pseudoinclusion which is bounded by a single membrane derived from the inner membrane of the nuclear envelope. Examples of such inclusions are presented later (pages 78-89). In this section we shall deal only with the common double-membrane-bound pseudoinclusion and the differences between such inclusions and true inclusions where the included material lies free in the nuclear matrix.

The morphology of pseudoinclusions is illustrated by two examples in *Plate 37* and by a diagram (*Plate 70, Fig. 1*), and it can be seen that an invagination in longitudinal section will appear as a pseudoinclusion in transverse section. Serial sections show that fusion of membranes in narrow-necked invagination can occur (Leduc and Wilson, 1959a), sequestrating the double-membrane-bound inclusion within the nucleus. At this stage one can argue that the included material is still not truly within the nucleus and hence such inclusions should be regarded as pseudoinclusions. However, dissolution of the covering membranes may occur and ultimately convert a pseudoinclusion into a true inclusion where the included material mingles with the nuclear matrix. Characteristically, pseudoinclusions are lined by the two membranes of the nuclear envelope and, as one would expect, the inner membrane is studded with ribosomes just like the outer membrane of the nuclear envelope, while condensed chromatin may be seen lying around the outer membrane of the inclusion as it does along the inner membrane of the nuclear envelope.

Pseudoinclusions show marked variations in size. Very large inclusions, as large as normal nuclei, were noted in the enlarged hepatocytes of mice fed a methionine-rich diet to which bentonite was added (Leduc and Wilson, 1959a, b). An extreme example of this has been reported by Bloom (1967), where virtually the entire cytoplasmic mass with its organelles and inclusions formed an inclusion within the nucleus, which was reduced to a thin shell lying just under the cell membrane. The number of inclusions seen in a single nucleus is also variable. Occasionally, the entire nucleus is studded with multiple inclusions (*Plate 2, Fig. 2*).

Plate 37

Fig. 1. Human synovial intimal cell showing an irregular nucleus (nucleus N; cytoplasm, C). An invagination such as that seen at A will appear as a pseudoinclusion (B) in transverse section. The characteristic double membrane lining such inclusions can barely be discerned at this low magnification. × 33 000 (*From Ghadially and Roy, 1969a*)

Fig. 2. Acute leukaemic cell from peripheral blood, showing an invagination (I) and a pseudoinclusion containing a mitochrondrion (M) with longitudinally orientated cristae. A few ribosomes can be seen along the inner membrane of the inclusion (arrow). × 42 000

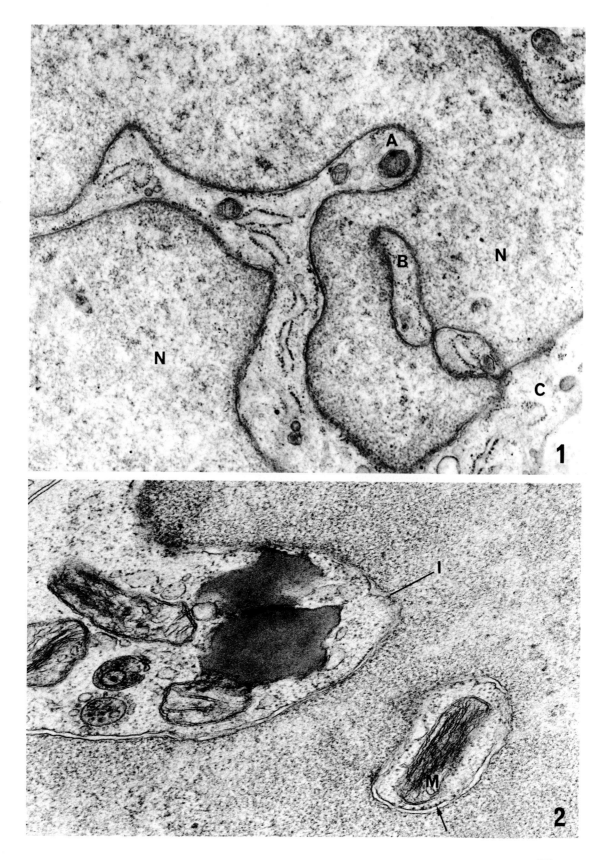

Changes often occur in the structures trapped in a pseudoinclusion (*Plate 38, Fig. 1*). Organelles such as rough endoplasmic reticulum and mitochondria frequently show degenerative changes which lead to the formation of membranous whorls and myelin figures. It would appear that such changes are more likely to occur when the invagination has a narrow opening or when the opening is occluded, and it has been suggested that normal structures promptly degenerate in such an unfavourable environment (Kleinfeld *et al.*, 1956; Leduc and Wilson, 1959a).

A variety of drugs which cause toxic injury to cells can produce nuclear invaginations and inclusions, and Sobel *et al.* (1969a) have postulated that in most of these instances there is an increased cytoplasmic volume (swelling) which probably leads to the ingress of cytoplasmic material into the nucleus. In this respect the observations of Wessel (1958) are interesting, for they suggest that pseudoinclusions can be transient. In colchicine-injected mice he noted a swelling of hepatocytes and formation of intranuclear pseudoinclusions which regressed when the effect of the drug had worn off and the swelling had subsided.

A study of published data indicates that intranuclear pseudoinclusions are seen infrequently in young animals, including humans, but with advancing years there is an increase in the number of both hyperploid nuclei and inclusions. This is suggested by the work of : (1) Sobel *et al.* (1969a) on human material; (2) Olitsky and Casals (1945) who observed invaginations of the nuclear envelope in the livers of two strains of mice and found that they were more frequent in older animals; and (3) Andrew *et al.* (1943) who observed intranuclear pseudoinclusions more frequently in the livers of older mice and humans.

A variety of true inclusions (*Plate 38, Fig. 2*) occurs in the nucleus, besides those containing cytoplasmic components; for example, inclusions produced by viruses and lead. These and other true inclusions are dealt with in later sections of this chapter. However, it is worth making a few brief comments here about the manner in which cytoplasmic components may come to lie in the nuclear matrix. It has already been pointed out that dissolution of the membranes enclosing a pseudoinclusion can produce a true inclusion. Other theories have also been offered to explain how true inclusions may occur. For example, it has been suggested that organelles as large as mitochondria can gain access to the interior of the nucleus via enlarged nuclear pores, or that organelles may become accidentally incorporated within the nucleus during mitosis (Brandes *et al.*, 1965; Bucciarelli, 1966; Bloom, 1967). The latter event is particularly liable to occur with frequent or abnormal mitosis. Such a view is in keeping with the observation that nuclear inclusions are commonly encountered in tumours, but it should be noted that even in this example most of the inclusions are pseudoinclusions dependent upon irregularity of nuclear shape. (*See* pages 2–9 for further discussion on this topic.)

Inclusions have been seen in such a large variety of tumours that it would be impossible to list all instances. Perhaps of special interest are the human and experimentally produced melanomas, for true inclusions of pigment granules may be found in the nucleus. However, such inclusions have also been observed in naevi and in choroid of human and animal eyes (Ludford, 1924; Apitz, 1937a; Sobel *et al.*, 1969a).

Plate 38

Fig. 1. Hepatocyte nucleus showing a large double-membrane-bound pseudoinclusion containing lipid droplets (L) and organelles which have suffered degenerative changes. From the liver biopsy of a patient with gastric carcinoma. × 28 000

Fig. 2. Mitochondria (M) and vesicular structures are seen lying free in the nuclear matrix. From a normal human vas deferens. × 27 000

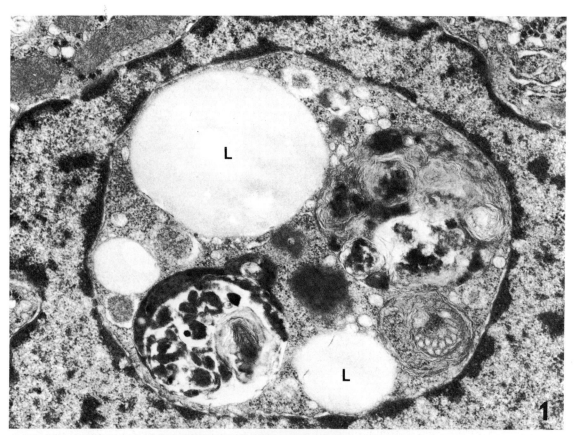

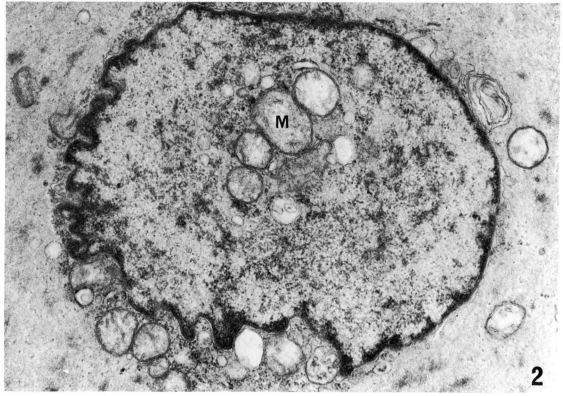

Intranuclear Russell bodies

In intranuclear Russell bodies we have an example of a single-membrane-bound pseudoinclusion (for other examples *see* pages 80-89. For mode of formation *see Plate 70, Fig. 1*), the single membrane being derived from the inner membrane of the nuclear envelope. This is in contrast to the common pseudoinclusion which is bounded by two membranes derived from the inner and outer membranes of the nuclear envelope (page 74). Intranuclear Russell bodies have been noted by many workers (Apitz, 1937b, Fruhling and Porte, 1958; Fruhling *et al.*, 1960; Bessis and Thiery, 1962; Brittin *et al.*, 1963; Maldonado *et al.*, 1966; Graham amd Bernier, 1975; Oikawa, 1975; Blom *et al.*, 1976; Djaldetti and Lewinski, 1978, Ghadially and Lalonde, 1979). The glycoprotein-rich Russell body develops within the rough endoplasmic reticulum and one may find one or a few large Russell bodies or numerous small Russell bodies within the dilated cisternae of the rough endoplasmic reticulum (*see Plate 239*). On rarer occasions, Russell bodies are also seen in the nucleus (*Plate 39*).

Brittin *et al.* (1963) suggested that Russell bodies may be synthesized in the nucleus but there is no reason to believe this. It takes little imagination to see that if a body lying in the perinuclear cistern were to enter the nucleus it would confront only the inner membrane of the nuclear envelope and would hence be bounded by only one membrane. Such an idea was put forward by Fruhling *et al.* (1960) and by Maldonado *et al.* (1966) and illustrations supporting such a contention have been presented by Blom *et al.* (1976) who show Russell bodies in the perinuclear cistern that appear to have forced the inner membrane of the envelope to protrude into the nucleus. Since the cisternae of the rough endoplasmic reticulum are continuous with the perinuclear cistern, one can envisage that a Russell body developing in a segment of the endoplasmic reticulum close to the perinuclear cistern would expand the membranes in this region, gain access to the perinuclear cistern, and then enter the nucleus as a single-membrane-bound pseudoinclusion derived from the inner membrane of the nuclear envelope.

For Russell bodies situated in more distal parts of the cisternae of the rough endoplasmic reticulum, the hypothesis proposed by Djaldetti and Lewinski (1978) is more attractive. These authors propose that a focal fusion of the outer membrane of the perinuclear cistern and the rough endoplasmic reticulum occurs and that later dissolution of the membranes in this region places the Russell body in a situation whereby it can enter the nucleus as a single-membrane-bound pseudoinclusion derived from the inner membrane of the nuclear envelope. In rare instances a Russell body may form a part of the contents of a double-membrane-bound pseudoinclusion, which besides the Russell body, contains other structures such as mitochondria and rough endoplasmic reticulum. An excellent example of this is shown in *Fig. 8* of the paper by Djaldetti and Lewinski (1978).

The idea that the membrane delimiting a classic pseudoinclusion may disintegrate and that a true inclusion may be formed in this way is now generally accepted (page 74). That the same is true about single-membrane-bound pseudoinclusions is evidenced in *Plate 39, Fig. 4*.

Plate 39

Fig. 1. The membrane (arrowheads) surrounding this large intranuclear Russell body (R) can be discerned in places. From a plasma cell found in a stomach biopsy from a case of hairy cell leukaemia. × 21 000 (*From Ghadially and Lalonde, 1979*)

Fig. 2. The nucleus of this plasma cell contains a single-membrane-bound (arrowheads) pseudoinclusion. Within it are seen numerous small Russell bodies(R) set in a flocculent, proteinaceous matrix of a texture similar to that found in the dilated cisternae of the rough endoplasmic reticulum. From same tissue as in *Fig. 1*. × 20 000 (*From Ghadially and Lalonde, 1979*)

Fig. 3. The membrane bounding this pseudoinclusion containing Russell bodies is difficult to visualize but heterochromatin aggregates (H) similar to those seen adjacent to the inner membrane of the nuclear envelope are evident. From the bronchial mucosa of a patient with bronchial carcinoma. × 27 000

Fig. 4. Appearances seen here suggest that the limiting membrane (arrowheads) of an inclusion containing Russell bodies has fragmented, releasing them into the nuclear matrix. From a plasma cell found in a haemartoma of the lung. × 23 000 (*From Ghadially and Lalonde, 1979*)

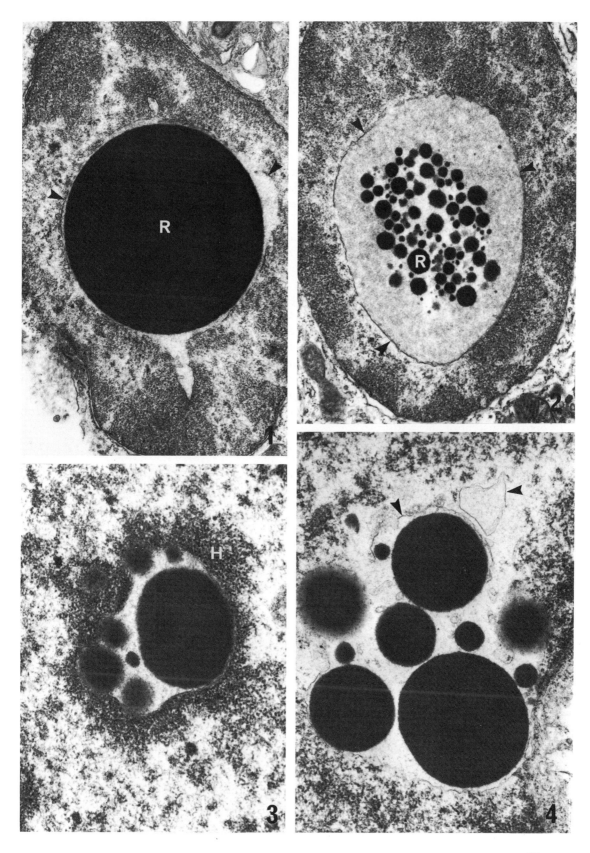

79

Intranuclear concentric laminated inclusions

Concentric laminated inclusions are examples of single-membrane-bound pseudoinclusions★. They present as alternating concentric shells of electron-dense and electron-lucent material. A single, smooth-surfaced, loose-fitting membrane usually separates the inclusion from the nuclear matrix (*Plates 40–42*).

Intranuclear laminated inclusions have been seen in: (1) oviduct epithelium of hens (Johnston, 1962); (2) mucus-secreting cells of human labial salivary glands (Tandler *et al.*, 1969); (3) acinar cell adenocarcinoma of parotid gland (Erlandson and Tandler, 1972); (4) parotid acinar cells from a patient with systemic lupus erythematosus (Itabashi *et al.*, 1976); (5) murine pulmonary adenomas and adenocarcinomas (Flaks and Flaks, 1970) (*Plate 40, Figs. 1–3*); (6) a synovial cell from an apparently normal human synovial membrane (*Plate 40, Fig. 4*); (7) a fibroblast† in a myxofibrosarcoma (Kindblom *et al.*, 1979); (8) pancreatic acinar cells from patients with insulinoma (Itabashi *et al.*, 1976; Ghadially and Lalonde, 1979, 1980) (*Plates 41* and *42*); (9) pancreatic acinar cells from cases of Reye's syndrome (Collins, 1974; Itabashi *et al.*, 1976); (10) renal proximal tubule cells of chickens (Mickwitz, 1972); (11) cells of an adrenal cortical adenoma (Conn's syndrome) (Propst, 1970); (12) fibroxanthosarcoma (Merkow *et al.*, 1971); and (13) adenoma of breast (Ghadially *et al.*, 1985) (page 86).

The bulk of the inclusions listed above seem to occur in cells capable of elaborating a mucoid or serous secretory product. Tandler *et al.* (1969) noted that such inclusions in labial glands occurred in immature mucous cells but not in cells containing abundant secretory products. Therefore these authors suggested that these inclusions may be related to the secretory cycle of mucus producing cells. In the hen's oviduct epithelium, Johnston (1962) found similar laminated inclusions both in the cytoplasm and nucleus and suggested that this might be a type of nuclear secretion. However, quite a few of the 'laminated bodies' portrayed in the cytoplasm are reminiscent of autolysosomes.

★The mechanisms of formation of single-membrane-bound inclusions are also described on pages 78 and 88. They are also explained with the aid of a diagram in *Plate 70*.
†The authors consider the cell to be a histiocyte, but it has no lysosomes and too much rough endoplasmic reticulum for a macrophage. Further, they describe the inclusion as a 'nuclear body', but I interpret it as a concentric laminated inclusion (bounded by a single membrane) in the nucleus of a fibroblast.

Plate 40

Figs. 1–3. Electron micrographs showing a variety of intranuclear concentric laminated inclusions found in pulmonary adenomas and adenocarcinomas of mice. × 16 000; × 25 000; × 21 000 (*From Flaks and Flaks, 1970*)

Fig. 4. An intranuclear concentric laminated inclusion found in an apparently normal human synovial cell. × 46 000 (*Ghadially and Roy, unpublished electron micrograph*)

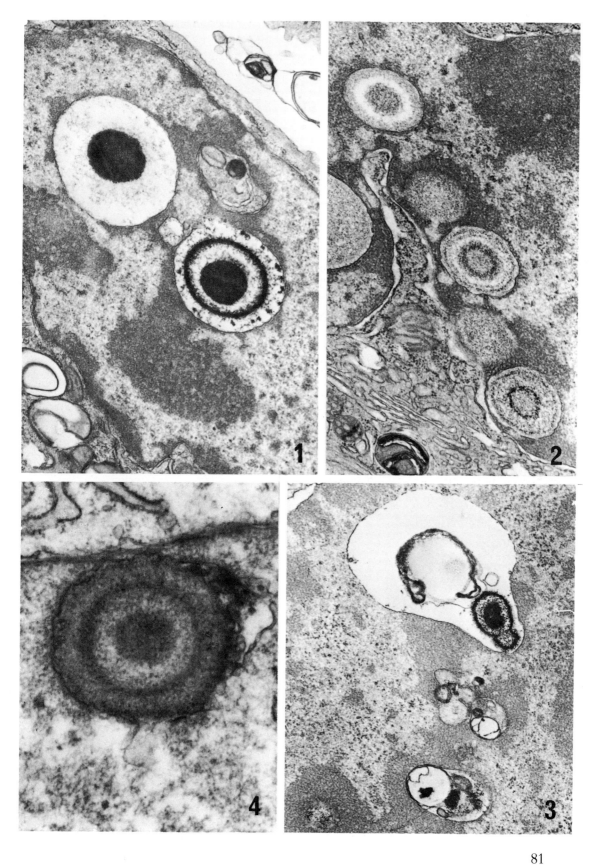

In the labial salivary glands (Tandler *et al.*, 1969) and in the murine tumours (Flaks and Flaks, 1970) electron-dense granules were at times seen within single-membrane-bound inclusions and the possibility that these might be lipidic in nature and that the concentric laminated inclusion may derive from this was considered (Tandler *et al.*, 1969).

In the pancreatic acinar cells we found single-membrane-bound inclusions containing electron-dense granules and laminated inclusions. Further, transitional stages between these were evident which suggest the manner in which these laminated inclusions develop (*Plates 41 and 42*).

Within the nuclei of some acinar cells we found single-membrane-bound inclusions containing one or two granules of a size and morphology identical to the zymogen granules in the cell cytoplasm (*Plate 41, Fig. 1*). This is probably the first stage in the formation of these laminated inclusions. In another group of inclusions the granule in the inclusion was no longer uniformly electron-dense but had a mottled appearance (*Plate 41, Fig. 2*), and such granules appeared to be somewhat larger than the zymogen granules in the cytoplasm. Mottled granules were not found in the cytoplasm. It would therefore appear that this is not a processing artefact and that the larger size and lucent zones indicate an influx of fluid into the granule. Appearances seen in *Plate 41, Figs. 3 and 4* may be looked upon as continuation of this process which leads to the formation of larger inclusions with an electron-dense lamina (*Plate 41, Fig. 3*) or laminae (*Plate 41, Fig. 4*). However, increasing hydration does not appear to be the only mechanism whereby these inclusions grow in size, for it would appear (*Plate 42, Figs. 1 and 2*) that an increase in size may occur by the fusion of two such inclusions within a single-membrane-bound space or by the addition of fresh granules to a well formed laminated inclusion (*Plate 42, Fig. 3*).

The inclusions found in the labial salivary gland were reported (Tandler *et al.*, 1969) to be eosinophilic but difficult to detect in H and E stained sections. Some stained with Nile blue

---

Plate 41

From human pancreatic tissue adjacent to an insulinoma. (*From Ghadially and Lalonde, 1980*)

Fig. 1. Pancreatic acinar cell showing zymogen granules (Z) in the cytoplasm and similar granules (Z) lying within single membrane-bound inclusion(s) in the nucleus. × 32 000

Fig. 2. A single-membrane-bound inclusion containing a mottled granule with a clear centre. × 50 000

Fig. 3. Two inclusions are seen in this nucleus. The one in the bottom left corner is tangentially cut and hence difficult to evaluate. The other inclusion bounded by a single membrane presents an electron-dense shell and a lucent centre containing flocculent material. × 42 000

Fig. 4. Single-membrane-bound laminated inclusions with a crenulated border. × 34 000

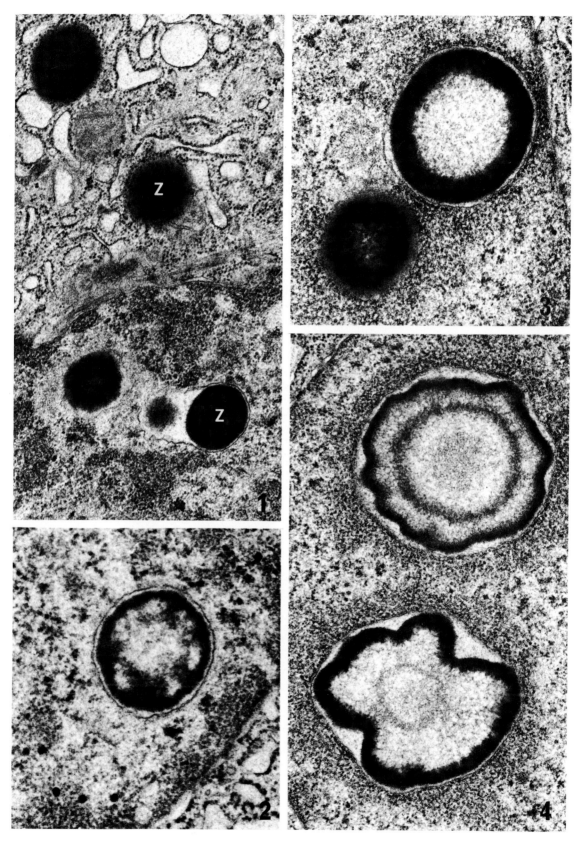

83

sulphate (neutral phospholipids) while others were PAS-positive but diastase-resistant. They were also Feulgen-negative.

The collective evidence now indicates that most but not all concentric laminated inclusions derive from single-membrane-bound pseudoinclusions containing either mucous or serous (including zymogenic) granules. One could argue that mucous granules are too 'pale' to produce the dense lamellae in the laminated inclusion. Therefore it is worth pointing out that not all mucous granules are of low electron density and that medium density granules and quite dense granules are also known to occur (*see Plates 152 and 153*).

Yet another intriguing feature of these inclusions is that they are bounded by a single membrane, in contrast to the common pseudoinclusion containing cytoplasmic material which is bounded by two membranes derived from the double-membraned nuclear envelope.

Zymogen granules are at times found in the cisternae of the rough endoplasmic reticulum (*see* page 530). Since this cisternal system is continuous with the perinuclear cistern one may envisage that a zymogen granule entering the nucleus by this route may carry before it the inner membrane of the nuclear envelope and thus form a single-membrane-bound inclusion★.

However the usual variety of zymogen granule seen in the cell cytoplasm is bounded by a membrane derived from the Golgi complex. For such a granule to form a single-membrane-bound inclusion one would have to speculate that a fusion of the membrane bounding the granule and the outer membrane of the nuclear envelope probably occurs and that dissolution of the membranes in the zone of fusion liberates the naked granule (i.e. not membrane-bound) into the perinuclear cistern whence it proceeds into the nucleus as a single-membrane-bound inclusion deriving its ensheathing membrane from the inner membrane of the nuclear envelope.

★Further discussion about single-membrane-bound pseudoinclusions is presented on page 78 where we deal with the intranuclear Russell body, which is another variety of intranuclear single-membrane-bound pseudoinclusion. The mode of formation of these inclusions is explained with the aid of a diagram in *Plate 70*.

Plate 42

From human pancreatic tissue adjacent to an insulinoma. Same case as *Plate 41*.

Fig. 1. Appearances seen here may be interpreted as two swollen zymogen granules which are fusing within an intranuclear inclusion. × 32 000 (*From Ghadially and Lalonde, 1979*)

Fig. 2. Fusion of included granules is suggested in this electron micrograph also. × 44 000 (*From Ghadially and Lalonde, 1980*)

Fig. 3. A laminated inclusion (L) and some dense granules acceptable as zymogen granules are seen in a single-membrane-bound space within the nucleus. One of the granules (G) appears to be fusing with the laminated inclusion. × 36 000 (*From Ghadially and Lalonde, 1980*)

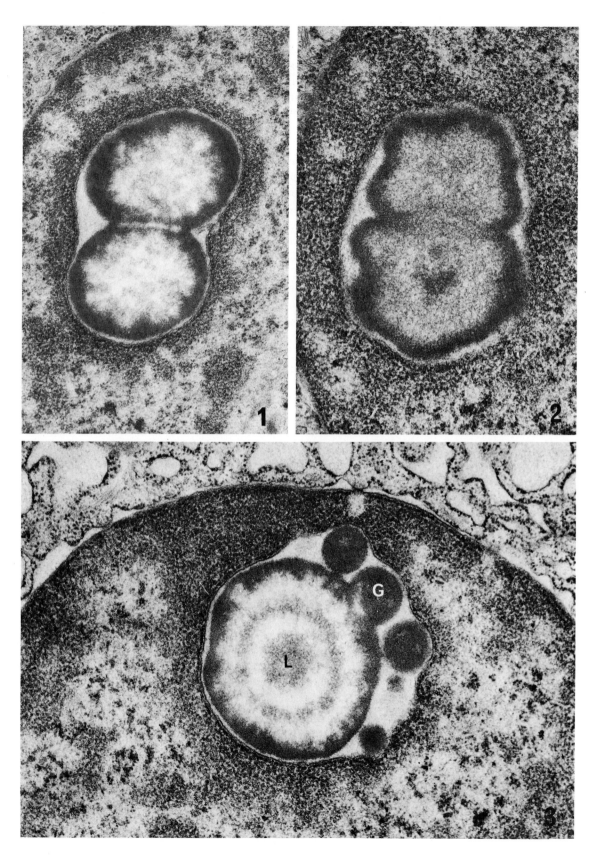

Intranuclear helioid inclusions

The term 'helioid inclusion' (Gk *helios* sun) was coined by us (Ghadially *et al.*, 1985c) to describe single-membrane-bound intranuclear inclusions which contain one or more rounded bodies (helioid bodies) with a corona of radiating filaments reminiscent of the rays emanating from the sun (*Plate 43, Fig. 1*). These inclusions were found in an adenoma of the breast removed from a woman aged 63 years. I am not aware of any other report in the literature where such bodies have been described.

The cytoplasm of a few tumour cells contained some electron-dense secretory granules (serous granules) about 0.25–0.45 μm in diameter. Granules of a similar size were not seen in intranuclear inclusions, but occasionally larger dense granules (about 0.5–1 μm) were seen and forms that could be interpreted as stages of evolution of dense granules into helioid bodies (*Plate 43, Figs. 2 and 3*).

In the nuclei of the epithelial cells we found several double-membrane-bound inclusions containing some cytoplasmic matrix and organelles but these did not contain helioid bodies except in one interesting instance where a helioid body was seen within dilated rough endoplasmic reticulum in a double-membrane-bound inclusion (*Plate 43, Fig. 4*). In the dilated rough endoplasmic reticulum of another such inclusion, we found a mass composed of numerous electron-lucent bodies set in a more dense granular matrix (*Plate 44, Fig. 1*).

Except for the above-mentioned instance (*Plate 43, Fig. 4*), helioid bodies were found only in single-membrane-bound inclusions in the nucleus. Usually only one such body was present in an inclusion, but at times several helioid bodies were present within a single-membrane-bound inclusion (*Plate 44, Fig. 2*). These bodies lay in a lucent pool containing flocculent material and a varying number of filaments (*Plate 44, Figs. 2–4*). Several inclusions were at times present in the nucleus and sometimes such inclusions were interconnected to produce large multiloculated inclusions (*Plate 44, Fig. 4*). Some profiles of single-membrane-bound inclusions contained only flocculent material and filaments set in a lucent matrix but such appearances may have been created by cuts through the peripheral part of an inclusion containing a helioid structure which did not lie in the plane of sectioning.

The core of the helioid body appeared either homogeneously electron-dense or had a laminated appearance. In some instances such variations could be real but in other instances such differences would be explicable on the basis of sectioning geometry (*Plate 44, Fig. 4*). The filaments emanating from the inclusion were quite straight and rigid-looking, but more distant from the inclusion they were undulating or reticulated (*Plate 44, Figs. 2 and 3*). Besides the helioid inclusions described above, some single-membrane-bound inclusions contained unilaminated or multilaminated bodies of the type described on page 80.

Plate 43

From an adenoma of the breast (*From Ghadially, Stinson, Payne and Leibovitz, 1985c*)

Fig. 1. Two intranuclear helioid inclusions are depicted here. They comprise helioid bodies lying in a lucent matrix (L) containing randomly oriented filaments. In this electron micrograph the helioid bodies present as structures with a dense core (D) (diameter of larger core is about 0.8 μm) and a corona of radiating filaments (F). Note that these are single-membrane-bound inclusions. The medium-density band (arrowheads) around the inclusion and at the periphery of the nucleus is the nuclear fibrous lamina. × 36 000

Fig. 2. The profiles seen here may be interpreted as sections through several single-membrane-bound inclusions, some of which may be connected to form a multiloculated inclusion or inclusions. Several profiles of dense granules are present. Some show a just discernible filamentous border, suggesting that a transformation from dense granules to helioid bodies may be occurring. If we ignore the granules which appear to be cut near the periphery rather than the centre, the diameter of the remainder ranges from about 0.5–1 μm. × 15 000

Fig. 3. The three bodies seen in this inclusion show a slender corona of radiating filaments around a relatively large dense core (about 0.5–0.7 μm in diameter). They could be regarded as newly formed helioid bodies where the radiating filaments are not fully developed. × 29 000

Fig. 4. A double-membrane-bound inclusion containing cytoplasmic structures (C) and a helioid body (H) lying in a dilated sac of rough endoplasmic reticulum (between arrows). × 25 000

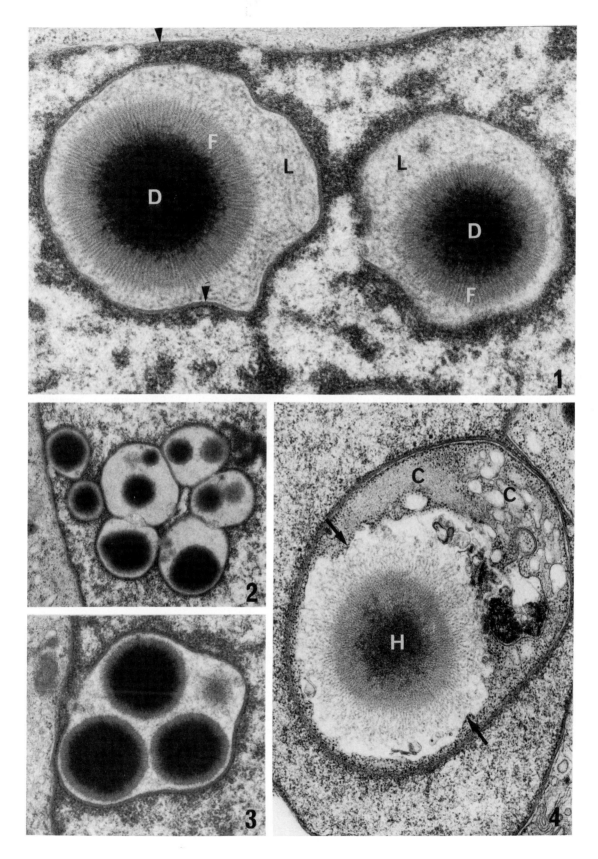

The genesis and mode of development of helioid inclusions is debatable. *A priori* one might argue that they evolve from secretory granules as do some concentric laminated inclusions★. Support for this thesis comes from the fact that dense granules and intermediate forms between such granules and helioid bodies were seen in intranuclear inclusions. Against this thesis is the fact that electron-dense secretory granules (i.e. serous granules) of a comparable size were found neither in the cell cytoplasm nor within the rough endoplasmic reticulum in the cytoplasm. However, since smaller serous granules were found in the cell cytoplasm one could speculate that: (1) the large granules in the intranuclear inclusions were probably formed by fusion of smaller cytoplasmic granules sequestered in inclusions; or (2) that large granules were present in the cell cytoplasm but they were so rare that they escaped detection in the small sample that can be examined with the electron microscope.

Be that as it may, another likely possibility worth considering would be that the contents of the perinuclear cistern or rough endoplasmic reticulum (these two are continuous systems *see* page 36) sequestered in an intranuclear inclusion condensed to form granules, laminated bodies and helioid bodies. *Plate 43, Fig. 4* gives credence to such a thesis for a helioid body is seen within a dilated sac of rough endoplasmic reticulum which forms part of a double-membrane-bound intranuclear inclusion. *Plate 44, Fig. 1* also supports this thesis, because it is difficult to see how this mottled inclusion could have derived from a dense granule, but it could easily be the product of precipitation of heterogeneous material in the rough endoplasmic reticulum in the inclusion.

It is well known that the contents of the rough endoplasmic reticulum can condense or crystallize to produce a bewildering variety of intracisternal inclusions, which may present as dense granules, reticulated granules, laminated bodies and crystals (*see* Chapter 5). Further, a large variety of filamentous and microtubular inclusions are also known to occur within the cisternae of the rough endoplasmic reticulum. It is therefore possible that the intranuclear helioid inclusion is but one more variation on this theme, whereby the products in the rough endoplasmic reticulum condense to form helioid bodies and associated filaments. The chemical composition of the helioid body and the associated filaments is obscure, but since they were produced in the rough endoplasmic reticulum one may speculate that they are principally proteinaceous in nature.

★The mechanisms involved in the formation of single-membrane-bound intranuclear inclusions, and the manner in which secretory granules sequestered in such inclusions turn into unilaminated and multilaminated inclusions is described on pages 80–85. The mode of formation of single-membrane-bound inclusions is explained with the aid of a diagram in *Plate 70.*

Plate 44

From an adenoma of the breast. Same case as *Plate 43.* (*From Ghadially, Stinson, Payne and Leibovitz, 1985c*)

Fig. 1. Within a dilated sac of rough endoplasmic reticulum (between arrowheads) in this inclusion lies a mass composed of numerous electron-lucent bodies (B) set in a medium-density granular matrix (M). × 14 000

Fig. 2. This single-membrane-bound inclusion contains profiles of six helioid bodies lying in a filamentous matrix. × 46 000

Fig. 3. This electron micrograph demonstrates the remarkable accumulation of well developed filaments found in some of these inclusions. Two profiles of peripherally cut helioid bodies are present. In some places the straight filaments emanating from these bodies appear to be continuous with the reticulated filaments in the matrix of the inclusions. × 33 000

Fig. 4. The profiles seen here show a multiloculated (trilobed) inclusion and two other inclusions above and below it. It It is possible that serial sections might show that all these are part of one large multiloculated inclusion. Two profiles contain only filaments set in a lucent matrix (M), three others contain also profiles of helioid bodies (A, B and C). The differences in appearance may be explained on the basis of sectioning geometry. The one marked 'A' may be looked upon as an equatorial section showing a laminated core and a corona of filaments: the one marked 'B' as a section through the dense peripheral part of the core; and the one marked 'C' as a cut that had missed the core entirely and just sectioned the radiating filaments. × 26 000

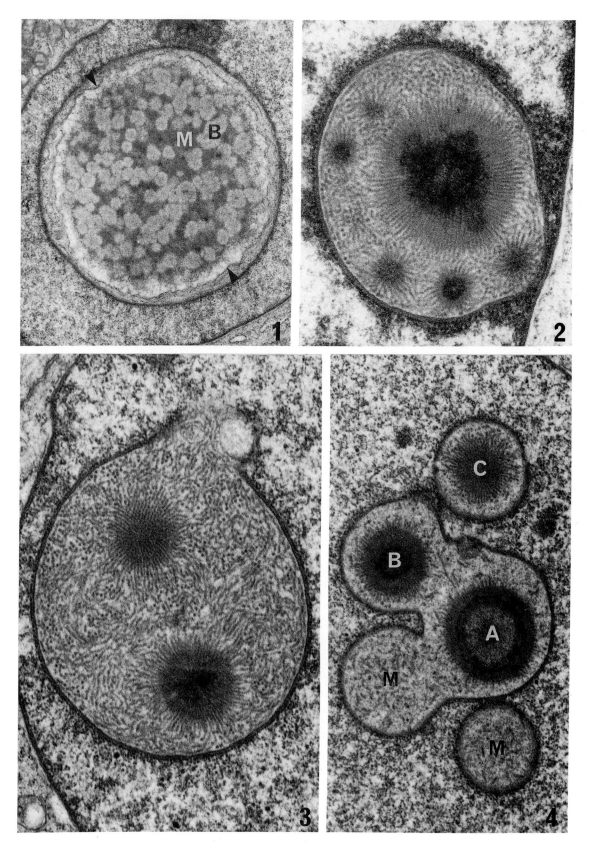

Intranuclear membranous lamellae, tubules and vesicles

Membranous profiles acceptable as sections through lamellae, tubules and vesicles have at times been found in nuclei; in many instances their origin from the inner membrane of the nuclear envelope has been convincingly demonstrated, as has continuity between the interior of such tubules or lamellae and the perinuclear cistern. The distinction between tubules and membranous lamellae can be made in favourable ultrathin sections on the basis that when tubules are present some of these are likely to be cut transversely and give the characteristic circular profile but membranous lamellae, being large flattened sac-like structures (i.e. cisterns), will appear like longitudinally sectioned tubules and circular profiles will be absent.

One of the most highly organized lamellar systems is that of the annulate lamellae, which usually occur in the cytoplasm but are sometimes seen also in the nucleus. Intranuclear annulate lamellae are derived from the inner membrane of the nuclear envelope, and indeed both intranuclear annulate lamellae and membranous formations of the type discussed in this section of the text can coexist in the same nucleus. However, intranuclear annulate lamellae are best considered later (Chapter 6).

The tubular inclusions (about 30–100 nm in diameter) described in this section (*Plates 45–47*) must not be confused with the microtubular★ inclusions (about 15–28 nm in diameter) such as those produced by some viruses (*Plate 68*) or forming a part of certain intranuclear crystals (*Plate 55*). Besides their size, a further point of distinction is that of the membranes comprising the tubular, vesicular and lamellar inclusions show the trilaminar structure characteristic of cytomembranes and plasma membranes, but the walls of microtubules do not show a trilaminar structure. Finally, it should be noted that lamellar and tubular systems arising from the inner membrane of the nuclear envelope may penetrate the nucleolus and ramify in this structure. This produces intranucleolar inclusions which are considered in the following section (page 98).

Intranuclear membranous structures (tubules, lamellae and vesicles) have been seen in: (1) Novikoff hepatoma (Novikoff, 1957; Babai *et al.*, 1969; Karasaki, 1970); (2) Yoshida ascites hepatoma (Hoshino, 1961; Locker *et al.*, 1968); (3) Morris hepatoma (Hruban *et al.*, 1972); (4) preneoplastic rat hepatocytes after administration of N,N-dimethyl-aminoazobenzene (Karasaki, 1973); (5) rat and mouse hepatocytes after exposure to sodium tetraphenyl boron (Parry, 1971); (6) mouse ascites lymphosarcoma (6C3HED) (Levine *et al.*, 1968); (7) Ehrlich's ascites tumour (Yasuzumi and Sugihara, 1965); (8) Rous sarcoma (Bucciarelli, 1966); (9) a cell from human acute leukaemia (*Plate 45, Fig. 1*); (10) pulmonary adenomas and adenocarcinomas of mice (Flaks and Flaks, 1970) (*Plate 45, Fig. 2*); (11) hyperplastic type II alveolar cells of patients

---

★For classification, nomenclature and differences between tubules and microtubules (*see* footnote on page 938).

Plate 45

Fig. 1. Nucleus of a leukaemic leucocyte showing intranuclear vesicles and/or tubules. The nuclear envelope is not clearly visualized because of tangential sectioning. However, infoldings of the inner membrane (arrow) depicting the probable manner in which these structures arise, can be discerned. × 44 000

Fig. 2. A group of intranuclear tubules, most cut longitudinally and some transversely (arrow), are seen in this electron micrograph. From murine pulmonary tumour. × 33 000 (*From Flaks and Flaks, 1970*)

Fig. 3. The membranous structures (arrows) in this nucleus represent sections through lamellae rather than tubules, as no circular profile of a transversely cut tubule is seen. Whether these lamellae are annulate or not is difficult to say. There are occasional interruptions along their length which could be interpreted as profiles of annuli. From monkey kidney cell culture infected with herpesvirus. × 24 000

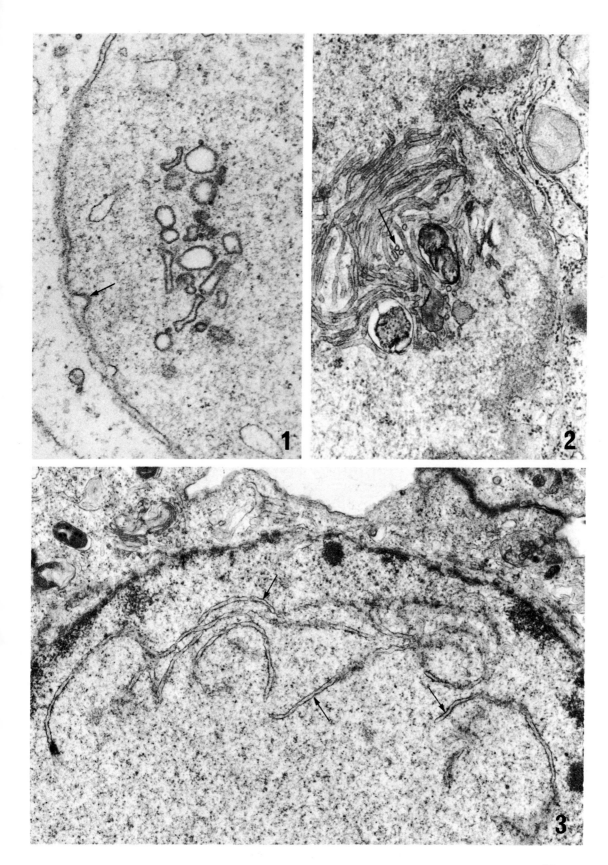

treated with busulphan and bleomycin (Gyorkey et al., 1980); (12) type II alveolar cells adjacent to a pulmonary leiomyoma (*Plate 46, Fig. 1*); (13) benign pulmonary adenomatosis in man (Kotoo et al., 1976); (14) metaplastic alveolar cells (derived from type II alveolar epithelial cells) from cases of fibrotic lung disease (Kawanami et al., 1979); (15) neoplastic type II alveolar cells in primary and secondary alveolar cell carcinoma and neoplastic or included★ type II alveolar cells in bronchiolo-alveolar carcinoma (Coalson et al., 1970; Kuhn, 1972; Torikata and Ishiwata, 1977; Ghadially et al., 1985a) (*Plate 46, Fig. 2* and *Plates 47* and *48*); (16) parosteal sarcoma (Murray et al., 1983); (17) cardiac muscle cells from cases of myocardial hypertrophy (Ferrans et al., 1975; Engedal et al., 1977); (18) calf adrenal cortex (Weber et al., 1964); (19) pituitary mammotrophs of mongolian gerbils (Nakayama and Nickerson, 1972; Nickerson, 1973, 1975a,b, 1977); (20) trophoblasts of rat and mouse chorioallantoic placenta (Carlson and Ollerich, 1969); and (21) herpesvirus-infected cells (*Plate 45, Fig. 3*). We have already seen (*Plates 21* and *22*) that in certain virus infections proliferations of the membranes of the nuclear envelope occur. While often quite complex structures are produced, sometimes the nucleus contains simpler lamellar inclusions (*Plate 45, Fig. 3*).

Intranuclear tubular inclusions or tubulovesicular inclusions vary much in size and complexity, some of the largest and most complex being those found in altered type II alveolar cells. Profiles seen in these inclusions suggest that the tubules may occur as: (1) solitary tubules meandering in the nucleus; (2) stacks of tubules in parallel arrays; (3) packed tubules showing a honeycomb pattern (when cross-cut); (4) loosely packed branching and ramifying tubules; and (5) tubules that have probably expanded to form vesicles. It will be noted from the list presented in the previous paragraph that in human material intranuclear tubular or tubulovesicular inclusions occur almost exclusively in hyperplastic or neoplastic type II alveolar cells. Therefore, in the correct histopathological setting they serve as a marker† for alveolar cell carcinoma.

The mode of origin and the significance of intranuclear membrane-bound structures are not well understood but certain points are worth commenting upon. One can envisage several possible sources from which these intranuclear membranous structures are derived: (1) cytomembranes (endoplasmic reticulum, Golgi complex, etc.) included in the nucleus, perhaps as a pseudoinclusion with later dissolution of the walls of the pseudoinclusion; (2) entrapment of cytomembranes in the nucleus during mitosis; (3) *de novo* synthesis of membranes in the nucleus; and (4) growth and invagination of the inner membrane of the nuclear envelope.

★Many tumours with a bronchiolo-alveolar pattern of growth contain a mixed population of cells such as type II alveolar cells, Clara cells and a few mucus cells. In such instances it is difficult to know whether all cell types are neoplastic and one is witnessing a stem cell tumour exhibiting multidirectional differentiation, or whether some of the cells are normal or hyperplastic cells 'accidentally included' in the tumour. (*See* Chapter 32 in Ghadially, 1985 for details of classification of bronchiolo-alveolar carcinoma and its subtypes.)

†This is illustrated by one of our cases (Ghadially et al., 1985a) where at autopsy on a male aged 67 years, a tumour mass involving the peripheral part of the lung and pleura (which was much thickened) was found, and also tumour deposits in mediastinal lymph nodes. The gross diagnosis was: 'probably a mesothelioma', the histological diagnosis was: 'adenocarcinoma or mesothelioma'. Ultrathin sections from the pleura showed tumour cells containing intranuclear tubular inclusions (*Plate 46, Figs. 2 and 3*), but no features supporting the diagnosis of mesothelioma. In the lymph node metastasis also, the prominent feature was the occurrence of numerous intranuclear tubular inclusions, and the occasional occurrence of material which reminded one of pulmonary surfactant. Only after diligent search in many blocks were cells containing several indubitable myelinosomes (i.e. secretory granules of type II alveolar cells) found and thus the diagnosis of alveolar cell carcinoma was established.

Plate 46

Fig. 1. From lung tissue adjacent to a leiomyoma. Nucleus of a type II alveolar cell showing an inclusion formed of loosely packed ramifying tubules. The structure between arrowheads seems to be derived by dilatation of tubules and apposition of the walls of adjacent tubules. × 35 000

Fig. 2. Pleural infiltrate from alveolar cell carcinoma (autopsy material). Three tubular inclusions are seen lying in the nucleus. × 25 000 (*From Ghadially, Harawi and Khan, 1985a*)

Fig. 3. Same block of tissue as *Fig. 2.* This intranuclear tubular inclusion presents as closely packed circular profiles arranged in a honeycomb-like pattern. They probably represent cross-cut tubules rather than sections through vesicles. Some solitary tubules are also evident (arrowheads) in the nucleus. × 58 000 (*From Ghadially, Harawi and Khan, 1985a*)

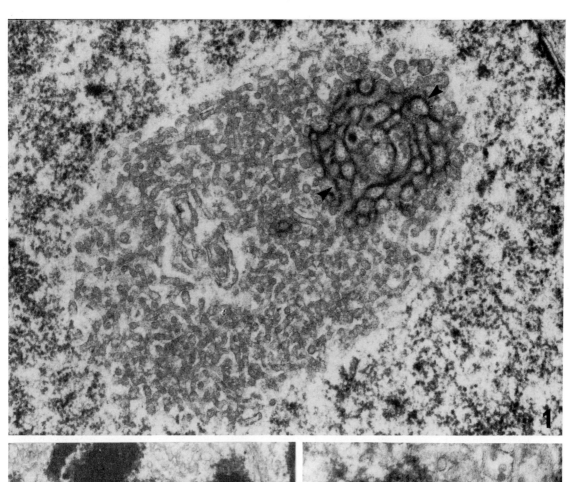

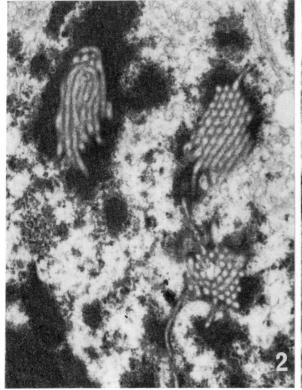

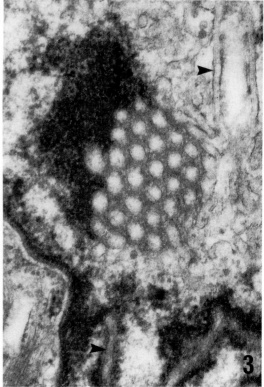

Regarding the mode of formation of intranuclear tubular inclusions in type II alveolar cells, there is little doubt that they derive by a process of proliferation of the inner membrane of the nuclear envelope (*Plate 70, Fig. 2*), because several studies (e.g. Gyorkey *et al.*, 1980) have shown that the tubules in these inclusions are continuous with the inner membrane of the nuclear envelope.

Murray *et al.* (1983) have described what they call 'undulating membrane complexes' which they found in the nuclei of cells of a parosteal sarcoma. I have seen a similar inclusion★ in a cell from a case of bronchiolo-alveolar carcinoma where an altered or neoplastic type II alveolar cell contained a large intranuclear inclusion, apparently composed entirely of undulating or pouched lamellae† formed by closely apposed paired membranes (*Plate 48, Fig. 2*). Several other type II alveolar cells in this tumour showed the characteristic intranuclear inclusions (similar to those shown in *Plates 46* and *47*) containing tubules deployed in various ways (random, parallel, reticular, ramifying, honeycomb). In a few of these one could discern small areas where the configuration suggested that undulating or pouched membranes rather than tubules were present (*Plate 48, Fig. 1*), and that as the tubules entered these areas they were transformed into undulating or pouched membranes.

The true three-dimensional morphology of these structures is difficult to ascertain but several possibilities regarding their genesis are worth considering: (1) that in rare instances the proliferation of the inner membrane of the nuclear envelope results not in the production of the usual tubules but of cisterns or membranous lamellae composed of closely apposed paired

★There is a close similarity between the measurements of the profiles seen in the intranuclear inclusion in the parosteal sarcoma and the bronchiolo-alveolar carcinoma described here. The actual figures are given in the legend to *Plate 48, Fig. 2*.

†An undulating membrane is rather like a corrugated galvanized iron sheet used for roofing. A pouched membrane is like an egg tray with multiple pouches to hold the eggs. Only in one plane of sectioning (across the corrugations) will the former give a wavy or undulating profile, the latter will give this profile whether it is cut longitudinally or transversely. In a plane of section parallel to the base of the egg tray the cross-cut pouches will give circular profiles. While a corrugated sheet will not normally give a circular profile, distortion of corrugations (from U-shaped to O-shaped) by applying lateral pressure may in fact do so. Circular profiles will also be produced if two adjacent undulating membranes are deployed in a manner whereby the peak or crest of one touches the trough of another. Thus in sectioned material it is not easy to say whether one is looking at an undulating membrane (i.e. like a corrugated sheet) or a pouched membrane (i.e. like an egg tray). (See also Plate 220, Figs. 3, 4 and 5.)

In the analogies presented above we have a single undulating or pouched membrane, but in the case of the intranuclear inclusions we are discussing we have paired membranous lamellae. Thus the cross-cut pouches (or distorted corrugations) will present profiles suggesting cross-cut double-membrane-bound tubules, and similarly the wavy or undulating profiles will also be composed of two parallel membranes. Such an appearance (i.e. double-membrane-bound cross-cut tubules) can also be produced by a superimposition of the images of two parallel, overlying, undulating tubules where the crest of one lies touching or overlapping the trough of another. Obviously in such a case the space between the two membranes will be the same as the diameter of the undulating tubules producing these profiles. This model is not applicable to the structures shown in *Plate 48* because the tubules of the intranuclear tubular inclusion (indicated by T and arrowhead in *Plate 48, Fig. 1*) are about 46 nm in diameter but the thickness of the wall of the profiles suggesting double-membrane-bound tubules (indicated by arrowheads *Plate 48, Fig. 2*) is only about 17.5 nm.

Plate 47
Intranuclear inclusions in type II alveolar cells from two different cases of bronchiolo-alveolar carcinoma.
Fig. 1. Most of the tubules in this inclusion are deployed more or less parallel to each other. × 43 000
Fig. 2. This tubulovesicular inclusion presents as a collection of tubular (T) and vesicular (V) profiles. × 60 000 (*From Ghadially, 1985*)

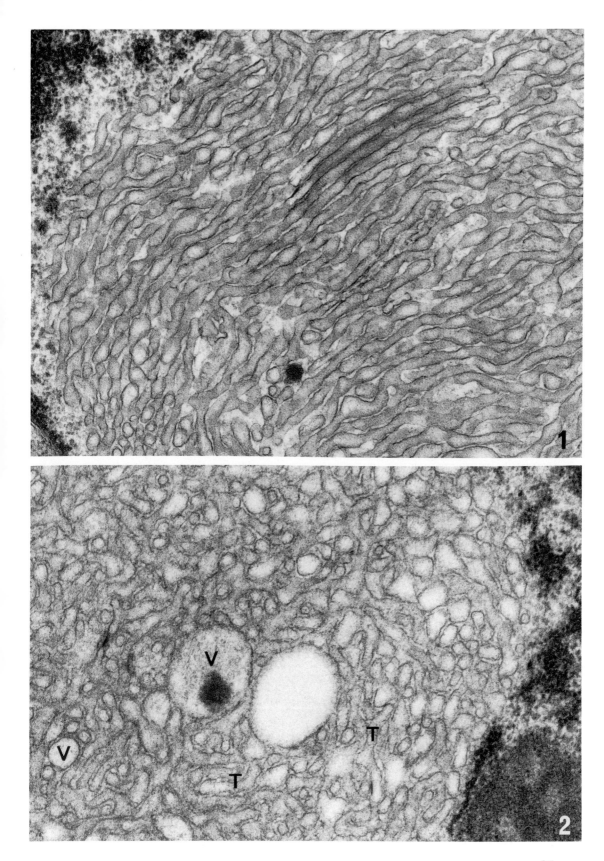

membranes which suffer close packing and undulation or pouching to produce the profiles we see; (2) that the appearance we call 'undulating or pouched membrane complex' is an illusion, created by a difficult to understand arrangement of closely packed ramifying tubules where the walls of adjacent tubules have come close together because the tubules are dilated; and (3) that a true transformation of tubules into flat (i.e. lamellar) cisternae occurs perhaps by compression and/or fusion of adjacent tubules, and that what we are looking at now are indeed undulating or pouched membranous lamellae derived from pre-existing tubules in the inclusion.

I am at a loss to choose between these alternatives, but since one can find inclusions where the tubules 'run into' foci presenting the undulating membrane image (*Plate 48, Fig.1*), I am inclined to discard the first hypothesis. It seems to me that what we are probably looking at are true undulating or pouched membranes derived from modified tubules. As such, I would suggest that until further studies elucidate the true three-dimensional morphology of these inclusions, we should classify them as 'paired membrane complexes' (this would include both the undulating and pouched variety) so as to distinguish them from the much commoner inclusions composed of obvious tubules.

The membranous formations found in Rous sarcoma by Bucciarelli (1966) bear a strong resemblance to the Golgi complex and no connections with the inner membrane of the nucleus are evident. Hence one is inclined to agree with the author that these are Golgi derived structures 'accidentally' included into the nucleus during mitosis.

There appear to be a group of intranuclear membranous formations (tubules and vacuoles) which are induced by hormonal stimuli (items 18 and 19 in the list in this section). Connections between these and the inner membrane of the nuclear envelope are not seen. There is no overwhelming proof that these are included cytomembranes except some illustrations in Nickerson (1975b, 1977) which are clearly pseudoinclusions. Hence one could argue that the membranous inclusions in this group are probably derived from included cytomembranes. An alternative hypothesis would be *de novo* synthesis of membranes in the nucleus but there is no proof that this actually ever occurs. In passing it is worth noting that the hormonally mediated intranucleolar tubular inclusion (nucleolar basket, page 98) found in the human endometrium is clearly derived from the inner membrane of the nuclear envelope and so are indeed most of the other inclusions listed in this section.

Thus it would appear that the cells in which intranuclear tubular, lamellar and vesicular inclusions occur are usually not dying cells but cells with a normal or heightened metabolic activity. Hence it has been frequently suggested that these membranous formations facilitate nucleocytoplasmic exchanges.

Plate 48

Fig. 1. Bronchiolo-alveolar carcinoma. Seen here is a small portion of a large intranuclear inclusion composed of ramifying tubules (T). The inclusion also contains two foci (F) where the profiles suggest that undulating or pouched membranes are present. Note how the tubules run into these foci. The diameter of the tubule indicated by an arrowhead is about 46 nm. × 70 000

Fig. 2. Same specimen as *Fig. 1.* Seen here is a small but representative sample of a large inclusion which occupied more than three-quarters of the nuclear profile. It is composed of profiles which suggest that undulating or pouched membranes rather than tubules are present. The thickness of the paired membranous lamellae is 17.5 nm, the width of each undulation is 74 nm. The periodicity ('wavelength') of the undulations is 99 nm. Note also the profiles which look like transverse sections through double-membrane-bound tubules (arrowheads). × 74 000

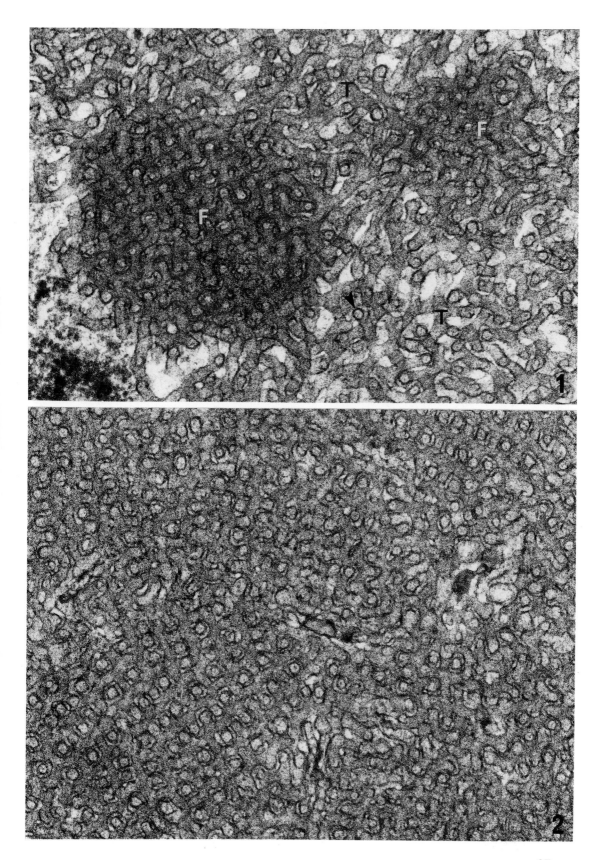

Intranucleolar membranous lamellae, tubules and vesicles

Membranous profiles interpretable as sections through lamellae, tubules and vesicles have at times been seen in the nucleolus. In some (but not all) instances their origin from the inner membrane of the nuclear envelope has been convincingly demonstrated, as has continuity between the interior of such tubules and lamellae with the perinuclear cistern.

It would appear that lamellar and tubular systems arising from the inner membrane of the nuclear envelope★ can come into close association with the nucleolus or penetrate and ramify in this structure. Examples of this have been seen in: (1) normal human endometrial cells during the early secretory phase of the menstrual cycle (Dubrauszky and Pohlmann, 1960a,b; Clyman, 1963; Moricard and Moricard, 1964; Ancla and De Brux, 1965; Terzakis, 1965; Roberts, 1967; Feldhaus *et al.*, 1977; More and McSeveney, 1980); (2) salamander and crayfish oocytes (Miller, 1966; Kessel and Beams, 1968); and (3) Novikoff hepatoma cells (Babai *et al.*, 1969; Karasaki, 1970).

Of the various intranucleolar lamellar or tubular inclusions, the one that occurs in the human endometrium (*Plate 49*) in the postovulatory half of the menstrual cycle has been most extensively studied. This inclusion was first described by Dubrauszky and Pohlmann (1960a,b). Later workers have used various terms to describe it such as the 'nucleolar basket' (Clyman, 1963), 'nucleolar channel system' (Terzakis, 1965), 'intranucleolar tubular structure' and 'intranuclear tubulate corpuscles' (Ancla and De Brux, 1965) and 'intranucleolar canalicular structure' (Roberts, 1967; Roberts *et al.*, 1975).

An examination of published electron micrographs leaves little doubt that this inclusion comprises an ordered array of tubules rather than lamellae, for circular profiles representing transverse sections through the tubules are clearly seen. Continuities between these tubules and the inner membrane of the nuclear envelope have also been convincingly demonstrated as has continuity between the interior of these tubules and the perinuclear cistern (Terzakis, 1965; Roberts, 1967). Thus it would appear that this inclusion arises by tubular invagination of the inner membrane of the nuclear envelope.

This inclusion has been described as 'unique' because it is found only in the human endometrium but not in the endometrium from other species. However, it is worth noting that some of the inclusions illustrated by Karasaki (1970) in Novikoff hepatoma cells are remarkably similar in appearance.

It is said that the nucleolar tubular system develops in the human endometrium only if ovulation has occurred and hence this may be a 'prerequisite to normal fertility in the human female' (Kohorn *et al.*, 1972). *In vivo* (Roberts *et al.*, 1975) and *in vitro* (Kohorn *et al.*, 1972) studies show that progesterone and medroxyprogesterone acetate can induce the formation of this intranucleolar tubular system (*Plate 49*). Screening with various steroids led Kohorn *et al.* (1972) to conclude that 'the acyl group in 17β position of the D ring of the progestational steroid is associated with nucleolar basket formation'. However, the true significance of this remarkable inclusion eludes us; the explanation usually given is that it assists nucleolar cytoplasmic exchanges.

★This section should be read in conjunction with the previous section (page 90) on intranuclear lamellar, tubular and vesicular inclusions.

Plate 49

Human secretory endometrium five days after medroxyprogesterone acetate (*Roberts, Horbelt, Powell and Walker, unpublished electron micrographs*)

Fig. 1. A nucleolus containing an intranucleolar tubular structure is seen adjacent to an invagination of the nuclear envelope. × 34 000

Fig. 2. A nucleolus containing an intranucleolar tubular structure. × 30 000

Fig. 3. High-power view of an intranucleolar tubular structure. × 110 000

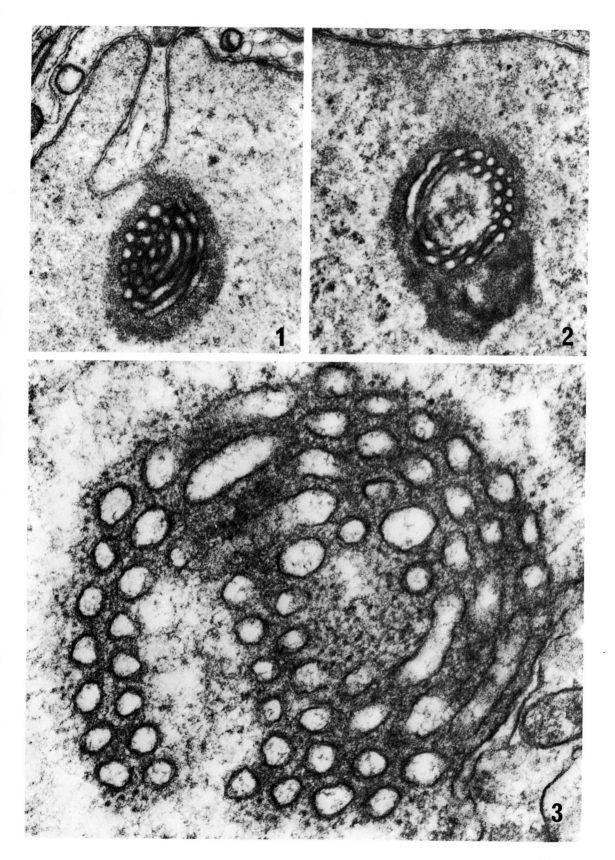

Intranuclear glycogen inclusions

Intranuclear glycogen deposits were first described by Ehrlich (1883) in the hepatocytes of patients suffering from diabetes mellitus. In routine histological sections such deposits present as clear vacuolar inclusions. With the electron microscope, characteristic plumbophilic electron–dense particles are seen. In most instances only monoparticulate glycogen is observed but in rarer instances rosettes or rosette-like formations have also been found.

Glycogen deposits may present as large irregular-shaped masses within the nucleus, or they may form a compact rounded mass surrounded by fibrillary material (*Plates 50* and *51*). Solitary glycogen particles or small groups of particles may also be seen lying free in the nuclear matrix. Invaginations of the nuclear envelope are not seen around these inclusions, so these deposits are regarded as true inclusions.

Intranuclear glycogen inclusions have been seen in: (1) hepatocytes in diabetes mellitus (Ehrlich, 1883; Chipps and Duff, 1942; Tanikawa and Igarashi, 1963; Caramia *et al.*, 1967, 1968; Schulz and Hahnel, 1969; Sobel *et al.*, 1969b); (2) hepatocytes in Graves' disease and Hodgkin's disease (Cazal and Mirouze, 1951); (3) hepatocytes in infective hepatitis (Biava, 1963; Wills, 1968); (4) hepatocytes in Wilson's disease and Gilbert's disease (Sobel *et al.*, 1969b); (5) hepatocytes in glycogen storage disease type I, but not in type II (Sheldon *et al.*, 1962; Baudhuin *et al.*, 1964); (6) hepatocytes in lupus erythematosus (Sparrow and Ashworth, 1965); (7) hepatocytes of a patient with carcinoma of the stomach (*Plates 50* and *51*); (8) hepatocytes of normal well-fed tadpoles (Himes and Pollister, 1962); (9) human myocardium obtained at open heart surgery but the reason for the occurrence of intranuclear glycogen could not be ascertained (Ghadially, 1975); (10) mouse (Shelton, 1955) and human hepatomas (Ghadially and Parry, 1966); (11) a chicken sarcoma (Binggeli, 1959); (12) Ehrlich ascites tumours (certain

---

Plate 50

From the liver biopsy of a patient with carcinoma of the stomach.

Fig. 1. Much of the glycogen in this inclusion in a hepatocyte nucleus is extracted; leaving behind a large electron-lucent area (A) containing poorly stained glycogen particles. This is the equivalent of the appearance seen with the light microscope where in formaldehyde fixed material intranuclear glycogen is usually represented by a clear 'vacuole' in the nucleus. Fixed in glutaraldehyde (phosphate buffer) followed by osmium; stained with uranium and lead. × 8900

Fig. 2. In this hepatocyte nucleus the glycogen inclusion presents as a small clear area (demarcated by arrowheads) containing poorly stained glycogen rosettes. Fixed and stained as in *Fig. 1.* × 11 500

Fig. 3. In this hepatocyte nucleus is seen a glycogen body (arrowhead) and glycogen particles (arrows) scattered in the nuclear matrix. Fixed in osmium (phosphate buffer), stained with uranium and lead. × 9000

Fig. 4. Glycogen particles (demarcated by arrowheads) are seen in the matrix of a hepatocyte nucleus. Fixed and stained as in *Fig. 3.* × 11 000

100

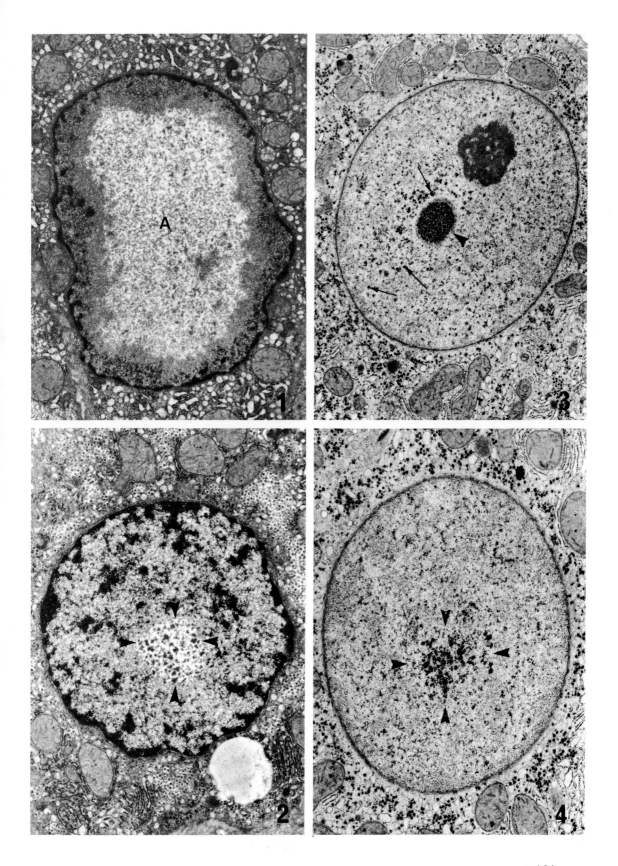

101

strains only) (Novikoff, 1957; Scholz and Paweletz, 1969; Granzow and Granzow, 1975; Zimmermann et al., 1976a,b); (13) Novikoff ascites rat hepatoma cells incubated with tritium-labelled D-glucose (Karasaki, 1971); (14) infantile type carcinoma of the pancreas (Frable et al., 1971); and (15) human rhabdomyosarcoma (Ghadially, 1985).

The idea that glycogen arrives in the nucleus via pseudoinclusions or that it enters the nucleus via the nuclear pores finds little support from published studies. Himes and Pollister (1962) suggested that glycogen in the nucleus may be synthesized in situ and this hypothesis is supported by the work of Karasaki (1971), who incubated hepatoma cells with tritium-labelled D-glucose and found that massive accumulations of glycogen can occur rapidly in nuclei without similar deposits in the cytoplasm at a period of active DNA synthesis when the nuclear envelope is intact. He noted an inverse relationship between deposits in the cytoplasm and nucleus, a point that has often also been made by those studying such deposits in human liver.

It is worth noting that focal glycogen deposits of the type illustrated in Plate 51, Fig. 2, can at times be confused with the fibrillogranular type of nuclear body as illustrated in Plate 78, Fig. 6. In this example distinction between the two is not too difficult because the glycogen forms pseudo-rosettes, but this is not always the case. Nuclear bodies that bear a remarkable resemblance to some examples of focal glycogen deposits (e.g. those observed by Caramia et al., 1967, 1968) are illustrated by Murad and Murthy (1970) in a chordoma, and by Wyatt et al. (1970) in a rhabdomyoma. In the latter example the bodies were PAS-positive but diastase-resistant. The focal deposits of glycogen, called 'glycogen bodies' by Caramia et al. (1967, 1968), were also PAS-positive but susceptible to diastase digestion. Thus it would appear that we are dealing with two distinct entities which may at times be difficult to distinguish on morphological grounds alone. Finally, it is worth noting that the term 'glycogen body' has also been used to describe glycogen membrane arrays in the cytoplasm (Plate 233), so this term should be avoided or the focal deposits of glycogen described more fully as the 'intranuclear glycogen body'.

Plate 51

Same case as *Plate 50*. Tissue fixed in osmium (phosphate buffer) stained with uranium and lead. Note that in this and the previous plate the glycogen is better preserved and stained when the primary fixation is with osmium in phosphate buffer. On the other hand the heterochromatin pattern is better visualized with glutaraldehyde.

Fig. 1. Hepatocyte nucleus showing a nucleolus (N) and monoparticulate glycogen (G). × 18 500

Fig. 2. A focal deposit of glycogen (G) surrounded by some fibrillary material is seen in this hepatocyte nucleus. Such a deposit is sometimes referred to as an intranuclear glycogen body. Smaller deposits of glycogen (arrows) are scattered in the nuclear matrix. × 57 000

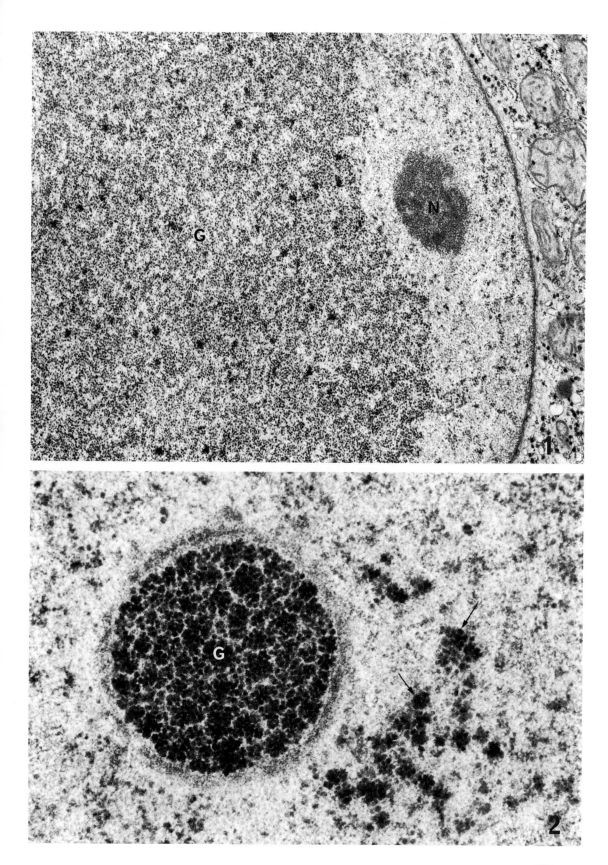

Intranuclear lipid inclusions

Both false and true lipid inclusions occur in the nucleus. In the former instance lipid forms but a part of a pseudoinclusion (*Plate 38, Fig. 1*) which also contains a variable amount of cytoplasm and often also some organelles. The true inclusion is seen as one or more lipid droplets lying free in the nuclear matrix (*Plate 52*). As a rule no membrane surrounds such droplets but at times a membrane or membrane-like structure (characteristic trilaminar structure has not been demonstrated) can be discerned closely applied to the lipid droplet (*Plate 52, Fig. 1*). However, it is unlikely that this is derived from the nuclear envelope, for a double membrane is not seen and at times cytoplasmic lipid also has such a 'membranous' structure around it. It is my experience that such 'membrane-bound' lipid droplets occur in the nucleus only when similar 'membrane-bound' lipid occurs in the cytoplasm.

The morphology of lipid droplets depends upon several factors such as the amount and degree of saturation of the fatty acids present, and the manner in which the tissue is processed. (For fuller discussion, *see* page 974.) Thus in electron micrographs lipid droplets show varying degrees of electron density ranging from very low to very high, or they may be totally removed during processing and appear as 'holes'. The contours of the lipid droplet may be smooth and round, ruffled or crenated. These are but a few of the many variations of lipid droplet morphology that one observes in electron micrographs. However, all such variations of morphology seen in cytoplasmic lipid are also seen in intranuclear lipid inclusions, and there is usually a close similarity between the two in any given specimen.

It would be futile to attempt to list all instances in which intranuclear lipid inclusions have been sighted, for lipid inclusions are perhaps the commonest form of true intranuclear inclusions. An occasional such inclusion may be encountered in a variety of normal tissues, particularly where lipid droplets normally occur in the cytoplasm. Thus an occasional intranuclear lipid inclusion is found in normal liver but they occur more frequently in situations where there is an increase in cytoplasmic lipid droplets. In normal synovial intimal cells lipid has not been seen in the nucleus, but in lipohaemarthrosis the synovial cells are loaded with lipid droplets and intranuclear lipid inclusions also occur (Ghadially and Roy, 1969b). Intranuclear lipid inclusions have often been noted in a variety of tumours. Passing mention of the occurrence of intranuclear lipid inclusions abound in the literature, but detailed description or comment about the mechanism by which such inclusions arise is made in only a few instances.

Plate 52

Fig. 1. A nucleus from an adenocarcinoma of the human stomach showing 'membrane-bound' crenated lipid inclusions (L). × 31 000

Fig. 2. Leukaemic lymphocyte from human peripheral blood. An electron-dense crenated lipid droplet (L) is seen in the nucleus. × 32 000

Fig. 3. Nucleus from small intestinal epithelial cell of a rat bearing a subcutaneous sarcoma showing a medium density lipid droplet (L) in the nucleus. × 48 000

Fig. 4. Human hepatoma cell nucleus showing a vacuolar electron-lucent area (L) which could be interpreted as lipid removed during tissue processing. × 49 000

104

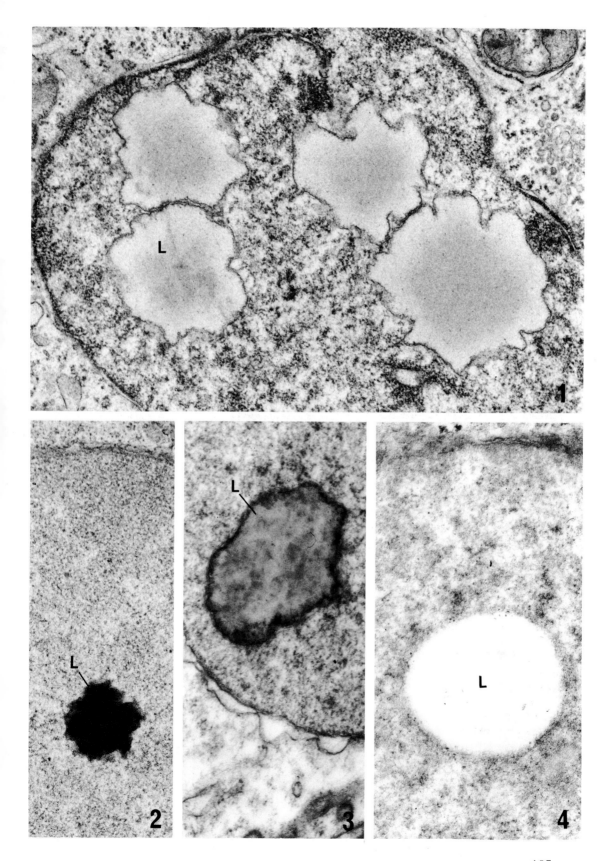

Such studies deal mainly with hepatomas, and liver cells, after various treatments such as partial hepatectomy and thioacetamide treatment (Kleinfeld and Von Haam, 1959; Leduc and Wilson, 1959a, b; Rouiller and Simon, 1962; Hruban *et al.*, 1965; Toker and Trevino, 1966; Smith *et al.*, 1968).

Regarding the mechanism of production of intranuclear lipid inclusions, the findings of Leduc and Wilson, (1959a) are of interest. They found numerous pseudoinclusions containing lipid and variable amounts of cytoplasmic material. As long as there was cytoplasmic material present separating the lipid droplet from the invaginated nuclear envelope the characteristic double membrane lining of such inclusions could be easily identified, but when lipid alone was present no surrounding membrane could be seen. About such lipidic inclusions studied in serial sections they comment: 'although double membranes could not be resolved around the inclusions that were entirely occupied by a lipid droplet, one such inclusion well within the nucleus was found to which the double membrane extended, then disappeared as if obscured by or dissolved in the lipid'. In this connection it is worth noting that when close association of lipid and mitochondria occurs (page 294) the outer mitochondrial membrane also seems to disappear as if obscured by or dissolved in the lipid.

My observations on intranuclear lipid inclusions seen in many situations support the idea that lipid droplets enter the nucleus at least in some instances in a manner similar to pseudoinclusions, but alterations and dissolutions of the membranes of the invaginating nuclear envelope occur during this process, thus liberating the lipid into the nuclear matrix. This point is made in *Plate 53*, which depicts the probable sequence of events.

Plate 53

Fig. 1. Cell from ascitic effusion in a case of ovarian carcinoma. Intranuclear lipid inclusions and cytoplasmic lipid droplets were of frequent occurrence in many cells. Appearances seen in this electron micrograph may be interpreted as an early stage of formation of intranuclear lipid inclusions. Three lipid droplets are seen, two of which have indented the nucleus. Probable dissolution of nuclear envelope is seen at one point (arrow), while at other points (arrowheads) the envelope appears altered and dense. × 31 500

Fig. 2. Acute leukaemic cell from peripheral blood. Lipid droplets were plentiful in both cytoplasm and nucleus and could be detected also in smears examined with the light microscope. Appearances seen here may be interpreted as a lipid droplet in the process of entering the nucleus. The expected double membrane is not seen around the lipid droplet but electron-dense material probably derived from it is seen on the surface of the lipid. Invaginated inner membrane of the nuclear envelope can just be discerned at the neck of the inclusion (arrow). × 40 000

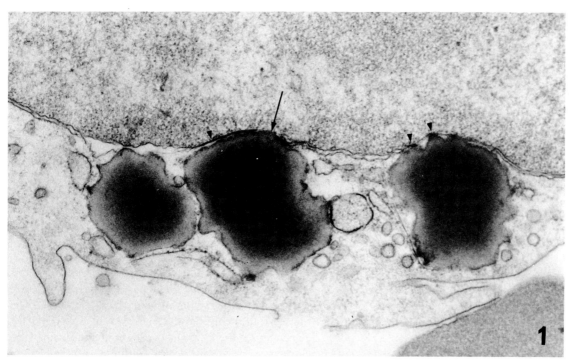

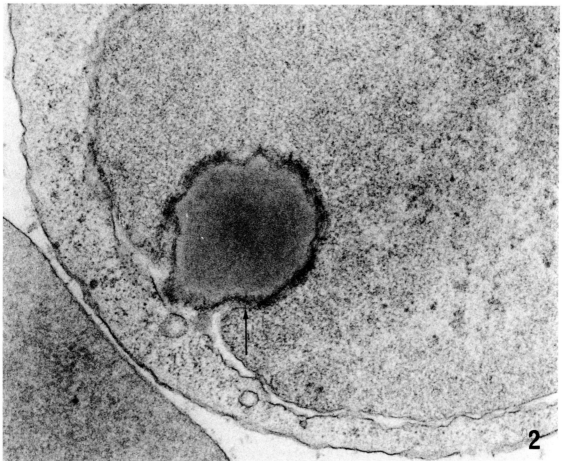

107

Intranuclear filamentous and crystalline inclusions

Intranuclear inclusions composed mainly or entirely of bundles of closely packed filaments have been seen in the nuclei of a large variety of cells; in both normal and pathological states. These inclusions often present as a band-shaped or rod-shaped body in the nucleus. At times a crystalline or paracrystalline lattice (presumably formed by crossing arrays of filaments overlapping in the section thickness) is seen. Occasionally microtubules are incorporated in these inclusions.

When filaments occur in more or less parallel or semi-ordered arrays the term 'paracrystalline inclusion' or 'crystalloid inclusion' is used rather than just 'filamentous inclusion'. However, the degree of order needed before one calls a filamentous inclusion a paracrystalline inclusion remains a matter of observer bias and opinion. Hence, the term filamentous inclusion is often used to cover both filamentous and paracrystalline inclusions. Substantially different, however, are the true crystalline inclusions, which have a clearly defined, often quite characteristic periodic structure stemming from a highly ordered arrangement of subunits be they filaments, microtubules, plates, or globules. (For further details on nomenclature and morphology of crystals *see* page 298.)

Analysis of filamentous and crystalline inclusions in various sites have led to the conclusion that they contain largely or entirely protein★, but only in rare instances has the protein been characterized. Virtually all the inclusions we are considering here are true intranuclear inclusions which are assembled in the nucleus, but whether the protein is actually produced in the nucleus or elsewhere is debatable†. However, rare examples of double-membrane-bound pseudoinclusions containing filaments also do occur (e.g. Merkow *et al.* 1971) (*Plate 54*).

Filamentous and crystalline inclusions of the type we are dealing with now have been seen in virus infected cells. These crystals must not be confused with viral crystals produced by arrays of virus particles (e.g. adenovirus *Plate 66, Fig. 1*). These do not concern us here. We are dealing in this section with a heterogeneous collection of inclusions which have been the subject of numerous reports. It is therefore essential to classify these into manageable and meaningful groups.

A large number of reports deal with the occurrence of these inclusions in various cells in the nervous system (mainly in the neurons). Light microscopists have been aware of these inclusions for over 90 years; they referred to them as 'rodlets' or 'battonets' (Mann, 1894; Roncoroni, 1895; Lenhossék, 1897; Prenant, 1897; Holmgren, 1899). Cajal (1909, 1911) demonstrated these structures in the neurons of various mammals with his elegant silver

★However, not all proteinaceous inclusions are filamentous or crystalline. For example globular intranuclear inclusions containing glycoproteins (major components with molecular weights which ranged from 10 000 to 100 000) have been found in the midgut cells of an insect (*Carausius morosus*) (Thomas and Gouranton, 1978, 1980; Thompson *et al.*, 1979) and morphologically similar intranuclear inclusions containing cystine-rich protein have been observed in the rostellar gland cells of the tapeworm (*Echinococcus granulosus*) (Thompson *et al.*, 1979).

†All reliable evidence now seems to indicate that no protein synthesis occurs in the nucleus, but polymerization of protein subunits to form filaments and microtubules can occur at this site. The thickness of several intranuclear filaments suggest that these are actin filaments, while the diameter of the intranuclear microtubules is in keeping with the idea that these are tubulin microtubules. Hence one may surmise that G-actin (globular actin) polymerizes to form F-actin (actin filaments) while tubulin polymerizes to form microtubules. One may further presume that G-actin and tubulin produced by polyribosomes in the cytoplasm reach the nucleus via the nuclear pores.

Plate 54

Fig. 1. Smooth muscle cell from human vas deferens. Myofilaments with focal densities (arrowheads) similar to those seen in the cell cytoplasm (arrowheads) are seen lying within pseudoinclusions in the nucleus. × 18 000

Fig. 2. Nucleus of cell from the lymph node of a case of follicular lymphoma showing a filamentous intranuclear inclusion (F). It is difficult to be certain whether this is a true inclusion or a pseudoinclusion. Although a double membrane is not seen around the inclusion, it is bounded by heterochromatin suggesting that the failure to visualize the membranes may be due to an unfavourable plane of sectioning. On the other hand the idea that this is a pseudoinclusion is difficult to reconcile with the fact that there were virtually no filaments in the cell cytoplasm. × 56 000

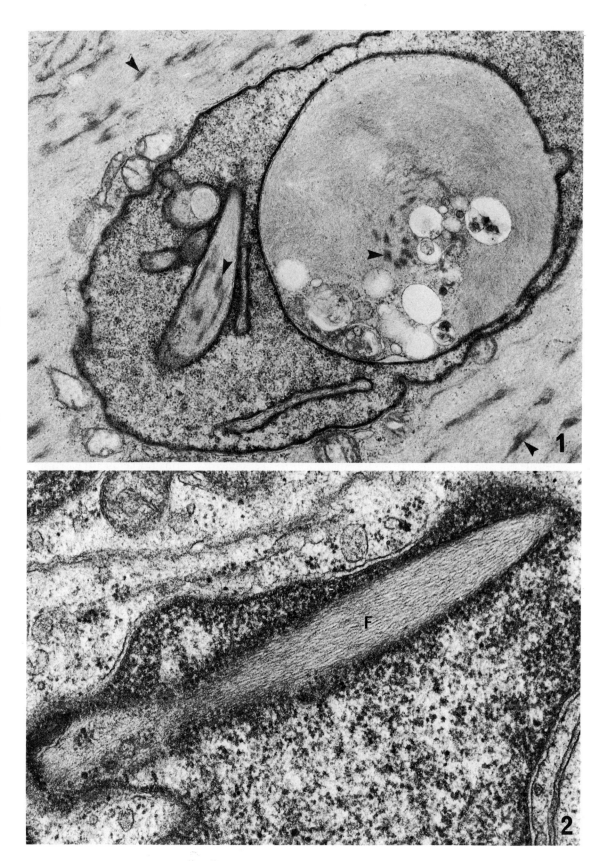

staining techniques and called them the 'rodlets of Roncoroni'★ although Mann (1894) appears to have been the first to observe these inclusions. Electron microscopic studies have demonstrated that the rodlets are composed of filaments. The filaments of the rodlet may form a slender fibril (more or less parallel filaments) or the rodlet may show a paracrystalline or crystalline structure.

Such rodlets, broader filamentous bands (i.e. wider fibrils) and rarely also crystalloids or crystals (wider than the crystalline rodlets). (All these are collectively referred to in the text that follows as filamentous and crystalline inclusions) (*Plate 55*) have been found in the normal neurons (of animals including man) of: (1) nervous tissue of planarian (*Dendrocoelum lacteum, Dugesia gonocephala* and *Polycelis tenuis*) (Le Moigne and Monnot-Sauzin, 1971); (2) central nervous system of molluscs (*Vaginulus borellianus* (Colosi) and *Milax gagates* (Draparnaud) (Quattrini, 1966); (3) ganglia of leech (*Hirudo medicinalis*) (Gray and Guillery, 1963); (4) cerebral cortex of hagfish (*Myxine glutinosa* (L)) (Mugnaini, 1967); (5) spinal and cranial ganglia of fish (Cyprinid species) (large cuboidal crystals 2–4 μm) (Hoover *et al.*, 1981); (6) cerebral cortex and sympathetic ganglia of chicken (Dahl, 1970; Masurovsky *et al.*, 1970); (7) cerebral cortex of mouse (Gambetti and Gonatas, 1967; Andrews and Sekhon, 1969); (8) parietal cortex of ageing mice (more frequent in older animals) (Field and Peat, 1971); (9) cerebral cortex, lateral geniculate nucleus, ciliary body, retina (bipolar ganglion cells), lateral vestibular nucleus, cochlear nucleus, hypothalamus and medulla oblongata of rat (Karlsson, 1966; Gambetti and Gonatas, 1967; Magalhães, 1967; Sotelo and Palay, 1968; Meier, 1969; Feldman and Peters, 1972; Johnson and Miquel, 1974; Lafarga and Palacios, 1977, 1979; Sëite *et al.*, 1977a; David and Nathaniel, 1978); (10) cerebral cortex, cerebellar cortex, olfactory bulb, ciliary body, retina (bipolar and ganglion cells) cervical ganglia and hypothalamus of rabbit (Siegesmund *et al.*, 1964; Magalhães, 1967; Dixon, 1970; Clattenburg *et al.*, 1972); (11) olfactory nucleus, olfactory bulb, prepyriform cortex, stellate ganglion, superior cervical ganglion, coeliac ganglion, nucleus lateralis of the periaqueductal grey matter, and face (motor neurons) of cat (Willey and Schultz, 1971; Sëite, 1970; Sëite *et al.*, 1971, 1973, 1975, 1977b, 1979; Vuillet-Luciani *et al.*, 1979; Liu and Hamilton, 1978; Kayahara, 1979); (12) olfactory bulb and cerebellar cortex of squirrel monkey (*Saimiri sciureus*) (Siegesmund *et al.*, 1964); and (13) cerebral cortex of man (Cragg, 1976).

These filamentous and crystalline inclusions have also been seen in neurons (of animals, including humans) in various pathological states and experimental situations. This includes neurons in: (1) mouse cerebral cortex injected with puromycin (Gambetti and Gonatas, 1967); (2) cerebral cortex of Wobbler (wr) mutant mouse (Andrews and Sekhon, 1969); (3) brain of mice with experimental amoebic (*Naegleria fowleri*) meningo-encephalitis (Schuster and Dunneback, 1977); (4) cerebral cortex of hamster implanted with the carcinogen 1,2,5,6-dibenzanthracine (Popoff and Stewart, 1968); (5) degenerating olfactory bulb and chromatolytic cervical ganglia of rabbit (Dixon, 1970; Pinching and Powell, 1971); (6) parietal cortex of

---

★Roncoroni also described Y-shaped or branching rodlets. Ultrastructural studies have failed to confirm this. It seems that Roncoroni must have mistaken invaginations of the nuclear envelope for rodlets.

Plate 55

Intranuclear inclusions from sympathetic neurons of the cat.

Fig. 1. A spindle-shaped filamentous intranuclear inclusion (arrow) and nucleolus (N). × 20 000 (*From Sëite, Mei and Vuillet-Luciani, 1973*)

Fig. 2. An inclusion composed of a central core of parallel filaments bounded by transversely cut microtubules. Another microtubular inclusion (arrow) is also present. × 150 000 (*From Sëite, Leonetti, Luciani-Vuillet and Vio, 1977a*)

Fig. 3. Layers of longitudinally cut and transversely cut filaments are seen in the core of this crystalline inclusion. Microtubules (arrows) are seen on either side of the inclusion. Nucleolus (N). × 80 000 (*From Sëite, Escaig, Luciani-Vuillet and Zerbib, 1975*)

Fig. 4. A crystalline inclusion. Microtubules (arrows) are seen at the periphery of the inclusion. × 40 000 (*From Sëite, Escaig and Couineau, 1971*)

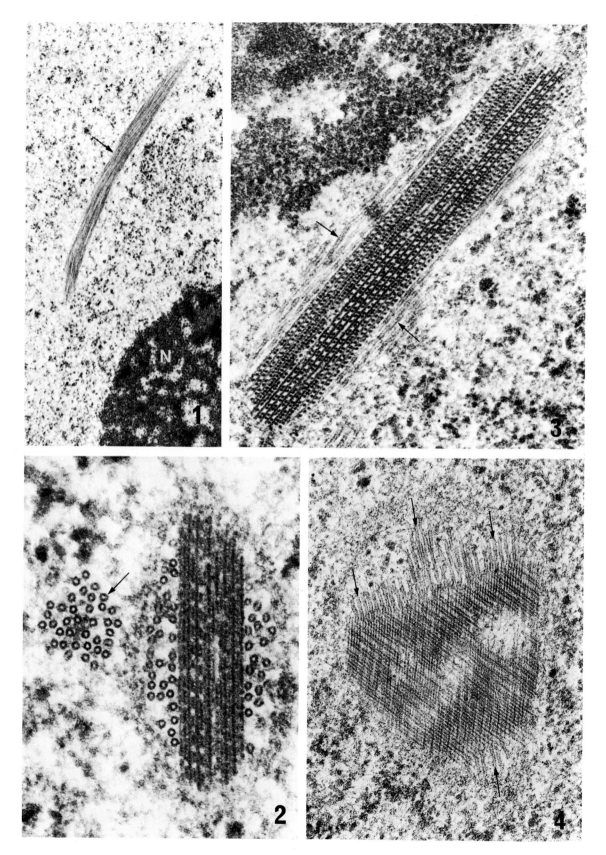

111

chronic ethanol intoxicated rats (Volk and Maletz, 1985); (7) sympathetic ganglia of the cat after electrical stimulation (Sëite *et al.*, 1973); (8) sympathetic ganglia of the cat after treatment with cyclic AMP (Sëite *et al.*, 1977c); (9) parietal cortex of four patients with Alzheimer's disease and in a case of post-traumatic hydrocephalus (Toper *et al.*, 1980); (10) human stellate ganglion in an unusual degenerative disorder (Sung, 1980); (11) human temporal gyri in Reye's syndrome (Partin *et al.*, 1975); (12) human frontal cortex in degenerative encephalopathies (Gambetti and Gonatas, 1967); (13) human frontal cortex in epilepsy (Brown *et al.*, 1968); and (14) human frontal cortex in multiple sclerosis (Raine and Field, 1968).

These filamentous and crystalline intranuclear inclusions have also been found in other cells (i.e. besides neurons) in normal and pathological neural tissues such as: (1) glial cells of normal hagfish (*Myxine glutinosa*(L)) (Mugnaini, 1967); (2) glial cells of normal rabbit (Weindl *et al.*, 1967); (3) oligodendrocytes of human frontal cortex in myoclonus epilepsy (Brown *et al.*, 1968); (4) foamy macrophages infiltrating human brain in multiple sclerosis (Raine *et al.*, 1974); (5) ependymal cells of normal lateral ventricle and third ventricle of rat (Hirano and Zimmerman, 1967; Warchol, 1978); (6) endothelial cells of normal cerebral cortex of mouse and rat (Gambetti and Gonatas, 1967).

The rodlets in the neurons can measure up to about 10 μm in length and vary in width from about 0.1–0.5 μm. In sympathetic neurons of the cat some of the inclusions are composed entirely of filaments but others contain microtubules as well (Sëite *et al.*, 1977c) (*Plate 55*). However, the inclusions in the sympathetic neurons of the chick are devoid of microtubules.

The significance of the intranuclear rodlet is not known, and its distribution in the nervous system gives no clue to its function. However, there seems to be some correlation between their number and the physiological activity of the neuron. An increase in the number of rodlets occurs after electrical stimulation (Sëite *et al.*, 1973) or treatment with cyclic AMP (Sëite *et al.*, 1977c), and (in the rabbit) they are said to disappear after coitus (Clattenburg *et al.*, 1972). Since the increase in rodlets and crystals (after electrical stimulation) is not inhibited by cyclohexamide (a potent inhibitor of protein synthesis) one may conclude (Sëite *et al.*, 1973) that the filaments and microtubules are not produced by *de novo* synthesis of proteins but by polymerization of existing protein subunits. Thus the formation and disappearances of rodlets and crystals appears to be a dynamic phenomenon related to physiological activity.

Neuroendocrine cells share several biological properties with neurons, therefore they are sometimes called 'paraneurons'. It is interesting to note that filamentous and crystalline inclusions have also been found in the nuclei of these cells. Such examples include neuroendocrine cells in: (1) parathyroid gland of frog (*Rana temporaria*) (Lange and Brehm, 1963); (2) pituitary gland of rabbit (Salazar, 1963; Buttner and Horstmann, 1968); (3) stomach of rabbit (Tusques and Pradal, 1968; Muller and Ratzenhofer, 1971); (4) endocrine pancreas (β-cells) (Boquist, 1969); (5) pulmonary neuroepithelial body of rabbit (El-Bermani *et al.*, 1981); (6) epidermis (Merkel cell) of rabbit and human oral mucosa (Merkel cell) (Straile *et al.*, 1975; Fortman and Winkelmann, 1977); and (7) alimentary tract (gastroenteropancreatic cells) of birds (quail, pigeon, gull, kite) (Iwanaga *et al.*, 1981).

Perhaps the most important group of intranuclear filamentous and crystalline inclusions are those found in virus infected cells and viral diseases. Such inclusions (which in some instances were histochemically characterized as protein) have been seen in the nuclei of: (1) HeLa cells infected with adenovirus (Morgan *et al.*, 1957); (2) cultured dog kidney cells and hepatocytes of

---

Plate 56

Fig. 1. Intranuclear paracrystalline filamentous inclusion found in the cerebral neuron of a case of subacute sclerosing panencephalitis. × 78 000 (*Grodums, unpublished electron micrograph*)

Fig. 2. A crystalline inclusion found in the neuron of a Coxsackie virus infected brain of a squirrel (*Citellus lateralis*). × 97 000 (*Grodums, unpublished electron micrograph*)

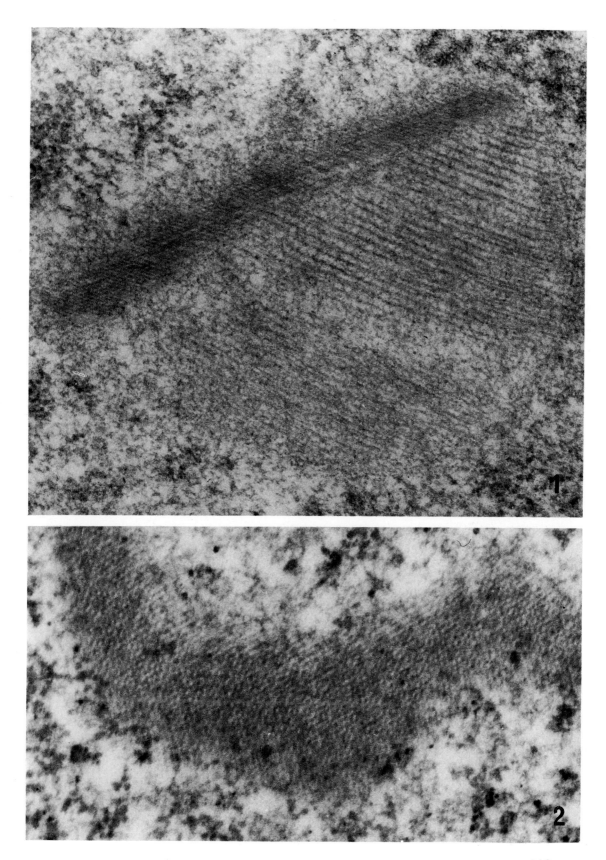

dogs infected with canine hepatitis virus (Givan and Jézéquel, 1969); (3) cultured human embryonic lung cells infected with Coxsackie virus (Jézéquel and Steiner, 1966); (4) cultured BHK 21 cells infected with Colorado tick fever virus (Murphy *et al.*, 1968); (5) cultured monkey kidney cells infected with herpesvirus (*Plate 65, Fig. 2*); (6) hepatocytes of mice infected with FV$_3$ (frog virus 3) (Bingen and Kirn, 1973); (7) lung tissue from a case of influenzal pneumonia (Tamura and Aronson, 1978); (8) neurons and glial cells from cases of sclerosing panencephalitis (Martinez *et al.*, 1974; Ishihara *et al.*, 1978) (*Plate 56*); and (9) virus-infected brain of a squirrel (*Citellus lateralis*) (*Plate 56, Fig. 2*).

Crystals have also been reported to occur in the hepatocyte nuclei of foxes, jackals and apparently normal dogs and it has been suggested that they too may indicate latent viral infection (Jézéquel and Steiner, 1966; Givan and Jézéquel, 1969). Structures designated as 'unusual intranuclear filaments', 'paramyxovirus-like intranuclear filaments' and 'filamentous tubular structures' have been reported in a variety of neurological and muscular disorders. These resemble the viral microtubules of measles (*Plate 68*) and other paramyxoviridae. Their nature and significance is discussed in page 136.

It would appear that filaments and crystals are seen in quite a variety of virus infections in various cell types, both *in vitro* and *in vivo*. It seems likely that these structures comprise host protein, not viral proteins and it has been suggested (Jézéquel and Steiner, 1966) that excessive protein production probably occurs in the nucleus (*see* second footnote on page 108) and when a critical concentration is reached filaments or crystal formation ensues.

Because of the frequent association of filaments and crystalline inclusions with viral infection, some workers regard them as 'viral footprints' or the 'hall-mark' of a viral infection. Such an attitude is not strictly speaking justifiable for as we have noted such inclusions are also found in normal cells and in pathological states where there is no evidence of a viral aetiology.

Besides the several aforementioned instances, filamentous and crystalline inclusions have been seen in some miscellaneous sites and in quite a number of tumours. This includes: (1) actinomycin D-treated oocytes (Lane, 1969); (2) thyroid follicular cells in normal woodchuck (Frink *et al.*, 1978); (3) various myopathies (for references *see* Oteruelo, 1976); (4) pleural mesothelial cells in an infant with a cardiac anomaly (Wang, 1974); (5) giant cells in Paget's disease of bone★ (Rebel *et al.*, 1974, 1976; LeCharpentier *et al.*, 1977; Schulz *et al.*, 1977); (6) human endometrial cells after administration of medroxyprogesterone acetate (*Plate 57*) (Roberts *et al.*, 1975); (7) human endometrial cells in: (a) first and second trimester spontaneous abortions; (b) term pregnancies; (c) uterus containing choriocarcinoma; (d) foci of endometriosis; and (e) caesarean scars (Mazur *et al.*, 1983; Sobel *et al.*, 1984); (8) fibroblast-like cells in a biopsy of superficial peroneal nerve (Vallat *et al.*, 1983); (9) eosinophilic myelocytes from a 2-year-old child with chronic benign neutropenia (rhomboidal crystals up to 3 µm long)

★Often described as inclusions composed of 15 nm thick filaments but many of them are clearly microtubules. Whether they are viral microtubules or not is the subject of continuing debate. Howatson and Fornasier (1982) find that in all specimens of pagetic bone, the nuclei of osteoclasts contain striated microtubules resembling the nucleocapsids of viruses of the Paramyxoviridae family. According to these authors viral antigens have been demonstrated in pagetic osteoclasts, but the exact identity of the virus is uncertain. The most likely candidates are measles virus and respiratory syncytial virus. Howatson and Fornasier (1982) have found that the external diameter of the microtubules in Paget's disease is 12.4 ± 0.4, measles virus 14.1 ± 0.3 and respiratory syncytial virus 12.4 ± 0.6.

Plate 57

Intranuclear filamentous inclusions (F) found in human endometrial cells ten days after administration of medroxyprogesterone acetate × 10 000 (*From Roberts, Horbelt and Powell, 1975*)

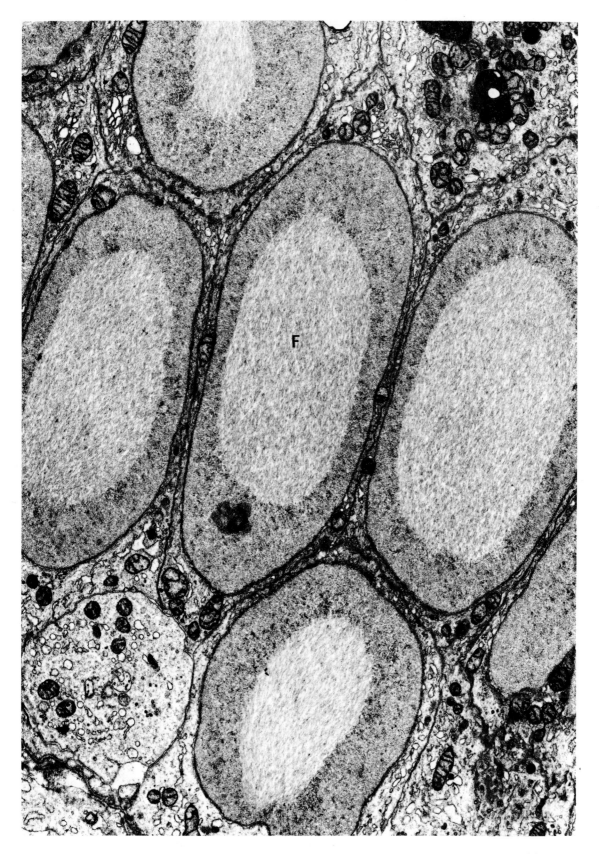

115

(Parmley *et al.*, 1981); (10) cells of a human insulinoma (Ohtsuki *et al.*, 1972); (11) pancreatic islet cell tumour (Bencosme *et al.*, 1963); (12) epithelial cells of a pulmonary hamartoma (Incze and Lui, 1977); (13) infantile haemangiopericytoma (Eimoto, 1977); (14) normal and leukaemic monocytes and lymphocytes (including a Sézary cell in the skin lesion) and the plasma cells in multiple myeloma (Stefani and Tonaki, 1970; Bessis, 1973; Smetana *et al.*, 1973, 1977; Oikawa, 1975) (*Plate 58, Fig. 1*); (15) splenic histiocytes from a case of malignant histiocytosis (*Plate 58, Fig. 2*); (16) proliferative histiocytic lesion (histiocytosis X ?) (Hou-Jensen *et al.*, 1973); (17) gliomas (Robertson and Maclean, 1965; Tani *et al.*, 1971; Erlandson, 1981); (18) synovial sarcoma (*Plate 58, Fig. 3*); (19) carcinoma of rectum (*Plate 58, Fig. 4*); (20) intrathyroid adenoma associated with hyperparathyroidism (Sherwin *et al.*, 1977); (21) undifferentiated soft tissue sarcoma (Gonzalez-Crussi *et al.*, 1978); (22) adenocarcinoma and squamous cell carcinoma of lung (Henderson and Papadimitriou, 1982); (23) malignant extracranial neuroepithelioma (Payne and Nagle, 1983); and (24) experimentally produced ependymoma in the mouse (Rubin, 1966 quoted by Hirano and Zimmermann, 1967).

It will be noted from the list presented above that intranuclear filamentous, paracrystalline and crystalline inclusions have been seen in tumours. It would appear that these inclusions constitute a rather rare type of inclusion but one which may be found in quite a variety of tumours. Hence these inclusions are of little or no diagnostic value. Erlandson (1981) expresses a similar opinion about intranuclear filamentous inclusions. However, Payne and Nagle (1983) found intranuclear rodlets in 5 per cent of the cells of a malignant extracranial neuroepithelioma and suggest that 'A quantitative evaluation of rodlets in conjunction with other diagnostic ultrastructural features may prove to be a useful marker in the diagnosis of poorly differentiated neoplasms'.

One of the best known and most extensively studied crystals is the crystal of Reinke (*see Plate 415*) found in the cytoplasm of the interstitial cells (Leydig cells) of the human testis after puberty. It is thought to be composed of hexagonal microtubules. Occasionally, this crystal is also seen as a true inclusion in the nucleus of the interstitial cell. It has been suggested (Yasuzumi *et al.*, 1967; DeKretser, 1967, 1968) that the intranuclear crystal is produced in the nucleus, because microtubular inclusions similar to those from which the cytoplasmic crystal develops are also seen in the nucleus. This does not provide proof of protein synthesis in the nucleus but it does support the idea that polymerization occurs at this site.

Plate 58

Fig. 1. Circulating monocyte from the blood of an apparently healthy technician who donated blood for an unrelated experiment. Two nuclear profiles (suggesting a section through a horseshoe-shaped nucleus) were present in the cell, one of which contained rigid-looking fibrils composed of fine filaments. × 18 000

Fig. 2. Splenic histiocyte from a case of malignant histiocytosis (histiocytic medullary reticulosis). The nucleus contains a fibril composed of filaments which are not clearly resolved. × 13 000

Fig. 3. Synovial sarcoma. The nucleus contains a rounded inclusion composed of parallel filaments. One could refer to this as a 'paracrystalline inclusion'. × 87 000

Fig. 4. Carcinoma of the rectum. This intranuclear crystalline inclusion is composed of alternating layers of filaments deployed at right angles to each other (between arrowheads). The other appearances seen are explicable on the basis of sectioning geometry. A portion of the inclusion (arrow) has a cross-striated appearance. The periodicity of the striations is 17 nm. The highly ordered pattern seen here justifies the use of the term 'crystalline inclusion'. × 63 000

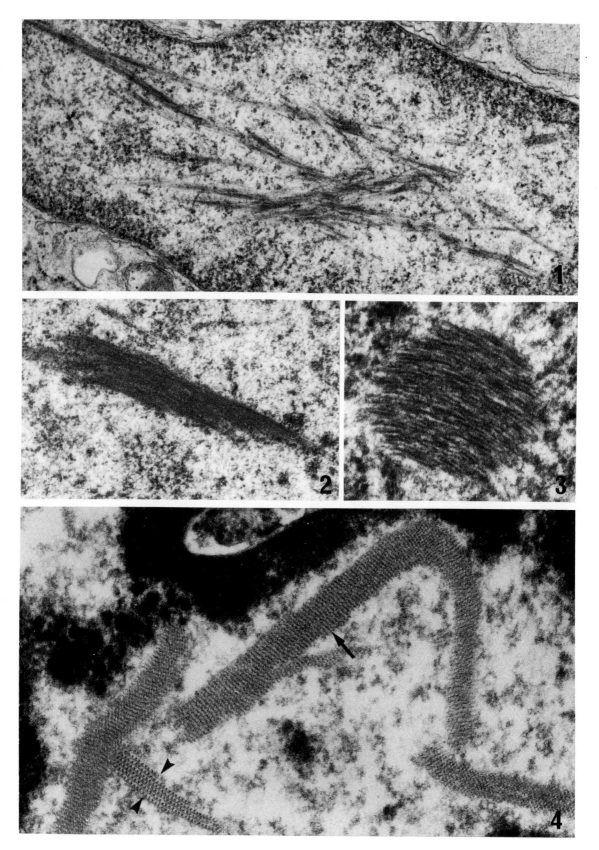

117

Rarer than the Reinke crystal and not too well known is the crystalloid of Lubarsch found in the cytoplasm of spermatogonia of the human testis, and this crystalloid composed of filaments has also been seen in the nucleus (Sohval et al., 1971). In the stallion crystalline inclusions composed of stacked flat plates have been found in the nucleus of the cauda epididymis but not in the cytoplasm. However, filamentous crystals are found both in the nucleus and cytoplasm of the dog cauda epididymis (Gouranton et al., 1979). Intranuclear crystals have also been found in the phagocytic cells of ovarian tissues in echinoderms. However, in Arbacia punctulata the crystal is said to be composed of spherical units 10 nm in diameter, and cytochemical studies show that it is rich in iron (Karasaki, 1963).

Intranuclear filaments and crystals have been seen in a variety of plant cells (Arsanto, 1973; Weintraub et al., 1971; Oliveira, 1976; Thomas and Gouranton, 1979). Of particular interest is the study by Fukui (1978) who showed that intranuclear bundles of filaments develop in the cells of the slime mould, Dictyostelium, after exposure to dimethyl sulphoxide and that these filaments are actin filaments. Ultrastructural and immunofluorescence studies have shown that contractile proteins exist in the nucleus as a major component of non-histone proteins. For example, in the nuclei of rat liver various proteins such as myosin, actin, tubulin and tropomyosin have been identified (Douvas et al., 1975).

On the basis of such observations one may speculate that as a result of altered physiological activity (e.g. in neurons) viral infection (in various cell types) or the action of some chemical agents (e.g. actinomycin D in oocytes and dimethyl sulphoxide in slime mould) certain nuclear proteins in the native state may be transformed into arrays of filaments or crystals; an excessive production of such protein may also contribute to this phenomenon.

Two theories exist regarding the source of proteins found in intranuclear crystals: (1) that they are synthesized in the nucleolus or nucleus; and (2) that they are synthesized by the polyribosomes in the cytoplasm and that the protein then migrates to the nucleus.

In the midgut cells of the whirligig (Gyrinus marinus Gyll) (Plate 59) numerous quite large polygonal crystals occur. Kinetic studies (Gouranton and Thomas, 1974) of labelling after injection of tritiated lysine showed radioactivity first in the cytoplasm and then in the crystals. This transfer of radioactivity strongly suggests a synthesis of crystal protein in the cytoplasm and its subsequent migration to the nucleus where it presumably crystallizes. Whether similar or different mechanisms operate in the formation of other crystals in other sites remains to be determined.

Plate 59

Intranuclear crystals found in the differentiated midgut cells of the whirligig (*Gyrinus marinus* Gyll) (*From Gouranton and Thomas, 1974*)

Fig. 1. A low-power view showing crystals (C) in the nucleus. × 14 500

Fig. 2. High-power view showing crystal lattice. × 140 000

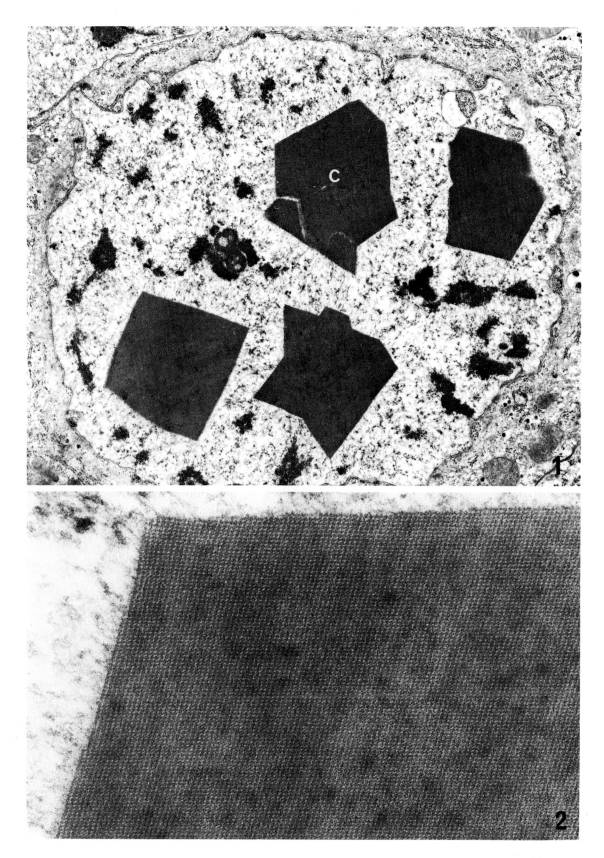

Intranuclear haemoglobin inclusions

Haemoglobin is usually thought to be localized in the cytoplasm of erythroid cells. Its occurrence in the nucleus has in the past been doubted or denied (e.g. Maximow and Bloom, 1948). Perhaps the first convincing evidence of the presence of intranuclear haemoglobin stems from the analysis of isolated avian erythrocyte nuclei by Stern *et al.* (1951).

Intranuclear deposits of haemoglobin present as areas of moderate electron density with an appearance similar to the haemoglobin-containing cytoplasm of the erythroid cells. In suitable specimens an uninterrupted continuity of intracytoplasmic and intranuclear haemoglobin is seen via the nuclear pores (*Plate 60*). Usually the deposits are lighter than the condensed chromatin masses, but if the chromatin is not well condensed or stained and the cell is well haemoglobinized the densities are reversed (*see*, for example, *Figs. 16* and *17* in Fawcett and Witebsky, 1964).

Intranuclear haemoglobin has been reported to occur in: (1) the erythrocytes of lower vertebrates such as fish, amphibians, reptiles and birds (Stern *et al.*, 1951; O'Brien, 1960; Davies, 1961; Tooze and Davies, 1963; Fawcett and Witebsky, 1964); and (2) erythroblasts (normoblasts) of mammals such as rabbit, dog and man (Jones, 1959; Davies, 1961; Grasso *et al.*, 1962; Simpson and Kling, 1967) in hepatic and adult medullary phases of erythropoiesis (Firkin, 1969).

However, evidence for the presence of intranuclear haemoglobin in human material and also other mammals is somewhat scanty, and rests solely on the occasional demonstration of areas within the nucleus of a density and texture similar to that of the haemoglobinized cytoplasm.

It is generally thought that haemoglobin probably migrates from the cytoplasm into the nucleus via the nuclear pores in the later stages of erythropoiesis as the nucleus becomes pyknotic. The converse possibility, however, is not denied. At least in the case of the chick embryo, histochemical studies suggest that during erythropoiesis haemoglobin first appears in the nucleus (O'Brien, 1960), and immunological and electrophoretic studies (Wilt, 1967) on haemoglobin from isolated nuclei have shown that it consists of only one of the three haemoglobins of the embryonic chicken. Whether intranuclear haemoglobin synthesis occurs in man and other mammals, and whether such synthesis contributes a particular type of haemoglobin, remains to be determined.

Plate 60

Erythrocyte from peripheral blood of a canary, showing intranuclear haemoglobin (*). The similarity of texture and density between the haemoglobinized cytoplasm and the included material is evident, as is continuity between the two (arrow). × 37 000

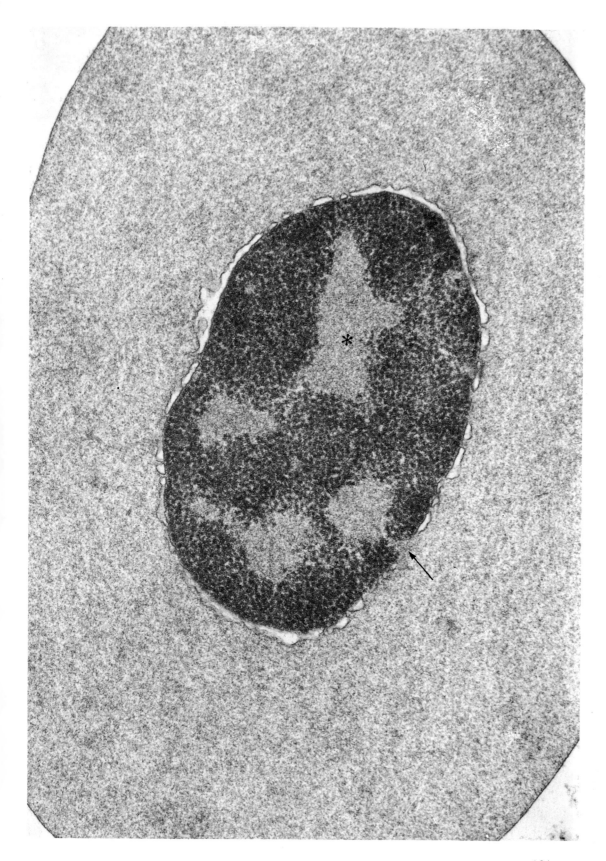

121

Intranuclear lead inclusions

The toxicity of lead has been recognized since the time of Hippocrates, but the characteristic intranuclear inclusions that occur were first described in 1936 by Blackman. In the rat such inclusions occur in the proximal tubular epithelial cells of the kidney (*Plates 61* and *62*), but in other animals such as the pig, rabbit and man, both kidney and liver contain such inclusions. The extensive early literature on lead poisoning has been reviewed by Calvery (1938). Many papers dealing with the morphology and chemistry of intranuclear lead inclusions have been published (Blackman, 1936; Finner and Calvery, 1939; Wachstein, 1949; Bracken *et al.*, 1958; Landing and Nakai, 1959; Beaver, 1961; Gueft and Molnar, 1961; Angevine *et al.*, 1962; Watrach and Vatter, 1962; Dallenbach, 1964, 1965; Goyer, 1968; Richter *et al.*, 1968; Goyer *et al.*, 1970). Intranuclear inclusions presumably containing lead have also been produced in cultured kidney cells exposed to lead salts (Walton, 1974), but the morphology of these *in vitro* inclusions is different from that seen *in vivo*.

Only two metals★ are known to produce large electron-dense intranuclear inclusions – lead and bismuth. They can be distinguished on the basis of their morphology. The bismuth inclusion is round and has a sharp margin (*see Plates 63* and *64*) while the typical lead inclusion presents as a body with a dense central core enveloped in a cortex of matted and radiating filaments. The early lesion starts in a zone between the nucleolus and the nuclear envelope and is clearly not derived from these structures. As the lesion increases in size it displaces the nucleolus and assumes a central position, and at light microscopy it could be mistaken for a viral inclusion. Numerous conflicting reports on the histochemistry of these lesions have been published, but it seems reasonably certain now that these inclusions are acid-fast to carbol fuschin (indicating the presence of proteins rich in sulphydryl groups), contain little or no lipid or carbohydrate, and probably no DNA or RNA either. About the latter (DNA, RNA), however, there is much uncertainty in the literature. The presence of protein has been confirmed by enzyme digestion studies on epon-embedded material (Richter *et al.*, 1968) and on inclusions isolated from tissue homogenates (Goyer *et al.*, 1970). The fibrillary cortex soon disappears after such treatment. On the other hand, chelating agents completely remove lead from these inclusions leaving behind an amorphous residue (Moore *et al.*, 1973).

★Neither mercury nor selenium produces intranuclear inclusions, but combined administration of salts of these metals produces clusters of small spherical electron-dense inclusions in the nuclei of renal tubular epithelial cells (Groth *et al.*, 1976). Hg and Se have been demonstrated in these inclusions by electron-probe x-ray analysis (Carmichael and Fowler, 1980). Small amounts of selenium protect against mercury toxicity and this is associated with the formation of electron-dense inclusions.

Plate 61

Figs. 1 and 2. Renal tubular epithelial cells from a rat that had received 0.5 per cent lead acetate in drinking water for two months. The large electron-dense lead inclusions (L) in the nucleus are not connected with the nucleolus (N). × 6500 and × 14 000

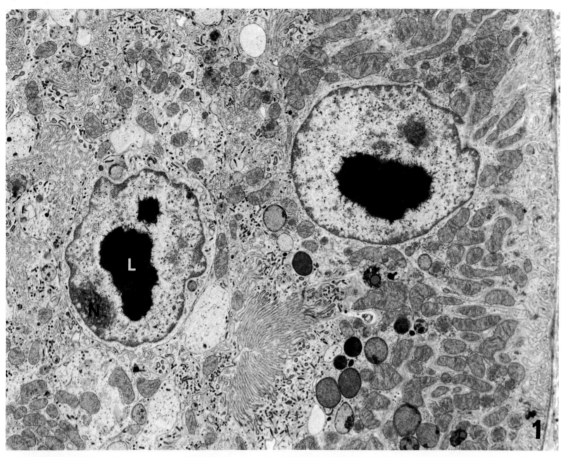

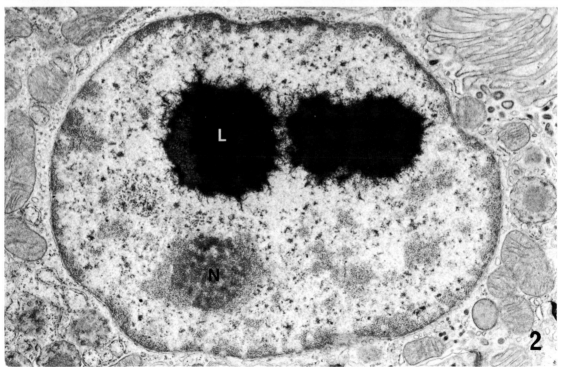

Although the presence of lead in these inclusions has long been suspected, unequivocal demonstration of this had to await the work of Dallenbach (1965) who, by autoradiography, demonstrated the presence of lead in the inclusions of animals that had received radioactive lead. Goyer et al. (1970) isolated and analysed these inclusions and they report that the lead is bound to protein, in a relatively constant ratio. They found that about 80–90 per cent of the renal lead resides in the nucleus and that at least 50 per cent can be recovered with the inclusions. They postulate that 'the inclusion body may therefore function as a store or a depot for intracellular lead'.

At one time it was thought that intranuclear lead inclusions were pathognomonic of chronic lead intoxication but it is now apparent that similar inclusions are produced as early as 24 hours after a single intraperitoneal injection of lead (Choie and Richter, 1972; Richter, 1976).

The accumulation of lead in vegetation as a result of environmental pollution has become a subject of concern in recent years. Ultrastructural and electron-probe x-ray analytical studies have now shown intranuclear lead inclusions in leaves of moss (*Rhytidiadelphus squarrosus* Hedw. Warnst.) collected from a park close to a busy road (Skaar *et al.*, 1973; Gullvåg *et al.*, 1974; Ophus and Gullvåg, 1974), and it appears that the lead is derived from the exhaust gases of motor traffic. Lead inclusions also develop in moss watered with lead acetate solution.

Plate 62

From the same specimen as *Plate 61*.

Figs 1–3. Intranuclear lead inclusions. The differences in appearances seen here probably relate to the plane of sectioning and the maturity of the inclusions. The one shown in *Fig. 1* is an equatorial section where one can clearly discern the dense core and fibrous cortex. × 40 000, × 33 000 and × 38 000

124

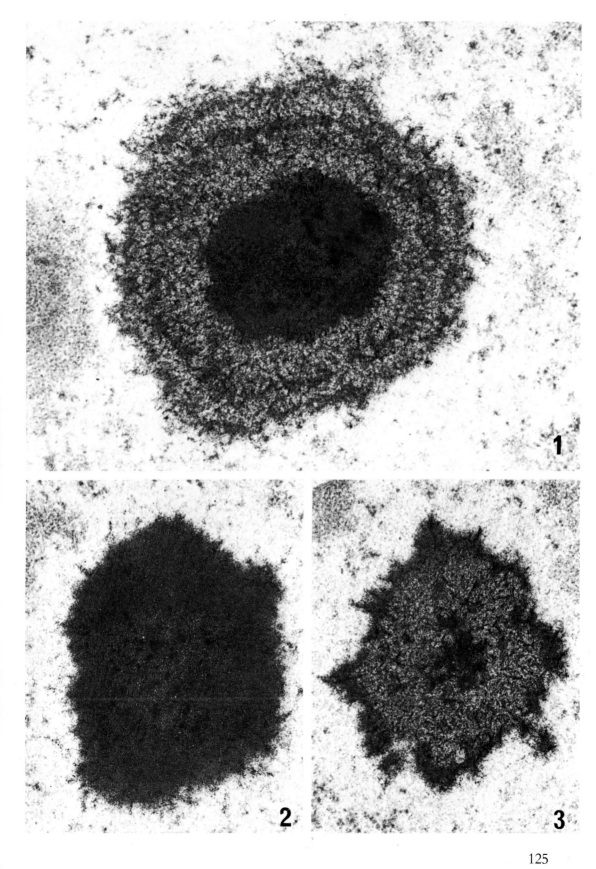

Intranuclear bismuth inclusions

In 1885 Langhans reported the occurrence of large spherical intranuclear inclusions and occasional similar intracytoplasmic inclusions in the renal tubular epithelial cells of rabbits that had been injected with bismuth subnitrate. Since this observation antedated the widespread use of bismuth for antisyphilitic therapy by several decades, it was soon forgotten and lost in the literature. As a result the origin of the mysterious 'Wismuthzellen' found in the urinary sediment of syphilitic patients after bismuth therapy (Kollert *et al.*, 1923; Grünblatt, 1925; Heimann-Trosien, 1925; Brytscheff, 1926) was not understood (Beaver and Burr, 1963a). Pappenheimer and Maechling (1934), unaware of Langhan's findings 'rediscovered' these renal inclusions in syphilitic patients treated with bismuth and were able to produce similar lesions in rats.

Histochemical studies failed to establish unequivocally the composition of these inclusions; even the presence or absence of bismuth in these inclusions was disputed (Pappenheimer and Maechling, 1934; Wachstein and Zak, 1946; Wachstein, 1949). Spectrographic analysis of the human kidney (Beaver and Burr, 1963b) and microchemical analysis of isolated bismuth-induced inclusions from the rabbit kidney also failed to reveal the presence of bismuth (Burr *et al.*, 1965) even though the limit of detectability of bismuth by this procedure was 0.1 parts per million.

However the problem has now been solved with the aid of electron probe x-ray analysis. With this technique Fowler and Goyer (1975) found bismuth★ in experimentally produced intranuclear inclusions in the rat kidney while we (Ghadially and Yong, 1976) demonstrated both bismuth and sulphur in the intranuclear inclusions produced in the rabbit kidney after injections of bismuth subnitrate.

It is interesting to note that these quite large (up to about 5 μm in our experience) spherical intranuclear inclusions (*Plates 63* and *64*) develop within a few days to a week in rat and rabbit kidney, but apparently in no other organ, after administration of bismuth salts. Similar inclusions are also occasionally seen lying free in the cytoplasmic matrix. At times the lysosomes of the tubular epithelial cells also contain markedly electron-dense material, but whether bismuth is present in these sites remains to be determined.

Ultrastructural studies (Beaver and Burr, 1963a; Ghadially and Yong, 1976) show that there is no connection between the inclusion and the nucleolus which remains distinct and well preserved (*Plates 63* and *64, Fig. 1*). The shape of virtually all inclusions is spherical but in rare instances oval or elongated inclusions are seen. Also rare is the occurrence of bipartite inclusions (*Plate 64, Fig. 2*) suggesting that a fusion of two inclusions is occurring or that an inclusion is dividing. Although in most instances only a single inclusion is found in the nucleus, on rare occasions two inclusions may be found within a single nucleus.

★Examination of the x-ray spectrum presented in *Fig. 4* of Fowler and Goyer (1975) shows that sulphur is also present, but because of peak overlap problems this was missed. For a detailed critique, *see* Ghadially and Yong, 1976.

Plate 63

Intranuclear bismuth inclusions (B) produced in the rabbit kidney by subcutaneous injections of bismuth subnitrate. The well developed brush border indicates that these are proximal tubule cells. × 10 500 (*From Ghadially and Yong, 1976*)

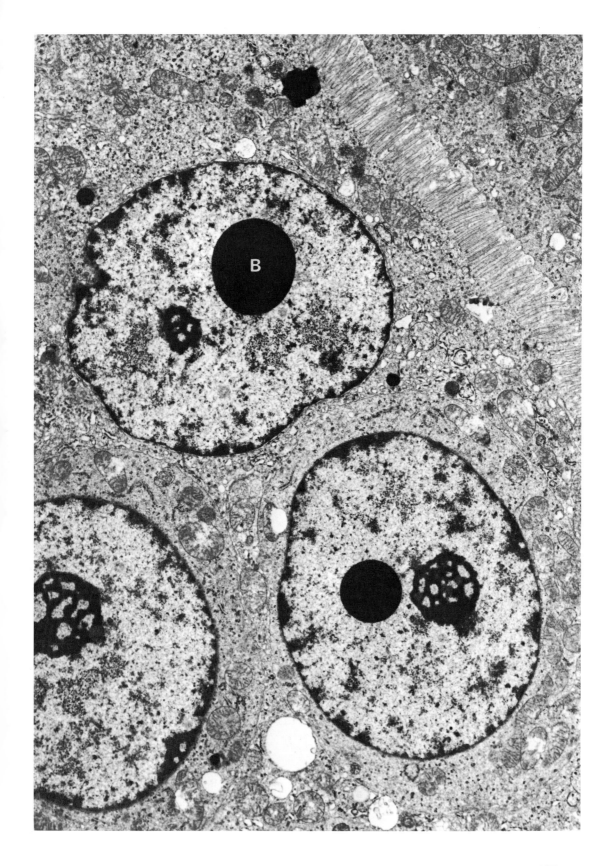

127

In glutaraldehyde fixed material the inclusions have a homogeneous highly electron-dense appearance and a remarkably sharp margin. This homogeneous appearance is also evident in quite a few of the inclusions found in osmium fixed material but in many instances (particularly when the sections are quite thin) a granular substructure is revealed. This ranges from a barely discernible granularity to instances where the granularity is quite obvious (*Plate 64, Fig. 3*). At high magnifications such inclusions show electron-dense granules (probably bismuth) and filamentous material (probably protein) set in a lucent matrix (*Plate 64, Fig. 4*).

An interesting phenomenon which we (Ghadially and Yong, 1976) have called the 'vanishing inclusion phenomenon' was witnessed when rather thick (150–300 nm) unstained sections from from unosmicated tissues (i.e. fixed in glutaraldehyde but not post-fixed in osmium) were examined in the electron microscope. With the condenser de-focused (to illuminate the entire viewing screen) the inclusions were readily detected because of their inherent electron density, presumably due to the presence of bismuth. However, when the illumination was increased by focusing the beam on the inclusion it vanished from view (i.e. it lost its electron density). This phenomenon is explicable on the basis of the presence of bismuth in these inclusions. It is common knowledge that specimens examined in the electron microscope heat up and that materials are lost by volatilization in the electron beam. For example, it has been shown (Dudley and Spiro, 1961; Ghadially and Mehta, 1970) that volatilization of lead (from stain) can occur from ultrathin sections and that this can shower down on the section and selectively reprecipitate as fine particles on collagen fibrils giving a false impression that these are sites of early mineralization.

Bismuth is a metal similar to lead, indeed in early times it was confused with tin and lead. It has a low melting point (271.3°C) and its thermal conductivity is lower than any other metal except mercury. It has a high electrical resistance and when placed in a magnetic field it shows an increase in electrical resistance greater than any other metal (Weast, 1975). Properties such as these are likely to lead to electrical charging and more than the usual increase in temperature of the specimen in areas where bismuth is present (e.g. in the inclusion) and this in turn could lead to volatilization of the bismuth from the inclusion.

The 'vanishing inclusion' phenomenon is not seen in lead- or uranium-stained sections or even in unstained sections from osmicated tissues. The fact that introducing such metals into the specimen stabilizes the inclusions and prevents the volatilization of bismuth is explicable on the basis of the improved electrical and thermal conductivity that would be produced by such manoeuvres.

Plate 64

Fig. 1. Intranuclear bismuth inclusion and a nucleolus. Note the absence of continuity between these structures. In this material fixed in glutaraldehyde (cacodylate buffer), post-fixed in osmium and stained with uranium and lead, the inclusion has a homogeneous electron-dense appearance. × 26 500 (*From Ghadially and Yong, 1976*)

Fig. 2. A bipartite inclusion, fixed and stained as in *Fig. 1*. Note the remarkably sharp margin. × 18 000 (*From Ghadially and Yong, 1976*)

Fig. 3. A markedly granular inclusion found in osmium-fixed material (cacodylate buffer) stained with uranium and lead. × 19 000 (*From Ghadially and Yong, 1976*)

Fig. 4. High-power view of inclusion shown in *Fig. 3*. Filamentous and granular material set in an electron-lucent matrix are evident × 160 000 (*From Ghadially and Yong, 1976*)

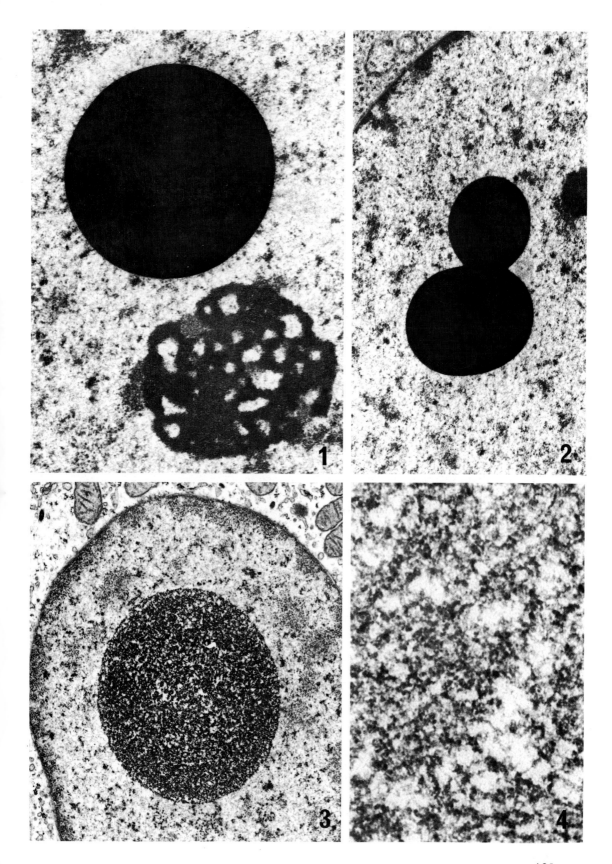

Intranuclear viral inclusions and virus–like particles

Viruses may be assembled in the nucleus and/or cytoplasm. Most DNA viruses such as adeno, papova and herpes are synthesized in the nucleus but some, such as pox viruses, are produced in the cytoplasm. Almost all RNA viruses are assembled in the cytoplasm, but some (e.g. myxoviruses) involve both nucleus and cytoplasm. It is beyond the scope of this work to illustrate and discuss the morphological changes produced in the nucleus by the large number of known viruses. Here we shall deal briefly with the intranuclear inclusions produced by three DNA viruses (herpes simplex virus, adenovirus and papilloma virus) and one RNA virus (measles virus). Later we shall deal with various structures which are mistaken for virus.

Various types of inclusions are seen in the nuclei of virus-infected cells. These include viral particles, precursors of such particles, malformed viral components and also structures derived by alterations of nuclear components. In herpesvirus and adenovirus infections such viral particles may be found scattered randomly in the nucleus or aligned close to the nuclear envelope. The particles may be solitary, in clusters, in linear arrays or in crystalline formations. Herpesvirus (*Plate 65*) rarely forms crystalline structures but large viral crystals are quite common with adenovirus (*Plate 66*). In human warts*, the viral particles (human papilloma virus†) may be randomly scattered or form crystalline arrays in nuclei from one and the same specimen (*Plate 67*).

Intranuclear herpesvirus particles usually present as a DNA-containing core and a protein envelope called the capsid. The two are separated by a less dense interval. The core measures 35–50 nm in diameter and is usually rounded, but it may be bar-shaped and appear 'solid' or 'hollow'. To a large extent the appearance depends upon the type of fixation. Thus the bar-shaped and solid cores are frequent after permanganate fixation, while hollow cores are said to be characteristic of osmium fixation. Some capsids appear empty. This is because cores are absent; it is not a sectioning artefact (Swanson *et al.*, 1966). The capsids often appear spherical. However, the pentagonal or hexagonal shape expected from sections through these viral particles which are known to have an icosahedral symmetry can at times be discerned in

---

*Human papilloma virus (HPV) is found in the nuclei of keratinocytes in the stratum granulosum, the basal cell layer is spared. In the more superficial layers of the skin the liberated virus is seen in the cell cytoplasm and lying free within the keratin.
†Several types and subtypes of HPV are now known to occur and there appears to be some correlation between the clinical types of warts and types of HPV. Thus HPV1 and HPV4 are associated with palmo-plantar warts, HPV6 with genital warts, and HPV7 with common or butchers' warts (for references and details *see* Bunney, 1982). The HPV types are identified by restriction enzyme analysis, molecular hybridization and immunofluorescence techniques but not by electron microscopy.

Plate 65

From monkey kidney cells in culture infected with herpes simplex virus. Fixed in glutaraldehyde, post-fixed in osmium and stained with uranium and lead.

Fig. 1. A group of nucleocapsids (about 103 nm in diameter) are seen lying in the nucleus adjacent to the marginated chromatin (M). Various morophological variations are depicted here. Thus we can see dense or 'solid' cores (S), 'hollow' cores (H) and capsids (C) without cores. × 58 000

Fig. 2. Beside a chromatin aggregate (C) lie numerous malformed capsids (M), occasional nucleocapsids and a filamentous paracrystalline inclusion (P). × 42 000

Fig. 3. Vermicellar bodies (V) are seen in the nucleus of this herpesvirus-infected cell. × 28 000

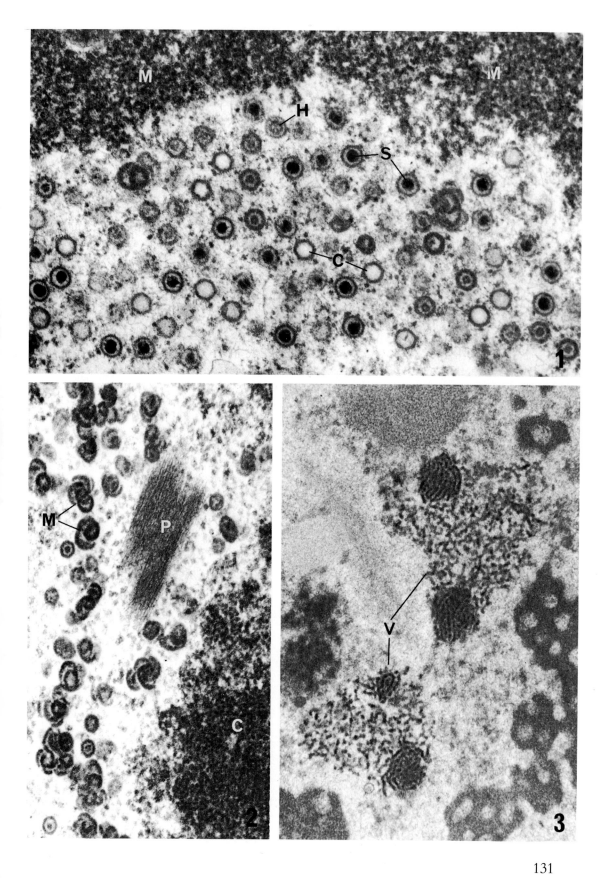

131

ultrathin sections. Herpesvirus particles are singularly resistant to a variety of treatments that cause gross disruption of cellular architecture. Thus such particles have been demonstrated in autopsy material, paraffin-embedded material and in tisues kept in formaldehyde for many years (Roy and Wolman, 1969).

In measles-infected cells the situation is quite different, for the virus presents as an aggregate of microtubules* composed of viral nucleoprotein (*Plate 68*). Such aggregates may be focal and rounded or quite large and almost entirely fill the nucleus, leaving little besides occasional clumps of marginated chromatin. Such aggregates of microtubules occur also in the cytoplasm and, while budding from the cell surface, become enveloped in cell membrane to form measles virions. The intranuclear microtubules, however, appear to be trapped in the nucleus. Few or none succeed in maturing into measles virions (Nakai *et al.*, 1969).

As mentioned earlier, the nucleus of the virus-infected cell contains other inclusions besides viral particles. Thus crystals or paracrystalline inclusions are at times seen in a variety of virus-infected cells. It seems likely that this is host protein, not viral protein (page 114). In herpes-infected cells collections of malformed capsids are at times encountered (*Plate 65, Fig. 2*), or a characteristic but rather rare inclusion called the vermicellar body (*Plate 65, Fig. 3*) may be found. This body is made up of intertwining thread-like or rod-like elements. The morphology of this plexiform inclusion is better appreciated in relatively thick sections, for in very thin sections it presents as dense granules, which may be confused with disintegrating and clumped nuclear and nucleolar material. The diameter of the vermicellar rods is of the same order as the diameter of viral cores and the staining reaction is also similar. Therefore, the vermicellar body might be looked upon as the site of core production, but one could argue that, since this structure is so rarely seen, this is not the way cores are normally produced, and that the vermicellar body probably represents deranged or frustrated core production.

In adenovirus-infected cells†, it has been shown (Yamamoto and Shahrabadi 1971; Hoenig *et al.*, 1974) that viral DNA is synthesized in ring-shaped inclusions which develop within a few hours after infection (*Plate 66, Fig. 2*). Such inclusions readily incorporate tritiated thymidine into DNA and later the labelled DNA is found incorporated in viral particles.

*These microtubules (about 14–15 nm in diameter) show faint striations, hence they are sometimes referred to as 'striated microtubules'. They are also at times referred to as 'viral microtubules' and 'nucleocapsids of measles virus'. *See also* footnote on page 114.
†The adenoviridae are non-enveloped and have an icosahedral symmetry.

Plate 66
From a culture of canine kidney cell line infected with canine adenovirus.
Fig. 1. Nucleus showing crystalline arrays of adenovirus. The viral particles measure about 67 nm in diameter. × 37 000 (*From Yamamoto, 1969*)
Fig. 2. Nucleus showing inclusions presenting ring-shaped profiles. × 24 000 (*Yamamoto, unpublished electron micrograph*)

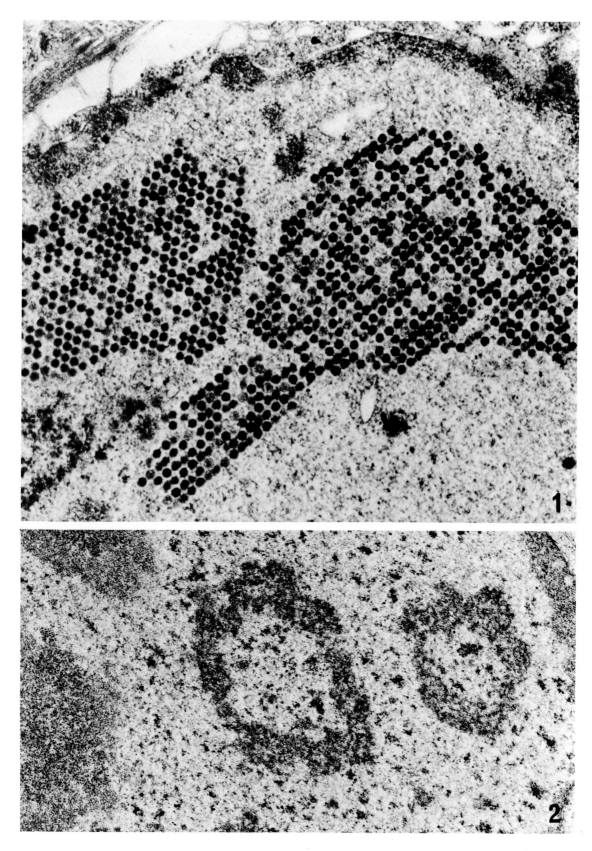

Many of the changes that occur in the nucleus of virus-infected cells, particularly herpesvirus-infected cells, have already been described (page 42). Such changes include thickening and reduplication of the nuclear envelope, margination of chromatin, increase in interchromatin and perichromatin granules, and segregation and scattering of nucleolar components. Other, mostly later, changes include rupture of nuclear membranes, chromatin dispersion and degeneration, disappearance of interchromatin and perichromatin granules, absence of a recognizable nucleolus, but presence of granular or fibrillar structures reminiscent of nucleolar material. Such alterations produce a variety of intranuclear bodies, the precise origin and nature of which it is at times difficult to be certain.

The electron microscope has proved of great value in discerning the fine structure of viruses and in the search for viral particles in cells. Some of these studies have been remarkably fruitful but others have become a source of perennial aggravation and controversy. For example, with this technique viruses were first demonstrated in subacute sclerosing panencephalitis (Bouteille et al., 1965; Tellez-Nagel and Harter, 1966; Shaw et al., 1967) and progressive multifocal leukoencephalopathy (ZuRhein and Chou, 1965; Silverman and Rubinstein, 1965) and later the precise identity of the agents involved was established by virological techniques (Chen et al., 1969; Horta-Barbosa et al., 1969; Padgett et al., 1971; Weiner et al., 1972).

On the other hand, the literature has been inundated by reports of 'virus-like particles' or 'VLPs' in cells, which range from the highly dubious to those which merit serious thought and

---

Plate 67

Papilloma virus in nuclei of keratinocytes in a plantar wart. These viral particles are said to be 50–55 nm in diameter, and so they are in negatively stained preparations. The size of the particles (calculated by me) in published electron micrographs (of sectioned warts) and in the ones presented here are smaller. Needless to say only distinct particles cut through the equator (identified by larger size and sharper margin) must be used for measurements.

Fig. 1. Nucleus showing crystalline arrays of human papilloma virus. The viral particle indicated by an arrow measures about 43 nm in diameter. × 35 000

Fig. 2. Nucleus showing randomly scattered viral particles. The particle indicated by an arrow measures about 46 nm. × 54 000

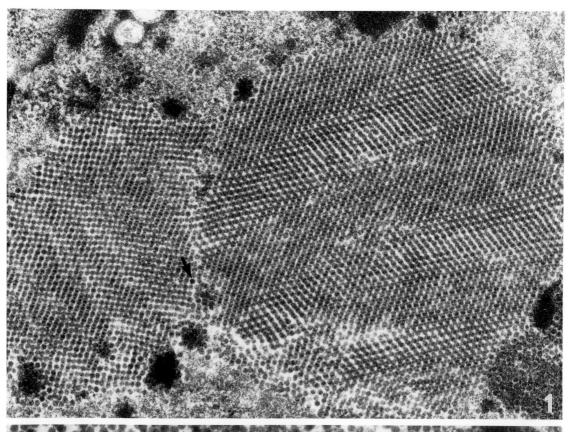

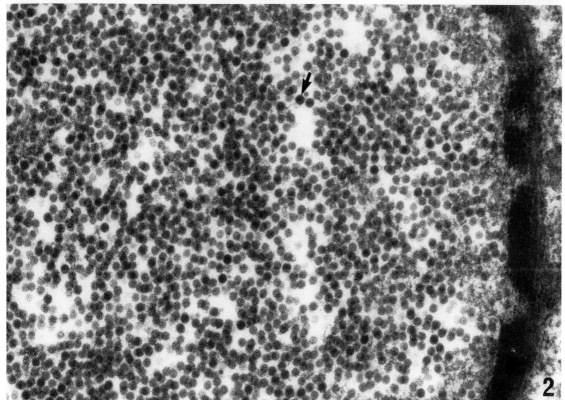

study by other techniques. Considerable interest and controversy has centred around reports of the occurrence of intranuclear structures designated by various terms such as 'paramyxovirus-like intranuclear filaments' and 'unusual intranuclear filaments' which bear some resemblance to the viral microtubules shown in *Plate 68, Fig. 2*. After parainfluenza Type I virus was isolated from cultured brain cells of two patients with multiple sclerosis (terMeulen *et al.*, 1972) quite a few reports describing such structures in mononuclear cells from the brain of cases with multiple sclerosis have been published (Prineas, 1972; Watanabe and Okazaki, 1973; Dubois-Dalcq *et al.*, 1973; Raine *et al.*, 1974; Tanaka *et al.*, 1974, 1976). However, it has been shown subsequently (Blinzinger *et al.*, 1974; Shaw and Sumi, 1975; Raine *et al.*, 1975) that such inclusions are found in a variety of neurological disorders, and it has been suggested by Shaw and Sumi (1975) that 'these structures are probably not viral but chromatin fibres'. Electron microscopy alone cannot resolve this controversy; it can only point to areas where further study by other techniques is indicated.

Nevertheless there is little doubt that most of these so-called 'paramyxovirus-like filaments'* are an artefact (Wills, 1983; Couvreur *et al.*, 1984) which is at times seen in the nuclei of a variety of cells in various organs. In my experience, this artefact is only occasionally seen in well collected and properly processed biopsy material (*Plate 69*). It is much more likely to be found in specimens where fixation is delayed for prolonged periods and postmortem material, particularly if the tissue is subjected to hypotonic stress by rinsing in water or fixing in unbuffered formalin. Such 'filament-containing' nuclei have a swollen appearance and at times the nuclear envelope is ruptured and its contents have spilled out into the cytoplasm. It will be recalled (page 16) that the technique widely employed by students of chromatin is to subject nuclei to a condition of low salinity. When this is done the compact chromatin unravels and presents a thread-like or a beads-on-a-string-like appearance. It seems to me that the production of the so-called 'paramyxovirus-like filaments' is a similar phenomenon and that these structures, which are often loosely referred to as 'viral filaments' by some are chromatin fibres and not viral microtubules.

*This is a peculiar term. Paramyxoviruses are microtubular, not filamentous.

Plate 68

Intranuclear inclusions produced by measles virus. (*From Nakai, Shand and Howatson, 1969*)

Fig. 1. A focal aggregate of viral microtubules in the nucleus of a BSC-1 cell (a cell line derived from green monkey kidney). × 110 000

Fig. 2. Extensive formation of viral microtubules has replaced the normal nuclear contents. From a primary culture of Rhesus monkey kidney. × 47 000

Fig. 3. Part of an intranuclear aggregate of viral microtubules is shown here at a higher magnification. × 140 000

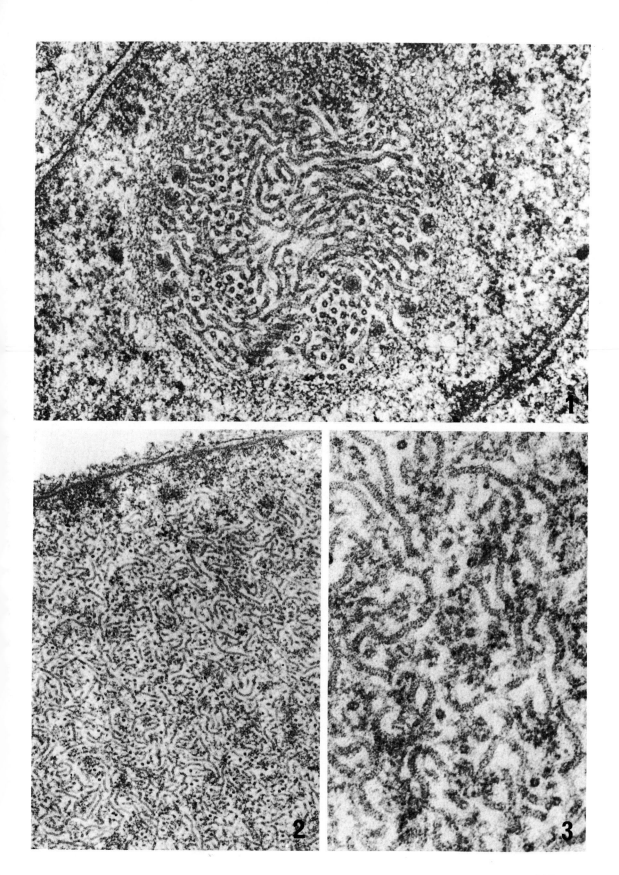

Distinction between the true paramyxovirus inclusions and chromatin fibres should not be too difficult, because the paramyxovirus inclusions are composed of striated microtubules about 14–18 nm in diameter, while the chromatin fibres★ are somewhat thicker (about 25 nm in diameter), more electron-dense, and have a fuzzy appearance. True striations are not seen, but at times these fibres have a beaded appearance. Almost invariably they are 'solid' or fibrous and not 'hollow' or microtubular, but on rare occasions (presumably due to vagaries of staining) they may look hollow.

Although this chapter is devoted to the nucleus, it is important and essential to digress a little and list all structures, be they within or outside the nucleus, which have at one time or the other been mistaken for viral inclusions or suspected of being viral particles by one or more authors. To name and criticize each author and paper would be a horrendously lengthy and traumatic procedure, suffice to say that just about every electron-dense particle or granule, filament or vesicle and some not too frequently encountered normal or near normal structures have been so misinterpreted or are likely to be misinterpreted by the novice. Structures mistakenly interpreted as virus or as virus-like particles include: (1) perichromatin granules; (2) nuclear bodies; (3) glycogen particles; (4) intranuclear filamentous inclusions; (5) altered chromatin (*Plate 69*); (6) nuclear pores (tangentially cut); (7) secretory granules; (8) micropinocytotic vesicles; (9) multivesicular bodies; (10) cross-cut microvilli; (11) glycocalyceal bodies; (12) spherical microparticles; (13) ribosome-lamella complex; (14) annulate lamellae; (15) microtubuloreticular complexes; and (16) cross-cut poorly stained collagen fibrils where only the periphery is stained (so-called 'hollow collagen', 'tubular collagen' or 'negatively stained collagen').

Such errors were made and at times are still made, principally by novices and by over-zealous but not too well-informed workers hunting for viruses in diseased tissues where a viral aetiology is suspected. Anybody with a modicum of knowledge about cell fine structure and with standard reference works at hand can avoid such pitfalls. All the structures mentioned above are amply illustrated and described in this book; familiarity with them should preclude the possibility of error.

★One does not as a rule call a 25 nm thick thread-like structure a 'fibre' but in the case of chromatin we are forced to make an exception (*see* footnote on page 14 and pages 1215–1221).

Plate 69
Fig. 1. From a biopsy of spinal astrocytoma. The entire nuclear contents are transformed into a mass of ill-defined chromatin fibres. Very few nuclei showing this change were detected in this tissue. × 27 000
Fig. 2. Same tumour as *Fig. 1.* Showing chromatin fibres (from another nucleus) at a higher magnification. The diameter of these poorly defined fibres is difficult to determine, but measurements on cross-cut fibres suggests that the diameter is about 24 nm. × 42 000

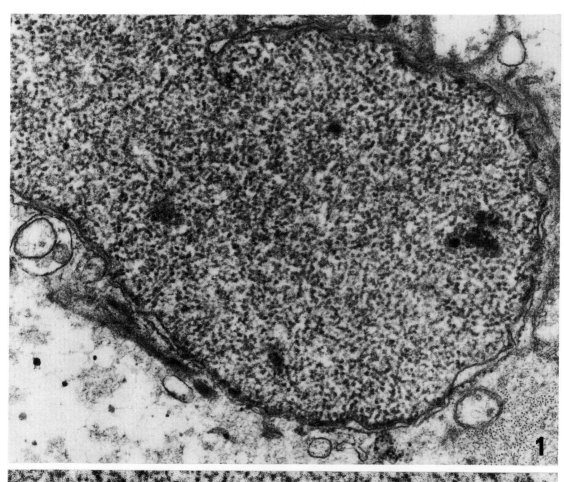

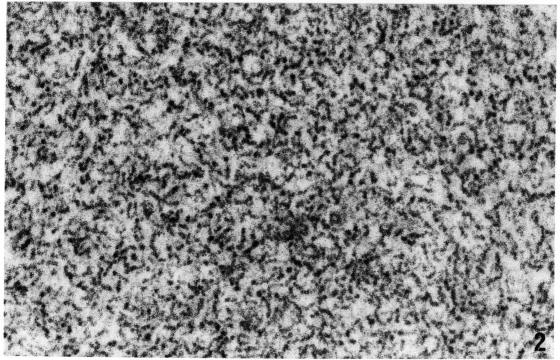

139

Nuclear projections, pockets, loops, satellites and clefts

Nuclear projections may present as a sessile or pedunculated nodule, tag, filament, club or drumstick arising from the surface of the nucleus. Such projections are best noted in whole cells examined with the light microscope. They have been seen more frequently in neutrophil polymorphonuclear leucocytes than in other cell types. In an ultrathin section the chance of encountering, say, a solitary filament or drumstick (e.g. the well-known drumstick containing chromatin of the XX chromosome pair in the human female) is small, and even more remote is the possibility of cutting such structures along their entire length so that their shape can be recognized. Thus, when an object resembling a drumstick is seen in an ultrathin section, it is much more likely to be a section through a sheet-like, or hood or cowl-like, formation with a thickened edge or margin. It is now thought that such formations (*Plates 70* and *71*) are an early stage of nuclear pocket formation (*see below*).

At a casual glance some nuclear pockets (*Plate 72*) may resemble a pseudoinclusion lying adjacent to the nuclear envelope. However, they have a different mode of genesis (*Plate 70*) and

---

Plate 70

Diagrams comparing the morphology and mode of formation of some intranuclear inclusions and nuclear pockets.

Fig. 1. Double-membrane-bound and single-membrane-bound pseudoinclusions (compare with *Plates 37, 39, 41* and *43*). In longitudinal section (L), the double-membrane-bound inclusion is seen to arise as an invagination of the nuclear envelope containing cytoplasmic material. (In this case a portion of cytoplasm containing a dense structure (S) which is meant to represent a secretory granule, lysosome or some other cytoplasmic organelle or inclusion.) A transverse section (T) through such an invagination (L) will present as a double-membrane-bound pseudoinclusion. Note how the ribosome-studded outer membrane of the nuclear envelope forms the inner membrane of the inclusion.

There are at least two ways (S1, S2) in which single-membrane-bound inclusions may form. The first possibility is that a dense body or granule (G) (this could be an intracisternal zymogen granule or a Russell body) travels along (as indicated by arrows) a cistern of the rough endoplasmic reticulum, impinges on the inner membrane of the nuclear envelope and enters the nucleus as a single-membrane-bound inclusion (S1). Besides the granule, the inclusion will contain a pool of flocculent material representing the contents of the perinuclear cistern. The second possibility is that a membrane-bound-granule (MG) (e.g. a serous or zymogen granule) lying in the cytoplasm travels (path indicated by arrows) to the nucleus where a fusion of the membrane bounding the granule and the outer membrane of the nucleus occurs and then dissolution of the membranes in the zone of fusion liberates a naked (i.e. no longer membrane-bound) granule into the perinuclear cistern. The granule then proceeds into the nucleus as a single-membrane-bound inclusion deriving its ensheathing membrane from the inner membrane of the nuclear envelope. As is to be expected, besides the granule, the inclusion contains a pool of flocculent material representing the contents of the perinuclear cistern.

Fig. 2. Intranuclear tubular or tubulovesicular inclusions (compare with *Plates 46* and *47*). These inclusions arise by a proliferation of the inner membrane (M) of the nuclear envelope which leads to the formation of tubules (T). A collection of these tubules comprise a tubular inclusion (between arrows). Segments of tubules may expand to form an inclusion composed of quite wide tubules and/or vesicles, i.e. a tubulovesicular inclusion (between arrowheads).

Fig. 3. Type 1 nuclear pocket (compare with *Plate 72, Fig. 2* and *Plate 73, Fig. 1*). The manner in which cytoplasmic material is sequestrated in the type 1 pocket is quite different from the manner in which cytoplasmic material is sequestrated in pseudoinclusions. The type 1 pocket commences as a fold (F) or ruffle (containing a chromatin band (B)), shaped like a hood or a cowl which springs from the surface of the nucleus partially trapping cytoplasmic material (C). This is followed by fusion of the margin of the fold with the nuclear surface. This leads to complete sequestration of cytoplasmic material (c) in a pocket demarcated by a chromatin band (b).

Fig. 4. Type 2 nuclear pocket and clefts (compare with *Plate 73, Fig. 5* and *Plates 74* and *76*). The type 2 nuclear pocket commences as a proliferation of the inner membrane of the nuclear envelope forming a microcleft (arrowheads) which invades the nucleus. The microcleft then curls and its margin ultimately fuses (at the point indicated by an arrow) with itself along its length or the inner membrane of the nuclear envelope to sequestrate a rounded mass of nuclear material (N). The chromatin band (C) is formed by the microcleft running parallel to, and separated from, the inner membrane of the nuclear envelope by a width of about 40 nm. It takes little imagination to see (bottom part of diagram) that if the structure depicted here (top part of illustration) rises above the nuclear surface it would present as a type 2 nuclear pocket demarcated by a chromatin band (C) and containing nuclear material (N). Also shown here is a double-membrane-bound macrocleft (M) which cleaves the nucleus. This is the cleft seen with the light microscope, the microcleft which creates the type 2 pocket is too slender to be resolved by this instrument.

140

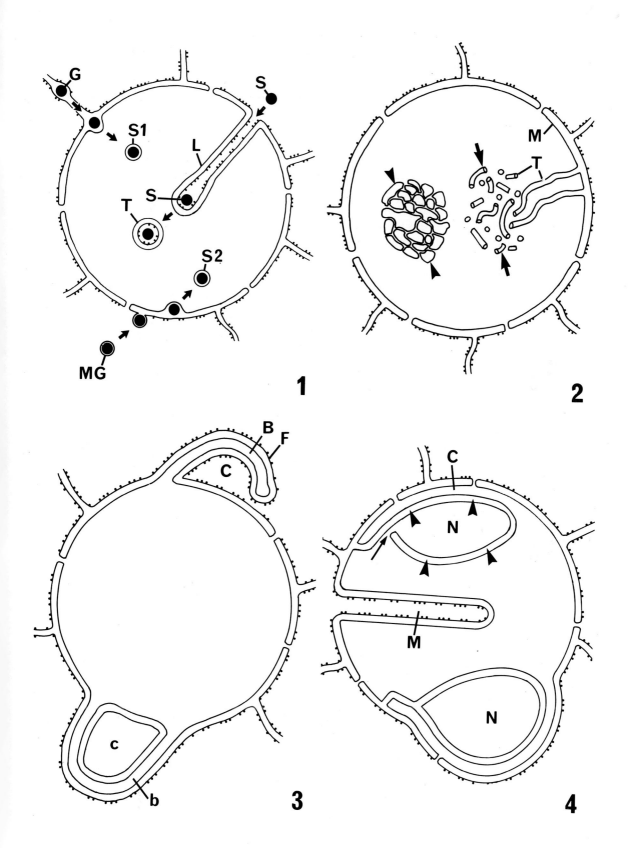

1

2

3

4

141

they can be distinguished from intranuclear pseudoinclusions by the fact that the nuclear pockets are bounded by one or more bands of chromatin about 40 nm wide (range 30–50 nm). In 1975 Ghadially drew attention to the fact that two varieties of nuclear pockets are seen in electron micrographs – those containing cytoplasmic material and those containing nuclear material (*Plates 70–73*). At first it was not clear whether they were two distinct and different morphological lesions or whether they were stages of evolution of but a single basic lesion. However, our serial section studies (Senoo *et al.*, 1984; Ghadially *et al.*, 1985b) have now shown that although both types of pockets may at times be found in one and the same specimen or nucleus (*Plate 73, Fig. 8*), they are in fact quite distinct and different lesions, each with its own mode of genesis, and that one does not evolve from the other. Thus two types of nuclear pockets occur, a common variety containing cytoplasmic material, which may be designated 'type 1 nuclear pocket' and a rarer variety containing nuclear material which may be designated 'type 2 nuclear pocket' (Ghadially *et al.*, 1985b).

Nuclear pockets are often erroneously called nuclear 'blebs' or 'blisters'. The latter terms have long been used by light microscopists to describe blebbing of the nucleus (and cytoplasm) seen at times in cultured cells. Such largely fluid-filled nuclear blebs and blisters (bounded by one or two membranes) have also been described in cultured cells, and cells in tissues, by electron microscopists (page 48). Both common sense and the principle of priority in scientific nomenclature dictate that we should not use these terms 'blebs' and 'blisters' to describe the totally different structures we are discussing here. The nuclear pocket is clearly and unequivocally distinguished from other nuclear anomalies (e.g. intranuclear pseudoinclusions (*Plate 37* and *Plate 38, Fig. 1*), blebs, blisters (*Plate 24*) and pocket-like structures (*Plate 23*)) by the presence of a chromatin band (or bands) – if no chromatin band (delineated by membranes) is present the structure must not be called a 'nuclear pocket'.

As pointed out above, confusion exists regarding the nomenclature of nuclear pockets. This makes the listing of sites and situations where they have been seen a bit difficult but bearing this difficulty in mind one can state that nuclear pockets have been observed in: (1) a variety of lymphomas and leukaemias of man (leukaemic cells and cultures derived from them) (Epstein and Achong, 1965; Achong and Epstein, 1966; Anderson, 1966; McDuffie, 1967; Mollo and Stramignoni, 1967; Dorfman, 1968; Freeman and Journey, 1971; Bessis, 1973; Ahearn *et al.*,

---

Plate 71
Polymorphonuclear neutrophil leucocytes from an ascitic effusion in a patient with adenocarcinoma of the ovary.
Fig. 1. One might at first think that what we are seeing here is the well-known drumstick-shaped projection (P) one sees with the light microscope in neutrophil leucocytes, but as explained in the text this is highly unlikely. The image seen here is almost certainly a stage in the formation of a type 1 pocket where cytoplasmic material (⋆) is about to be trapped by a hood or cowl-like formation springing from the nucleus. (A similar structure is shown in a lymphocyte from a lymphoma in *Plate 73, Fig. 1*). Note also the chromatin loop surrounding cytoplasmic material (C). × 32 000
Fig. 2. Nuclear pocket. The material in the pocket (C) shows an intermediate electron-density when compared with the nucleus and cytoplasm. However, the presence of vesicles and a paucity of particles that could be regarded as chromatin, favours the idea that this is a type 1 pocket containing cytoplasmic material (C). The inner (I) and outer (O) membranes of the nuclear envelope are continued over the surface of the pocket. The inner surface of the pocket under the chromatin band (B) is similarly lined. Note that the perinuclear cistern (P) is seen on both the outer and inner side of the band of chromatin (B) demarcating the nuclear pocket. The former is a portion of the perinuclear cistern surrounding the nucleus, the latter represents the portion of the perinuclear cistern which was sequestrated when the pocket formed. × 60 000

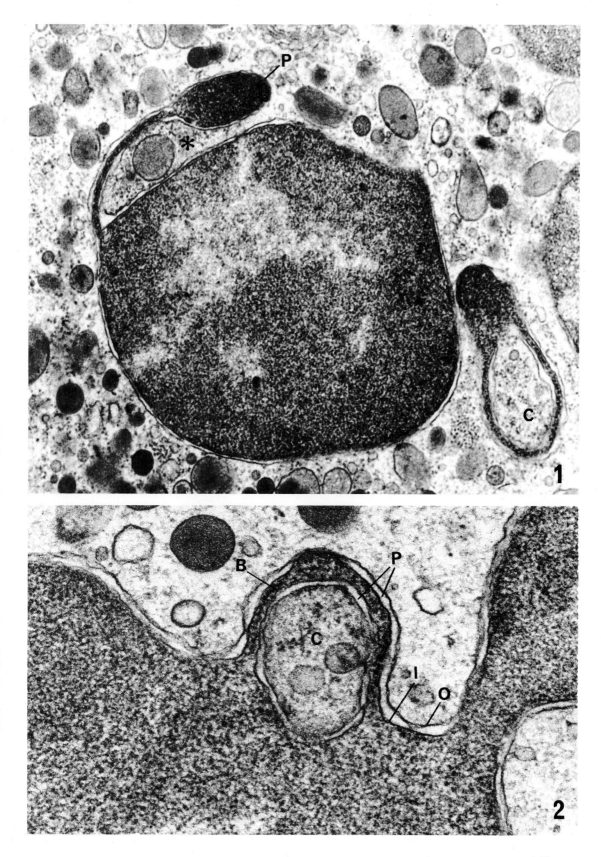

143

1974, 1978; Levine and Dorfman, 1975; Glick *et al.*, 1978; McKenna *et al.*, 1979; Smith *et al.*, 1982; Senoo *et al.*, 1984; Ghadially, 1985; Ghadially *et al.*, 1985b) (*Plates 72* and *73*); (2) avian lymphomatosis (Marek's disease) (Fujimoto *et al.*, 1970; Doak *et al.*, 1973); (3) swine leukosis (Ito *et al.*, 1973); (4) canine lymphoma (Parker *et al.*, 1967); (5) murine lymphoma (Papadimitriou, 1966); (6) bovine lymphoma and leukaemia (Knocke, 1964; Miller *et al.*, 1969; Urbaneck and Schulze, 1969; Weber *et al.*, 1969; Pomeroy *et al.*, 1977); (7) thymocytes of fetal guinea-pig and man (Sebuwufu, 1966; Toro and Olah, 1966); (8) granulocytes of patients treated with cystosine arabinoside (Ahearn *et al.*, 1967) and fluorouracil (Stalzer *et al.*, 1965); (9) granulocytes of pernicious anaemia patients (Stalzer *et al.*, 1965); (10) neutrophils and eosinophils of children with D_1 (13–15) trisomy and partial C trisomy (Huehns *et al.*, 1964; Lutzner and Hecht, 1966); (11) circulating neutrophils of four persons with bronchial cancer (Clausen and Von Haam, 1969) (6–16 per cent of neutrophils showed nuclear pockets in the cancer patients, but only one nuclear pocket was seen from the blood of five normal individuals); (12) neutrophils and monocytes in malignant ascites resulting from an ovarian carcinoma (*Plate 71*); (13) on rare occasions (about 1 per cent) neutrophils, lymphocytes and monocytes of apparently healthy individuals (Huhn, 1967; Smith and O'Hara 1967; Bessis, 1973); (14) normoblasts of patients with preleukaemia and leukaemia patients with dyserythropoietic anaemia and rats with dyserythropoieses experimentally induced with phenylhydrazine and lead (for references *see* Maldonado *et al.*, 1976); (15) human retinoblastoma (Popoff and Ellsworth, 1971); and (16) piscine melanoma (Vielkind and Vielkind, 1970).

This list is by no means complete, my experience is that on rare occasions a pocket or two may be found in a variety of tumours, but an abundance of pockets (*Plate 72*) is virtually diagnostic of lymphoma and leukaemia. Ultrastructurally lymphomas and leukaemias are distinguished from other tumours (e.g. anaplastic carcinoma) by the absence of specific features (e.g. desmosomes between tumour cells) known to occur in other tumours. Since it is impossible to prove a 'negative', this becomes quite a tiresome and worrisome process. In such a situation, the finding of nuclear pockets is a great relief. I can recall at least three cases where nuclear pockets helped to establish a diagnosis. Conversely, however one has to point out that nuclear pockets are of limited value in diagnosis because only some cases of lymphomas and leukaemias show pockets.

Plate 72
Lymph node from the groin of a case of follicular lymphoma.
Fig. 1. Neoplastic cells showing numerous nuclear pockets (arrows). × 6700
Fig. 2. Higher-power view showing that the pockets contain cytoplasmic material. × 40 000

144

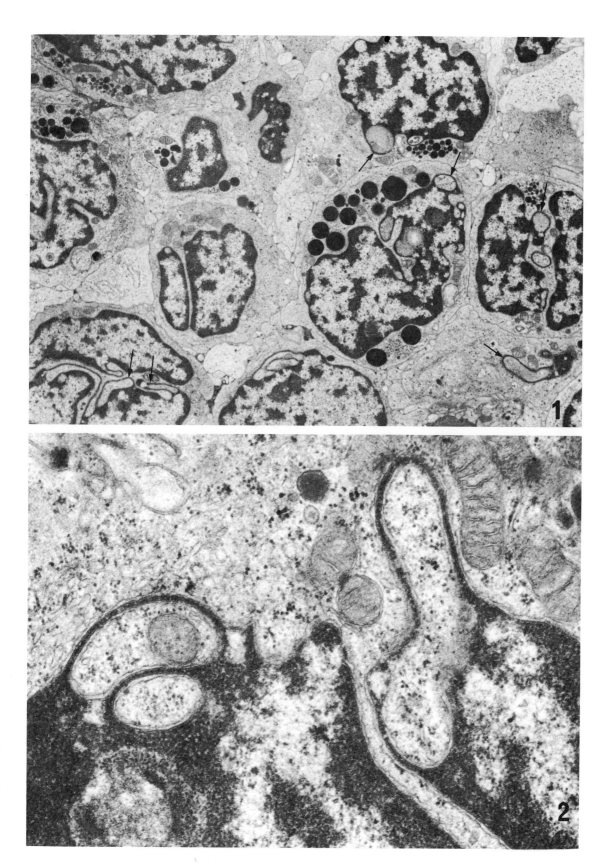

145

On the basis of their observations and a review of the literature on the incidence of nuclear pockets (which they call 'blebs') in various states Clausen and Von Haam (1969) point out that, 'There is a strong correlation between the reported occurrence of nuclear blebs and chromosomal abnormalities, either unusual numbers, breakage or a defect in nucleoprotein synthesis', and that 'blebs may be the morphologic expression of chromatin dislocation resulting from such chromosomal abnormalities'. Subsequent studies (Ahearn *et al.*, 1974) on human acute leukaemic cells have shown a close correlation between the occurrence of aneuploidy and a high frequency of nuclear pockets. Successful therapy produces a reduction or total disappearance of these abnormalities, while impending relapse is heralded by their reappearance. Ahearn *et al.* (1974) therefore think that this might provide a useful tool for monitoring therapy.

The number of pockets seen in cases of lymphomas and leukaemias is quite variable. As mentioned earlier, in some cases no pockets are detected, but when present, it is usually not difficult to find half a dozen or more pockets. At the other end of the scale was a lymphoma of the stomach which we studied (Senoo *et al.*, 1984) where in random sections about 90 per cent of the nuclei bore (one or more) type 1 nuclear pockets, and serial sections showed that every single tumour cell nucleus bore type 1 nuclear pockets (10–50 pockets per nucleus), but they were not homogeneously distributed over the surface of the nucleus. Most pockets were demarcated by a single chromatin band, but at times pockets bounded by two or three (*Plate 73, Fig. 3*) bands were seen and in rare instances one pocket was seen lying on top of another (*Plate 73, Fig. 4*). In some pockets the cytoplasmic structures were well preserved but in others they were degenerate. Serial sections showed that while some pockets were closed (i.e. contained completely sequestrated cytoplasmic material), other were open at one point. Very few type 2 pockets containing nuclear material were seen in this lymphoma.

Plate 73

Figs. 1–4 are from a lymphoma of the stomach. *Figs. 5, 7 and 8* are from acute lymphoblastic leukaemia. *Fig. 6* is from chronic lymphocytic leukaemia. As is to be expected the chromatin in this nucleus is markedly condensed, while that in the leukaemic lymphoblasts is more dispersed.

Fig. 1. The drumstick-like profile (containing one chromatin band) shown here is interpreted as a section through a fold or a hood-like structure springing from the nuclear surface. × 19 500 (*From Senoo, Fuse and Ghadially, 1984*)

Fig. 2. Seen here is a section through a fold or hood-like structure containing a doubled-up chromatin band. × 19 500 (*From Senoo, Fuse and Ghadially, 1984*)

Fig. 3. Three chromatin bands (between arrowheads) are seen demarcating a type 1 nuclear pocket containing cytoplasmic material (C). × 24 000 (*From Senoo, Fuse and Ghadially, 1984*)

Fig. 4. Seen here are two type 1 nuclear pockets (containing cytoplasmic material (C)), one lying on top of the other. × 25 000 (*From Senoo, Fuse and Ghadially, 1984*)

Fig. 5. This type 2 nuclear pocket containing nuclear material (N) is demarcated by a single chromatin band (arrow). × 33 000

Fig. 6. Two chromatin bands demarcate this type 2 nuclear pocket containing nuclear material (N). One of the chromatin bands expands out into a bulbous (B) mass. × 26 500 (*From Ghadially, Senoo and Fuse, 1985b*)

Fig. 7. A type 2 nuclear pocket demarcated by two chromatin bands (arrowheads). Three masses of nuclear material are present in the pocket. × 44 000 (*From Ghadially, Senoo and Fuse, 1985b*)

Fig. 8. This illustration demonstrates that a type 1 nuclear pocket (arrow) and a type 2 nuclear pocket (arrowhead) can occur in one and the same nucleus. × 27 000 (*From Ghadially, Senoo and Fuse, 1985b*)

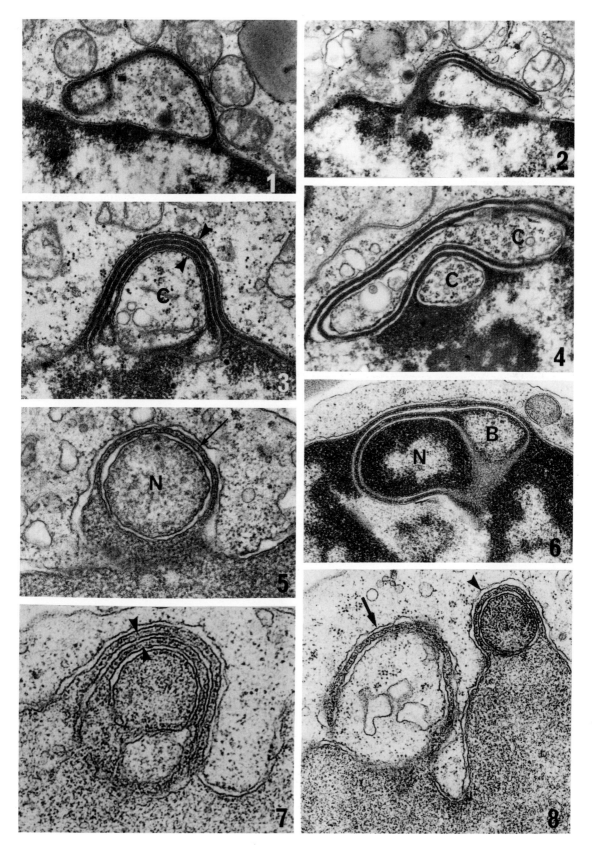

As mentioned earlier type 2 pockets are less frequently seen in lymphomas and leukaemias than type 1 pockets, and it would appear that even when present they are not quite as abundant. We studied the peripheral blood samples from a case (Case 1) of acute lymphoblastic leukaemia and a case (Case 2) of chronic lymphocytic leukaemia. In random sections about 21 per cent of the nuclei in Case 1 bore type 2 nuclear pockets, while in Case 2 about 41 per cent of the nuclei bore type 2 nuclear pockets. However, a study of serial sections showed that about 47 per cent of the nuclei in Case 1 and about 82 per cent in Case 2 bore type 2 nuclear pockets.

The type 2 nuclear pockets are usually demarcated by a single chromatin band (Plate 73, Fig. 5), but in rare instances two bands are present (Plate 73, Figs. 6 and 7). Usually a single rounded nuclear mass is seen in a pocket, but at times two or three such masses may be present. Our serial section studies show that in some instances the nuclear material in the pocket is connected with the main nuclear mass, while in other instances no such connection is detectable and the nuclear material in the pocket is completely sequestrated from the main nuclear mass.

As mentioned earlier, type 1 pockets bear some resemblance to intranuclear pseudoinclusions, but the manner in which they form is quite different (Plate 70). The well-known common double-membrane-bound intranuclear pseudoinclusion containing cytoplasmic material is derived by an invagination of the nuclear envelope. Later fusion of membranes in a narrow-necked invagination can occur (see pages 76 and 77) leading to a complete sequestration of the double-membrane-bound cytoplasmic material in the nucleus and degeneration of sequestrated organelles ensues.

In contrast to this, the type 1 nuclear pocket develops (Plate 70, Fig. 3) as a fold or ruffle (containing a chromatin band), shaped like a hood or a cowl which springs from the nuclear surface and entraps cytoplasmic material (Plate 73, Fig. 1). Sometimes a fold containing a doubled up chromatin band is seen (Plate 73, Fig. 2), usually the fold has an expanded drumstick-like end (Plate 71, Fig. 1 and Plate 73, Fig. 1). Fusion of the margin of the fold with the nuclear surface leads to sequestration of cytoplasmic material in the pocket.

The manner in which type 2 nuclear pockets develop is markedly different (Plates 70 and 74) from the manner in which type 1 pockets develop. The basic mechanism here seems to be a proliferation of the inner membrane of the nuclear envelope leading to the formation of a sheet-like invagination of the perinuclear cistern into the nucleus. In favourably sectioned material this presents as a single-membrane-bound channel or microcleft* whose contents are

*I have coined the term 'microclefts' to describe the very slender single-membrane-bound clefts, which meander in the nucleus to produce type 2 pockets. These microclefts (about 0.04 μm wide) are beyond the resolving power of the light microscope. The clefts at times seen in lymphocytic cells with the light microscope are about 0.3–1 μm in width. In order to avoid confusion we will call them 'macroclefts'. Elongation of the macrocleft splits or cleaves the nucleus into two portions. Such macroclefts are double-membrane-bound (Plate 76).

Plate 74

Leukaemic cells from the peripheral blood of a case of chronic lymphocytic leukaemia.

Fig. 1. At the bottom of this straight microcleft lies a double-membrane-bound pseudoinclusion (P), but the microcleft itself appears to be lined by a single membrane. × 40 000

Fig. 2. A meandering microcleft has demarcated a band of chromatin (arrowhead). The deep end of the microcleft expands into a double-membrane-bound pseudoinclusion (P). The single membrane lining the microcleft can be discerned in places, but in other places it is not visualized because of oblique sectioning. × 37 000

Fig. 3. Two microclefts are seen here, one has sequestrated nuclear material (N), the other nuclear material and a pseudoinclusion containing cytoplasmic material (C). × 37 000

Fig. 4. Appearances seen here could be interpreted as three microclefts that have sequestrated nuclear material. The one at the top (arrow) has only to be raised a little above the nuclear surface to form a typical nuclear pocket. The appearances seen here could be explained by assuming that the section has passed through the base or deep part of type 2 nuclear pockets. × 29 000

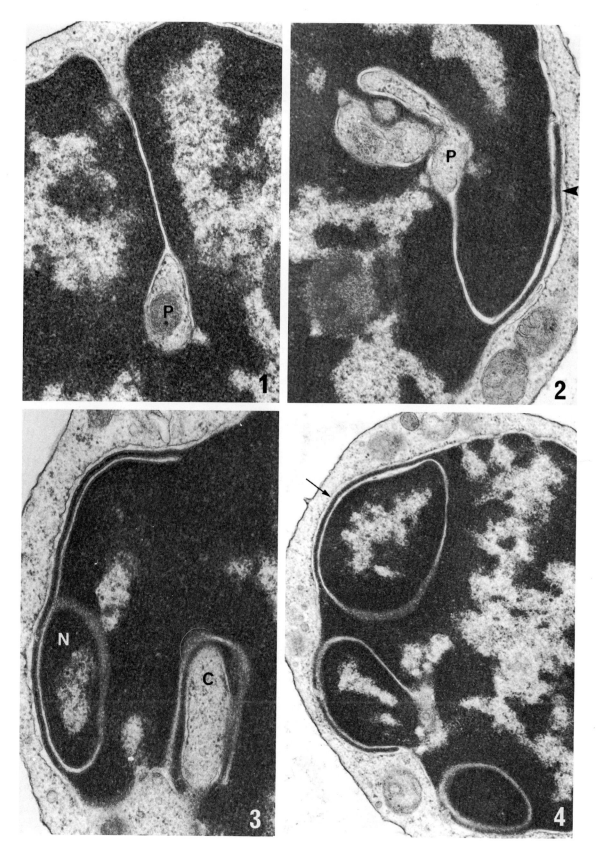

149

continuous with that in the perinuclear cistern. The membrane lining the microcleft is continuous with the inner membrane of the nuclear envelope. It is easy to see that if such an invagination or microcleft were to curl and its margin fuse with itself along its length or the inner membrane of the nuclear envelope, a rounded mass of nuclear material would be sequestrated from the main nuclear mass, but this mechanism on its own leaves unexplained how the chromatin band forms. (For illustrations depicting this, *see* Ghadially *et al.*, 1985b).

It would appear that the formation of the chromatin band is engendered when the microcleft formed by the invaginating perinuclear cistern runs parallel to, and separated from, the inner membrane of the nuclear envelope by a width of about 40 nm (*Plate 74, Fig. 2*). Two chromatin bands are formed when two invaginations of the perinuclear cistern set side by side invade the nucleus. Thus the nuclear material in the chromatin band or bands remains continuous with the main mass of nuclear material. Curling of the invading cistern demarcates material destined for sequestration, while fusion of the leading edge with the nuclear envelope or the invaginating cistern itself leads to sequestration of the nuclear material in the type 2 nuclear pocket (*Plate 70*).

Some doubt has been expressed (Smith *et al.*, 1982) as to whether nuclear material is ever completely cut-off or sequestrated in type 2 nuclear pockets or whether such appearances are the product of sectioning geometry. Our serial section study (Ghadially *et al.*, 1985b) dispels such doubts and shows that in some instances the pocket is closed and the included nuclear material is completely separated from the main nuclear mass. On the other hand, one also finds open pockets where continuity between the material in the pocket and nucleus is demonstrable. It is well known (page 76) that when material in an intranuclear pseudoinclusion suffers complete sequestration it shows degenerative changes. We have seen images which could be interpreted as a degenerative change or a breakdown or fragmentation of material in both type 1 and type 2 nuclear pockets.

Structures referred to as 'nuclear loops' or 'chromatin loops' and structures referred to as 'satellite nuclei' are seen in cells showing nuclear pockets and it has been debated whether such images represent structures truly detached from the main nuclear mass or whether such images are the product of sectioning geometry (*Plate 75*). Our serial section studies support the latter idea because a truly detached chromatin loop or satellite nucleus was not found (Senoo *et al.*, 1984).

Plate 75

Figs. 1–6. This set of serial sections demonstrates that what appears as chromatin loops lying free (i.e. detached from the nucleus) in the cytoplasm are in fact sections through nuclear pockets. Three of these structures (a, b and c) are seen in *Figs. 1–3* as chromatin loops lying free in the cytoplasm, but *Figs. 4–6* show that they are connected with the nucleus in another plane of sectioning. × 5700 (*From Senoo, Fuse and Ghadially, 1984*)

Figs. 7–12. Profiles suggesting that a satellite nucleus is present are seen in *Figs. 7–9*, but *Figs. 10–12* show that these profiles are in fact continuous with the profiles of a type 2 nuclear pocket. Thus it is apparent that there is in fact no satellite nucleus present, only the illusion of one created by fortuitous sectioning. × 30 000 (*From Ghadially, Senoo and Fuse, 1985b*)

150

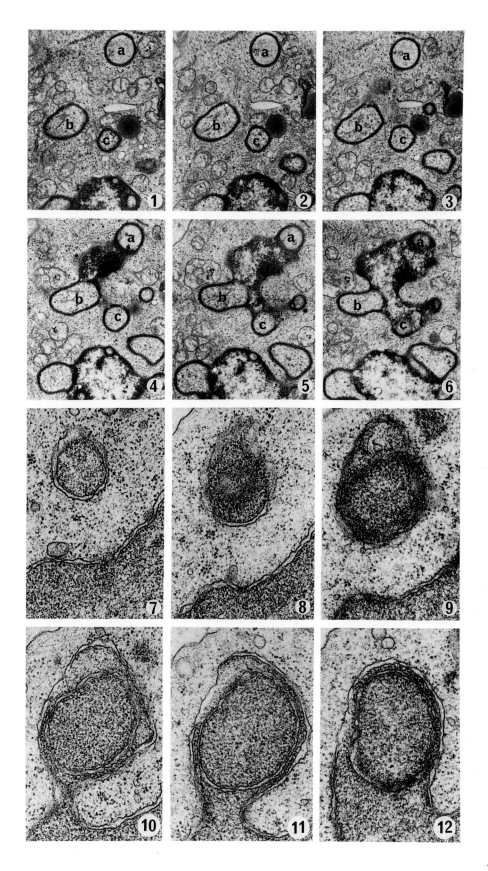

In specimens containing nuclei bearing nuclear pockets one also at times finds cleaved or clefted nuclei, and indeed both these nuclear abnormalities may be found in one and the same nucleus. A few cleaved nuclei may be found in the perifollicular zone of normal lymph nodes, but much larger numbers are seen in some lymphomas and leukaemias (*Plate 76*). In sectioned material, profiles of the cleaved nuclei seen with the light microscope, suggest that a deep cleft (henceforth referred to as 'macrocleft', *see* footnote on page 148) develops in the nucleus and ultimately divides it into two portions. The electron microscope reveals profiles which suggest that these macroclefts commence as double-membrane-bound invaginations of the nuclear envelope which, as they elongate, cleave the nucleus.

One is not surprised to find cytoplasmic material lying in or at the bottom (leading edge) of a double-membrane-bound macrocleft but at times a paradoxical image is seen, where cytoplasmic material (in the form of a double-membrane-bound inclusion) lies at the bottom of a single-membrane-bound microcleft (*Plate 74, Figs. 1 and 2*).

Our serial section study showed (*see Fig. 9a–o in Ghadially et al., 1985b*) that this type of double-membrane-bound cytoplasmic inclusion lying at the bottom (leading edge) of a single-membrane-bound microcleft (similar to that shown in *Plate 74, Fig. 1*) is continuous (in another plane of sectioning) with cytoplasmic material in an adjacent double-membrane-bound macrocleft (similar to that shown in *Plate 76, Fig. 1*). Thus in such instances the microcleft may be regarded as a lateral extension★ derived from the outer membrane (which in turn is derived from the inner membrane of the nuclear envelope) of the macrocleft. Thus it appears that at times there is a membrane-continuity between microclefts and macroclefts which produces images (profiles) that are difficult to interpret. Be that as it may, the basic lesion in these neoplastic lymphocyte nuclei seems to be a proliferation of a membrane or membranes of the nuclear envelope, which can then lead to the formation of macroclefts, microclefts and type 1 and type 2 pockets. Little wonder then that one or more of these morphologically complex structures are seen in a given nucleus.

★The concept of lateral extension arising from a double-membrane-bound inclusion is not unique to this situation. Intranuclear annulate lamellae often arise in this fashion. This is clearly demonstrated in *Plate 251*.

Plate 76

Leukaemic cells from the peripheral blood of a case of chronic lymphocytic leukaemia.

Figs. 1 and 2. Double-membrane-bound macroclefts (i.e. invaginations of the nuclear envelope) containing cytoplasmic material (C). × 27 000, × 29 000

Fig. 3. The profile seen here suggests that a macrocleft has just completely cleaved the nucleus, but serial sections would be needed to prove this. The separation (★) of the nucleus and cytoplasm is a preparative artefact. × 26 000

Fig. 4. The nuclear profiles seen here suggest that a macrocleft has completely cleaved a nucleus into two separate portions, but serial sections would be needed to prove this. × 27 000

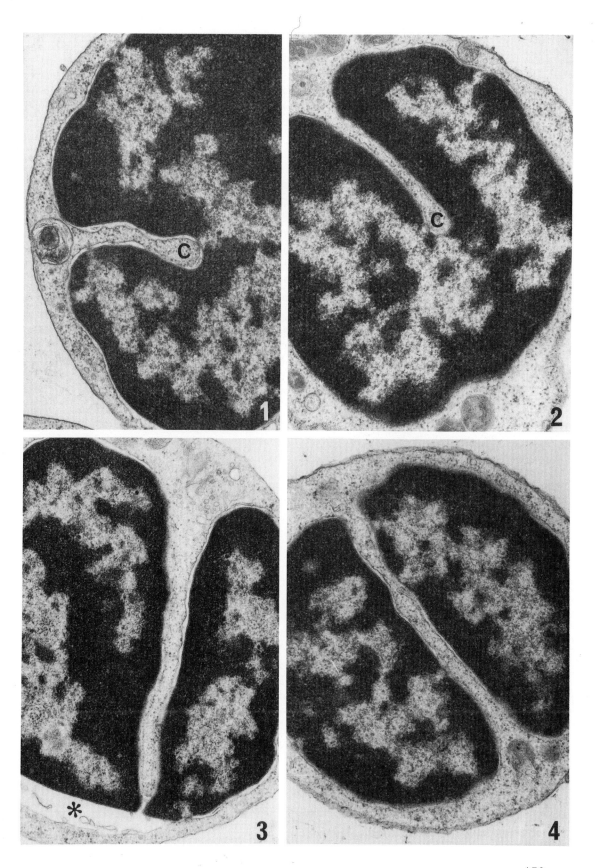

153

Nuclear bodies

The term 'nuclear bodies' is used to describe a group of intranuclear structures of diverse morphology (*Plates* 77 and 78). Several attempts have been made to classify nuclear bodies on the basis of their ultrastructural appearance. For example, Bouteille *et al.* (1967) divided them into types I to V, Vazquez *et al.* (1970) into types I to IV, Popoff and Stewart (1968) into types I to III, and Krishan *et al.* (1967) into groups a, b and c. Little is gained by this exercise, and therefore in this text will be used the descriptive terms which, although cumbersome at times, convey the meaning more clearly.

The simplest type of nuclear body is composed of filaments (5–7 nm thick) which may be randomly orientated or orientated to form concentric or annular fibrils. More than one such body may occur in a nucleus and they are easily spotted because there is usually a clear halo around them (*Plate* 77). Another variety of nuclear body is composed of fibrils and granules. Such fibrillogranular bodies may contain only a few granules set in a fibrillary matrix or there may be many granules surrounded by a fibrillary cortex (*Plate* 78). Some examples of these are likely to be confused with focal glycogen deposits in the nucleus (*see* page 102). Occasionally, one encounters nuclear bodies which contain microtubules or vesicles surrounded by a fibrillary cortex. Finally, there is a complex group of large nuclear bodies which, besides the usual fibrils and perhaps some small granules, may also contain one or more structures such as vesicles, large electron-dense masses and lipid. Such bodies are of rarer occurrence. Only the simpler varieties of nuclear bodies, that is to say the fibrillar and small varieties of fibrillogranular bodies with sparse granules, are commonly encountered in normal tissues of plants and animals.

Nuclear bodies have been reported to occur in the following situations: (1) normal plants (LaFontaine, 1965; Sankaranarayanan and Hyde, 1965; Büttner, 1968); (2) normal animal tissues (Farquhar and Palade, 1962; Horstmann, 1962, 1965; Horstmann *et al.*, 1966; Latta and Maunsbach, 1962a, b; Weber and Frommes, 1963; Ishikawa, 1964; Nicander, 1964; Brooks and Siegel, 1967; Henry and Petts, 1969; Misrabi, 1969; Dixon, 1970; Masurovsky *et al.*, 1970; Van Noord *et al.*, 1972; Yasuzumi *et al.*, 1975; Ryder *et al.*, 1979); (3) a variety of tumours, such as Shope papilloma, papillary carcinoma of the thyroid, bronchial carcinoid and carcinoma, ependymomas, gliomas, meningiomas, leukaemias, Hodgkin's disease, Waldenström's macroglobulinaemia, squamous cell carcinoma, melanoma, rhabdomyoma, and tumours of salivary gland (De The *et al.*, 1960; Hinglais-Guillaud *et al.*, 1961; Bessis and Thiery, 1962; Ogawa, 1962; Bernhard and Granboulan, 1963; Bessis *et al.*, 1963; Robertson, 1964; Robertson and Maclean, 1965; Brooks and Siegel, 1967; Bouteille *et al.*, 1967; Krishan *et al.*, 1967; Kuhn, 1967; Kierszenbaum, 1968; Vazquez *et al.*, 1970; Wyatt *et al.*, 1970; Sobrinho-Simões and Gonçalves, 1974, 1978; Schulze, 1979); (4) in tissues or cultures infected with adenovirus, herpes zoster and herpes simplex, human cytomegalovirus, polyoma, SV40, Shope papilloma, varicella, vaccinia and wart virus (Granboulan *et al.*, 1963; Patrizi and Middlekamp, 1969; Takeichi *et al.*, 1977); (5) drug action (Torack, 1961; Swanbeck and Thyresson, 1964; Simard, 1966; Ulrich and Kidd, 1966); (6) immunological stimulation (Simar, 1969; Dumont and Roberts, 1971); and (7) hormonal stimulation (Lemaire, 1963; Weber *et al.*, 1964; Horstmann, 1965; Simar and Lemaire, 1966; Dahl, 1970; Santibanez and Lafarga, 1979).

Plate 77

Nucleus of a cell from human bronchial mucosa, showing fibrillary nuclear bodies surrounded by a clear halo (arrows). × 32 000

154

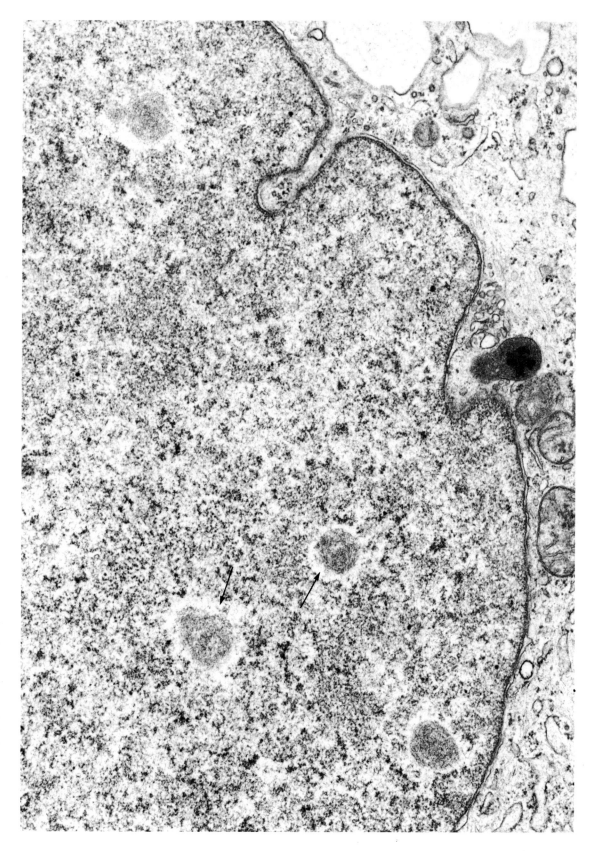

Nuclear bodies have been observed in such a wide variety of tissues that many authors now consider them to be a normal constituent of the nucleus, and probably of universal occurrence. A review of the literature also indicates that when cells are stimulated to activity by a variety of means an increase in numbers, size and complexity of the nuclear bodies is observed. Thus in the zona fasciculata of the calf adrenal after ACTH stimulation the fibrillogranular nuclear body transforms into a large multiloculated vesicular structure (Weber et al., 1964). Numerous nuclear bodies occur in the epithelium of the dog epididymis, but these are absent or less frequent in the young, castrated or oestrogen-treated animal (Lemaire, 1963; Simar and Lemaire, 1966). Horstmann (1962) has noted a close relationship between the differentiation of nuclear bodies and maturation of the epididymis in man. An increase in the number and size of nuclear bodies is reported by Dahl (1970) in ovarian tissue after clomiphene or gonadotrophin treatment.

Similarly, there are experiments which indicate that nuclear bodies increase in size, number and complexity in inflammation and after immunological stimulation. For example, it has been found that after intravenous injection of various micro-organisms in hamsters the peritoneal macrophages contain large complex nuclear bodies (Dumont and Roberts, 1971). When to this is added the fact that most of the larger nuclear bodies are seen in tumours, and that cells in culture and virus-infected cells show abundant nuclear bodies, one has to concede that these bodies are a sign of stimulated or metabolically active cells.

Despite numerous studies the nature and function of these bodies remain obscure. There is also much doubt about their chemical composition, for conflicting reports abound in the literature. For example, the fibrillogranular body which can at times be large enough to locate with the light microscope, has been reported to be basophilic by some authors and eosinophilic by others (Wyatt et al., 1970). Cytochemical studies have not revealed DNA or RNA in the simpler nuclear bodies, and the fibrillary nuclear body is said to contain only protein (Krishan et al., 1967). However, in larger complex bodies enzyme digestion studies suggest that the fibrillary component contains RNA while the dense granular component contains DNA (Sankaranarayanan and Hyde, 1965; Simar, 1969). This is in keeping with the observation of Vazquez et al. (1970), that the granules of the large fibrillogranular bodies in gliomas are Feulgen-positive. The idea that the fibrillary component of nuclear bodies contains RNA is supported also by the autoradiographic studies of Yasuzumi et al. (1975), who found that labelled uridine locates in the fibrillar component of the nuclear body and nucleolus of normal mouse leucocytes. They therefore conclude that 'the nuclear body appearing in the normal leucocytes active in protein synthesis may cooperate with a nucleolus in the formation of ribosomes'.

The idea that nuclear bodies are derived from the nucleolus (and hence contain RNA) is supported also by the work of Vagner-Capodano et al. (1980) on cultured thyroid cells stimulated by thyrotropin. After stimulation a phenomenon of nucleolar budding occurs. A series of convincing electron micrographs are presented by these authors showing how such budded nucleolar material transforms into fibrillogranular or granular nuclear bodies.

Plate 78

Fig. 1. A nuclear body with a concentric arrangement of its components. From full-term human placenta. × 77 000

Fig. 2. A nuclear body with a fibrillary cortex and some microtubules. From bronchial mucosa of heavy smoker. × 40 000

Fig. 3. A fibrillary nuclear body with an annular configuration. From liver of phenobarbitone-treated hamster. × 48 000

Fig. 4. From the same nucleus as *Fig. 3.* More annular fibrillary nuclear bodies and also one that could be a compact spherical body as in *Plate 77,* or a tangential cut through an annular one. × 42 000

Fig. 5. A nuclear body containing vesicles. From human chronic lymphocytic leukaemia. × 66 000

Fig. 6. Fibrillogranular nuclear body from the same case as *Fig. 2.* × 55 000

Fig. 7. A nuclear body containing a lipid droplet, numerous dense structures with paler centres and a fibrillary cortex. From liver of phenobarbitone-treated hamster. × 65 000

156

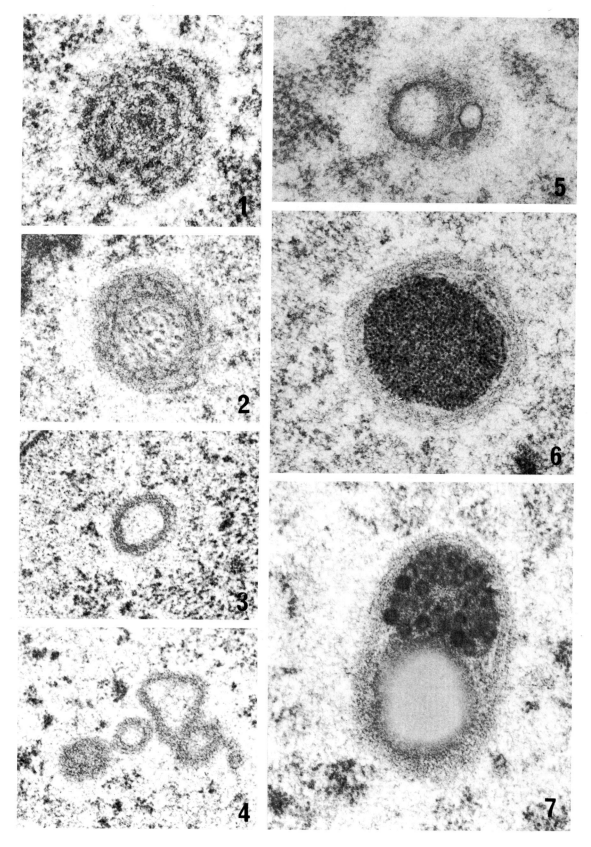

157

References

Abuelo, J. G. and Moore, D. E. (1969). The human chromosome. Electron microscopic observations on chromatin fiber organization. *J. Cell Biol.* **41,** 73

Achong, B. G. and Epstein, M. A. (1966). Fine structure of the Burkitt tumor. *J. natn Cancer Inst.* **36,** 877

Afzelius, B. A. (1955). The ultrastructure of the nuclear membrane of the sea urchin oocyte as studied with the electron microscope. *Exp. Cell Res.* **8,** 147

Agutter, P. S. and Richardson, J. C. W. (1980). Nuclear non-chromatin proteinaceous structures: their role in the organization and function of the interphase nucleus. *J. Cell Sci.* **44,** 395

Ahearn, M. J., Lewis, C. W. and Campbell, L. A. (1967). Nuclear bleb formation in human bone marrow cells during cytosine arabinoside therapy. *Nature, Lond.* **215,** 196

Ahearn, M. J., Trujillo, J. M., Cork, A., Fowler, A. and Hart J. S. (1974). The association of nuclear blebs with aneuploidy in human acute leukemia. *Cancer Res.* **34,** 2887

Ahearn, M. J., Trujillo, J. M. and Dicke, K. A. (1978). Electron microscope identification of leukemic cells in human bone marrow colonies. *Prevention & Detection of Cancer, Part II, Vol. 1.* pp. 1102. USA: Marcel Dekker

Ahmed, M. M. and Mukherjee, D. K. (1974). Virus-like particles in human laryngeal papilloma. An ultrastructural study. *Experientia,* **30,** 361

Akhtar, M. and Miller, R. M. (1977). Ultrastructure of elastofibroma. *Cancer,* **40,** 728

Albrecht, R. and Küttner, K. (1970). Zur ultrastruktur der juvenilen Nasenrachenfibrome. *Z. Laryngol. Rhinol.* **49,** 653

Alguacil-Garcia, A., Unni, K. K. and Goellner, J. R. (1978). Histogenesis of dermatofibrosarcoma protuberans. An ultrastructural study. *Am. J. clin. Path.* **69,** 427

Ancla, M. and De Brux, J. (1965). Occurrence of intranuclear tubular structures in the human endometrium during the secretory phase, and of annulate lamellae in hyperestrogenic states. *Obstet. Gynec.* **26,** 23

Anderson, D. R. (1966). Ultrastructure of normal and leukemic leukocytes in human peripheral blood. *J. Ultrastruct. Res.* (Suppl. 9), 26

Andrew, W. (1955). Amitotic division in senile tissues as a probable means of self-preservation of cells. *J. Gerontol.* **10,** 1

Andrew, W. (1962). An electron microscope study of age changes in the liver of the mouse. *Am. J. Anat.* **110,** 1

Andrew, W., Brown, H. M. and Johnson, J. (1943). Senile changes in the liver of mouse and man, with special reference to the similarity of the nuclear alterations. *Am. J. Anat.* **72,** 199

Andrews, J. M. and Sekhon, S. S. (1969). Varieties of intranuclear filamentous aggregates in cerebral neurons. *Bull. Los Angeles Neurol. Soc.* **34,** 163

Angevine, J. M., Kappas, A., DeGowin, R. L. and Spargo, B. H. (1962). Renal tubular nuclear inclusions in lead poisoning. A clinical and experimental study. *Archs Path.* **73,** 486

Apitz, K. (1937a). Über die pigmentbildung in den zellkernen melanotischer geschwulste: I. Beitrag zur pathologie des zellkernes. *Virchows Arch. path. Anat. Physiol.* **300,** 89

Apitz, K. (1937b). Über die Bildung Russellscher Körperchen in den Plasmazellen multipler Myelome. 2. Beitrag zur Pathologie des Zellkernes. *Virchows Arch. path. Anat.* **300,** 113

Arsanto, J. P. (1973). Nature protéique des structures paracristallines intranucléaires dans les tissus des jeunes frondes de l'Asplenium fontanum (Polypodiacée). *C. R. Acad. Sci. Paris Series D* **276,** 1345

Babai, F., Tremblay, G. and Dumont, A. (1969). Intranuclear and intranucleolar tubular structures in Novikoff hepatoma cells. *J. Ultrastruct. Res.* **28,** 125

Banner, B. F., Alroy, J., Pauli, B. U. and Carpenter, J. L. (1978). An ultrastructural study of acinic cell carcinoma of the canine pancreas. *Am. J. Path.* **93,** 165

Barnes, B. G. and Davis, J. M. (1959). The structure of nuclear pores in mammalian tissue. *J. Ultrastruct. Res.* **3,** 131

Barnett, C. H., Cochrane, W. and Palfrey, A. J. (1963). Age changes in articular cartilage of rabbits. *Ann. rheum. Dis.* **22,** 389

Basler, J. W., David, J. D. and Agris, P. F. (1979). Deteriorating collagen synthesis and cell ultrastructure accompanying senescence of human normal and Werner's syndrome fibroblast cell strains. *Exp. cell Res.* **118,** 73

Baud, C. A. (1963). Nuclear membrane and permeability. In *Intracellular Membrane Structure,* p. 323. Ed. by S. Seno and E. V. Cowdry. Okayama: Chugoku Press

Baudhuin, P., Hers, H. G. and Loeb, H. (1964). An electron microscopic and biochemical study of type II glycogenosis. *Lab. Invest.* **13,** 1139

158

Beams, H. W., Tahmisian, T. N., Devine, R. and Anderson, E. (1957). Ultrastructure of the nuclear membrane of a Gregarine parasitic in grasshoppers. *Exp. Cell Res.* **13**, 200

Beaver, D. L. (1961). The ultrastructure of the kidney in lead intoxication with particular reference to intranuclear inclusions. *Am. J. Path.* **39**, 195

Beaver, D. L. and Burr, R. E. (1963a). Electron microscopy of bismuth inclusions. *Am. J. Path.* **42**, 609

Beaver, D. L. and Burr, R. E. (1963b). Bismuth inclusions in the human kidney. *Arch. Path.* **76**, 89

Beçak, M. L. and Fukuda, K. (1979). Arrangement of nucleosomes in condensed chromatin fibres. *Experientia* **35**, 24

Beltran, G. and Stuckey, W. J. (1972). Nuclear lobulation and cytoplasmic fibrils in leukemic plasma cells. *Am. J. clin. Path.* **58**, 159

Bencosme, S. A., Allen, R. A. and Latta, H. (1963). Functioning pancreatic islet cell tumors studied electron microscopically. *Am. J. Pathol.* **42**, 1

Berezney, R. and Coffey, D. S. (1977). Nuclear matrix. Isolation and characterization of a framework structure from rat liver nuclei. *J. Cell Biol.* **73**, 616

Bernhard, W. (1966). Ultrastructural aspects of the normal and pathological nucleolus in mammalian cells. *Natn. Cancer Inst. Monogr.* **23**, 13

Bernhard, W. and Granboulan, N. (1963). The fine structure of the cancer cell nucleus. *Exp. Cell Res.* (Suppl. 9), 19

Bernhard, W. and Granboulan, N. (1968). Electron microscopy of the nucleolus in vertebrate cells. In *The Nucleus.* Ed. by A. Dalton and F. Haguenau. New York: Academic Press

Bessis, M. C. (1961). Ultrastructure of lymphoid and plasma cells in relation to globulin and antibody formation. *Lab. Invest.* **10**, 1040

Bessis, M. (1973). *Living blood cells and their ultrastructure.* New York, Heidelberg, Berlin: Springer-Verlag

Bessis, M. and Breton-Gorius, J. (1965). Rôle des fibrilles cytoplasmiques dans la lobulation du noyau cellulaire (Formation de Cellules de Rieder). *C. R. Acad. Sci. Paris* **261**, 1392

Bessis, M. and Thiery, J.-P. (1962). Étude au microscope électronique de hémosarcomes humains. III. Leucémies à cellules-souches. Érythrémies, Réticulo-lympho-sarcomes, Maladie de Hodgkin, Plasmocytomes. *Nouv. Rev. Fr. Hematol.* **2**, 577

Bessis, M. S. and Thiery, J. P. (1962). Études au microscope électronique sur les leucemies humains. II. Les leucemies lymphocytaires. Comparison avec la leucemie de la souris de souche A. K. *Nouv. Rev. Fr. Hematol.* **2**, 387

Bessis, M. S., Breton-Gorius, J. and Binet, J. L. (1963). Etude comparee du plasmocytome et du syndrome de Waldenstrom. Examen au microscope electronique. *Nouv. Rev. Fr. Hematol.* **3**, 159

Biava, C. (1963). Identification and structural forms of human particulate glycogen. *Lab. Invest.* **12**, 1179

Bingen, A. and Kirn, A. (1973). Modifications ultrastructurales précoces des noyaux des hépatocytes de souris au cours de l'hépatite dégénérative aiguë provoquée par le FV$_3$ (Frog Virus 3). *J. Ultrastruct. Res.* **45**, 343

Binggeli, M. F. (1959). Abnormal intranuclear and cytoplasmic formations associated with a chemically induced transplantable chicken sarcoma. *J. biophys. biochem. Cytol.* **5**, 143

Birge, W. J. and Doolin, P. F. (1974). The ultrastructural differentiation of the endoplasmic reticulum in choroidal epithelial cells of the chick embryo. *Tissue & Cell* **6**, 335

Blackburn, W. R. and Vinijchaikul, K. (1969). The pancreas in kwashiorkor. An electron microscopic study. *Lab. Invest.* **20**, 305

Blackman, S. S. Jr. (1936). Intranuclear inclusion bodies in kidney and liver caused by lead poisoning. *Bull. Johns Hopkins Hosp.* **58**, 384

Blinzinger, K., Anzil, A. P. and Jellinger, K. (1974). On so-called 'virus-like' intranuclear filaments in brain autopsy material: A reappraisal on hand of two fatal cases of tick borne encephalitis. *Acta Neuropathol.* **28**, 69

Blom, J., Mansa, B. and Wiik, A. (1976). A study of Russell bodies in human monoclonal plasma cells by means of immunofluorescence and electron microscopy. *Acta path. microbiol. scand. Sect. A.* **84**, 335

Bloom, G. D. (1967). A nucleus with cytoplasmic features. *J. Cell Biol.* **35**, 266

Bloom, S. and Cancilla, P. A. (1969). Conformational changes in myocardial nuclei of rats. *Circulat. Res.* **24**, 189

Boquist, L. (1969). Intranuclear rods in pancreatic islet β-cells. *J. Cell Biol.* **43**, 377

Bourgeois, C. A., Hemon, D. and Bouteille, M. (1979). Structural relationship between the nucleolus and the nuclear envelope. *J. Ultrastruct. Res.* **68**, 328

Bouteille, M. (1972). Ultrastructural localization of proteins and nucleoproteins in the interphase nucleus. Karolinska symposia on research methods in endocrinology. 5th Symposium May 29–31. Gene transcription in reproductive tissue

Bouteille, M., Fontaine, C., Vedrenne, Cl. and Delarue, J. (1965). Sur un cas d'encéphalite subaiguë à inclusions. Etude anatomo-clinique et ultrastructurale. *Revue Neurol.* **113**, 454

Bouteille, M., Kalifat, S. R. and Delarue, J. (1967). Ultrastructural variations of nuclear bodies in human diseases. *J. Ultrastruct. Res.* **19**, 474

Boyle, W. F., McCoy, E. G. and Fogarty, W. A. (1971). Electron microscopic identification of virus-like particles in laryngeal papilloma. *Ann. Otol. Rhinol. Laryngol.* **80**, 693

Bracken, E. C., Beaver, D. L. and Randall, C. C. (1958). Histochemical studies of viral and lead-induced intranuclear bodies. *J. Path. Bact.* **75**, 253

Brandes, D., Schofield, B. H. and Anton, E. (1965). Nuclear mitochondria? *Science,* **149**, 1373

Brinkley, B. R. (1965). The fine structure of the nucleolus in mitotic divisions of Chinese hamster cells *in vitro. J. Cell Biol.* **27**, 411

Brittin, G. M., Tanaka, Y. and Brecher, G. (1963). Intranuclear inclusions in multiple myeloma and macroglobulinemia. *Blood* **21**, 335

Brock, M. A. and Hay, R. J. (1971). Comparative ultrastructure of chick fibroblasts *in vitro* at early and late stages during their growth span. *J. Ultrastruct. Res.* **36**, 291

Brooks, R. E. and Siegel, B. V. (1967). Nuclear bodies of normal and pathological human lymph node cells. An electron microscopic study. *Blood* **29**, 269

Brown, D. D. and Gurdon, J. B. (1964). Absence of ribosomal RNA synthesis in the anucleolate mutant of *Xenopus laevis. Proc. Natn. Acad. Sci., USA* **51**, 139

Brown, W. J., Kotorii, K. and Riehl, J.-L. (1968). Ultrastructural studies in myoclonus epilepsy (Clinical Unverricht-Lafora's disease). *Neurology* **18**, 427

Brytscheff, A. A. (1926). Die Wismutbehandlung der Syphilis mit dem russischen Präparat Bijochinol. *Zbl. Haut Geschlkr.* **18**, 433

Bucciarelli, E. (1966). Intranuclear cisternae resembling structures of the Golgi complex. *J. Cell Biol.* **30**, 664

Bunney, M. H. (1982). *Viral warts: their biology and treatment.* New York: Oxford University Press

Burr, R. E., Gotto, A. M. and Beaver, D. L. (1965). Isolation and analysis of renal bismuth inclusions. *Toxicol. appl. Pharmacol.* **7**, 588

Busch, H. and Smetana, K. (1970). *The Nucleolus.* New York & London: Academic Press

Busch, H., Byvoet, P. and Smetana, K. (1963). The nucleolus of the cancer cell: a review. *Cancer Res.* **23**, 313

Büttner, D. W. (1968). Elektronenmikroskopische Beobachtung von Sphaeridien im karyoplasma der pauropsidenzelle. *Z. Zellforsch. Mikrosk. Anat.* **85**, 527

Büttner, D. W. and Horstmann, E. (1968). Stabförmige Strukturen im Interphasenkern von Epithelgeweben. *Exp. Cell Res.* **49**, 686

Cajal, R. Y. S. (1909). Histologie du système nerveux de l'homme et des vertebrés. Madrid: Edition Francaise par l Azoulay, Consejo Superior de Investigaciones Cientificas

Cajal, R. Y. S. (1911). *Histologie du système nerveux de l'homme et des vertebrés.* II Trans L. Azoulay. Paris: Maloine

Calvery, H. O. (1938). Chronic effects of ingested lead and arsenic; a review and correlation. *J. Am. med. Ass.* **111**, 1722

Cameron, I. L., Pavlat, W. A. and Jeter, J. R. Jr. (1979). Chromatin substructure: An electron microscopic study of thin-sectioned chromatin subjected to sequential protein extraction and water swelling procedures. *Anat. Rec.* **194**, 547

Cammermeyer, J. (1963). Cytological manifestations of aging in rabbit and chinchilla brains. *J. Gerontol.* **18**, 41

Caramia, F., Ghergo, F. G. and Menghini, C. (1967). A glycogen body in liver nuclei. *J. Ultrastruct. Res.* **19**, 573

Caramia, F. Ghergo, F. G., Branciari, C. and Menghini, C. (1968). New aspect of hepatic nuclear glycogenosis in diabetes. *J. clin. Path.* **21**, 19

Carlson, E. C. and Ollerich, D. A. (1969). Intranuclear tubules in Trophoblast III of rat and mouse chorioallantoic placenta. *J. Ultrastruct. Res.* **28**, 150

Carmichael, N. G. and Fowler, B. A. (1980). Separate and combined chronic mercuric chloride and sodium selenate administration in rats: Histological, ultrastructural and x-ray microanalytical studies of liver and kidney. *J. Environ. Path. & Toxicol.* **3**, 399

Caspersson, T. (1950). *Cell Growth and Cell Function: a cytochemical study.* New York: W. W. Norton

Caspersson, T. and Santesson, L. (1942). Studies on protein metabolism in the cells of epithelial tumors. *Acta Radiol. (Suppl.)* **46**, 1

Caspersson, T. and Schultz, J. (1940). Ribonucleic acids in both nucleus and cytoplasm and the function of the nucleolus. *Proc. Natn Acad. Sci. USA* **26**, 507

Cawley, J. C. (1972). The microtubules of leukaemic Rieder cells. An ultrastructural study. *Scand. J. Haemat.* **9**, 417

160

Cazal, P. and Mirouze, J. (1951). Une anomalie mal connue des cellules hépatiques: les noyaux vacuolaires et leur signification physiopathologique probable dans le syndrome d'adaptation. *Presse méd.* **59,** 571

Cervera, J. (1979). Effects of thermic shock on HEp-2 cells. *J. Ultrastruct. Res.* **66,** 182

Chaly, N., Lord, A. and Lafontaine, J. G. (1977). A light and electron microscope study of nuclear structure throughout the cell cycle in the Euglenoid *Astasia longa* (Jahn). *J. Cell Sci.* **27,** 23

Chen, T. T., Watanabe, I., Zeman, W. and Mealey, J. (1969). Subacute sclerosing panencephalitis: propagation of measles virus from brain biopsy in tissue culture. *Science* **163,** 1193

Chiga, M., Kume, F. and Millar, R. C. (1966). Nucleolar alteration produced by actinomycin D and the delayed onset of hepatic regeneration in rats. *Lab. Invest.* **15,** 1403

Chipps, H. D. and Duff, G. L. (1942). Glycogen infiltration of liver cell nuclei. *Am. J. Path.* **18,** 645

Choie, D. D. and Richter, G. W. (1972). Lead poisoning: Rapid formation of intranuclear inclusions. *Science* **177,** 1194

Cinti, S., Enzi, G., Cigolini, M. and Bosello, O. (1983). Ultrastructural features of cultured mature adipocyte precursors from adipose tissue in multiple symmetric lipomatosis. *Ultrastruct. Path.* **5,** 145

Cinti, S., Balercia, G., Osculati, F., Dantchev, D. and Mathé,G. (1985). Ultrastructural appearance of malignant non-Hodgkin's lymphomas and lymphoid leukemias. *Biomed. Pharmacother.* **39,** 123

Clark, W. H. (1960). Electron microscope studies of nuclear extrusions in pancreatic acinar cells of the rat. *J. biophys. biochem. Cytol.* **7,** 345

Clattenburg, R. E., Singh, R. P. and Montemurro, D. G. (1972). Intranuclear filamentous inclusions in neurons of the rabbit hypothalamus. *J. Ultrastruct. Res.* **39,** 549

Clausen, K. P. and Von Haam, E. (1969). Fine structure of malignancy-associated changes (MAC) in peripheral human leukocytes. *Acta cytol.* **13,** 435

Clyman, M. J. (1963). A new structure observed in the nucleolus of the human endometrial epithelial cell. *Am. J. Obstet. Gynec.* **86,** 430

Coalson, J. J., Mohr, J. A., Pirtle, J. K., Dee, A. L. and Rhoades, E. R. (1970). Electron microscopy of neoplasms in the lung with special emphasis on the alveolar cell carcinoma. *Am. Rev. resp. Dis.* **101,** 181

Coggeshall, R. E. and Fawcett, D. W. (1964). The fine structure of the central nervous system of the leech *Hirudo medicinalis. J. Neurophysiol.* **27,** 229

Coggeshall, R. E., Coulter, J. D. and Willis, W. D. Jr. (1974). Unmyelinated axons in the ventral roots of the cat lumbosacral enlargement. *J. comp. Neur.* **153,** 39

Cohen, A. H. and Sundeen, J. R. (1976). The nuclear fibrous lamina in human cells: Studies on its appearance and distribution. *Anat. Rec.* **186,** 471

Collins, D. N. (1974). Ultrastructural study of intranuclear inclusions in the exocrine pancreas in Reye's syndrome. *Lab. Invest.* **30,** 333

Cooper, N. S. (1956). Early cytologic changes produced by carcinogens. *Bull. N. Y. med. Soc.* **32,** 79

Couvreur, Y., Leeman, M. and Ketelbant, P. (1984). 'Viral' intranuclear inclusions. *Ultrastruct. Path.* **7,** 67

Cowdry, E. V. and Paletta, F. X. (1941). Changes in cellular, nuclear and nucleolar sizes during methylcholanthrene epidermal carcinogenesis. *J. Natn. Cancer. Inst.* **1,** 745

Cragg, B. G. (1976). Ultrastructural features of human cerebral cortex. *J. Anat.* **121,** 331

Crissman, R. S., Lane, R. D., Didio, L. J. A. and Johnson, R. C. (1978). The relationship of myofilaments and T-tubules to the nuclei of canine myocardium studied by scanning and transmission electron microscopy. *J. Submicr. Cytol.* **10,** 155

Dahl, E. (1970). The fine structure of nuclear inclusions. *J. Anat.* **106,** 255

Dahl, E. (1970). Studies of the fine structure of ovarian interstitial tissue. 6. Effects of clomiphene on the thecal gland of the domestic fowl. *Z. Zellforsch. mikrosk. Anat.* **109,** 227

Dallenbach, F. D. (1964). Phenolrotausscheidung und trypanblauspeicherung bei der Blei-Nephropathie der ratte. *Virchows Arch. path. Anat. Physiol.* **338,** 91

Dallenbach, F. D. (1965). Uptake of radioactive lead by tubular epithelium of the kidney. *Verh. deutsch. Ges. Path.* **49,** 179

Dardick, I., Setterfield, G., Hall, R., Bladon, T., Little, J. and Kaplan, G. (1981). Nuclear alterations during lymphocyte transformation. *Am. J. Pathol.* **103,** 10

Darlington, R. W. and Moss, L. H. (1968). Herpes virus envelopment. *J. Virol.* **2,** 48

Daskal, Y., Prestayko, A. W. and Busch, H. (1974). Ultrastructural and biochemical studies of the isolated fibrillar component of nucleoli from Novikoff hepatoma ascites cells. *Exp. Cell Res.* **88,** 1

Daskal, I., Merski, J. A., Hughes, B. B. and Busch, H. (1975). The effects of cycloheximide on the ultrastructure of rat liver cells. *Exp. Cell Res.* **93,** 935

Daskal, Y., Woodard, C., Crooke, S. T. and Busch, H. (1978). Comparative ultrastructural studies of nucleoli of tumor cells treated with adriamycin and the newer anthracyclines, carminomycin and marcellomycin. *Cancer Res.* **38,** 467

David, S. and Nathaniel, E. J. H. (1978). Intranuclear inclusions in the developing neurons of the rat cuneate nuclei. *Cell Tiss. Res.* **193,** 525

Davies, H. G. (1961). Structure in nucleated erythrocytes. *J. biophys. biochem. Cytol.* **9,** 671

De Kretser, D. M. (1967). Changes in the fine structure of the human testicular interstitial cells after treatment with human gonadotrophins. *Z. Zellforsch. Mikrosk. Anat.* **83,** 344

De Kretser, D. M. (1968). Crystals of Reinke in the nuclei of human testicular interstitial cells. *Experientia* **24,** 587

De Man, J. C. H. and Noorduyn, N. J. (1967). Light and electron microscopic radioautography of hepatic cell nucleoli in mice treated with actinomycin D. *J. Cell Biol.* **33,** 489

Derenzini, M. and Bonetti, E. (1975). Cycloheximide-induced ultrastructural changes in hepatocyte nuclei in partially hepatectomized rats. *Virchows Arch. B Cell Path.* **19,** 115

Derenzini, M. and Moyne, G. (1978). The nucleolar origin of certain perichromatin-like granules: A study with α-Amanitine. *J. Ultrastruct. Res.* **62,** 213

Derenzini, M., Marinozzi, V. and Novello, F. (1976). Effects of α-Amanitine on chromatin in regenerating rat hepatocytes. A biochemical and morphologic study. *Virchows Arch. B Cell Path.* **20,** 307

De Robertis, E. (1956). Electron microscopic observations on the submicroscopic morphology of the meiotic nucleus and chromosomes. *J. biophys. biochem. Cytol.* **2,** 785

De The, G., Riviere, M. and Bernhard, W. (1960). Examen au microscope electronique de la tumeur VX 2 du lapin domestique derivee du papillome de Shope. *Bull. Cancer* **47,** 569

Dixon, J. S. (1970). Nuclear bodies in normal and chromatolytic sympathetic neurons. *Anat. Rec.* **168,** 179

Djaldetti, M. and Lewinski, U. H. (1978). Origin of intranuclear inclusions in myeloma cells. *Scand. J. Haematol.* **20,** 200

Djaldetti, M., Bessler, H., Fishman, P, and Machtey, I. (1975). Functional and ultrastructural studies of Sézary cells. *Nouv. Rev. Fr. Hémat.* **15,** 567

Doak, R. L., Munnell, J. F. and Ragland, W. L. (1973). Ultrastructure of tumor cells in Marek's disease virus-infected chickens. *Am. J. Vet. Res.* **34,** 1063

Dorfman, R. F. (1968). Diagnosis of Burkitt's tumor in the United States. *Cancer* **21,** 563

Dorn, A., Nowak, R., Dietzel, K. and Reichel, A. (1971). Untersuchungen am Juvenilen Nasenrachenfibrom. *Acta Histochem. (Jena).* **39,** 162

Douvas, A. S., Harrington, C. A. and Bonner, J. (1975). Major nonhistone proteins of rat liver chromatin: Preliminary identification of myosin, actin, tubulin and tropomyosin. *Proc. Nat. Acad. Sci. USA* **72,** 3902

Dubois-Dalcq, M., Schumacher, G. and Sever, J. L. (1973). Acute multiple sclerosis: Electron-microscopic evidence for and against a viral agent in the plaques. *Lancet* **2,** 1408

Dubrauszky, V. and Pohlmann, G. (1960a). Strukturveranderungen am Nukleolus von Korpusendometriumzellen während der Sekretionsphase. *Naturwissenschaften* **47,** 523

Dubrauszky, V. and Pohlmann, G. (1960b). Veränderlungen der submikroskopischen struktur von Drüsenzellen der Corpusmucosa während des Zyklus. *Proceedings of the European Conference on Electron Microscopy* Vol II, p. 862

Dudley, H. R. and Spiro, D. (1961). The fine structure of bone cells. *J. biophys. biochem. Cytol.* **11,** 627

Dumont, A. and Roberts, A. (1971). Ultrastructure of complex nuclear bodies produced experimentally in hamster peritoneal macrophages. *J. Ultrastruct. Res.* **36,** 483

Duryee, W. K. (1956). Precancer cells in amphibian adenocarcinoma. *Ann. N. Y. Acad. Sci.* **63,** 1280

Duryee, W. K. and Doherty, J. R. (1954). Nuclear and cytoplasmic organoids in the living cell. *Ann. N. Y. Acad. Sci.* **58,** 1210

Dwyer, N. and Blobel, G. (1976). A modified procedure for the isolation of a pore complex-lamina fraction from rat liver nuclei. *J. Cell Biol.* **70,** 581

Edstrom, J. E. Grampp, W. and Schor, N. (1961). The intracellular distribution and heterogeneity of ribonucleic acid in starfish oocytes. *J. biophys. biochem. Cytol.* **11,** 549

Ehrlich, P. (1883). Ueber das Vorkommen von Glykogen in Diabetischen und in normalen organismus. *Z. klin. Med.* **6,** 33

Eimoto, T. (1977). Ultrastructure of an infantile hemangiopericytoma. *Cancer* **40,** 2161

El-Bermani, Al-W. I., Montvilo, J. A. and Bloomquist, E. I. (1981). Intranuclear rodlets in a pulmonary neuroepithelial body of a rabbit. *Cell Tiss. Res.* **220,** 439

Emura, M. (1978). Morphological studies on the development of tracheal epithelium in the Syrian golden hamster. IV. Electron microscopy: Blebbing of nuclear membrane. *Z. Versuchstierk. Bd.* **20,** S 163

Engedal, H., Jensen, H. and Saetersdal, T. S. (1977). Ultrastructure of abnormal membrane inclusions in nuclei of human myocardial cells. *Br. Heart J.* **39,** 145

Engel, E., McGee, B. J. and Harris, H. (1969). Cytogenic and nuclear studies on A9 and B82 cells fused together by Sendai virus: The early phase. *J. Cell Sci.* **8,** 93

Epstein, M.A. (1962). Observations on the mode of release of herpes virus from infected HeLa cells. *J. Cell Biol.* **12,** 589

Epstein, M. A. and Achong, B. G. (1965). Fine structural organization of human lymphoblasts of a tissue culture strain (EB1) from Burkitt's lymphoma. *J. Natl Cancer Inst.* **34**, 241

Erlandson, R. A. (1981). *Diagnostic Transmission Electron Microscopy of Human Tumors.* New York: Masson Publishing USA

Erlandson, R. A. and Tandler, B. (1972). Ultrastructure of acinic cell carcinoma of the parotid gland. *Archs Path.* **93**, 130

Farquhar, M. G. and Palade, G. E. (1962). Functional evidence for the existence of a third cell type in the renal glomerulus. Phagocytosis of filtration residues by a distinctive 'third' cell. *J. Cell Biol.* **13**, 55

Fawcett, D. W. (1981). *The Cell,* 2nd Edn. Philadelphia and London: Saunders

Fawcett, D. W. (1966). On the occurrence of a fibrous lamina on the inner aspect of the nuclear envelope in certain cells of vertebrates. *Am. J. Anat.* **119**, 129

Fawcett, D. W. and Witebsky, F. (1964). Observations on the ultrastructure of nucleated erythrocytes and thrombocytes, with particular reference to the structural basis of their discoidal shape. *Z. Zellforsch. Mikrosk. Anat.* **62**, 785

Feldhaus, F. J., Themann, H., Wagner, H. and Verhagen, A. (1977). Feinstrukturelle Untersuchungen über das Nuclear-Channel-System im menschlichen Endometrium. *Arch. Gynäk.* **223**, 195–204

Feldherr, C. M. (1962). The nuclear annuli as pathways for nucleocytoplasmic exchanges. *J. Cell Biol.* **14**, 65

Feldherr, C. M. (1972). Structure and function of the nuclear envelope. *Advances in Cell and Molecular Biology,* Vol. 2, 273, Ed. by E. J. DuPraw. New York & London: Academic Press

Feldman, M. L. and Peters, A. (1972). Intranuclear rods and sheets in rat cochlear nucleus. *J. Neurocytol.* **1**, 109

Ferenczy, A. (1976). The ultrastructural morphology of gynecologic neoplasms. *Cancer* **38**, 463

Ferrans, V. J., Jones, M., Maron, B. J. and Roberts, W. C. (1975). The nuclear membranes in hypertrophied human cardiac muscle cells. *Am. J. Path.* **78**, 427

Field, E. J. and Peat, A. (1971). Intranuclear inclusions in neurones and glia: a study in the ageing mouse. *Gerontologia* **17**, 129

Finch, J. T. and Klug, A. (1976). Solonoidal model for superstructure in chromatin. *Natl. Acad Sci. Proc. USA* **73**, 1897

Finner, L. L. and Calvery, H. O. (1939). Pathologic changes in rats and in dogs fed diets containing lead and arsenic compounds. *Archs. Path.* **27**, 433

Firkin, B. G. (1969). The fine structure and chemistry of haemopoietic tissue. In *The Biological Basis of Medicine,* Vol. 3. Ed. by E. E. Bittar and N. Bittar. New York and London: Academic Press

Fisher, H. W. and Cooper, T. W. (1967). Electron microscope observations on the nuclear pores of HeLa cells. *J. Cell Biol.* **35**, p. 40A, Abstract No. 79

Flaks, B. and Flaks, A. (1970). Fine structure of nuclear inclusions in murine pulmonary tumour cells. *Cancer Res.* **30**, 1437

Flaxman, B. A., Zelazny, G., VanScott, E. J. (1971). Nonspecificity of characteristic cells in mycosis fungiodes. *Arch. Dermatol.* **104**, 141

Fletcher, V., Zackheim, H. S. and Beckstead, J. H. (1984). Circulating Sézary cells. *Arch. Path. Lab. Med.* **108**, 954

Fortman, G. J. and Winkelmann, R. K. (1977). The Merkel cell in oral human mucosa. *J. Dent. Res.* **56**, 1303

Fowler, B. A. and Goyer, R. A. (1975). Bismuth localization within nuclear inclusions by x-ray micro-analysis. Effects of accelerating voltage. *J. Histochem. Cytochem.* **23**, 722

Frable, W. J., Still, W. J. S. and Kay, S. (1971). Carcinoma of the pancreas, infantile type. A light and electron microscopic study. *Cancer* **27**, 667

Franke, W. W. (1967). Zur Feinstruktur isolierter Kernmembranen aus tierischen Zellen. *Zeitschrift fur Zellforschung* **80**, 585

Franke, W. W. (1970a). Attachment of muscle filaments to the outer membrane of the nuclear envelope. *Z. Zellforsch.* **III**, 143

Franke, W. W. (1970b). On the universality of nuclear pore complex structure. *Z. Zellforsch.* **105**, 405

Franke, W. W. and Schinko, W. (1969). Nuclear shape in muscle cells. *J. Cell Biol.* **42**, 326

Frasca, J. M., Auerbach, O., Parks, V. and Stoeckenius, W. (1965). Electron microscope observations of nuclear evaginations in bronchial epithelium. *Exp. Molec. Path.* **4**, 340

Freeman, A. I. and Journey, L. J. (1971). Ultrastructural studies on monocytic leukaemia. *Br. J. Haematol.* **20**, 225

Frenster, J. H. (1974). Ultrastructure and function of heterochromatin and euchromatin. *The Cell Nucleus* Vol. I. Ed. by H. Busch. New York, London: Academic Press

Frink, R., Krupp, P. P. and Young, R. A. (1978). Intranuclear rodlets in woodchuck thyroid follicular cells. *Cell Tiss. Res.* **193**, 561

163

Fruhling, L. and Porte, A. (1958). Contribution de la microscopic électronique à l'étude d'un sarcome plasmocytaire. *Ann. Anat. Pathol.* **3,** 538

Fruhling, L., Porte, A. and Kempf, J. (1960). Stockage de glycoprotéines dans la citerne périnucléaire avec formation d'inclusions dans le noyau de cellules plasmocytaires. *C. R. Acad. Sci.* **251,** 794

Fujimoto, Y., Okada, M. and Okada, K. (1970). Electron microscopic studies on Marek's disease. V. Light and electron microscopic observations on skeletal muscle lesions. Proc. 70th Meet. of Jap. Soc. Vet. *Jap. J. vet. Sci.* **32,** 221

Fukui, Y. (1978). Intranuclear actin bundles induced by dimethyl sulfoxide in interphase nucleus of *Dictyostelium. J. Cell Biol.* **76,** 146

Gajkowska, B., Puvion, E. and Bernhard, W. (1977). Unusual perinuclear accumulation of ribonucleoprotein granules induced by Camptothecin in isolated liver cells. *J. Ultrastruct. Res.* **60,** 335

Gambetti, P. and Gonatas, N. K. (1967). Fibrils and lattice-like intranuclear structures in nuclei of neurons. *Riv. Patol. Nerv. Ment.* **88,** 188

Gay, H. (1956). Chromosome-nuclear membrane-cytoplasmic interrelations in Drosophila. *J. biophys. biochem. Cytol.* **2,** No. 4 Suppl., 407

Gerace, L., Blum, A. and Blobel, G. (1978). Immunocytochemical localization of the major polypeptides of the nuclear pore complex-lamina fraction. *J. Cell Biol.* **79,** 546

Ghadially, F. N. (1958). Comparative morphological study of keratoacanthoma of man and similar experimentally produced lesions in rabbit. *J. Path. Bact.* **75,** 441

Ghadially, F. N. (1961). The role of the hair follicle in the origin and evolution of some cutaneous neoplasms of man and experimental animals. *Cancer* **14,** 801

Ghadially, F. N. (1971). Keratoacanthoma. In *Dermatology in General Medicine*, p. 425. Ed. by T. B. Fitzpatrick and D. P. Johnson. New York and Maidenhead: McGraw-Hill

Ghadially, F. N. (1975). *Ultrastructural Pathology of the Cell,* 1st Edn. London: Butterworths

Ghadially, F. N. (1980). *Diagnostic Electron Microscopy of Tumours.* London: Butterworths

Ghadially, F. N. (1985). *Diagnostic Electron Microscopy of Tumours,* 2nd Edn. London: Butterworths

Ghadially, F. N. and Lalonde, J.-M. A. (1979). Single-membrane-bound pseudoinclusions in the nucleus. *J. Submicr. Cytol.* **11,** 413

Ghadially, F. N. and Lalonde, J.-M. A. (1980). Genesis of concentric laminated inclusions in the nucleus. *Experientia* **36,** 59

Ghadially, F. N. and Mehta, P. N. (1970). Ultrastructure of osteogenic sarcoma. *Cancer* **25,** 1457

Ghadially, F. N. and Parry, E. W. (1966). Ultrastructure of a human hepatocellular carcinoma and surrounding non-neoplastic liver. *Cancer* **19,** 1989

Ghadially, F. N. and Roy, S. (1969a). *Ultrastructure of Synovial Joints in Health and Disease.* London: Butterworths

Ghadially, F. N. and Roy, S. (1969b). Ultrastructural changes in the synovial membrane in lipohaemarthrosis. *Ann. rheum. Dis.* **28,** 529

Ghadially, F. N. and Yong, N. K. (1976). Ultrastructural and x-ray analytical studies on intranuclear bismuth inclusions. *Virchows Arch. B. Cell Path.* **21,** 45

Ghadially, F. N., Barton, B. W. and Kerridge, D. F. (1963). The etiology of keratoacanthoma. *Cancer* **16,** 603

Ghadially, F. N., Bhatnager, R. and Fuller, J. A. (1972). Waxing and waning of nuclear fibrous lamina. *Archs Path.* **94,** 303

Ghadially, F. N., Dick, C. E. and Lalonde, J.-M. A. (1980a). Thickening of the nuclear lamina in injured human semilunar cartilages. *J. Anat.* **131,** 717

Ghadially, F. N., Fuller, J. A. and Kirkaldy-Willis, W. H. (1971). Ultrastructure of full-thickness defects in articular cartilage. *Archs Path.* **92,** 356

Ghadially, F. N., Harawi, S. and Khan, W. (1985a). Diagnostic ultrastructural markers in alveolar cell carcinoma. *J. Submicrosc. Cytol.* **17,** 269

Ghadially, F. N., Lalonde, J.-M. A. and Yong, N. K. (1980b). Myofibroblasts and intracellular collagen in torn semilunar cartilages. *J. Submicrosc. Cytol.* **12,** 447

Ghadially, F. N., Meachim, G. and Collins, D. H. (1965). Extracellular lipid in the matrix of human articular cartilage. *Ann. rheum. Dis.* **24,** 136

Ghadially, F. N., Oryschak, A. F. and Mitchell, D. M. (1974). Nuclear fibrous lamina in pathological human synovial membrane. *Virchows Arch. Abt. B Zellpath.* **15,** 223

Ghadially, F. N., Senoo, A. and Fuse, Y. (1985b). A serial section study of nuclear pockets containing nuclear material. *J Submicrosc. Cytol.* **17,** 687

Ghadially, F. N., Stinson, J. C., Payne, C. M. and Leibovitz, A. (1985c). Intranuclear helioid inclusions. *J. Submicrosc. Cytol.* **17,** 469

Givan, K. F. and Jézéquel, A. M. (1969). Infectious canine hepatitis: a virologic and ultrastructural study. *Lab. Invest.* **20,** 36

Glick, A. D., Vestal, B. K., Flexner, J. M. and Collins, R. D. (1978). Ultrastructural study of acute lymphocytic leukemia: Comparison with immunologic studies. *Blood* **52,** 311

Goessens, G. and LePoint, A. (1974). The fine structure of the nucleolus during interphase and mitosis in Ehrlich tumour cellls cultivated *in vitro*. *Exp. Cell Res.* **87,** 63

Goldblatt, P. J., Sullivan, R. J. and Farber, E. (1969a). Morpholic and metabolic alterations in hepatic cell nucleoli induced by varying doses of actinomycin D. *Cancer Res.* **29,** 124

Goldblatt, P. J., Sullivan, R. J. and Farber, E. (1969b). Induction of partial nucleolar segregation in hepatic parenchymal cells by actinomycin D, following inhibition of ribonucleic acid synthesis by ethionine. *Lab. Invest.* **20,** 283

Golomb, H. M. and Bahr, G. F. (1971). Scanning electron microscopic observations of surface structure of isolated human chromosomes. *Science* **171,** 1024

Golomb, H. M., Bahr, G. F. and Borgaonkar, D. S. (1971). Analysis of human chromosomal variants by quantitative electron microscopy. I. Group D chromosome with giant satellites. *Genetics* **69,** 123

Gonzalez-Crussi, F., Hull, M. T. and Mirkin, D. L. (1978). Intranuclear filaments in a soft tissue sarcoma. *Human Pathol.* **9,** 189

Gouranton, J. and Thomas, D. (1974). Cytochemical, ultrastructural, and autoradiographic study of the intranuclear crystals in the midgut cells of *Gyrinus marinus* Gyll. *J. Ultrastruct. Res.* **48,** 227

Gouranton, J., Folliot, R. and Thomas, D. (1979). Fine structure and nature of the crystalloid intranuclear and intracytoplasmic inclusions in dog cauda epididymidis. *J. Ultrastruct. Res.* **69,** 273

Goyer, R. A. (1968). The renal tubule in lead poisoning. 1. Mitochondrial swelling and aminoaciduria. *Lab. Invest.* **19,** 71

Goyer, R. A., May, P., Cates, M. M. and Krigman, M. R. (1970). Lead and protein content of isolated intranuclear inclusion bodies from kidneys of lead-poisoned rats. *Lab. Invest.* **22,** 245

Graham, R. C. and Bernier, G. M. (1975). The bone marrow in multiple myeloma: correlation of plasma cell ultrastructure and clinical state. *Medicine* **54,** 225

Granboulan, N. and Bernhard, W. (1961). Cytochimie ultrastructurale. Exploration des structures nucleaires par digestion enzymatique. *C. r. Soc. Biol.* **155,** 1767

Granboulan, N., Tournier, P., Wicker, R. and Bernhard, W. (1963). An electron microscope study of the development of SV40 virus. *J. Cell Biol.* **17,** 423

Granboulan, N. and Granboulan, P. (1964). Cytochimie ultrastructurale du nucleole. I. Mise en evidence de chromatine a l'interieur du nucleole. *Exp. Cell. Res.* **34,** 71

Granzow, C. and Granzow, V. (1975). Glycogen synthesis by two Ehrlich ascites tumour cell strains *in vitro*. *Virchows Arch. B Cell Path.* **18,** 281

Grasso, J. A., Swift, H. and Ackerman, G. A. (1962). Observations on the development of erythrocytes in mammalian fetal liver. *J. Cell. Biol.* **14,** 235

Gray, E. G. and Guillery, R. W. (1963). On nuclear structure in the ventral nerve cord of the leech *Hirudo medicinalis*. *Z. Zelforsch. mikrosk. Anat.* **59,** 738

Greenstein, J. P. (1954). Chemistry of the tumour-bearing host. In *Biochemistry of Cancer,* p. 507. New York: Academic Press

Gregg, M. B. and Morgan, C. (1959). Reduplication of nuclear membranes in HeLa cells infected with adenoviruses. *J. biophys. biochem. Cytol.* **6,** 539

Groth, D. H., Stettler, L. and Mackay, G. (1976). Interactions of mercury, cadmium, selenium, tellurium, arsenic and beryllium. In *Effects and Dose-Response Relationships of Toxic Metals.* Ed. by G. F. Nordberg, pp. 527–543. Amsterdam: Elsevier Scientific Publishing Co

Grünblatt, G. N. (1925). Zur Frage der Mikrosopie und Mikrochemie der Harnsedimente bei Wismutbehandlung. *Zbl Haut Geschlke* **16,** 725

Gueft, B. and Molnar, J. J. (1961). The lead poisoned liver cell under the electron microscope. In *Abstracts of the 58th Annual Meeting of the American Association of Pathologists and Bacteriologists,* p. 45. Chicago, Ill.

Gullvåg, B. M., Skaar, H. and Ophus, E. M. (1974). An ultrastructural study of lead accumulation within leaves of *Rhytidiadelphus squarrosus* (Hedw.) Warnst. A comparison between experimental and environmental poisoning. *J. Bryol.* **8,** 117

Gyorkey, F., Gyorkey, P. and Sinkovics, J. G. (1980). Origin and significance of intranuclear tubular inclusions in type II pulmonary alveolar epithelial cells of patients with bleomycin and busulfan toxicity. *Ultrastruct. Path.* **1,** 211

Hadek, R. and Swift, H. (1962). Nuclear extrusion and intracisternal inclusions in the rabbit blastocyst. *J. Cell Biol.* **13,** 445

Haggis, G. H. and Bond, E. F. (1978). Three-dimensional view of the chromatin in freeze-fractured chicken erythrocyte nuclei. *J. Microscopy* **115,** 225

Harris, C., Grady, H. and Svoboda, D. (1968). Alterations in pancreatic and hepatic ultrastructure following acute cyclohexamide intoxication. *J. Ultrastruct. Res.* **22,** 240

Hashimoto, K., Brownstein, M. H. and Jakobiec, F. A. (1974). Dermatofibrosarcoma protuberans. A tumor with perineural and endoneural cell features. *Arch. Dermatol.* **110,** 874

Hay, E. D. (1968). Structure and function of the nucleolus in developing cells. In *The Nucleus,* pp. 2–79. Ed. by A. Dalton and F. Haguenau. New York: Academic Press

Hay, E. D. and Revel, J. P. (1962). The DNA component of the nucleolus studied in autoradiographs viewed with the electron microscope. In *Fifth Int. Congr. Electron Microscopy, Philadelphia.* Vol. 2, pp. 1–7. New York: Academic Press

Hay, E. D. and Revel, J. P. (1963). The fine structure of the DNP-component of the nucleus. An electron microscopic study utilizing autoradiography to localize DNA synthesis. *J. Cell Biol.* **16,** 29

Hayhoe, F. G. J., Quaglino, D. and Doll, R. (1964). *The Cytology and Cytochemistry of Acute Leukaemia,* p. 73. London: Her Majesty's Stationery Office

Heath, J. C. (1954). The effect of cobalt on mitosis in tissue culture. *Exp. Cell Res.* **6,** 311

Heimann-Trosien, A. (1925). Über Gewöhnungser-scheinungen an der Niere bei Wismut-Behandlung. *Klin. Eschr.* **4,** 1963

Heine, U., Severak, L., Kondratic, J. and Bonar, R. A. (1971). The behaviour of HeLa-S$_3$ cells under the influence of supranormal temperatures. *J. Ultrastruct. Res.* **34,** 375

Henderson, D. W. and Papadimitriou, J. M. (1982). *Ultrastructural Appearances of Tumours.* London, Melbourne, New York: Churchill Livingstone

Henry, K. and Petts, V. (1969). Nuclear bodies in human thymus. *J. Ultrastruct. Res.* **27,** 330

Hill, D. L. (1985). Morphology of nasopharyngeal angiofibroma. An electron microscopic study. *J. Submicrosc. Cytol.* **17,** 443

Himes, M. M. and Pollister, A. W. (1962). Glycogen accumulation in the nucleus. *J. Histochem. Cytochem.* **10,** 175

Hinglais-Guillaud, N., Moricard, R. and Bernhard, W. (1961). Ultrastructure des cancers pavimenteux invasip du col uterin chez la femme. *Bull. Cancer* **49,** 283

Hirano, A. and Zimmerman, H. M. (1967). Some new cytological observations of the normal rat ependymal cell. *Anat. Rec.* **158,** 293

Hoenig, E. M., Margolis, G. and Kilham, L. (1974). Experimental adenovirus infection of the mouse adrenal gland. II. Electron microscopic observations. *Am. J. Path.* **75,** 375

Holmgren, E. (1899). Weitere Mitteilungen über den Bau der Nervenzellen. *Anat. Anz.* **16,** 388

Hoover, K. L., Harshbarger, J. C., Lee, C. W., Banfield, W. and Chang, S. C. (1981). Intranuclear inclusion bodies within neurons of spinal and cranial ganglia in three cyprinid species. *Cell Tiss. Res.* **218,** 529

Horstmann, E. (1962). Elektronenmikroskopie des menschlichen nebenhodenepithels. *Z. Zellforsch. mikrosk. Anat.* **57,** 692

Horstmann, E. (1965). Die Kerneinschlüsse im nebenhodenepithel des hundes. *Z. Zellforsch. mikrosk. Anat.* **65,** 770

Horstmann, E., Richter, R. and Roosen-Runge, E. (1966). Zur elektronenmikroskopie der kerneinschlüsse im menschlichen nebenhodenepithel. *Z. Zellforsch. mikrosk. Anat.* **69,** 69

Horta-Barbosa, L., Fuccillo, D. A. and Sever, J. L. (1969). Subacute sclerosing panencephalitis: isolation of measles virus from a brain biopsy. *Nature* **221,** 974

Hoshino, M. (1961). The deep invagination of the inner nuclear membrane into the nucleoplasm in the ascites hepatoma cells. *Exp. Cell Res.* **24,** 606

Hou-Jensen, K., Rawlinson, D. G. and Hendrickson, M. (1973). Proliferating histiocytic lesion (histioctyosis X ?). *Cancer* **32,** 809

Howatson, A. F. and Fournasier, V. L. (1982). Microtubules in Paget's disease of bone. *J. Microscop. Soc. (Canada)* **9,** 36

Hozier, J., Renz, M. and Nehls, P. (1977). The chromosome fiber: evidence for an ordered superstructure of nucleosomes. *Chromosoma (Berl.)* **62,** 301

Hruban, Z., Swift, H. and Recheigl, M., Jr. (1965). Fine structure of transplantable hepatomas of the rat. *J. natn. Cancer Inst.* **35,** 459

Hruban, Z., Mochizuki, Y., Slesers, A. and Morris, H. P. (1972). Comparative study of cellular organelles of Morris hepatomas. *Cancer Res.* **32,** 853

Hsu, T. C. and Lou, T. Y. (1959). Nuclear extrusions in cells of Cloudman melanoma *in vitro.* In *Pigment Cell Biology,* pp. 315–325. Ed. by M. Gordon. New York: Academic Press

Hsu, T. C., Humphrey, R. M. and Somers, C. E. (1964). Persistent nucleoli in animal cells following treatments with fluorodeoxyuridine and thymidine. *Exp. Cell Res.* **33,** 74

Hsu, T. C., Arrighi, F. E., Klevecz, R. R. and Brinkley, B. R. (1965). The nucleoli in mitotic divisions of mammalian cells *in vitro. J. Cell Biol.* **26,** 539

Huehns, E. R., Lutzner, M. and Hecht, F. (1964). Nuclear abnormalities of the neutrophils in the D$_1$(13–15) trisomy syndrome. *Lancet* **1,** 589

166

Huhn, D. (1967). Nuclear pockets in normal monocytes. *Nature, Lond.* **216,** 1240

Huxley, H. E. and Zubay, G. (1961). Preferential staining of nucleic acid-containing structures for electron microscopy. *J. biophys. biochem. Cytol.* **11,** 273

Hyde, B. B., Sankaranarayanan, K. and Birnstiel, M. L. (1965). Observations on fine structure in pea nucleoli *in situ* and isolated. *J. Ultrastruct. Res.* **12,** 652

Hyden, H. (1943). Die funktion des kernkörperchens bei der Eiweibbildung in Nervenzellen. *Z. mikrosk.-anat. Forsch.* **54,** 96

Incze, J. S. and Lui, P. S. (1977). Morphology of the epithelial component of human lung hamartomas. *Human Pathol.* **8,** 411

Ishihara, T., Uchino, F., Kamei, T., Yokota, T., Nakamura, H., Etoh, H., Suzuki, E., Konishi, S. and Matsumoto, N. (1978). Subacute sclerosing panencephalitis with special reference to the ultrastructure of inclusions in the brain and lung. *Acta Path. Jap.* **28,** 139

Ishikawa, H. (1964). Peculiar intranuclear structures in sympathetic ganglion cells of a dog. *Z. Zellforsch. mikrosk. Anat.* **62,** 822

Itabashi, M., Hruban, Z., Wong, T.-W. and Chou, S.-F. (1976). Concentric nuclear inclusions. *Virchows Arch. B Cell Path.* **20,** 103

Ito, S. (1974). Study on the *in vitro* Rieder Cell. *Scand. J. Haemat.* **12,** 355

Ito, S. and Hattori, A. (1974). Study on the fibrillar formation surrounding the nuclear bridge in some types of leukaemic cells. *Scand. J. Haemat.* **12,** 321

Ito, T., Miura, S., Ohshima, K-I., Numakunai, S. and Tanimura, I. (1973). Pathological studies on swine leukosis. Fine structure of reticulum cell sarcoma and lymphosarcoma. *Jap. J. Vet. Sci.* **35,** 97

Iwanaga, T., Yamada, J., Yamashita, T. and Misu, M. (1981). Intranuclear filamentous inclusions in the gastro-entero-pancreatic (GEP) endocrine cells of birds. *Cell Tiss. Res.* **217,** 283

Janssen, M. and Johnston, W. H. (1978). Anaplastic seminoma of the testis. *Cancer* **41,** 538

Jézéquel, A. M. and Marinozzi, V. (1963). A propos de certains composants granulaires du noyau reveles par la fixation aux aldehydes. *J. Microscopie* **2,** 34 (abstract)

Jézéquel, A. M. and Steiner, J. W. (1966). Some ultrastructural and histochemical aspects of coxsackie virus-cell interactions. *Lab. Invest.* **15,** 1055

Jézéquel, A. M., Shreeve, M. M. and Steiner, J. W. (1967). Segregation of nucleolar components in mycoplasma-infected cells. *Lab. Invest.* **16,** 287

Johannessen, J. V. (1977). Use of paraffin material for electron microscopy. *Path. Ann.* **12,** 189. Ed. by S. C. Sommers and P. P. Rosen. Appleton-Century-Crofts

Johnson, J. E. Jr. and Miquel, J. (1974). Fine structural changes in the lateral vestibular nucleus of ageing rats. *Mechanisms of Ageing and Development* **3,** 203

Johnston, H. S. (1962). Nuclear inclusions in the epithelium of the hens oviduct. *Zellforsch. mikrosk. Anat.* **57,** 385

Jones, O. P. (1959). Formation of erythroblasts in the fetal liver and their destruction by macrophages and hepatic cells. *Anat. Rec.* **133,** 294

Jordan, E. G. and Chapman, J. M. (1973). Nucleolar and nuclear envelope ultrastructure in relation to cell activity in discs of carrot root (*Daucus carota* L.). *J. exp. Botany* **24,** 197

Kalifat, S. R., Bouteille, M. and Delarue, J. (1967). Etude ultrastructurale de la lamelle dense observée au contact de la membrane nucleaire interne. *J. Microscopie* **6,** 1019

Kalimo, H., Garcia, J. H., Kamijyo, Y., Tanaka, J. and Trump, B. F. (1977). The ultrastructure of 'Brain Death'. II. Electron microscopy of feline cortex after complete ischemia. *Virchows Arch. B Cell Path.* **25,** 207

Karasaki, S. (1963). Studies on amphibian yolk. I. The ultrastructure of the yolk platelet. *J. Cell Biol.* **18,** 135

Karasaki, S. (1970). An electron microscope study of intranuclear canaliculi in Novikoff hepatoma cells. *Cancer Res.* **30,** 1736

Karasaki, S. (1971). Cytoplasmic and nuclear glycogen synthesis in Novikoff ascites hepatoma cells. *J. Ultrastruct. Res.* **35,** 181

Karasaki, S. (1973). Passage of cytoplasmic liquid into interphase nuclei in preneoplastic rat liver. *J. Ultrastruct. Res.* **42,** 463

Karásek, J., Smetana, K., Hrdlička, A., Dubinin, I., Horňák, O. and Ohelert, W. (1972). Nuclear and nucleolar ultrastructure during the late stages of normal human keratinoctye maturation. *Br. J. Derm.* **86,** 601

Karlsson, U. (1966). Three-dimensional studies of neurons in the lateral geniculate nucleus of the rat. *J. Ultrastruct. Res.* **16,** 429

Kawanami, O., Ferrans, V. J., Fulmer, J. D. and Crystal, R. G. (1979). Nuclear inclusions in alveolar epithelium of patients with fibrotic lung disorders. *Am. J. Pathol.* **94,** 301

Kayahara, T. (1979). Intranuclear inclusions in facial motor neurons of the cat. *Mie Med.* **29**, 37

Kaye, J. S. (1969). The ultrastructure of chromatin in nuclei of interphase cells and in spermatids. In *Handbook of Molecular Cytology*, p. 362. Ed. by A. Lima-de-Faria. Amsterdam and London: North Holland Publ.

Kessel, R. G. and Beams, H. W. (1968). Intranucleolar membranes and nuclear-cytoplasmic exchanges in young crayfish oocytes. *J. Cell Biol.* **39**, 735

Kierszenbaum, A. L. (1968). The ultrastructure of human mixed salivary tumors. *Lab. Invest.* **18**, 391

Kindblom, L. -G., Merck, C. and Angervall, L. (1979). The ultrastructure of myxofibrosarcoma. A study of 11 cases. *Virchows Arch. A Path. Anat. Histol.* **381**, 121

Kirschner, R. H., Rusli, M. and Martin, T. E. (1977). Characterization of the nuclear envelope, pore complexes, and dense lamina of mouse liver nuclei by high resolution scanning electron microscopy. *J. Cell Biol.* **72**, 118

Kleinfeld, R. and Koulish, S. (1957). Cytological aspects of mouse and rat liver containing nuclear inclusions. *Anat. Rec.* **128**, 433

Kleinfeld, R. and Von Haam, E. (1959). Effect of thioacetamide on rat liver regeneration. II. Nuclear RNA in mitosis. *J. biophys. biochem. Cytol.* **6**, 393

Kleinfeld, R., Greider, M. H. and Frajola, W. J. (1956). Electron microscopy of intranuclear inclusions found in human and rat liver parenchymal cells. *J. biophys. biochem. Cytol.*(Suppl. 4) **2**, 435

Knocke, K. W.(1964). Elektronenmikroskopische Befunde an Lymphozyten und Lymphoidzellen des peripherischen Blutes bei der Leukose des Rindes. *Zbl. VetMed.* **11**, 1

Kohorn, E. I., Rice, S. I., Hemperly, S. and Gordon, M. (1972). The relation of the structure of progestational steroids to nucleolar differentiation in human endometrium. *J. clin. endocr. Metab.* **34**, 257

Kollert, V., Strasser, U. and Rosner, R. (1923). Trépol und Niere. *Wien. Klin. Wschr.* **36**, 49

Koshiba, K., Smetana, K. and Busch, H. (1970). On the ultrastructural cytochemistry of nuclear pores in Novikoff hepatoma cells. *Exp. Cell Res.* **60**, 199

Kotoo, Y., Horie, A. and Kurita, Y. (1976). Fine structure of benign pulmonary adenomatosis. *J. clin. electron Microsc. (Japan)* **9**, 445

Krishan, A., Uzman, B. G. and Hedley-Whyte, E. T. (1967). Nuclear bodies, a component of cell nuclei in hamster tissues and human tumors. *J. Ultrastruct. Res.* **19**, 563

Kuhn, C. H. (1967). Nuclear bodies and intranuclear globulin inclusions in Waldenstrom's macroglobulinemia. *Lab. Invest.* **17**, 404

Kuhn, C. (1972). Fine structure of bronchiolo-alveolar cell carcinoma. *Cancer* **30**, 1107

Kume, F., Maruyama, S., D'Agostino, A. N. and Chiga, M. (1967). Nucleolar change produced by mithramycin in rat hepatic cell. *Exp. molec. Path.* **6**, 254

Kumegawa, M., Rose, G. G., Cattoni, M., Luna, M. A. and Stimson, P. G. (1969). Electron microscopy of intranuclear inclusions in a mixed tumor. *Am. Acad. Oral Path.* **28**, 89

Kyte, J. (1964). Nuclear extrusion in dissociated rat heart cell. *Z. Zellforsch. mikrosk. Anat.* **62**, 495

Lafarga, M. and Palacios, G. (1977). Intranuclear rodlets in retrochiasmatic area neurons of the hypothalamus of the rat. *Experientia* **33**, 1368

Lafarga, M. and Palacios, G. (1979). Nuclear inclusions in paraventricular nucleus neurons of the rat hypothalamus. *Cell Tiss. Res.* **203**, 223

LaFontaine, J. G. (1965). A light and electron microscope study on small, spherical nuclear bodies in meristematic cells of *Allium cepa, Vicia faba* and *Raphanus sativus*. *J. Cell Biol.* **26**, 1

Landing, B. H. and Nakai, H. (1959). Histochemical properties of renal lead-inclusions and their demonstration in urinary sediment. *Am. J. clin. Path.* **31**, 499

Lane, B. P. (1965). Alterations in the cytologic detail of intestinal smooth muscle cells in various stages of contraction. *J. Cell Biol.* **27**, 199

Lane, N. J. (1969). Intranuclear fibrillar bodies in actinomycin D-treated oocytes. *J. Cell Biol.* **40**, 286

Lange, R. and Brehm, H. V. (1963). Über Kristallartige und Fibrilläre Zellkerneinschlüsse in der Glandula Parathyreoidea von *Rana temporaria*. *Z.Zellforsch.* **60**, 755

Langhans (1885). Pathologisch-anatomische Befunde bei mit Bismuthum subnitricum vergifteten Thieren. *Z. Chir.* **22**, 575

Lantos, P. L. (1971). The effect of a single dose of N-Ethyl-N-Nitrosourea on the fine structure of the brain of the rat. *Experientia* **27**, 1322

Lapis, K. and Bernhard, W. (1965). The effect of mitomycin C on the nucleolar fine structure of KB cells in cell culture. *Cancer Res.* **25**, 628

Latta, H. and Maunsbach, A. B. (1962a). The juxtaglomerular apparatus as studied electron microscopically. *J. Ultrastruct. Res.* **6**, 547

Latta, H. and Maunsbach, A. B. (1962b). Relations of the centrolobular region of the glomerulus to the juxtaglomerular apparatus. *J. Ultrastruct. Res.* **6**, 562

Lazarus, S. S., Vethamany, V. G., Shapiro, S. H. and Amsterdam, D. (1966). Histochemistry and fine structure of 4-nitroquinoline-N-oxide-induced nuclear inclusions. *Cancer Res.* **26**, 2229

LeCharpentier, Y., LeCharpentier, M., Forest, M., Daudet-Monsac, M., Lavenu-Vacher, M.-C., Louvel, A., Sedel, L. and Abelanet, R. (1977). Inclusions intranucléaires dans une tumeur osseuse a cellules géantes. Mise en évidence au microscope électronique. *Nouv. Presse med.* **6**, 259

Leduc, E. H. and Wilson, J. W. (1959a). An electron microscope study of intranuclear inclusions in mouse liver and hepatoma. *J. biophys. biochem. Cytol.* **6**, 427

Leduc, E. H. and Wilson, J. W. (1959b). A histochemical study of intranuclear inclusions in mouse liver and hepatoma. *J. Histochem. Cytochem.* **7**, 8

Leeson, T. S. and Leeson, C. R. (1968). The fine structure of Brunner's glands in man. *J.Anat.* **103**, 263

Leestma, J. E., Bornstein, M. B., Sheppard, R. D. and Feldman, L. S. (1969). Ultrastructural aspects of herpes simplex virus infection in organized cultures of mammalian nervous tissue. *Lab. Invest.* **20**, 70

Lemaire, R. (1963). Recherches morphologiques, cytochimiques et experimentales sur les inclusions nucleaires dans l'epididyme du chien. *Arch. Biol.* **3**, 342

LeMoigne, A. and Monnot-Sauzin, M-J. (1971). Etude au microscope électronique d'inclusions nucléaires chez des planaires (turbellariés, triclades). *J. Microscopie* **10**, 107

Lenhossék, M. (1897). Beiträge zur Kenntniss der Zwischenzellen des Hodens. *Arch. Anat. Physiol. (Anat. Abt.)* **20**, 65

Levine, A. S., Nesbit, M. E., White, J. G. and Yarbro, J. W. (1968). Effects of fractionated histones on nucleic acid synthesis in 6C3HED mouse ascites tumor cells and in normal spleen cells. *Cancer Res.* **28**, 831

Levine, G. D. (1973). Primary thymic seminoma–a neoplasm ultrastructurally similar to testicular seminoma and distinct from epithelial thymoma. *Cancer* **31**, 729

Levine, G. D. and Dorfman, R. F. (1975). Nodular lymphoma: An ultrastructural study of its relationship to germinal centers and a correlation of light and electron microscopic findings. *Cancer* **35**, 148

Levinson, W. (1967). Fragmentation of the nucleus in Rous sarcoma virus-infected chick embryo cells. *Virology* **32**, 74

Levinson, W. (1970). Fragmentation of the nucleus in Rous sarcoma virus-infected chick embryo cells. II. Structural and metabolic studies. *U.S. J. Natl. Cancer Inst.* **44**, 151

Litovitz, T. L. and Lutzner, M. A. (1974). Quantitative measurements of blood lymphocytes from patients with chronic lymphocytic leukemia and the Sézary syndrome. *J. Natl. Cancer Inst. (USA)* **53**, 75

Liu, R. P. C. and Hamilton, B. L. (1978). Intranuclear bodies in neurons of the periaqueductal gray matter in the cat. *Am. J. Anat.* **147**, 139

Liu, T. P. and Davies, D. M. (1972). Ultrastructure of the nuclear envelope from black-fly, fat-body cells with and without microsporidan infection. *J. intervert. Path.* **20**, 176

Locker, J., Goldblatt, P. J. and Leighton, J. (1968). Some ultrastructural features of Yoshida ascites hepatoma. *Cancer Res.* **28**, 2039

Loewenstein, W. R. and Kanno, Y. (1963). Some electrical properties of a nuclear membrane examined with a micro-electrode. *J. gen. Physiol.* **46**, 1123

Long, M. E. and Sommers, S. C. (1969). Staging, grading and histochemistry of ovarian epithelial tumors. *Clin. Obstet. Gynecol.* **12**, 937

Lord, A. and LaFontaine, J. G. (1969). The organization of the nucleolus in meristematic plant cells. A cytochemical study. *J. Cell Biol.* **40**, 633

Love, R. and Soriano, R. Z. (1971). Correlation of nucleolini with fine structural nucleolar constituents of cultured normal and neoplastic cells. *Cancer Res.* **31**, 1030

Lozinski, P. (1911). I. Wissenschaftliche mitteilungen. 1. Uber die Malpighischen gefabe der Myrmeleonidenlarven als Spinndrusen. *Zool. Anz.* **38**, 401

Ludford, R. J. (1924). Nuclear activity during melanosis. *J. Roy. Micro. Soc.* **13**, 13

Lung, B. (1972). Ultrastucture and chromatin disaggregation of human sperm head with thioglycolate treatment. *J. Cell Biol.* **52**, 179

Lutzner, M. A. and Hecht, F. (1966). Nuclear anomalies of the neutrophil in a chromosomal triplication. The D_1 (13–15) trisomy syndrome. *Lab. Invest.* **15**, 597

Lutzner, M. A. and Jordan, H. W. (1968). The ultrastructure of an abnormal cell in Sézary's syndrome. *Blood* **31**, 719

Lutzner, M. A., Hobbs, J. W. and Horvath, P. (1971). Ultrastructure of abnormal cells. In Sézary syndrome, mycosis fungoides and parapsoriasis en plaque. *Arch. Dermatol.* **103**, 375

MacCarty, W. C. (1937). Further observations on the macronucleolus of cancer. *Am. J. Cancer* **31**, 104

McDuffie, N. G. (1967). Nuclear blebs in human leukaemic cells. *Nature, Lond.* **214**, 1341

MacGregor, H. C. and Mackie, J. B. (1967). Fine structure of the cytoplasm in salivary glands of *Simulium*. *J. Cell Sci.* **2**, 137

McKenna, R. W., Parkin, J. and Brunning, R. D. (1979). Morphologic and ultrastructural characteristics of T-cell acute lymphoblastic leukemia. *Cancer* **44,** 1290

Magalhães, M. C. and Magalhães, M. M. (1980). Induction of nucleolar segregation in adrenal fasciculata cells by actinomycin D. *Experientia* **36,** 345

Magalhães, M. C. and Magalhães, M. M. (1985). The effects of α-amanitin on the fine structure of adrenal fasciculata cells in the young rat. *Tissue and Cell* **17,** 27

Magalhães, M. M. (1967). Intranuclear bodies in cells of rabbit and rat retina. *Exp. Cell Res.* **47,** 628

Majno, G., La Gattuta, M. and Thompson, T. E. (1960). Cellular death and necrosis. Chemical, physical and morphologic changes in rat liver. *Virchows Arch. path. Anat. Physiol.* **333,** 421

Majno, G., Gabbiani, G., Joris, I. and Ryan, G. B. (1970). Contraction of nonmuscular cells: Endothelium and fibroblasts. *J. Cell Biol.* **47,** 127

Maldonado, J. E., Maigne, J. and Lecoq, D. (1976). Comparative electron-microscopic study of the erythrocytic line in refractory anemia (preleukemia) and myelomonocytic leukemia. *Blood Cells* **2,** 167

Maldonado, J. E., Brown, A. L., Bayrd, E. D. and Pease, G. L. (1966). Cytoplasmic and intranuclear electron-dense bodies in the myeloma cell. *Arch. Path.* **81,** 484

Mann, D. M. A., Neary, D., Yates, P. O., Lincoln, J., Snowden, J. S. and Stanworth, P. (1981). Neurofibrillary pathology and protein synthetic capability in nerve cells in Alzheimer's disease. *Neuropath. & Appl. Neurobiol.* **7,** 37

Mann, G. (1894). Histochemical changes induced in sympathetic, motor and sensory nerve cells by functional activity. *J. Anat., Lond.* **29,** 100

Marinozzi, V. (1964). Cytochimie ultrastructurale du nucleole-RNA et proteines intranucleolaires. *J. Ultrastruct. Res.* **10,** 433

Marinozzi, V. and Bernhard, W. (1964). Presence dans le nucleole de deux types de ribonucleoproteines morphologiquement distinctes. *Exp. Cell Res.* **32,** 595

Marinozzi, V. and Fiume, L. (1971). Effects of α-Amanitin on mouse and rat liver cell nuclei. *Exp. Cell Res.* **67,** 311

Markesbery, W. R., Brooks, W. H., Milsow, L. and Mortara, R. H. (1976). Ultrastructural study of the pineal germinoma *in vivo* and *in vitro*. *Cancer* **37,** 327

Markovics, J., Glass, L. and Maul, G. G. (1974). Pore patterns on nuclear membranes. *Exp. Cell Res.* **85,** 443

Martinez, A. J., Ohya, T., Jabbour, J. T. and Dueñas, D. (1974). Subacute sclerosing panencephalitis (SSPE) reappraisal of nuclear, cytoplasmic and axonal inclusions. Ultrastructural study of eight cases. *Acta Neuropath. (Berl.)* **28,** 1

Masurovsky, E. B., Benitez, H. H., Kim, S. U. and Murray, M. R. (1970). Origin, development and nature of intranuclear rodlets and associated bodies in chicken sympathetic neurons. *J. Cell Biol.* **44,** 172

Maul, G. G. and Deaven, L. (1977). Quantitive determination of nuclear pore complexes in cycling cells with differing DNA content. *J. Cell Biol.* **73,** 748

Maul, G. G., Price, J. W. and Lieberman, M. W. (1971). Formation and distribution of nuclear pore complexes in interphase. *J. Cell Biol.* **51,** 405

Maximow, A. and Bloom, W. (1948). *Textbook of Histology*. Philadelphia and London: Saunders

Mazur, M. T., Hendrickson, M. R. and Kempson, R. L. (1983). Optically clear nuclei. *Am. J. Surg. Path.* **7,** 415

Meier, C. (1969). Intranukleäre Einschlusskörper in neuronen alternder Ratten. *Experientia* **25,** 294

Mercer, E. H. (1959). An electron microscopic study of *Amoeba proteus*. *Proc. R. Soc. B.* **150,** 216

Merkow, L. P., Frich, J. C., Slifkin, M., Kyreages, C. G. and Pardo, M. (1971). Ultrastructure of a fibroxanthrosarcoma (malignant fibroxanthoma). *Cancer* **28,** 372

Merriam, R. W. (1962). Some dynamic aspects of the nuclear envelope. *J. Cell Biol.* **12,** 79

Merski, J. A., Daskal, I. and Busch, H. (1976). Effects of adriamycin on ultrastructure of nucleoli in the heart and liver cells of the rat. *Cancer Res.* **36,** 1580

Mickwitz, C.-U. v. (1972). Konzentrisch geschichtete Kerneinschlüsse im Nierenepithel beim Küken. *Zbl. allg. Path. Bd.* **116,** 191

Miller, J. M., Miller, L. D., Gillette, K. G. and Olson, C. (1969). Incidence of lymphocytic nuclear projections in bovine lymphosarcoma. *J. Natl. Cancer Inst.* **43,** 719

Miller, L. and Gonzales, F. (1976). The relationship of ribosomal RNA synthesis to the formation of segregated nucleoli and nucleolus bodies. *J. Cell Biol.* **71,** 939

Miller, O. L., Jr. (1966). Structure and composition of peripheral nucleoli of salamander oocytes. *Natn Cancer Inst. Monogr.* **23,** 53

Miller, O. L., Jr. and Beatty, Barbara R. (1969). Nucleolar structure and function. In *Handbook of Molecular Cytology*. Ed. by A. Lima-de-Faria. Amsterdam and London: North Holland Publ. Company.

Mirsky, A. E. and Osawa, S. (1961). The interphase nucleus. In *The Cell*, Vol.2, p.677. Ed. by J. Brachet and A. E. Mirsky. New York: Academic Press

Misrabi, M. (1969). Intranuclear inclusions in neurons and glial cells in the spiral cord of foetal, neonatal and adult rats. *J. Anat.* **104**, 588

Miyai, K. and Steiner, J. W. (1965). Fine structure of interphase liver cells nuclei in subacute ethionine intoxication. *Exp. Molec. Path.* **4**, 525

Miyai, K. and Steiner, J. W. (1967). Fine structure of interphase liver cell nuclei in acute ethionine intoxication. *Lab. Invest.* **16**, 677

Mollo, F. and Stramignoni, A. (1967). Nuclear projections in blood and lymph node cells of human leukaemias and Hodgkin's disease and in lymphocytes cultured with phytohaemagglutinin. *Br. J. Cancer* **21**, 519

Montella, G. (1954). Lo studio del nucleo cellulare nei tumori. *Tumorii* **40**, 232

Montgomery, P. O'B., Reynolds, R. C. and Cook, J. E. (1966). Nucleolar 'caps' induced by flying spot ultraviolet nuclear irradiation. *Am. J. Path.* **49**, 555

Moor, H. and Mühlethaler, K. (1963). Fine structure in frozen-etched yeast cells. *J. Cell Biol.* **17**, 609

Moore, G. E. and Pickren, J. W. (1967). Study of a virus-containing hematopoietic cell line and a melanoma cell line derived from a patient with a leukemoid reaction. *Lab. Invest.* **16**, 882

Moore, J. F., Goyer, R. A. and Wilson, M. (1973). Lead-induced inclusion bodies: solubility, amino acid content, and relationship to residual acidic nuclear proteins. *Lab. Invest.* **29**, 488

More, I. A. R. and McSeveney, D. (1980). The three dimensional structure of the nucleolar channel system in the endometrial glandular cell: serial sectioning and high voltage electron microscopic studies. *J. Anat.* **130**, 673

Morgan, C., Godman, G. C., Rose, H. M., Howe, C. and Huang, J. S. (1957). Electron microscopic and histochemical studies of an unusual crystalline protein occuring in cells infected by type 5 adenovirus. Preliminary observations. *J. biophys. biochem. Cytol.* **3**, 505

Moricard, R. and Moricard, F. (1964). Modifications cytoplasmiques et nucleaires ultrastructurales uterines au cours de l'état folliculuteinique à glycogene massif. *Gynec. Obstet.* **63**, 203

Moses, M. J. (1956). Studies on nuclei using correlated cytochemical, light and electron microscope techniques. *J. biophys. biochem. Cytol.* **2**, No. 4 Suppl., 397

Moses, M. J. (1960). Patterns of organization in the fine structure of chromosomes. In *4th Int. Congr. Electron Microscopy,* Vol. 2, p. 199. Berlin: Springer-Verlag

Mugnaini, E. (1967). On the occurrence of filamentous rodlets in neurons and glia cells of *Myxine glutinosa* (L). *Sarsia* **29**, 221

Müller, O. and Ratzenhofer, M. (1971). Intranukleäre Einschlüsse in endokrinen Zellen des Kaninchenmagens. *Z. Zellforsch.* **117**, 526

Munnell, J. F. and Getty, R. (1968). Nuclear lobulation and amitotic division associated with increasing cell size in the aging canine myocardium. *J. Gerontol.* **23**, 363

Murad, T. M. and Murthy, M. S. N. (1970). Ultrastructure of a chordoma. *Cancer* **25**, 1204

Murad, T. M. and Scarpelli, D. G. (1967). The ultrastructure of medullary and scirrhous mammary duct carcinoma. *Am. J. Path.* **50**, 335

Murphy, F. A., Coleman, P. H., Harrison, A. K. and Gary, G. W. Jr. (1968). Colorado tick fever virus: an electron microscopic study. *Virology* **35**, 28

Murray, A. B., Büscher, H. and Erfle, V. (1983). Intranuclear undulating membranous structures in cells of a human parosteal osteosarcoma. *Ultrastruct. Path.* **5**, 163

Myagkaya, G. L., van Veen, H. and James, K. (1985). Quantitative analysis of mitochondrial flocculent densities in rat hepatocytes during normothermic and hypthermic ischemia *in vitro*. *Virchows Arch. B Cell Path.* **49**, 61

Nagl, W. and Hiersche, H.-D. (1983). Condensed chromatin in the cell nuclei of the human uterine cervix: Squamous and columnar epithelium, non-pregnant and pregnant state, and adenocarcinomata. *J. Submicrosc. Cytol.* **15**, 1065

Nakai, T., Shand, F. L. and Howatson, A. F. (1969). Development of measles virus *in vitro*. *Virology* **38**, 50

Nakayama, I. and Nickerson, P. A. (1972). Intranuclear inclusions in mammotrophs of the female Mongolian gerbil. *Am. J. Anat.* **135**, 93

Nicander, L. (1964). Fine structure and cytochemistry of nuclear inclusions in the dog epididymis. *Exp. Cell Res.* **34**, 533

Nickerson, P. A. (1973). Induction of intranuclear inclusions by estrogen in mammotrophs of the Mongolian gerbil. *J. Ultrastruct. Res.* **44**, 41

Nickerson, P. A. (1975a). Effect of partial thyroidectomy, propylthiouracil or thyroxine on estrogen-induced intranuclear inclusions in mammotrophs of the Mongolian gerbil. *Tissue & Cell* **7**, 763

Nickerson, P. A. (1975b). Intranuclear inclusions in mammotrophs of the Mongolian gerbil: Effect of low doses of estradiol benzoate and a study of females before weaning. *Tissue & Cell* **7**, 773

Nickerson, P. A. (1977). Effect of stimulation (reserpine) or suppression (bromocriptin) on intranuclear inclusions in mammotrophs of the Mongolian gerbil. *Biol. Cell (Paris)* **29**, 149

Nii, S. and Kamahora, J. (1963). High frequency appearance of amitotic nuclear divisions in PS cells induced by Herpes Simplex virus. *Biken j.* **6**, 33

Nii, S., Morgan, C. and Rose, H. M. (1968). Electron microscopy of herpes simplex virus. II. Sequence of development. *J. Virol.* **2**, 517

Nii, S., Morgan, C., Rose, H. M. and Rosenkranz, H. S. (1966). Analytical studies of the development of herpes simplex virus. In *Proceedings of the 6th International Congress of Electron Microscopy*. Vol. 2, p. 201. Ed. by R. Uyeda. Tokyo: Maruzen

Norberg, B. (1969). Cytoplasmic microtubules and radial-segmented nuclei (Rieder Cells). *Scand. J. Haemat.* **6**, 312

Norberg, B. (1970). Cytoplasmic microtubules and radial-segmented nuclei (Rieder cells). Ultrastructural studies. *Scand. J. Haemat.* **7**, 445

Norberg, B. (1971). Contractile processes in human lymphocytes and monocytes from peripheral blood. *Scand. J. Haematol.* **14** (Suppl.) 1

Norberg, B. and Söderström, N. (1967). The effect of demecolcine on the oxalate-induced formation of radial-segmented nuclei. (Rieder Cells). *Scand. J. Haemat.* **4**, 161

Norton, W. N., Daskal, I., Savage, H. E., Seibert, R. A., Busch, H. and Lane, M. (1977). Effects of Galactoflavin-induced riboflavin deficiency upon rat hepatic cell ultrastructure. *Virchows Arch. B Cell Path.* **23**, 353

Novikoff, A. B. (1957). A transplantable rat liver tumor induced by 4-dimethylaminoazobenzene. *Cancer Res.* **17**, 1010

Oberling, Ch. and Bernhard, W. (1961). The morphology of the cancer cells. In *The Cell*, Vol. 5, p. 405. Ed. by J. Brachet and A. E. Mirsky. New York: Academic Press

O'Brien, B. R. A. (1960). The presence of hemoglobin within the nucleus of the embryonic chick erythroblast. *Exp. Cell Res.* **21**, 226

Oda, A. and Chiga, M. (1965). Effect of actinomycin D on the hepatic cells of partially hepatectomised rats: an electron microscopic study. *Lab. Invest.* **14**, 1419

Ogawa, K. (1962). Elektronenoptische untersuchungen bei eunem fall von sogenannten Hodgkensarkom. *Frankfurt Z. Path.* **71**, 677

Ohtsuki, Y., Ohmori, M. and Ogawa, K. (1972). Intranuclear fibrillar bundles in functioning β-Cell adenoma of pancreas. *Acta Med. Okayama* **26**, 149

Oikawa, K. (1975). Electron microscopic observation of inclusion bodies in plasma cells in multiple myeloma and Waldenström's macroglobulinemia. *Tohoku J. exp. Med.* **117**, 257

Olitsky, P. K. and Casals, J. (1945). Certain affections of the liver that arise spontaneously in so-called normal stock albino mice. *Proc. Soc. exp. Biol Med.* **60**, 48

Oliveira, L. (1976). Ultrastructural, cytochemical and experimental studies on the cytoplasmic and nucleoplasmic inclusions of root meristematic cells of *A. triticale*. *J. Submicr. Cytol.* **8**, 29

Ophus, E. M. and Gullvåg, B. M. (1974). Localization of lead within leaf cells of *Rhytidiadelphus squarrosus* (Hedw.) Warnst. by means of transmission electron microscopy and x-ray microanalysis. *Cytobios.* **10**, 45

Oryschak, A. F., Ghadially, F. N. and Bhatnager, R. (1974). Nuclear fibrous lamina in the chondrocytes of articular cartilage. *J. Anat.* **118**, 511

Oryschak, A. F., Mitchell, D. M. and Ghadially, F. N. (1976). Nuclear fibrous lamina in the rheumatoid synovium. *Arch. Path. Lab. Med.* **100**, 218

Oteruelo, F. T. (1976). Intranuclear inclusions in a myopathy of late onset. *Virchows Arch. B Cell Path.* **20**, 319

Padgett, B. L., Walker, D. L., ZuRhein, G. M. and Eckroade, R. J. (1971). Cultivation of papova-like virus from human brain with progressive multifocal leucoencephalopathy. *Lancet* **1**, 1257

Panner, B. J. and Honig, C. R. (1967). Filament ultrastructure and organization in vertebrate smooth muscle. Contraction hypothesis based on localization of actin and myosin. *J. Cell Biol.* **35**, 303

Papadimitriou, J. M. (1966). Electron microscopic findings of a murine lymphoma associated with reovirus Type 3 infection. *Proc. Soc. exp. Biol. Med.* **121**, 93

Pappas, G. D. (1956). The fine structure of the nuclear envelope of *Amoeba proteus*. *J. biophys. biochem. Cytol. Suppl.* **4**, 431

Pappenheimer, A. M. and Maechling, E. H. (1934). Inclusions in renal epithelial cells following the use of certain bismuth preparations. *Am. J. Path.* **10**, 577

Parker, J. W., Wakasa, H. and Lukes, R. J. (1967). Canine and Burkitt's lymphomas. (Letter.) *Lancet*, January 28, 214

Parmley, R. T., Crist, W. M., Roper, M., Takagi, M. and Austin, R. L. (1981). Intranuclear crystalloids associated with abnormal granules in eosinophilic leukocytes. *Blood* **58**, 1134

Parry, E. W. (1971). Membrane-bounded intranuclear structures in hepatocytes after exposure to sodium tetraphenyl boron. *J. Path.* **104,** 210

Parry, E. W. and Ghadially, F. N. (1967). Ultrastructure of the livers of rats bearing transplanted tumours. *J. Path. Bact.* **93,** 295

Partin, J. C., Partin, J. S., Schubert, W. K. and McLaurin, R. L. (1975). Brain ultrastructure in Reye's syndrome (encephalopathy and fatty alteration of the viscera). *J. Neuropath. & Exp. Neurol.* **34,** 325

Patrizi, G. and Middelkamp, J. N. (1969). *In vivo* and *in vitro* demonstration of nuclear bodies in vaccinia infected cells. *J. Ultrastruct. Res.* **28,** 275

Patrizi, G. and Poger, M. (1967). The ultrastructure of the nuclear periphery. The zonula nucleum limitans. *J. Ultrastruct. Res.* **17,** 127

Patrizi, G., Middelkamp, J. N. and Reed, C. A. (1967). Reduplication of nuclear membranes in tissue culture cells infected with guinea pig cytomegalovirus. *Am. J. Path.* **50,** 779

Payne, C. M. and Nagle R. B. (1983). An ultrastructural study of intranuclear rodlets in a malignant extracranial neuroepithelial neoplasm. *Ultrastruct. Path.* **5,** 1

Payne, C. M., Nagle, R. B. and Lynch, P. J. (1984). Quantitative electron microscopy in the diagnosis of mycosis fungoides. *Arch. Derm.* **120,** 63

Payne, C. M., Hicks, M. J. and Kim, A. (1985). Ultrastructural morphometric analysis of normal human lymphocytes stimulated *in vitro* with mitogens and antigens. *Am. J. Path.* **120,** 263

Pedro, N., Carmo-Fonseca, M. and Fernandes, P. (1984). Quantitative analysis of pore patterns on rat prostate nuclei using spatial statistics methods. *J. Microscopy* **134,** 271

Perry, R. P. (1964). Role of the nucleolus in ribonucleic acid metabolism and other cellular processes. *Natn. Cancer Inst. Monogr.* **14,** 73

Perry, R. P. (1966). On ribosome biogenesis. *Natn. Cancer Inst. Monogr.* **23,** 527

Perry, R. P. (1969). Nucleoli: the cellular sites of ribosome production. In *Handbook of Molecular Cytology.* Ed. by A. Lima-de-Faria. Amsterdam and London: North Holland Publ.

Pianese, G. (1896). Beitrag zur histologie und aetiologie des carcinoms. Histologische und experimentelle untersuchungen. Aus dem Italieneschen ubersetzt von R. Teuscher. I–II. Histologische unter-suchungen. *Ziegler's Beitr.* **142,** Suppl. 1, 1

Pierce, G. B. (1966). Ultrastructure of human testicular tumors. *Cancer* **19,** 1963

Pinching, A. J. and Powell, T. P. S. (1971). Ultrastructural features of transneuronal cell degeneration in the olfactory system. *J. Cell Sci.* **8,** 253

Pomerat, C. M., Lefeber, C. G. and Smith, McD. (1954). Quantitative cine analysis of cell organoid activity. *Ann. N. Y. Acad. Sci.* **58,** 1311

Pomeroy, K. A., Paul, P. S., Weber, A. F., Sorensen, D. K. and Johnson, D. W. (1977). Evidence that B-lymphocytes carry the nuclear pocket abnormality associated with bovine leukemia virus infection: Brief communication. *J. Natl. Cancer Inst.* **59,** 281

Popoff, N. A. and Ellsworth, R. M. (1971). The fine structure of retinoblastoma. *In vivo* and *in vitro* observations. *Lab. Invest.* **25,** 389

Popoff, N. and Stewart, S. E. (1968). The fine structure of nuclear inclusions in the brain of experimental golden hamsters. *J. Ultrastruct. Res.* **23,** 347

Porter, K. R. (1960). Problems in the study of nuclear fine structure. In *4th Int. Congr. Electron Microscopy,* Vol. 2, p. 186. Berlin: Springer-Verlag

Prenant, A. (1897). Cristalloides intranucléaires des cellules nerveuses sympathiques chez les mammifères. *Arch. Anat. micr. Morph. exp.* **1,** 336

Prineas, J. (1972). Paramyxovirus-like particles associated with acute demyelination in chronic relapsing multiple sclerosis. *Science* **178,** 760

Propst, A. (1970). Über konzentrisch geschichtete Kerneinschlüsse in einem menschlichen Nebennieren-rindenadenom. *Virchows Arch. Abt. B. Zellpath.* **4,** 263

Puvion-Dutilleul, F. and Puvion, E. (1981). Relationship between chromatin and perichromatin granules in cadmium-treated isolated hepatocytes. *J. Ultrastruct. Res.* **74,** 341

Puvion, E., Bachellerie, J.-P. and Burglen, M.-J. (1979). Nucleolar perichromatin granules induced by dichlorobenzimidazole riboside. *J. Ultrastruct. Res.* **69,** 1

Puvion, E., Moyne, G. and Bernhard, W. (1976). Action of 3'deoxyadenosine (cordycepin) on nuclear ribonucleoproteins of isolated liver cells. *J. Microsc. Biol. Cell.* **25,** 17

Quattrini, D. (1966). Un altro reperto di fibrille endonucleari nelle cellule nervose dei molluschi gasteropodi. Osservazioni in *Vaginulus borellianus* (Colosi). *Caryologia* **19,** 41

Raine, C. S. and Field E. J. (1968). Nuclear structures in nerve cells in multiple sclerosis. *Brain Res.* **10,** 266

Raine, C. S., Powers, J. M. and Suzuki, K. (1974). Acute multiple sclerosis. Confirmation of 'paramyxovirus-like' intranuclear inclusions. *Arch. Neurol.* **30,** 39

Raine, C. S., Schaumberg, H. H., Snyder, D. H. and Suzuki, K. (1975). Intranuclear 'paramyxovirus-like' material in multiple sclerosis, adrenoleukodystrophy and Kuf's disease. *J. Neurol. Sci.* **25,** 29

Ramos, C. V., Gillespie, W. and Narconis, R. J. (1978). Elastofibroma. A pseudotumor of myofibroblasts. *Arch. Pathol. Lab. Med.* **102,** 538

Ramsey, H. J. (1965). Ultrastructure of a pineal tumor. *Cancer* **18,** 1014

Rattner, J. B and Hamkalo, B. A. (1979). Nucleosome packing in interphase chromatin. *J. Cell Biol.* **81,** 453

Rebel, A., Malkani, K., Baslé, M. and Bregeon, Ch. (1976). Osteoclast ultrastructure in Paget's disease. *Calcif. Tiss. Res.* **20,** 187

Rebel, A., Malkani, K., Baslé, M., Bregeon, Ch., Le Patezour, A. and Filmon, R. (1974). Particularités ultrastructurales des ostéoclastes de la maladie de Paget. *Revue du Rhumatisme* **41,** 767

Recher, L., Briggs, L. G. and Parry, N. T. (1971). A re-evaluation of nuclear and nucleolar changes induced *in vitro* by actinomycin D. *Cancer Res.* **31,** 140

Recher, L., Whitescarver, J. and Briggs, L. (1970). A cytochemical and radioautographic study of human tissue culture cell nucleoli. *J. Cell Biol.* **45,** 479

Reddy, J. and Svoboda, D. J. (1968). The relationship of nucleolar segregation to ribonucleic acid synthesis following the administration of selected hepatocarcinogens. *Lab. Invest.* **19,** 132

Ree, K., Rugstad, H. E. and Bakka, A. (1982). Ultrastructural changes in the nucleus of a human epithelial cell line exposed to cytotoxic agents. *Acta path. microbiol. immunol. scand. Sect A.* **90,** 427

Reider, H. (1893). *Atlas der klinischen Mikroskopie des Blutes.* Leipzig: Vogel

Rejthar, A. and Blumajer, J. (1974). Difference in density of nuclear pores in normal and malignant fibroblasts of Syrian hamster. *Neoplasma* **21,** 479

Reynolds, R. C. and Montgomery, P. O'B. (1967). Nucleolar pathology produced by acridine orange and proflavine. *Am. J. Path.* **51,** 323

Reynolds, R. C., Montgomery, P. O'B. and Karney, D. H. (1963). Nucleolar 'caps' a morphologic entity produced by the carcinogen 4-nitroquinoline-N-oxide. *Cancer Res* **23,** 535

Rhodin, J. A. G. (1963). *An Atlas of Ultrastructure.* Philadelphia, Pa: Saunders

Richter, G. W. (1976). Evolution of cytoplasmic fibrillar bodies induced by lead in rat and mouse kidneys. *Am. J. Path.* **83,** 135

Richter, G. W., Kress, Y. and Cornwall, C. C. (1968). Another look at lead inclusion bodies. *Am. J. Path.* **53,** 189

Rifkin, B. R. and Heijl, L. (1979). The nuclear fibrous lamina of alveolar bone cells. *J. Periodontal Res.* **14,** 132

Ris, H. (1956). A study of chromosomes with the electron microscope. *J. biophys. biochem. Cytol.* **2,** Supp. **4,** 385

Ris, H. (1962). Interpretation of ultrastructure in the cell nucleus. In *The Interpretation of Ultrastructure,* Vol.1, p.69. Ed. by R. J. Harris. New York: Academic Press.

Ris, H. (1978). Higher order structures in chromosomes. In *9th International Congress on Electron Microscopy, Toronto* **3,** 545

Risueño, M. C., Galán-Cano, J. and Giménez-Martín, G. (1975). Ultrastructure of the nuclear envelope in the covering tissues of the ovule and another beginning of meiosis. *Mikroskopie Bd.* **31,** 5

Roberts, D. K. (1967). Canalicular structures in the nucleus of human endometrium: A three-dimensional study. *J. Cell Biol.* **35,** 114A, Abstract 237

Roberts, D. K., Horbelt, D. V. and Powell, L. C. (1975). The ultrastructural response of human endometrium to medroxyprogesterone acetate. *Am. J. Obstet. & Gynecol.* **123,** 811

Robertson, D. M. (1964). Electron microscopic studies of nuclear inclusions in meningiomas. *Am. J. Path.* **45,** 835

Robertson, D. M. and Maclean, J. D. (1965). Nuclear inclusions in malignant gliomas. *Archs Neurol., Chicago* **13,** 287

Roncoroni, L. (1895). Su un nuovo reperto nel nucleo delle cellule nervose. *Arch. Psychiat.* **16,** 447

Rouiller, C. and Simon, G. (1962). Contribution de la microscopie electronique au progres de nos connaissances en cytologie et en histo-pathologie hepatique. *Revue int. Hépat.* **12,** 167

Roy, S. and Wolman, L. (1969). Electron microscopic observations on the virus particles in *Herpes simplex* encephalitis. *J. clin. Path.* **22,** 51

Roy-Taranger, M., Mayaud, G. and Davydoff-Alibert, S. (1965). Lymphocytes binucléés dans le sang d'individus irradiés a faible dose. *Rev. franc. Étud. clin. biol.* **10,** 958

Rubin, R. C. (1966). Personal communication. Quoted by Hirano, A. and Zimmerman, H. M., *Anat. Rec.* (1967) **158,** 293

Rudzinska, M. A. (1961a). The use of a protozoan for studies on ageing: 1. Differences between young and old organisms of *Tokophyra infusionum* as revealed by light and electron microscopy. *J. Gerontol.* **16,** 213

Rudzinska, M. A. (1961b). The use of a protozoan for studies on ageing: 11. The macronucleus in young and old organisms of *Tokophyra infusionum*. Light and electron microscope observations. *J. Gerontol.* **16**, 326

Ryan, G. B., Cliff, W. J., Gabbiani, G., Irle, C., Statkov, P. R. and Majno, G. B. (1973). Myofibroblasts in an avascular fibrous tissue. *Lab. Invest.* **29**, 197

Ryder, D. R., Horvath, E. and Kovacs, K. (1979). Nuclear inclusions in the human adenohypophysis. *Acta Anat.* **105**, 273

Salazar, H. (1963). The pars distalis of the female rabbit hypophysis: An electron microscopic study. *Anat. Rec.* **147**, 469

Sanel, F. T. and Lepore, M. J. (1968). Granular and crystalline deposits in perinuclear and ergastoplasmic cisternae of human lamina propria cells. *Exp. Molec. Path.* **9**, 110

Sankaranarayanan, K. and Hyde, B. B. (1965). Ultrastructural studies of a nuclear body in peas with characteristics of both chromatin and nucleoli. *J. Ultrastruct. Res.* **12**, 748

Santibanez, G. P. and Lafarga, M. (1979). Nuclear bodies in the rat adrenal glomerular zone in normal and experimental conditions. *Z. mikrosh.-anat. Forsch., Leipzig* **93**, 951

Schoefl, G. I. (1964). The effect of actinomycin D on the fine structure of the nucleolus. *J. Ultrastruct. Res.* **10**, 224

Scholz, W. and Paweletz, N. (1969). Glykogenablagerung in zellkernen des Ehrlich-ascites-tumors. *Z. Krebsforsch.* **72**, 211

Schrek, R. (1972). Ultrastructure of blood lymphocytes from chronic lymphocytic and lymphosarcoma cell leukemia. *J. Natl. Cancer Inst. (USA)* **48**, 51

Schulz, A., Delling, G., Ringe, J.-D. and Ziegler, R. (1977). Morbus Paget des Knochens. Untersuchungen zue Ultrastruktur der Osteoclasten und ihrer Cytopathogenese. *Virchows Arch. A Path. Anat. Histol.* **376**, 309

Schulz, H. and Hahnel, E. (1969). Die ultrastruktur des Glykogens in Lochkernen der menschlichen Leberepithelzellen bei Diabetes mellitus. *Virchows Arch. Abt. B. Zellpath.* **3**, 282

Schulze, C. (1979). Giant nuclear bodies (Sphaeridia) in Sertoli cells of patients with testicular tumors. *J. Ultrastruct. Res.* **67**, 267

Schumacher, H. R., Szekely, I. E., Park, S. A. and Fisher, D. R. (1973). Ultrastructural studies on the acute leukemic lymphoblast. *Blut Zeitschrift fur die Gesamte Blutforschung* **27**, 396

Schuster, F. L. and Dunnebacke, T. H. (1977). Ultrastructural observations of experimental Naegleria meningoencephalitis in mice: Intranuclear inclusions in amebae and host cells. *J. Protozool.* **24**, 489

Schwartz, R. A. and Bangert, J. L. (1979). Use of electron microscopy in mycosis fungoides and other cutaneous oncologic conditions. *Arizona Med.* **36**, 344

Sebuwufu, P. H. (1966). Nuclear blebs in the human foetal thymus. *Nature, Lond.* **212**, 1382

Seifert, K. (1971). Elektronenmikroskopische untersuchungen am juvenilen Nasenrachenfibrom. *Arch. Klin. Exp. Ohr. Nas-u. Kehlk. Heilk.* **198**, 215

Seîte, R. (1970). Etude ultrastructurale de divers types d'inclusions nucléaires dans les neurones sympathiques du Chat. *J. Ultrastruct. Res.* **30**, 152

Seîte, R., Escaig, J. and Couineau, S. (1971). Microfilaments et microtubules nucléaires et organisation ultrastructurale des batonnets intranucléaires des neurones sympathiques. *J. Ultrastruct. Res.* **37**, 449

Seîte, R., Mei, N. and Vuillet-Luciani, J. (1973). Effect of electrical stimulation on nuclear microfilaments and microtubules of sympathetic neurons submitted to cycloheximide. *Brain. Res.* **50**, 419

Seîte, R., Escaig, J., Luciani-Vuillet, J. and Zerbib, R. (1975). Microtubules et microfilaments nucléaires: organisation ultrastructurale de cristalloides annulaires dans les neurones sympathiques. *J. Microscopie Biol. Cell.* **24**, 387

Seîte, R., Vuillet-Luciani, J., Vio, M. and Cataldo, C. (1977a). Sur la présence d'inclusions nucléaires dans certains neurones du noyau caudé du rat: répartition, fréquence et organisation ultrastructurale. *Extrait de la Revue Biologie Cellulaire* **30**, 73

Seîte, R., Zerbib, R., Vuillet-Luciani, J. and Vio, M. (1977b). Nuclear inclusions in sympathetic neurons: A quantitive and ultrastructural study in the superior cervical and celiac ganglia of the cat. *J. Ultrastruct. Res.* **61**, 254

Seîte, R., Leonetti, J., Luciani-Vuillet, J. and Vio, M. (1977c). Cyclic AMP and ultrastructural organization of the nerve cell nucleus: stimulation of nuclear microtubules and microfilaments assembly in sympathetic neurons. *Brain Res.* **124**, 41

Seîte, R., Vuillet-Luciani, J., Zerbib, R., Cataldo, C., Escaig, J., Pebusque, M. J. and Autillo-Touati, A. (1979). Three-dimensional organization of tubular and filamentous nuclear inclusions and associated structures in sympathetic neurons as revealed by serial sections and tilting experiments. *J. Ultrastruct. Res.* **69**, 211

Senoo, A., Fuse, Y. and Ghadially, F. N. (1984). A serial section study on nuclear pockets and loops. *J. Submicrosc. Cytol.* **16**, 379

175

Severs, N. J. and Jordan, E. G. (1978). Nuclear pores. Can they expand and contract to regulate nucleocytoplasmic exchange? *Experientia* **34,** 1007

Severs, N. J., Jordan, E. G. and Williamson, D. H. (1976). Nuclear pore absence from areas of close association between nucleus and vacuole in synchronous yeast cultures. *J. Ultrastruct. Res.* **54,** 374

Sézary, A. (1949). La réticulose maligne leucémique a histo-monocytes monstreux et a forme d'érythrodermie eodémateuse et pigmentée. *Ann. Derm. Syph.* **9,** 5

Shaw, C. -M. and Sumi, S. M. (1975). Nonviral intranuclear filamentous inclusions. *Arch. Neurol.* **32,** 428

Shaw, C. -M., Buchan, G. C. and Carlson, C. B. (1967). Myxovirus as a possible etiologic agent in subacute inclusion-body encephalitis. *New Engl. J. Med.* **277,** 511

Sheldon, H., Silverberg, M. and Kerner, I. (1962). On the differing appearance of intranuclear and cytoplasmic glycogen in liver cells in glycogen storage disease. *J. Cell Biol.* **13,** 468

Shelton, E. (1955). Hepatomas in mice: factors affecting rapid induction of a high incidence of hepatomas by *o*-amino-azotoluene. *J. Natn. Cancer Inst.* **16,** 107

Shepard, D. C. (1964). Production and elimination of excess DNA in ultraviolet- irradiated Tetrahymena. *J. Cell Biol.* **23,** Abstr. No. 178,86A

Sherwin, R. P., Kaufman, C., Dermer, G. R. and Monroe, S. A. (1977). Intranuclear rodlets in an intrathyroid tumor associated with hyperparathyroidism. *Cancer* **39,** 178

Shinozuka, H., Goldblatt, P. J. and Farber, E. (1968). The disorganization of hepatic cell nucleoli induced by ethionine and its reversal by adenine. *J. Cell Biol.* **36,** 313

Shipkey, F. H., Erlandson, R. A., Bailey, R. B., Babcock, V. I. and Southam, C. V. (1967). Virus biographies II. Growth of *Herpes simplex* virus in tissue culture. *Exp. Molec. Path.* **6,** 39

Siegesmund, K. A., Dutta, C. R. and Fox, C. A. (1964). The ultrastructure of the intranuclear rodlet in certain nerve cells. *J. Anat. (Lond.)* **98,** 93

Silverman, L. and Rubinstein, L. J. (1965). Electron microscopic observations on a case of progressive multifocal leucoencephalopathy. *Acta Neuropathol.* **5,** 215

Simar, L. J. (1969). Ultrastructure et constitution des corps nucleaires dans les plasmocytes. *Z. Zellforsch. Mikrosk. Anat.* **99,** 235

Simar, L. J. and Lemaire, R. (1966). Etude ultrastructurale des inclusions nucleaires de l'epididyme du chien. *C. R. Acad. Sci., Paris* **262,** 1455

Simard, R. (1966). Specific nuclear and nucleolar ultrastructural lesions induced by proflavin and similarly acting antimetabolites in tissue culture. *Cancer Res.* **26,** 2316

Simard, R. and Bernhard, W. (1966). Le phenoméne de la segregation nucleolaire specificité d'action de certains antimetabolites. *Int. J. Cancer* **1,** 463

Siminoff, P. and Menefee, M. G. (1966). Normal and 5-bromo-deoxyuridine inhibited development of *Herpes simplex* virus. *Exp. Cell Res.* **44,** 241

Simpson, C. F. and Kling, J. M. (1967). The mechanism of denucleation in circulating erythroblasts. *J. Cell Biol.* **35,** 237

Sirtori, C. and Bosisio, M. (1966). Oncolysis by *Herpes simplex*. *Lancet* **1,** 96

Skaar, H., Ophus, E. and Gullvåg, B. M. (1973). Lead accumulation within nuclei of moss leaf cells. *Nature* **241,** 215

Skinnider, L. F., Card, R. T. and Padmanabh, S. (1977). Chronic myelomonocytic leukemia. An ultrastructural study by transmission and scanning electron microscopy. *Am. J. clin. Path.* **67,** 339

Smetana, K. and Busch, H. (1964). Studies on the ultrastructure of the nucleoli of the Walker tumor and rat liver. *Cancer Res.* **24,** 537

Smetana, K., Gyorkey, F., Gyorkey, P. and Busch, H. (1970a). Studies on the ultrastructure of nucleoli in human smooth muscle cells. *Exp. cell Res.* **60,** 175

Smetana, K., Gyorkey, F., Gyorkey, P. and Busch, H. (1970b). Comparative studies on the ultrastructure of nucleoli in human lymphosarcoma cells and leukemic lymphocytes. *Cancer Res.* **30,** 1149

Smetana, K., Gyorkey, F., Gyorkey, P. and Busch, H. (1973). Ultrastructural studies on human myeloma plasmacytes. *Cancer Res.* **33,** 2300

Smetana, K., Daskal, Y., Gyorkey, F., Gyorkey, P., Lehane, D. E., Rudolph, A. H. and Busch, H. (1977). Nuclear and nucleolar ultrastructure of Sézary cells. *Cancer Res.* **37,** 2036

Smith, E. B., Nosanchuk, J. S., Schnitzer, B. and Swarm, R. (1968). Fatty inclusions and microcysts. Thioacetamide-induced fatty inclusions in nuclei of mouse liver cells and hepatoma cells. *Archs Path.* **85,** 175

Smith, G. F. and O'Hara, P. T. (1967). Nuclear pockets in normal leukocytes. *Nature, Lond.* **215,** 773

Smith, H., Collins, R. J., Martin, N. J. and Siskind, V. (1982). A questionable developmental characteristic of the ultrastructure of childhood leukaemic lymphoblasts. *Leuk. Res.* **6,** 675

Sobel, H. J., Marquet, E., Schwarz, R. and Mazur, M. T. (1984). Optically clear endometrial nuclei. *Ultrastruct. Path.* **6,** 229

Sobel, H. J., Schwarz, R. and Marquet, E. (1969a). Non-viral nuclear inclusions. 1. Cytoplasmic invaginations. *Archs Path.* **87,** 179

Sobel, H. J., Schwarz, R. and Marquet, E. (1969b). Non-viral nuclear inclusions. 2. Glycogen and lipid. *Lab. Invest.* **20,** 604 (abstract)

Sobhon, P., Tanphaichitr, N., Chutatape, C., Vongpayabal, P. and Panuwatsuk, W. (1982). Electron microscopic and biochemical analyses of the organization of human sperm chromatin decondensed with Sarkosyl and dithiothreitol. *J. Exp. Zool.* **223,** 277

Sobrinho-Simões, M. A. and Gonçalves, V. (1974). Nuclear bodies in papillary carcinomas of the human thyroid gland. *Arch. Pathol.* **98,** 94

Sobrinho-Simões, M. A. and Gonçalves, V. (1978). Nucleolar abnormalities in human papillary thyroid carcinomas. *Arch. Path. & Lab. Med.* **102,** 635

Sohval, A. R., Suzuki, Y., Gabrilove, J. L. and Churg, J. (1971). Ultrastructure of crystalloids in spermatogonia and Sertoli cells of normal human testis. *J. Ultrastruct. Res.* **34,** 83

Sotelo, C. and Palay, S. L. (1968). The fine structure of the lateral vestibular nucleus in the rat. *J. Cell Biol.* **36,** 151

Sparrow, W. T. and Ashworth, C. T. (1965). Electron microscopy of nuclear glycogenesis. *Archs Path.* **80,** 84

Stalzer, R. C., Kiely, J. M., Pease, G. L. and Brown, A. L. (1965). Effect of 5-fluorouracil on human hematopoiesis. *Cancer* **18,** 1071

Stefani, S. S. and Tonaki, H. (1970). Fibrillar bundles in the nucleus of blood lymphocytes from leukemic and nonleukemic patients. *Blood* **35,** 243

Steiner, G. C. (1979). Ultrastructure of benign cartilaginous tumors of intraosseous origin. *Human Path.* **10,** 71

Stelly, N., Stevens, B. J. and Andre, J. (1970). Étude cytochimique de la lamelle dense de l'enveloppe nucléaire. *J. Microsc.* **9,** 1015

Stenstam, M., Von Mecklenburg, C. and Norberg, B. (1975). The ultrastructure of spontaneous radial segmentation of the nuclei in bone marrow cells from 3 patients with acute myeloid leukaemia. *Scand. J. Haematol.* **15,** 63

Stern, H., Allfrey, V., Mirsky, A. E. and Saetren, H. (1951). Some enzymes of isolated nuclei. *J. gen. Physiol.* **35,** 559

Stevens, B. J. and Andre, J. (1969). The nuclear envelope. In *Handbook of Molecular Cytology*, p. 837. Ed. by A. Lima-de-Faria. Amsterdam and London: North-Holland Publ.

Stiller, D., Katenkamp, D. and Küttner, K. (1976). Cellular differentiations and structural characteristics in nasopharyngeal angiofibromas. An electron microscopic study. *Virchows Arch. A Pathol. Anat.* **371,** 273

Stowell, R. E. (1949). Alterations in nucleic acids during hepatoma formation in rats fed p-dimethylaminoazobenzene. *Cancer* **2,** 121

Straile, W. E., Tipnis, U. R., Mann, S. J. and Clark, W. H. (1975). Lattice and rodlet nuclear inclusions in Merkel cells in rabbit epidermis. *J. Invest. Derm.* **64,** 178

Sung, J. H. (1980). Light, fluorescence and electron microscopic features of neuronal intranuclear hyaline inclusions associated with multisystem atrophy. *Acta Neuropathol. (Berl.)* **50,** 115

Švejda, J., Vrba, M. and Blumajer, J. (1975). A freeze-etch study of occurrence of nuclear pores in normal and tumour cells. *Neoplasma* **22,** 385

Svoboda, D., Grady, H. J. and Higginson, J. (1966). Aflatoxin B₁ injury in rat and monkey liver. *Am. J. Path.* **49,** 1023

Svoboda, D. J. and Kirchner, F. (1966). Ultrastructure of nasopharyngeal angiofibromas. *Cancer* **19,** 1949

Svoboda, D., Racela, A. and Higginson, J. (1967). Variations in ultrastructural nuclear changes in hepatocarcinogenesis. *Biochem. Pharmac.* **16,** 651

Swanbeck, G. and Thyresson, N. (1964). Electron microscopy in intranuclear particles in lichen ruber planus. *Acta derm-vener.* **44,** 105

Swanson, J. L., Craighead, J. E. and Reynolds, E. S. (1966). Electron microscopic observations on *Herpes virus hominis* (*Herpes simplex* virus) encephalitis in man. *Lab. Invest.* **15,** 1966

Swift, H. (1959). Studies on nucleolar function. In *Symposium on Molecular Biology*, p. 266. Ed. by R. E. Zirkle. Chicago Ill.: University of Chicago Press

Swift, H. (1963). Cytochemical studies on nuclear fine structure. *Exp. Cell. Res.* Suppl. **9,** 54

Szollosi, D. (1965). Extrusion of nucleoli from pronuclei of the rat. *J. Cell Biol.* **25,** 545

Takeichi, S., Otsuka, H. and Kimura, S. (1977). Studies on tumors produced by cells transformed with herpes simplex virus type 2. *Gann* **68,** 653

Tamura, H. and Aronson, B. E. (1978). Intranuclear fibrillary inclusions in influenzal pneumonia. *Arch. Path. Lab. Med.* **102,** 252

177

Tan, H. K., Harrison, M. and Grainick, H. R. (1974). Nuclear topography in the abnormal cell of Sézary Syndrome: Observation by freeze-etch electron microscopy. *J. Natl. Cancer Inst.* **52**, 1367

Tanaka, R., Iwasaki, Y. and Koprowski, H. (1974). Unusual intranuclear filaments in multiple-sclerosis brain. *Lancet* **1**, 1236

Tanaka, R., Santoli, D. and Koprowski, H. (1976). Unusual intranuclear filaments in the circulating lymphocytes of patients with multiple sclerosis and optic neuritis. *Am. J. Path.* **83**, 245

Tandler, B., Denning, C. R., Mandel, I. D. and Kutscher, A. H. (1969). Ultrastructure of human labial salivary glands. II. Intranuclear inclusions in the acinar secretory cell. *Z. Zellforsch. mikrosk. Anat.* **94**, 555

Tani, E., Ametani, T., Ishijima, Y., Higashi, N. and Fujihara, E. (1971). Intranuclear paracrystalline fibrillar arrays in human glioma cells. *Cancer Res.* **31**, 1210

Tanikawa, K. and Igarashi, M. (1963). Electron microscopic observation of the liver in diabetes mellitus with special attention to the intranuclear glycogen of the liver cell. *J. Electron Micro.* **12**, 117

Tellez-Nagel, I. and Harter, D. H. (1966). Subacute sclerosing leukoencephalitis: Ultrastructure of intranuclear and intracytoplasmic inclusion. *Science* **154**, 899

TerMeulen, V., Koprowski, H., Iwasaki, Y., Käckell, Y. M. and Müller, D. (1972). Fusion of cultured multiple-sclerosis brain cells with indicator cells: Presence of nucleocapsids and virions and isolation of parainfluenza-type virus. *Lancet* **2**, 1

Terzakis, J. A. (1965). The nucleolar channel system of human endometrium. *J. Cell Biol.* **27**, 293

Thoma, F., Koller, Th., Klug, A. (1979). Involvement of histone HI in the organization of the nucleosome and of the salt-dependent superstructures of chromatin. *J. Cell Biol.* **83**, 403

Thomas, D. and Gouranton, J. (1978). Observations on globular intranuclear inclusions in the midgut cells of an insect. *Proceedings of the Ninth International Congress on Electron Microscopy Toronto, 1978.* Vol. II, p. 258

Thomas, D. and Gouranton, J. (1979). Ultrastructural and autoradiographic study of the intranuclear inclusions of *Pinguicula lusitanica L. Planta* **145**, 89

Thomas, D. and Gouranton, J. (1980). Globular intranuclear inclusions in the midgut cells of *Carausius morosus*: Ultrastructure, composition and kinetics of growth. *J. Ultrastruct. Res.* **70**, 137

Thompson, R. C. A., Dunsmore, J. D. and Hayton, A. R. (1979). *Echinococcus granulosus*: Secretory activity of the rostellum of the adult cestode *in situ* in the dog. *Exp. Parasitol.* **48**, 144

Toker, C. and Trevino, N. (1966). Ultrastructure of human primary hepatic carcinoma. *Cancer* **19**, 1594

Tooze, J. and Davies, H. G. (1963). The occurrence and possible significance of haemoglobin in the chromosomal regions of mature erythrocyte nuclei of the newt. *Triturus cristatus cristatus. J. Cell Biol.* **16**, 501

Toper, S., Bannister, C. M., Lincoln, J., Mann, D. M. A. and Yates, P. O. (1980). Nuclear inclusions in Alzheimer's disease. *Neuropath. & Appl. Neurobiology* **6**, 245

Topilko, A., Moyne, G. and Zakrzewski, A. (1981). Intranuclear dense granules in tumor cells of nasopharyngeal angiofibroma. Ultrastructure and submicroscopic cytochemistry. *Rev. Laryngol.* **102**, 491

Topilko, A., Zakrzewski, A., Pichard, E. and Viron, A. (1984). Ultrastructural cytochemistry of intranuclear dense granules in nasopharyngeal angiofibroma. *Ultrastruct. Path.* **6**, 221

Torack, R. M. (1961). Ultrastructure of capillary reaction to brain tumors. *Archs Neurol. Chicago* **5**, 416

Torikata, C. and Ishiwata, K. (1977). Intranuclear tubular structures observed in the cells of an alveolar cell carcinoma of the lung. *Cancer* **40**, 1194

Toro, I. and Olah, I. (1966). Nuclear blebs in the cells of the guinea-pig thymus. *Nature, Lond.* **212**, 315

Trump, B. F., Goldblatt, P. J. and Stowell, R. E. (1963). Nuclear and cytoplasmic changes during necrosis *in vitro* (autolysis); an electron microscopic study. *Am. J. Path.* **43**, 23a

Trump, B. F., Goldblatt, P. J. and Stowell, R. E. (1965a). Studies on necrosis of mouse liver *in vitro*. Ultrastructural alterations in the mitochondria of hepatic parenchymal cells. *Lab. Invest.* **14**, 343

Trump, B. F., Goldblatt, P. J. and Stowell, R. E. (1965b). Studies of necrosis *in vitro* of mouse hepatic parenchymal cells. Ultrastructural alterations in endoplasmic reticulum, Golgi's apparatus, plasma membrane and lipid droplets. *Lab. Invest.* **14**, 2000

Tusques, J. and Pradal, G. (1968). Inclusion d'aspect filamenteux, dans le noyau des cellules argyrophiles de la muqueuse gastrique du Lapin, mise en évidence en microscopie électronique. *C. R. Acad. Sci. (D). Paris* **267**, 1738

Ulrich, J. and Kidd, M. (1966). Subacute inclusion body encephalitis. A histological and electron microscopical study. *Acta neuropath.* **6**, 359

Undritz, E. (1952). *Sandoz Atlas of Haematology,* Fig. 140. Basle: Sandoz Ltd.

Urbaneck, D. and Schulze, P. (1969). Untersuchungen zur Pathologie und Pathogenese der enzootischen Rinderleukose. *Arch. Exper. Vet. Med.* **23**, 1103

Vagner-Capodano, A. M., Mauchamp, J., Stahl, A. and Lissitzky, S. (1980). Nucleolar budding and formation of nuclear bodies in cultured thyroid cells stimulated by Thyrotropin, Dibutyryl Cyclic AMP, and Prostaglandin E_2. *J. Ultrastruct. Res.* **70,** 37

Vallat, J. M., Leboutet, M. J., Loubet, A., Corvisier, N. and Dumas, M. (1983). Nonviral intranuclear inclusions in a nerve biopsy: an ultrastructural study. *Muscle and Nerve* **6,** 167

van der Putte, S. C. J., Schuurman, H. J., Rademakers, L. H. P. M., Kluin, Ph., and van Unnik, J. A. M. (1984). Malignant lymphoma of follicle centre cells with marked nuclear lobation. *Virchows Arch. B Cell Pathol.* **46,** 93

Van Noord, M. J., Van Pelt, Frida G., Hollander, C. F. and Daems, W. T. (1972). The development of ultrastructural glomerular alterations in *Praomys (mastomys) natalensis*. An electron microscopic study. *Lab. Invest.* **26,** 364

Vazquez, J. J., Ortuno, G. and Cervos-Navarro, J. (1970). An ultrastructural study of spheroidal nuclear bodies found in gliomas. *Virchows Arch. Abt. B Zellpath.* **5,** 288

Vasquez-Nin, G. and Bernhard, W. (1971). Comparative ultrastructural study of perichromatin- and Balbiani ring granules. *J. Ultrastruct. Res.* **36,** 842

Vielkind, U. and Vielkind, J. (1970). Nuclear pockets and projections in fish melanoma. *Nature* **226,** 655

Volk, B. and Maletz, J. (1985). Nuclear inclusions following chronic ethanol administration. *Acta Neuropathol., (Berl.)* **67,** 170

Vuillet-Luciani, J., Vio, M., Cataldo, C. and Sëite, R. (1979). Frequency and distribution of tubulo-filamentous nuclear inclusions in the celiac ganglion of the cat as revealed by serial sections. *Experientia* **35,** 394

Wachstein, M. (1949). Studies on inclusion bodies. 1. Acid fastness of nuclear inclusion bodies that are induced by ingestion of lead and bismuth. *Am. J. clin. Path.* **19,** 608

Wachstein, M. and Zak, F. G. (1946). Bismuth pigmentation. Its histochemical identification. *Am. J. Path.* **22,** 603

Walton, J. R. (1974). Intranuclear inclusions in the lead-poisoned cultured kidney cell. *J. Path.* **112,** 213

Wang, N-S. (1974). Fine structural alterations in mesothelial cells associated with cardiac anomaly. *Virchows Arch. Abt. B. Zellpath.* **15,** 217

Warchol, J. B. (1978). Intranuclear microfilament bundles in the ependymal cells of the third ventricle of the rat. *Cell Tiss. Res.* **194,** 353

Wassef, M. (1979). A cytochemical study of interchromatin granules. *J. Ultrastruct. Res.* **69,** 121

Watanabe, I. and Okazaki, H. (1973). Virus-like structure in multiple sclerosis. *Lancet* **2,** 569

Watrach, A. M. and Vatter, A. E., Jr. (1962). The nature of inclusion bodies in lead poisoning. In *Proc. Fifth Int. Congr. for Electron Microscopy*, p.VV-II. Ed. by S. S. Breese, New York: Academic Press

Watson, D. H. and Wildy, P. (1963). Some serological properties of *Herpes virus* particles studied with the electron microscope. *Virology* **21,** 100

Watson, M. L.(1955). The nuclear envelope. Its structure and relation to cytoplasmic membranes. *J. biophys. biochem. Cytol.* **1,** 257

Watson, M. L. (1959). Further observations on the nuclear envelope of the animal cell. *J. biophys. biochem. Cytol.* **6,** 147

Watson, M. L. (1962). Observations on a granule associated with chromatin in the nuclei of cells of rat and mouse. *J. Cell Biol.* **13,** 162

Weast, R. C. (1975). Ed. *Handbook of Chemistry and Physics*, 56th edition. Ohio: CRC Press

Weber, A., Andrews, J., Dickinson, B., Larson, V., Hammer, R., Dirks, V., Sorensen, D. and Frommes, S. (1969). Occurrence of nuclear pockets in lymphocytes of normal, persistent lymphocytotic and leukemic adult cattle. *J. Natl. Cancer Inst.* **43,** 1307

Weber, A. F. and Frommes, S. P. (1963). Nuclear bodies: their prevalence, location and ultrastructure in the calf. *Science* **141,** 912

Weber, A. F., Whipp, S., Usenik, E. and Frommes, S. (1964). Structural changes in the nuclear body in the adrenal zona fasciculata of the calf following the administration of ACTH. *J. Ultrastruct. Res.* **11,** 564

Weindl, A., Schwink, A. and Wetzstein, R. (1967). Intranucleäre Tubuli-Bündel im Gefäßorgan der lamina terminalis. *Naturwissenschaften* **54,** 473

Weiner, L. P., Herndon, R. M., Narayan, O., Johnson, R. T., Shah, K., Rubinstein, L. J., Preziosi, T. J. and Conley, F. K. (1972). Isolation of virus related to SV40 from patients with progressive multifocal leukoencephalopathy. *New Engl. J. Med.* **286,** 385

Weintraub, M., Ragetli, H. W. J. and Schroeder, B. (1971). The protein composition of nuclear crystals in leaf cells. *Am. J. Bot.* **58,** 182

Weiss, J. and Lansing, A. I. (1953). Age changes in the fine structure of anterior pituitary of the mouse. *Proc. Soc. Exp. Biol. Med.* **82,** 460

Weiss, M. and Meyer, J. (1972). Comparison of the effects of Coxsackie virus A9 and of actinomycin D on the nucleolar ultrastructure of the monkey kidney cells. *J. Ultrastruct. Res.* **38,** 411

Wessel, W. (1958). Electronenmikroskopische untersuchungen von intranuclearen einschlusskorpern. *Virchows Arch. path. Anat. Physiol.* **331,** 314

Wiener, J., Spiro, D. and Loewenstein, W. R. (1965). Ultrastructure and permeability of nuclear membranes. *J. Cell Biol.* **27,** 107

Willey, T. J. and Schultz, R. L. (1971). Intranuclear inclusions in neurons of the cat primary olfactory system. *Brain Res.* **29,** 31

Willison, J. H. M. and Rajaraman, R. (1976). 'Large' and 'small' nuclear pore complexes: the influence of glutaraldehyde. *J. Microscopy* **109,** 183

Wills, E. J. (1968). Acute infective hepatitis. *Archs Path.* **86,** 184

Wills, E. J. (1983). Ultrathin section electron microscopy in the diagnosis of viral infections. *Path Ann.* **18,** 139

Wilt, F. H. (1967). The control of embryonic hemoglobin synthesis. In *Advances in Morphogenesis,* Vol.6, p.89. Ed. by M. Abercrombie and T. Brachet. New York. Academic Press

Wischnitzer, S. (1958). An electron microscope study of the nuclear envelope in amphibian oocytes. *J. Ultrastruct. Res.* **1,** 201

Wischnitzer, S. (1973). The submicroscopic morphology of the interphase nucleus. In *International Review of Cytology.* Ed. by G. H. Bourne and J. F. Danielli. Vol. **34,** 1

Wischnitzer, S. (1974). The nuclear envelope: its ultrastructure and functional significance. *Endeavour* **33,** 137

Wiseman, G. and Ghadially, F. N. (1958). A biochemical concept of tumour growth, infiltration and cachexia. *Br. med. J.* **2,** 18

Woodcock, C. L. F., Frado, L. -L. Y., and Rattner, J. B. (1984). The higher-order structure of chromatin: Evidence for a helical ribbon arrangement. *J. Cell Biol.* **99,** 42

Wunderlich, F. and Franke, W. W. (1968). Structure of macronuclear envelopes of *Tetrahymena pyriformis* in the stationary phase of growth. *J. Cell Biol.* **38,** 458

Wunderlich, F. and Herlan, G. (1977). A reversibly contractile nuclear matrix. Its isolation, structure and composition. *J. Cell Biol.* **73,** 271

Wyatt, R. B., Schochet, S. S. and McCormick, W. F. (1970). Rhabdomyoma. Light and electron microscopic study of a case with intranuclear inclusions. *Archs Otolar.* **92,** 32

Yamamoto, T. (1969). Correlation of electron and light microscopy on the replication of a canine adenovirus. *Micro-biology* **1,** 371

Yamamoto, T. and Shahrabadi, M. S. (1971). Enzyme cytochemistry and autoradiography of adenovirus-infected cells as determined with the electron microscope. *Can. J. Microbiol.* **17,** 249

Yasuzumi, G. (1960). Licht und electronenmikroskopische studien an kernhaltigen erythrocyten. *Z. Zellforsch mikrosk. anat.* **51,** 325

Yasuzumi, G. and Sugihara, R. (1965). The fine structure of nuclei as revealed by electron microscopy. The fine structure of Ehrlich ascites tumor cell nuclei in preprophase. *Exp. Cell Res.* **37,** 207

Yasuzumi, G., Nakai, Y. and Ochiai, H. (1975). Electron microscopic autoradiographic studies on nuclear bodies appearing in normal leucocytes. *10th Int. Cong. Anat. Tokyo, 1975 Proceedings.* p. 470

Yasuzumi, G., Nakai, Y., Tsubo, I., Yasuda, M. and Sugioka, T. (1967). The fine structure of nuclei as revealed by electron microscopy, IV. The intranuclear inclusion formation in Leydig cells of ageing human testis. *Exp. Cell Res.* **45,** 261

Yeckley, J. A., Weston, W. L., Thorne, E. G. and Krueger, G. G. (1975). Production of Sézary-like cells from normal human lymphocytes. *Arch. Dermatol.* **111,** 29

Zichner, L. and Engel, D. (1971). Electron microscopical examination of the ultra-sonic effect on the rabbit's synovial membrane. *Z. ges. exp. Med.* **154,** 1

Zimmermann, H. -P., Granzow, V. and Granzow, C. (1976a). Ultrastructure and cytochemistry of Ehrlich ascites cells of the strain HD 33: Masked protein in glycogen deposits. *J. Ultrastruct. Res.* **57,** 140

Zimmermann, H. -P., Granzow, V. and Granzow, C. (1976b). Nuclear glycogen synthesis in Ehrlich ascites cells. *J. Ultrastruct. Res.* **54,** 115

Zina, A. M. and Bundino, S. (1979). Dermatofibrosarcoma protuberans. An ultrastructural study of five cases. *J. Cut. Path.* **6,** 265

Zucker-Franklin, D. (1968). Electron microscopic studies of human granulocytes: structural variations related to function. *Semin. Hemat.* **5,** 109

Zucker-Franklin, D., Melton, J. W., and Quagliata, F. (1974). Ultrastructural, immunologic and functional studies on Sézary cells: A neoplastic variant of thymus-derived (T) lymphocytes. *Proc. Nat. Acad. Sci. USA* **71,** 1877

ZuRhein, G. M. and Chou, S. -M. (1965). Particles resembling papova viruses in human cerebral demyelinating disease. *Science* **148,** 1477

180

2

Centrioles

Introduction

The existence of centrioles and their association with the process of mitosis has been recognized by light microscopists for many years (Van Beneden, 1876). In the historic work *The Cell in Development and Heredity*, Wilson (1925) described them as 'granules of extreme minuteness, staining intensely with iron haematoxylin, crystal violet, and some other dyes, and often hardly to be distinguished from a microsome save that it lies at the focus of astral rays'.

Another intracellular structure, the basal body of cilia and flagella, has long been observed by light microscopists and believed to be related to centrioles (Henneguy, 1897; Lenhossek, 1898). The ultrastructure of centrioles and basal bodies has been studied by several workers (De Harven and Bernhard, 1956; Sorokin, 1962; Renaud and Swift, 1964; Forer, 1965; Stubblefield and Brinkley, 1967) and it is now clear that the two structures are morphologically identical (Stubblefield and Brinkley, 1967) and that the basal body is no more than a centriole in another type of activity.

In suitably stained light microscopic preparations, a pair of centrioles is usually seen in a cell. These present in electron micrographs as short cylindrical bodies, usually lying at right angles to one another. Collectively they comprise the diplosome which usually lies in the juxtanuclear region partially surrounded by the Golgi complex. The region in which the centrioles lie is called the centrosome, and the line joining the centrosome to the centre of the nucleus is referred to as the cell axis. In some cells, such as those of certain epithelia, the diplosomal centrioles lie not in the juxtanuclear position but under the apical portion of the cell membrane.

Although in most instances only a single pair of centrioles is seen, it should be remembered that well before the cell enters mitosis the centrioles replicate (Mazia, 1961). At this stage four centrioles (i.e. two pairs) are seen. Each pair then migrates to the poles of the mitotic apparatus. The megakaryocyte, with its peculiar nucleus derived through cycles of division and fusion of daughter nuclei without cell division (cytokinesis), may contain as many as 40 centrioles. Neoplastic and other varieties of giant cells formed either by repeated division of the nucleus without cytokinesis or a fusion of cells also contain multiple centrioles (*Plate 79*).

Structure and function

Ultrastructural studies have demonstrated that centrioles are hollow cylindrical bodies usually about 0.1–0.25 μm in diameter and 0.3–0.7 μm in length★ (*Plates 79–82*). The cylindrical wall of the centriole is composed of nine longitudinally orientated, evenly spaced triplets of microtubules set in a dense matrix. The microtubules† of each triplet are designated A, B and C as indicated in *Plate 82, Fig.1*. When viewed in transverse section the triplets appear like the arms or vanes of a pyrotechnic Catherine wheel (pinwheel). The vane pitch (i.e. the angle which each triplet axis subtends to the radius of the centriole) varies from about 10 degrees at the proximal end of the centriole to about 57 degrees at the distal end of the centriole (Wheatley, 1982).

The end of the centriole or basal body from which the cilium arises is called the 'distal end'. In longitudinal section the proximal end has a clearer internum (i.e. material within the cylinder). A transverse section of the centriole can be viewed from the distal end or the proximal end (by turning the grid bearing the section upside down). In the former case the vanes of the pinwheel appear to rotate anti-clockwise, while in the latter situation they appear to rotate clockwise.

The detailed anatomy of the centriole is quite complex and difficult to discern. Rarely is a centriole cut exactly transversely or longitudinally. More frequent are oblique sections (*Plate 81, Fig. 3*), where the features mentioned above cannot be appreciated. Even in sections close to the transverse plane, all the microtubules are often not clearly visualized, because they follow a low-pitched helical course and not a course parallel to the long axis of the organelle. Excellent illustrations and a detailed account of the anatomy of the centriole as seen in cultured fibroblasts of the Chinese hamster may be found in Stubblefield and Brinkley's (1967) paper. Here only a brief description of some of these features will be presented.

★The size of centrioles is fairly constant in a given cell line, hence they can be used as internal standards (Wheatley, 1982). In human material the average centriole or basal body measures about 0.4 μm in length. The largest centriole we (Larsen and Ghadially, 1974) have found in human material was in a lupus kidney. It formed the basal body of a cilium (*Plate 506*). This centriole was about 2 μm in length, i.e. about five times the length of the usual centriole, hence we called it a 'giant centriole'. This, however, is by no means the largest centriole known to occur. Giant centrioles up to about 8 μm in length have been found in the testes of neuropteran insects by Friedlander and Wahrman (1966). In contrast to this, the centriole in the water mold *Allomyces arbusculus* is only about 0.16 μm long.

†Microtubule A appears circular in cross section; microtubules B and C present C-shaped profiles, because they share the walls of adjacent microtubules. Like most other microtubules (*see* page 937) microtubule A has 13 tubulin protofilaments but microtubules B and C each have only 10 tubulin protofilaments (Fawcett, 1981).

Plate 79
Poorly differentiated carcinoma of adrenal cortex. Depicted here is a giant cell containing several centrioles. Profiles 1–8 derive from centrioles cut in various planes. Profiles 9 and 10 are acceptable as cuts through the peripheral parts of centrioles. Also seen is an obliquely cut cilium (C) lying in a vacuole or a tunnel which probably communicates with the cell surface. (This phenomenon is explained on page 1178). The centriole acting as the basal body of this cilium lies outside the plane of this section. × 74 000

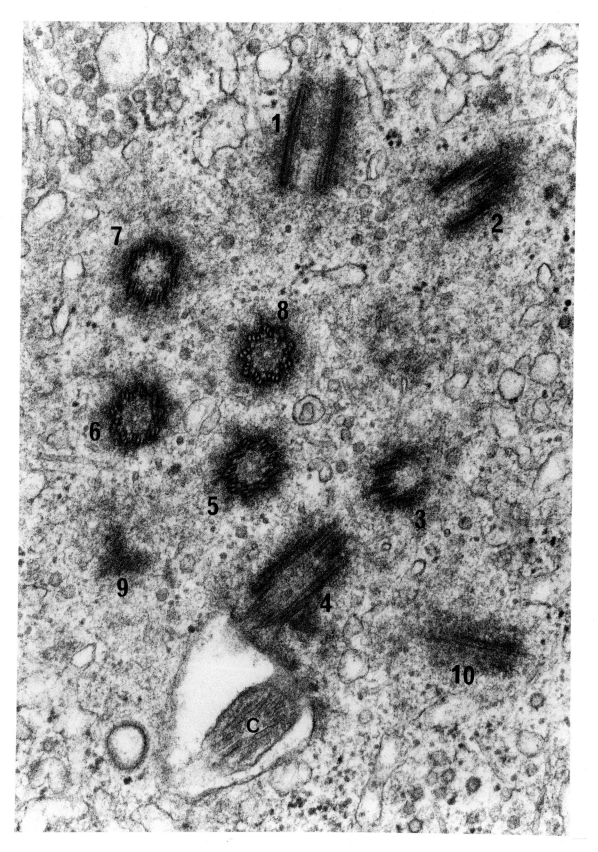

The 'cavity' within the hollow cylindrical centriole contains many interesting structures besides material resembling the cytoplasm. In sections (transverse, oblique or longitudinal) through the centriole a small vesicle 60 nm in diameter is sometimes seen (*Plate 81*). The significance and function of this structure are entirely unknown, but it has been seen in the centrioles of a wide variety of cells and is probably of universal occurrence. Another component which is singularly difficult to demonstrate is the internal helix which spirals the entire length of the cylinder just under the triplets (*Plate 80*).

Since the centriole has a rotational symmetry (ninefold), it is possible to perform a Markham analysis on this structure (Markham *et al.*, 1963). Briefly, this involves making a multiple exposure photograph from an electron micrograph of a transverse section of a centriole, rotated through a 40-degree angle between each of the nine exposures. Such treatment enhances structures that repeat at 40-degrees and tends to obliterate the randomly distributed structures and 'noise' in the electron micrograph. Using this technique, Stubblefield and Brinkley (1967) have shown a faint double structure, called the triplet base, on which the triplet blade rests. The innermost dense part of this structure forms a foot-like appendage continuous with the microtubule A (*Plate 82, Fig. 1*). On Markham analysis performed on thicker sections where a substantial part of the arc of the internal helix is included, it can be shown that this helical structure contacts the 'feet' mentioned above.

Markham analysis of transverse sections at one end of the centriole reveals another structure which has been called the cartwheel. This has been seen in the centrioles and basal bodies of several species (Gibbons and Grimstone, 1960; Gall, 1961). (In some protozoon centrioles more than one cartwheel is present.) The cartwheel has a ninefold symmetry and presents as nine radial spokes arising from a hub at the centre of the centriole and extending to the triplet base. A structure with eightfold symmetry, called the octagonal end structure, is seen in the end opposite to the cartwheel (Stubblefield and Brinkley, 1967). It is probably homologous to the basal plate of basal bodies.

Adjacent to, and at times continuous with, the centriole are seen various pericentriolar structures or satellites. They show numerous diverse forms, such as knob-like dense bodies, radial arms extending from one end of the centriole, or electron-dense granular and fibrillary masses quite separate from the centriole.

Plate 80

Two parent centrioles cut transversely are seen in company with immature daughter centrioles sectioned longitudinally. One of the parent centrioles is slightly obliquely sectioned so that a fairly large segment of the internal helix is revealed (arrow). Note also the numerous microtubules radiating from the centrosome. × 40 000 (*From Stubblefield and Brinkley, 1967*)

184

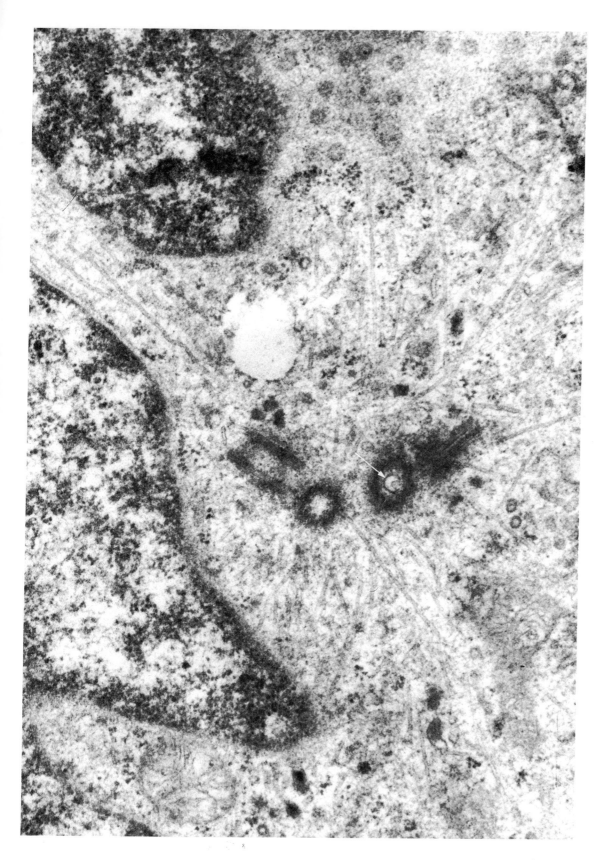

185

Microtubules are at times seen radiating from (usually at angles approaching 90 degrees to the centriolar wall) the centrosome (*Plates 80* and *81*), particularly in rapidly growing cells where a part of the mitotic apparatus persists during interphase. Many more microtubules are seen when the cell is entering the mitotic phase and during mitosis. Such appearances led to the belief that centrioles either produce tubulin dimers from which microtubules are formed or that they serve as nucleation sites and that microtubules are assembled and organized by centrioles from the pool of tubulin in the cytoplasm. However, careful examination of the diplosomal region has shown that few if any microtubules actually arise from the centriolar wall, and that in fact they arise from pericentriolar structures. Since centrioles are instruments of synthesis and/or organization of pericentriolar material, one may argue that they are at best only indirectly involved in microtubule assembly and spindle mechanics. Indeed one may contend that centrioles are not absolutely essential for spindle formation because in plants the typical mitotic spindle forms and mitosis proceeds in the absence of centrioles.

At an early stage of cell division the centrioles replicate and position themselves to form the poles of the future mitotic spindle. Ultrastructural studies have shown that the mitotic apparatus (comprising the spindle and astral rays of classic light microscopy) is not composed of 'fibres' (as believed by light microscopists) but of microtubules. With the condensation of chromosomes and the dissolution of the nuclear envelope, microtubules form by polymerization from the tubulin in the cytoplasmic pool. The microtubule bundles extend from pole-to-pole (equivalent of spindle fibres) and from chromosomes-to-poles (equivalent of astral rays). At anaphase the separation of the chromosomes is as a rule produced by two movements: (1) a movement of the chromosomes towards the poles; and (2) a movement of the poles away from each other (however, either may occur alone in some cells). The actual motive force which generates these movements remains controversial. Some investigators favour a sliding microtubule mechanism (as seen in cilia), while others favour the idea that polarized polymerization lengthens the pole-to-pole microtubules (this pushes the poles apart) and depolymerization shortens the pole-to-chromosome microtubules (this draws the chromosomes towards the poles).

Plate 81

Fig. 1. Cross-section of a centriole from a Chinese hamster fibroblast cultivated *in vitro.* × 120 000 (*From Stubblefield and Brinkley, 1967*)

Fig. 2. Longitudinal section of a centriole from a mitotic cell. Note the central vesicle (V) and adjacent cytoplasmic microtubules (arrows). × 140 000 (*From Stubblefield and Brinkley, 1967*)

Fig. 3. Obliquely sectioned centrioles from a rat sarcoma. The section has passed through the central vesicle (V) in one of the centrioles. × 102 000

186

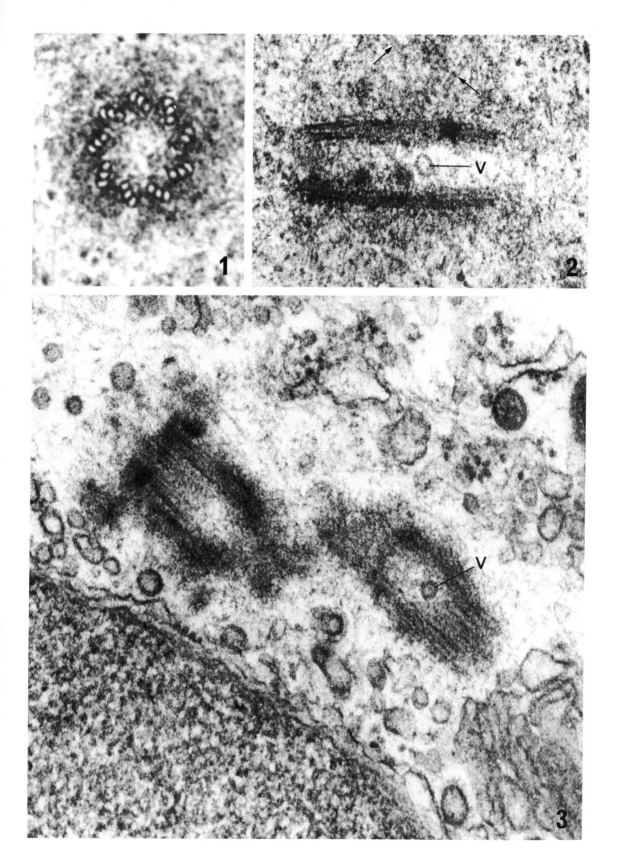

187

As mentioned before (page 181), the basal body of the cilium is no more than a centriole in another type of activity. During ciliogenesis newly formed single centrioles serve as the basal bodies of developing cilia. The nine peripheral doublets of the axial microtubule complex of cilia develop in continuity with the inner two microtubules (A and B) of the centriolar triplets (Gibbons and Grimstone, 1960). Thus in this instance the microtubules in the centriole do serve as nucleation sites for microtubular protein (i.e. tubulin dimers) to form the microtubules in cilia.

Centrioles are self-replicating organelles but the process involved is not one of fission whereby a structure divides to produce two equivalent daughter units, but a generative mechanism which involves the production of a procentriole from or near the end of the parent. The procentriole is a short cylindrical body with a structure similar to the parent centriole. Growth and lengthening of the procentriole at right angles to the parent produces a mature centriole (Plate 82, Fig. 2). According to some observers, basal bodies are also produced in a similar fashion from pre-existing centrioles (Gall, 1961; Mizukami and Gall, 1966; Steinman, 1968; Kalnins and Porter, 1969), but others claim that basal bodies arise also from the granular and filamentous bodies found in the neighbourhood of the centrioles and elsewhere in the cell (Dirksen and Crocker, 1965; Sorokin, 1968; Dirksen, 1971).

Since centrioles are self-replicating organelles it was at one time thought that like mitochondria they may have their own DNA. Early biochemical studies on isolated basal bodies (Seaman, 1960; Randall and Disbrey, 1965) gave credence to this idea but later work (Flavell and Jones, 1971) with better purified fractions does not support this thesis. However, several studies (Stubblefield and Brinkley, 1967; Brinkley and Stubblefield, 1970; Hartman et al., 1974; Dippell, 1976) support the idea that RNA is present in centrioles and their satellites.

Plate 82

Fig. 1. High-resolution photograph obtained by the Markham technique using the centriole image shown in *Plate 81, Fig. 1*. The microtubules A, B and C are clearly visualized, as are the triplet base and dense foot (circle). × 460 000 *(From Stubblefield and Brinkley, 1967)*

Fig. 2. A procentriole (arrow) is seen arising as a short cylindrical structure at right angles to a parent centriole. Numerous centriolar satellites are also present. × 48 000 *(From Stubblefield and Brinkley, 1967)*

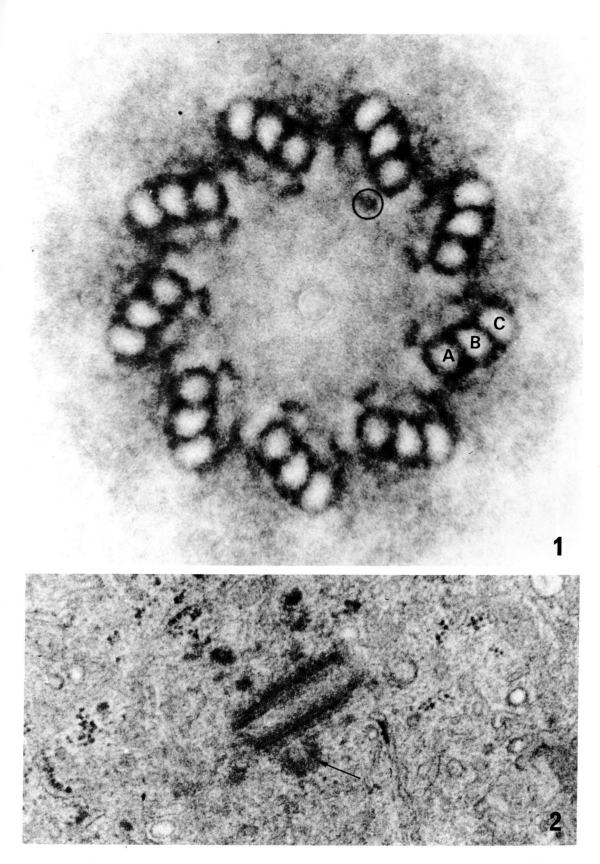

References

Brinkley, B. R. and Stubblefield, E. (1970). Ultrastructure and interaction of the kinetochore and centriole in mitosis and meiosis. In *Advances in Cell Biology*, Vol. 1. Ed. by D. M. Prescott. New York: Appleton-Century-Crofts

De Harven, E. and Bernhard, W. (1956). Etude au microscope electronique de l'ultrastructure du centriole chez les vertebres. *Z. Zellforsch. mikrosk. Anat.* **45**, 378

Dippell, R. V. (1976). Effects of nuclease and protease digestion on the ultrastructure of *Paramecium* basal bodies. *J. Cell Biol.* **69**, 622

Dirksen, E. R. (1971). Centriole morphogenesis in developing ciliated epithelium of the mouse oviduct. *J. Cell Biol.* **51**, 286

Dirksen, E. R. and Crocker, T. T. (1965). Centriole replication in differentiating ciliated cells of mammalian respiratory epithelium. An electron microscope study. *J. Microscopie* **5**, 629

Fawcett, D. W. (1981). *The Cell*, 2nd Edn. Philadelphia and London: Saunders

Flavell, R. A. and Jones, I. G. (1971). DNA from isolated pellicles of Tetrahymena. *J. Cell Sci.* **9**, 719

Forer, A. (1965). Local reduction of spindle fiber birefringence in living *Nephrotoma suturalis* (Loew) spermatocytes induced by ultraviolet microbeam irradiation. *J. Cell Biol.* **25**, 95

Friedlander, M. and Wahrman, J. (1966). Giant centrioles in neuropteran meiosis. *J. Cell Sci.* **1**, 129

Gall, J. G. (1961). Centriole replication. A study of spermatogenesis in the snail *Viviparus*. *J. biophys. biochem. Cytol.* **10**, 163

Gibbons, I. R. and Grimstone, A. V. (1960). On flagellar structure in certain flagellates. *J. biophys. biochem. Cytol.* **7**, 697

Hartman, H., Puma, J. D. and Gurney, T. (1974). Evidence for the association of RNA with the ciliary basal bodies of Tetrahymena. *J. Cell Sci.* **16**, 241

Henneguy, L. F. (1897). Les rapports des cils vibratilies avec les centrosomes. *Arch. anat. microscop.* **1**, 481

Kalnins, V. I. and Porter, K. R. (1969). Centriole replication during ciliogenesis in the chick tracheal epithelium. *Z. Zellforsch. mikrosk. Anat.* **100**, 1

Larsen, T. E. and Ghadially, F. N. (1974). Cilia in lupus nephritis. *J. Path.* **114**, 69

Lenhossek, M. von (1898). *Verhandl. dent. Anat. Ges. Jena* **12**, 106. Ueber Flimmerzellen

Markham, R., Frey, S. and Hills, G. J. (1963). Methods for the enhancement of image detail and accentuation of structure in electron microscopy. *Virology*, **20**, 88

Mazia, D. (1961). Mitosis and the physiology of cell division. In *The Cell*, Vol. III, p. 77. Ed. by J. Brachet and A. E. Mirsky. New York: Academic Press

Mizukami, I. and Gall, J. (1966). Centriole replication. II. Sperm formation in the fern Marsilea and the cycad Zamia. *J. Cell Biol.* **29**, 97

Randall, J. and Disbrey, C. (1965). Evidence for the presence of DNA at basal body sites in *Tetrahymena pyriformis*. *Proc. Roy. Soc. (Biol)* **162**, 473

Renaud, F. L. and Swift, H. (1964). The development of basal bodies and flagella in *Allomyces arbusculus*. *J. Cell Biol.* **23**, 339

Seaman, G. R. (1960). Large-scale isolation of kinetosomes from the ciliated protozoon *Tetrahymena pyriformis*. *Exp. Cell Res.* **21**, 292

Sorokin, S. P. (1962). Centrioles and the formation of rudimentary cilia by fibroblasts and smooth muscle cells. *J. Cell Biol.* **15**, 363

Sorokin, S. P. (1968). Reconstructions of centriole formation and ciliogenesis in mammalian lungs. *J. Cell Sci.* **3**, 207

Steinman, R. M. (1968). An electron microscopic study of ciliogenesis in developing epidermis and trachea in the embryo of *Xenopus laevis*. *Am. J. Anat.* **122**, 19

Stubblefield, E. and Brinkley, B. R. (1967). Architecture and function of the mammalian centriole. In *Formation and Fate of Cell Organelles*, Vol. 6, p. 175. Ed. by K. B. Warren. New York and London: Academic Press

Van Beneden, E. (1876). *Bull. acad. roy. med. Belg.* **42**, Ser. II, 35

Wheatley, D. N. (1982). *The Centriole: A Central Enigma of Cell Biology*. Amsterdam: Elsevier Biomedical Press

Wilson, E. B. (1925). *The Cell in Development and Heredity*, 3rd edn. New York: Macmillan

3
_____

Mitochondria

Introduction

The term 'mitochondrion' was introduced by Benda (1902) to describe certain thread-like or granular components seen in cells. In living cells these organelles are seen to make slow sinuous movements accompanied by changes in size and shape. They also appear to divide and recombine. Mitochondria show many variations in size, shape and fine structure, yet they are sufficiently characteristic to be distinguishable from other cell organelles in electron micrographs. Mitochondria are now known to occur in the cytoplasm of all aerobic eucaryotic cells. The main morphological features can be summarized by defining a mitochondrion as a double-membrane-bounded body containing matrix, a system of cristae and, frequently, some dense granules (Palade, 1952, 1953; Sjostrand, 1956; Dalton and Felix, 1957; Howatson and Ham, 1957; Rouiller, 1960; Lehninger, 1965). This highly characteristic pattern of organization is found to hold true for the mitochondria of vertebrates, invertebrates, protozoa and plants.

Although the basic morphology of the mitochondrion is so characteristic, innumerable variations on this central theme occur. Such variations can be considered in terms of species differences, tissue or organ differences, physiological and functional activity, and pathological states. It is now well established that the mitochondrion is the major source of cellular ATP. Since it supplies the cell with most of its usable energy it is considered to be the powerhouse or powerplant of the cell (Siekevitz, 1957; Lehninger, 1960, 1961, 1965; Racker, 1968). In cell fractions prepared by homogenization of eucaryotic cells, enzymes of the Krebs cycle, oxidative phosphorylation and respiratory chain are found to be largely confined to the mitochondrial fraction while the enzymes of anaerobic glycolysis occur in the unsedimented supernatant (cytoplasmic matrix or hyaloplasm).

Fractionation of disrupted mitochondria has shown that most of the Krebs cycle enzymes are located in the matrix and the electron transport and oxidative phosphorylation enzymes form molecular assemblies in or on the inner mitochondrial membrane covering the wall and cristae (*see also* page 192). Stalked spheres about 8.5 nm in diameter, covering the surface of the inner mitochondrial membrane facing the matrix, have been found in negatively stained preparations of ruptured mitochondria. The inner membrane and its spheres are thought to be the site of oxidative phosphorylation. The stalks of the inner membrane spheres are probably a preparation artefact. The idea that each sphere may be a complete 'respiratory assembly' has been abandoned because the spheres are too small to hold all the enzymes responsible for electron transport and associated phosphorylation. They are thought to represent the F_1 coupling factor for oxidative phosphorylation, a protein with a diameter of approximately 8 nm and molecular weight 280 000 (Kagawa *et al.*, 1966; Racker, 1968, 1969; Lehninger, 1970a).

Mitochondrial morphology and enzyme content

To demonstrate the ultrastructural anatomy of the mitochondrion and its component parts, I shall here employ a mitochondrion with lamellar or plate-like cristae (*Plate 83*) as this type of mitochondrion is the one most commonly encountered in a majority of the cells of higher animals.

This organelle is bounded by two membranes, an external limiting membrane (about 7 nm thick) and an inner membrane (about 5 nm thick) from which arise the cristae. These membranes enclose two chambers, which are not connected with each other. The outer chamber is the space between the two membranes. The inner or matrix chamber is bounded by the internal membrane, and contains the matrix which is usually more electron dense than the contents of the outer chamber.

The cristae mitochondriales are seen as a system of membranous laminae or plate-like structures lying within the mitochondrion. They arise from the inner membrane and traverse a variable distance across the width of the organelle. The cristae are infoldings of the inner membrane, enclosing a cleft-like space which is continuous with the outer chamber. In favourable sections the membranous layers of the cristae are seen to be continuous with the inner membrane of the mitochondrial envelope (*see also* page 196).

In ultrathin sections not all the cristae within a mitochondrion are visualized, for some of them are cut obliquely or tangentially. This is particularly so in long, thin mitochondria which are often slightly bent and sometimes quite tortuous. Here an appearance is created as if some parts of the mitochondrion are lacking in cristae. Since sectioning geometry can produce this kind of effect, it is extremely difficult to decide in a given example whether the cristae are truly missing or not in a particular segment of a mitochondrion.

In the mitochondria of most cells the matrix contains some electron-dense granules 20–50 nm in diameter. These are referred to by various terms such as 'dense granules', 'intramitochondrial granules' or 'matricial or matrix granules'.

It is now well established that the inner and outer mitochondrial membranes have different permeabilities and chemical compositions. For example, the outer membrane is permeable to sucrose but the inner membrane is not. The evolution of techniques which permit the separation of the outer membrane, inner membrane and matrix have made possible the direct chemical analysis of these components and indicated the locations of various mitochondrial enzymes. The results of these studies have been summarized lucidly by Lehninger (1970a). The localization of some mitochondrial enzymes according to this author is as follows: *Outer membrane*: monoamine oxidase, fatty acid thiokinases, kynurenine hydroxylase, and rotenone-insensitive cytochrome c reductase. *Space between the membranes*: adenylate kinase and nucleoside diphosphokinase. *Inner membrane*: respiratory chain enzymes, ATP-synthesizing enzymes, α-keto acid dehydrogenases, succinate dehydrogenase, D-β-hydroxybutyrate dehydrogenase and carnitine fatty acyl transferase. *Matrix*: citrate synthase, isocitrate dehydrogenase, fumarase, malate dehydrogenase, aconitase, glutamate dehydrogenase and fatty acid oxidation enzymes.

Plate 83

Mitochondria from kidney tubule of mouse, showing the double-membraned envelope (E), lamellar cristae (C), matrix (M) and dense granules (circle). At the base of a crista (arrow) continuity between the inner membrane of the mitochondrion and the membranes of the crista can be discerned. In some zones (⋆) the cristae are presumably tangentially cut and hence not visualized in the electron micrograph. × 90 000

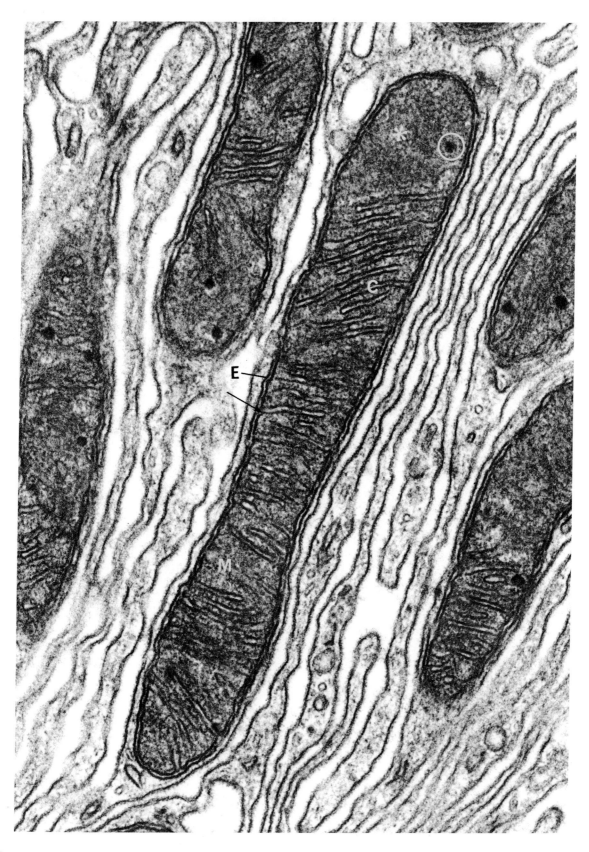

Concentration of cristae

It is widely held that there is a positive correlation between the metabolic activity of a tissue and the number and size of mitochondria and also the number, size, surface area and concentration of cristae. This point may be illustrated by comparing the mitochondria from two extreme examples (*Plate 84*), the high energy transforming (chemical to mechanical) flight muscle of the dragonfly, and the metabolically depressed liver of a frog collected in the winter.

The general validity of the thesis stated above is attested by many examples. Thus large mitochondria with abundant cristae occur in: (1) brown adipose tissue, where energy is required for the synthesis of lipid prior to storage, and later for the breakdown of lipid to yield heat and raise the body temperature during arousal from hibernation; (2) various epithelia where energy is needed for active transport of ions across membranes (e.g. kidney tubules); and (3) continuously active muscle tissue with a high energy demand, like that of the heart and diaphragm. Comparatively speaking, most examples of skeletal muscle and smooth muscle have fewer mitochondria with less abundant cristae. (For references, more details and further examples, *see* reviews by Rouiller, 1960; Novikoff, 1961; Lehninger, 1965.)

In the myocardium of birds, Slautterback (1965) has noted a relationship between heart rate and mitochondrial size and complexity of cristae structure. Similarly cardiac, uterine or skeletal muscle hypertrophy is accompanied or preceded by an increase in mitochondrial mass and also an increase in the concentration of cristae (*see also* page 254).

Exceptions or apparent exceptions to the thesis above have also been recorded. Leeson and Leeson (1969) found complex mitochondrial forms with abundant cristae in rat palatine muscle, and they note that 'mitochondrial concentrations in muscle fibres of the palate are much more extensive than those in the diaphragmatic (red) fibres'. The reason for this is not clear, for one would not expect palatine muscle to be more demanding in energy requirement than the diaphragm. However, as these authors suggest, it is conceivable that palatine muscle may possess hitherto unknown, peculiar or unusual physiological properties. In malignant tumours, the mitochondria are pleomorphic and examples of mitochondria with sparse or numerous cristae may be found in the same tumour and even in an individual tumour cell. The mitochondrial population is also quite variable but often the mitochondria appear to be too few and the cristae too sparse to support the obviously heightened metabolic activity and rapid growth rate. The historical work of Warberg (1956, 1962) showed the predominance of glycolysis over respiration in the energy metabolism of many tumours, and this may well explain the apparent paradox of this fast-growing tissue which as a rule is not particularly well endowed with mitochondria. (For more details about mitochondria in tumours *see* page 284.)

Plate 84

Fig. 1. Liver of a winter-starved frog, showing abundant glycogen deposits (G) and mitochondria (M) with sparse cristae. × 24 000

Fig. 2. Dragon-fly flight muscle, showing voluminous mitochondria (M) with abundant complex cristae. Note also the close association between the smooth endoplasmic reticulum (arrow) and the mitochondria (page 226). × 34 000

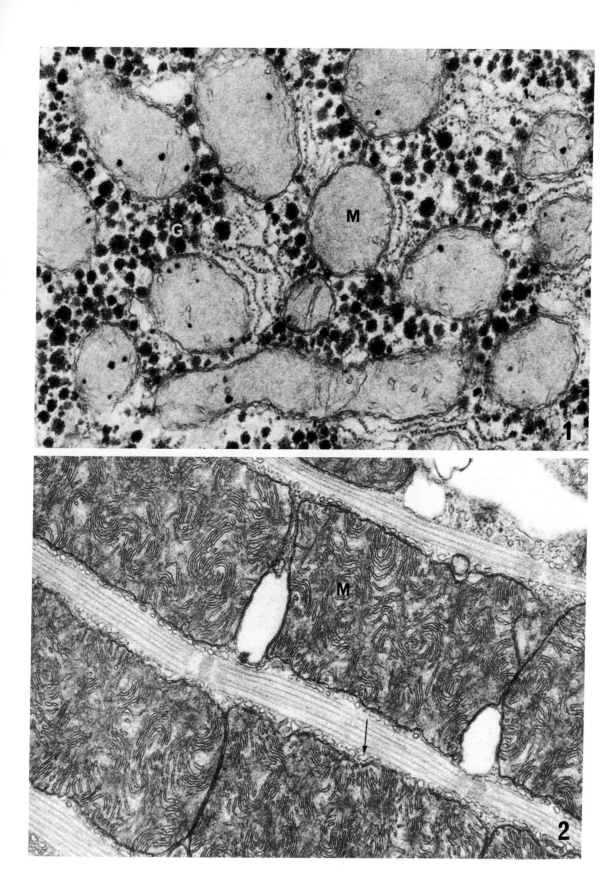

Lamellar, tubular and vesicular cristae

Mitochondria show many diverse variations of form and internal structure, most of which are dependent on the type and orientation of the cristae. As already noted (page 192), lamellar cristae are believed to arise from the inner mitochondrial membrane as thin plate-like or shelf-like infoldings extending a variable distance into the mitochondrial matrix (*Plate 83*). Continuity between the inner membrane of the mitochondrion and the membranes of the crista is occasionally demonstrable but since such images are rare it has been suggested that the failure to demonstrate such continuity more frequently, may be due to the vagaries of sectioning geometry and also because the base of attachment of the cristae to the inner membrane may be quite narrow*. Other alternatives have also been debated; namely, that not all cristae are attached to the inner membrane, or that they are detached during tissue preparation.

The length of the cristae and the extent to which they penetrate the mitochondrial matrix is quite variable. For example, in hepatocyte mitochondria many of the cristae barely reach the centre of the mitochondrion. In the mitochondria of muscle tissue and kidney tubules, they penetrate far deeper, often extending across almost the entire width of the organelle and at times they are seen to be continuous with the inner mitochondrial membrane on the opposite side†. The number of cristae per mitochondrion also varies greatly, and as a rule this is related to the metabolic activity of the tissue (*see* pages 194 and 254).

Tubular cristae also show many variations of morphological detail (*Plate 85*). In transverse section they show the circular profile expected of a tubular structure, but in longitudinal sections they may present as: (1) short blind-ending tubules (villous cristae); (2) irregular meandering or tortuous tubules; or (3) long tubules extending right across the width of the organelle, sometimes continuous with the inner mitochondrial membrane on the opposite side.

*On the basis of serial section studies, Daems and Wisse (1966) concluded that in mouse hepatocyte mitochondria, cristae are attached to the inner mitochondrial membrane by rounded stems which they call 'pediculi cristae'.
†Such an appearance is seen when a mitochondrion is about to divide. (*See Plate 95, Figs. 1 and 2* and *Plate 133, Fig. 3.* See also page 216 and footnote on page 244.)

Plate 85

Fig. 1. A group of mitochondria from *Amoeba proteus* showing tubular cristae. There is no reason to suppose that vesicular cristae are also present because the diameter of the circular profiles (transversely cut tubular cristae) are similar to the width of the longitudinally cut tubular cristae. × 42 000

Fig. 2. Suprarenal cortex from Cushing's syndrome. Both tubular and vesicular cristae are present. This is evidenced by the fact that some of the circular profiles are not acceptable as transverse section through tubular cristae because their diameter is much greater than the width of the longitudinally cut tubular cristae. × 35 000

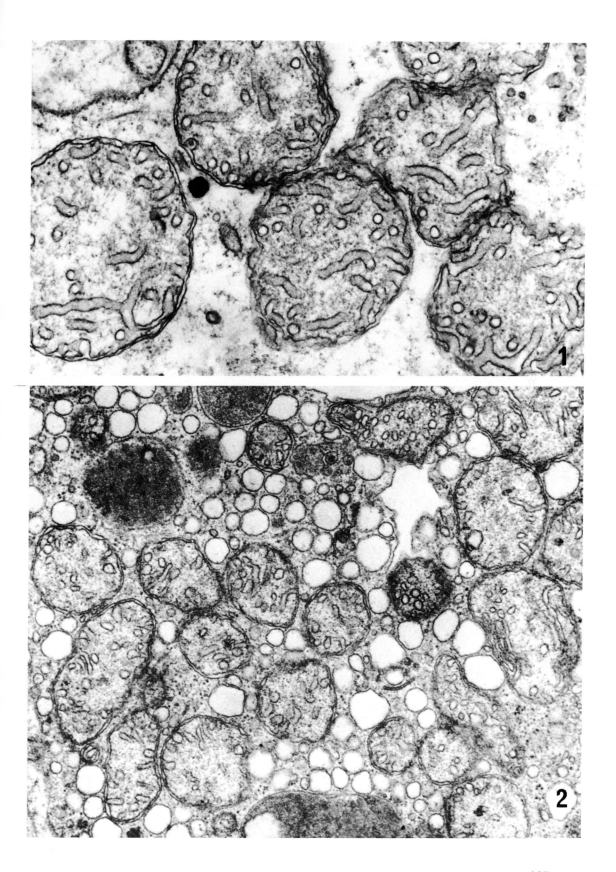

In certain protozoans and other lower forms, mitochondria with tubular cristae are of common occurrence (*Plate 85, Fig. 1*), but in higher animals including man mitochondria with tubular and/or vesicular cristae (*see Plates 85* and *86*) occur in cells which are involved in cholesterol metabolism and the production of steroids, such as the cells of the adrenal cortex, ovary and interstitial cells of the testis. It is interesting to note that all these cells are also well endowed with smooth endoplasmic reticulum★.

It is not always easy to decide whether the cristae in a given mitochondrion are lamellar or tubular. Lamellar cristae cut longitudinally or transversely present an appearance similar to a tubule cut longitudinally. Generally, the gap between the membranes of a lamellar crista is quite narrow and slit-like, while that in the tubular crista is somewhat wider. However, even when one sees this wider gap, one wonders whether this is 'genuine' or due to a slight influx of water (a phenomenon referred to as intracristal swelling; page 242). Thus it is only when one sees some circular profiles (besides the ones described above) acceptable as transverse sections through tubules that one can entertain the idea that tubular cristae are present. Needless to say, vesicles cut in any plane produce circular profiles. Therefore, if only such profiles are present, then one might surmise that vesicular cristae are present. Generally, such cristae are seen budding off the inner membrane of the mitochondrion or from the end of a tubular crista. When vesicular and tubular cristae are present in the same mitochondrion one usually finds that the circular profile produced by a vesicular crista is larger than that produced by a tubular crista. Such difficulties in distinguishing tubular cristae from vesicular cristae and the possibility that these two forms are interconvertible have led some authors to use the term 'tubulovesicular cristae', which seems an acceptable solution to this dilemma, particularly in circumstances where one is not certain as to whether vesicular and/or tubular cristae are present in a given mitochondrion.

★Cell types which have abundant rough endoplasmic reticulum usually have little smooth endoplasmic reticulum, and vice versa. An exception to this is the hepatocyte, where both forms of endoplasmic reticulum are fairly well represented and continuities between the two can be demonstrated. It is interesting to note that an occasional tubular crista is seen among the lamellar cristae in hepatocyte mitochondria.

Plate 86

Mitochondria from the adrenal cortex of a cow showing vesicular (V) cristae, some of which appear to be budding from the inner membrane of the mitochondrial envelope. Cristae which may be interpreted as lamellar (arrows) and tubular (T) are also present. × 52 000

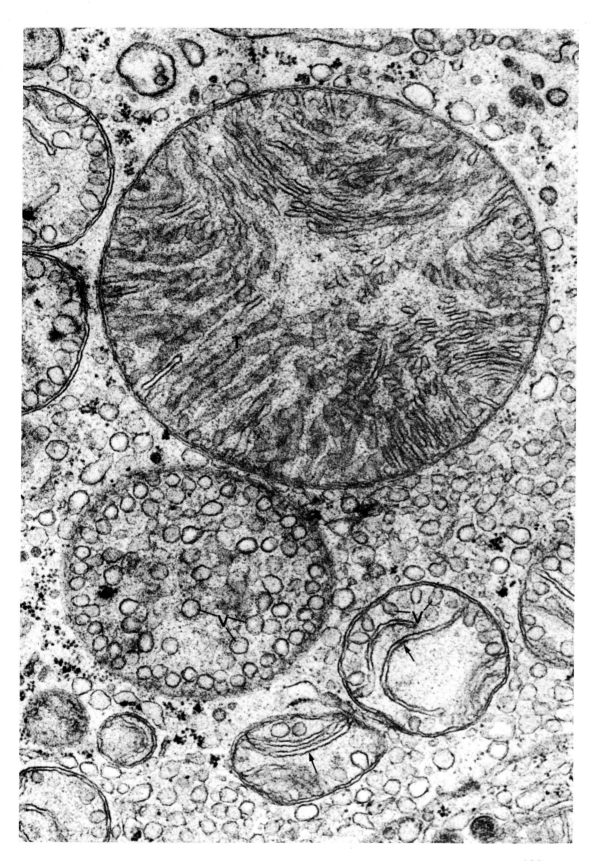

199

Concentric cristae

Mitochondria containing cristae which in ultrathin sections present crescentic, annular, spiral or concentric profiles have been noted to occur in certain normal and pathological tissues (*Plate 87*). Examples of both lamellar and tubular cristae showing this kind of orientation have been observed.

In ultrathin sections, mitochondria with concentric cristae are often found in company with mitochondria with stacked parallel cristae, and it is thought that in such instances the stacked cristae appearance may represent a longitudinal section through cristae which on transverse section would appear concentric (Leeson and Leeson, 1969; Hug and Schubert, 1970).

Mitochondria with concentric cristae have been reported to occur in: (1) axons of lobsters (Geren and Schmitt, 1954); (2) spermatids of snails (Beams and Tahmisian, 1954; Grasse *et al.*, 1956); (3) normal mammalian myocardium (on rare occasions) (Moore and Ruska, 1957; Stenger and Spiro, 1961); (4) hearts of birds such as the quail (quite frequently) (Slautterback, 1965); (5) soft palate of the normal rat (Leeson and Leeson, 1969); (6) a case of idiopathic cardiomyopathy (Hug and Schubert, 1970; this was associated with an increased myocardial glycogen phosphorylase activity, suggesting hypermetabolism); (7) a case of severe hypermetabolism of non-thyroid origin (Luft *et al.*, 1962); (8) cases of myopathy (Hulsmann *et al.*, 1967; D'Agostino *et al.*, 1968); (9) rhabdomyosarcoma (Polack *et al.*, 1971); and (10) Warthin's tumour (adenolymphoma of salivary gland) (Tandler and Shipkey, 1964).

Mitochondria with crescentic or concentrically arranged tubular cristae have been seen in the ovarian theca lutein cells of mouse (Rhodin, 1963) and in the rat adrenals after spironolactone administration (Fisher and Horvat, 1971). This transformation of adrenal mitochondrial morphology was regarded as an expression of increased or altered aldosterone production or secretion or both. Mitochondria with a few annular or concentric cristae may also be found in the adrenal cortex of the cow (*see Plate 127*).

An analysis of the above-mentioned examples indicates that mitochondria with concentric cristae occur in tissues with a naturally high metabolic activity or when metabolic activity is increased in disease or by experimental procedures. It is debatable, however, whether such mitochondria are in fact metabolically more active than others, or represent a sequence of change in the life-span of the mitochondrion, heralding degenerative changes leading ultimately to lysosomal degradation and myelin figure formation. The latter idea finds some support at least in the case of some pathologically altered tissues. For example, such a sequence is suggested by Hug and Schubert's (1970) observations in the mitochondria in cardiomyopathy and by the illustrations of mitochondria in rat adrenals after spironolactone administration (Fisher and Horvat, 1971). Furthermore, there is evidence that mitochondria in adenolymphoma (Tandler and Shipkey, 1964) may be biochemically defective, and in the patient studied by Luft *et al.* (1962) there was uncoupling of oxidative phosphorylation. In any case the two ideas are not mutually exclusive or incompatible, for it is conceivable that at some stage these mitochondria may be metabolically quite active, and later suffer degenerative changes.

Plate 87
Normal rat myocardium showing mitochondria with concentric cristae. × 41 000

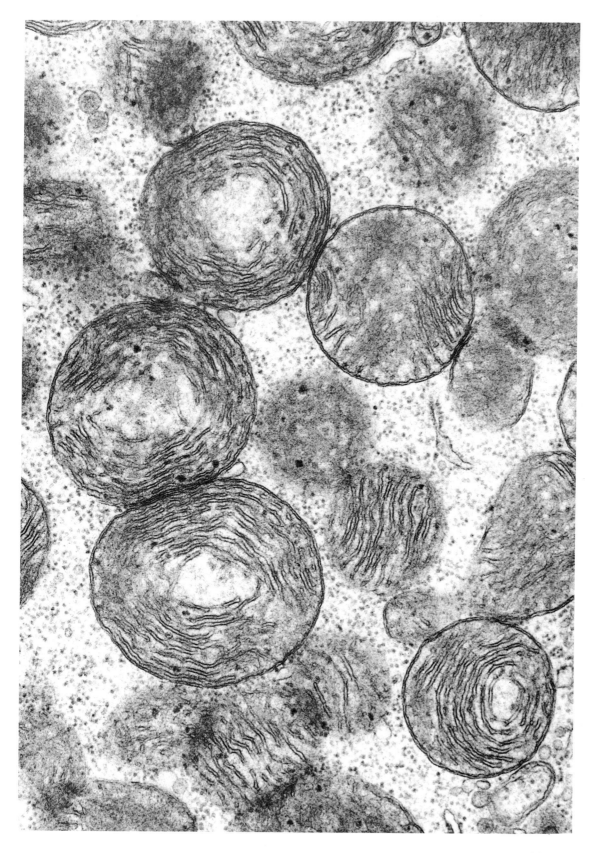

Zig-zag cristae

The term 'zig-zag' is applied to cristae which exhibit sharp angulations of their membranes, and pursue a zig-zag rather than the usual, more or less straight, course across the mitochondrion (*Plate 88*). Mitochondria with zig-zag cristae show many different patterns, depending upon the plane of sectioning and on whether the zig-zag courses of neighbouring cristae are in register or out of register. In the former instance they are easily recognized as zig-zag cristae, but in the latter instance when angulations of adjacent cristae make contact and probably fuse, a complex honeycomb pattern enclosing irregular or cylindrical compartments of matrix is produced (for illustrations depicting this phenomenon, *see* Fawcett, 1981). Frequently all the cristae in a mitochondrion show a zig-zag conformation, but at times only a few are so affected, the rest following a straight course.

Mitochondria with zig-zag or angulated cristae have been noted in various cells, such as: (1) giant amoeba, *Pelomyxa carolinensis*, Wilson, (*Chaos chaos* L.) (Pappas and Brandt, 1959); (2) chloride cells from the gills of *Fundulus heteroclitus* and granular cells from gastric mucosa of the frog (Revel *et al.*, 1963; Fawcett, 1966); (3) myocardium of the canary, and occasionally of sparrow hearts, but rarely in hearts of the zebra-finch, quail or goose (Slautterback, 1965); (4) ventricle and atrium of cats (Fawcett and McNutt, 1969; McNutt and Fawcett, 1969); (5) myocardium of adrenaline-treated rats and, on rare occasions, normal animals (Ferrans *et al.*, 1970); (6) dog heart preserved for 18 hours with plasma-dextran perfusate (Ferrans *et al.*, 1971); (7) hypertrophied human myocardium (*Plate 88*); (8) skeletal muscle from a man with severe hypermetabolism of non-thyroid origin (Luft *et al.*, 1962; Ernster and Luft, 1963); (9) skeletal muscle of rats treated with thyroxine (Gustafsson *et al.*, 1965); and (10) palatine muscle of the rat (Leeson and Leeson, 1969).

Mitochondria with zig-zag cristae have mostly been observed in metabolically active tissues. Since this type of configuration obviously results in an increase in membrane surface per unit volume of mitochondrion, it has been suggested (Pappas and Brandt, 1959) that this is a more efficient mitochondrion better suited to meet high metabolic needs.

Plate 88

Mitochondrion with zig-zag cristae. From a biopsy of hypertrophied human myocardium obtained during open-heart surgery. × 90 000

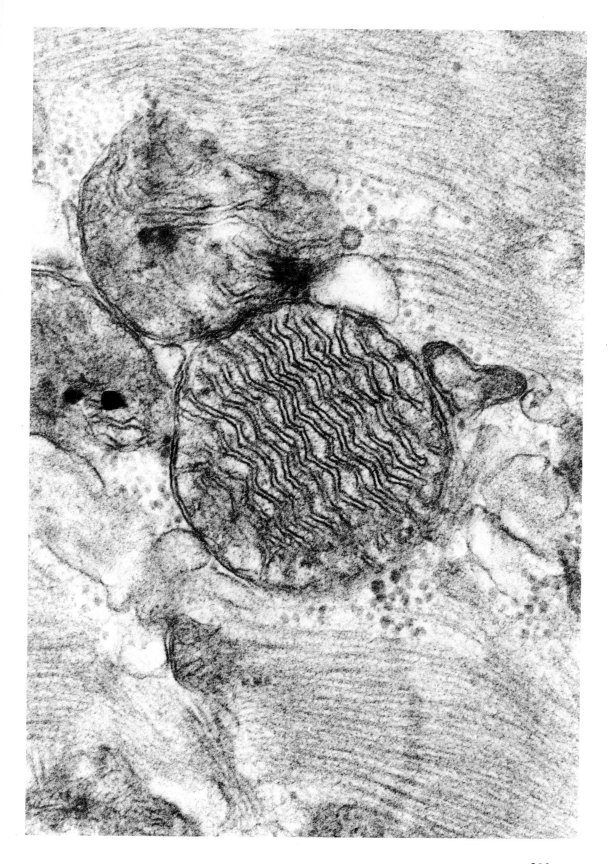

203

Fenestrated cristae

Mitochondria with fenestrated cristae seem to be of rare occurrence. Frequently such cristae occur in close-packed parallel arrays, and when sectioned transversely numerous discontinuities (fenestrations) may be noted along the course of such cristae (*Plate 89*). It is, however, in sections parallel to the surface of the cristae that the circular or nearly circular fenestrae are readily identified. This is particularly so when the fenestrae in adjacent cristae are in register, for in such instances clear matrix-filled channels traversing the mitochondrion at right angles to the cristae are formed.

The finest example of mitochondria with fenestrated cristae so far recorded (Smith, 1963) is that found in the flight muscle of the blowfly (*Calliphora erythrocephala*). Here the fenestrae are in perfect register and are evenly spaced over the cristae. Mitochondria with fenestrated cristae have also been seen: (1) in the myocardium of the shrew (Slautterback, 1961); (2) in birds such as canaries and sparrows (Slautterback, 1965); and (3) in the palatine muscle of the rat (Leeson and Leeson, 1969). In these instances, however, accurate juxtaposition of fenestrae in adjacent cristae is not evident as in the case of the blowfly.

Mitochondria with fenestrated cristae occur in metabolically active tissues and one may suggest that, in these mitochondria packed with cristae, continuity of the matrix chamber and short diffusion paths are achieved by the fenestrae in the cristae.

Plate 89

Mitochondria with fenestrated cristae from the myocardium of a canary.

Fig. 1. In two of the mitochondria where the cristae are sectioned transversely the fenestrae are seen as interruptions along the course of the cristae (arrow). Note that the fenestrae in adjacent cristae are out of register in most instances. × 42 000

Fig. 2. The section has passed parallel to the surface of the cristae in most of the mitochondria shown in this illustration. Mitochondrial matrix and dense granules are clearly seen lying within the fenestrae (circle) of the cristae. × 41 000

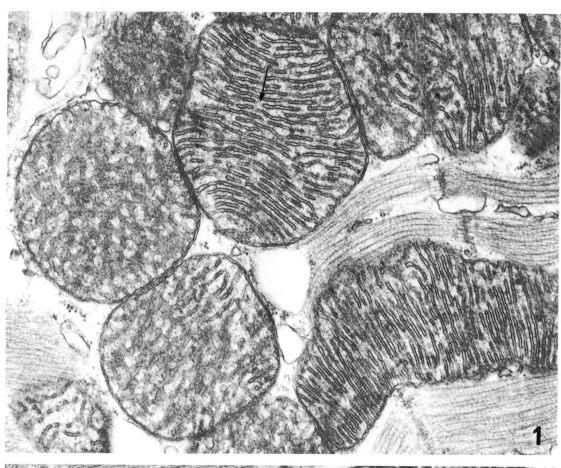

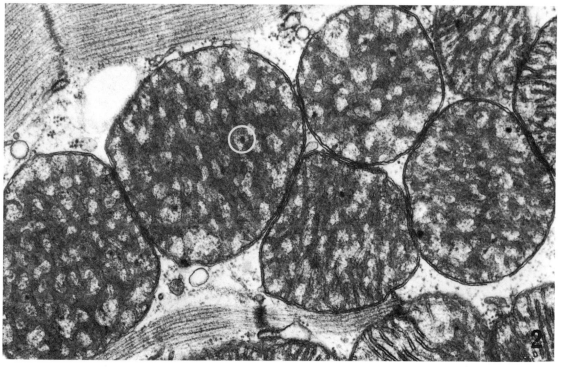

Longitudinally orientated cristae

Mitochondrial cristae usually pursue a transverse course, lying at right angles to the long axis of the mitochondrion, but in this interesting variation of mitochondrial inner structure, longitudinally orientated cristae lie parallel to the long axis of the mitochondrion (*Plate 90*). This transformation may be complete or incomplete. In the latter instance one or both poles of the mitochondrion contain transversely orientated cristae while in the remainder of the organelle the cristae are arranged longitudinally.

Some interesting correlations between this morphological transformation and altered mitochondrial enzyme content have been recorded. For example: (1) the cytochrome oxidase activity of the proximal kidney tubules of frogs (*Rana pipiens*) collected in the winter is greatly reduced compared with freshly caught summer frogs, and in these animals (winter frogs) many of the mitochondria in this region (*Plate 90, Fig. 1*) show partial or complete transformation of the cristae to a longitudinal orientation (Karnovsky, 1962 1963); (2) Luft *et al.* (1962) have reported a case of non-thyroid hypermetabolism where a partial uncoupling of oxidative phosphorylation was associated with complex alterations of mitochondrial morphology (some of the cristae could be regarded as longitudinally orientated); and (3) in rats exposed to high concentrations of oxygen, mitochondria with longitudinally orientated cristae develop in the type II alveolar cells of the lung (Rosenbaum *et al.*, 1969; Yamamoto *et al.*, 1970) and it is known from biochemical studies that high oxygen concentrations can act as an inhibitor of several kinds of enzymatic activity, including such exclusively mitochondrial enzymes as succinic dehydrogenase and cytochrome oxidase.

However, as Karnovsky has already pointed out, low cytochrome oxidase activity is not invariably associated with horizontally orientated cristae. Thus certain 'petite mutant' strains of yeast lack cytochrome oxidase (Ephrussi, 1953) but have unchanged mitochondria with transverse cristae (Yotsuyanagi, 1959), and in the urodele, *Necturus maculosus*, the proximal tubular cells lack cytochrome oxidase but have mitochondria with sparse transverse cristae (Himmelhoch and Karnovsky, 1961). There is lack of both mitochondria and cytochrome oxidase activity in yeast (*Torulopsis utilis*) grown anaerobically (Linnane *et al.*, 1962).

Plate 90

Fig. 1. Mitochondria with longitudinally orientated cristae from a kidney tubule of a winter-starved frog. × 56 000

Fig. 2. Human acute leukaemic cell. Three mitochondria with longitudinally arranged cristae are seen. One shows complete transformation (C), the other two partial transformation (P). × 45 000

Fig. 3. Human acute leukaemic cell, showing partially transformed mitochondria, one of which shows a C-shaped profile. × 41 000

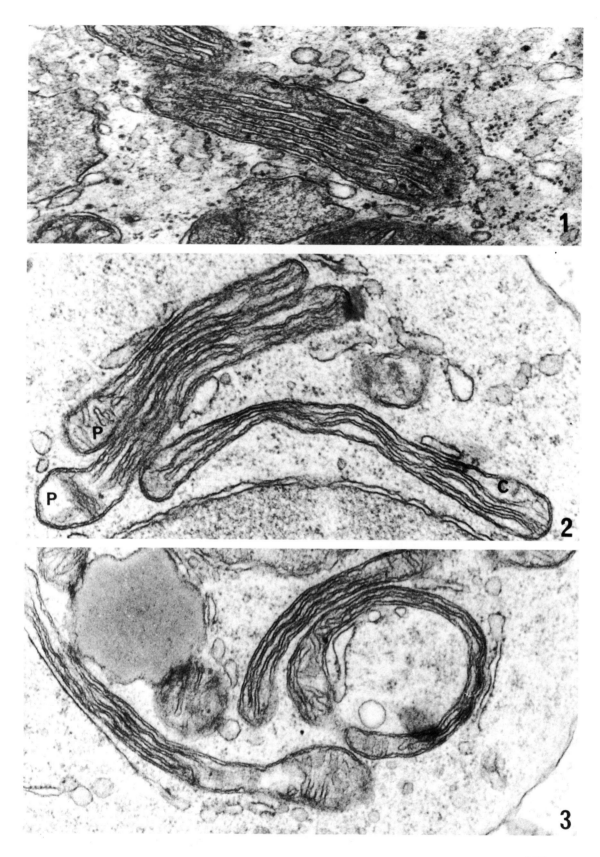

Besides the examples mentioned earlier mitochondria with longitudinally orientated cristae have been seen in: (1) the liver of thyrotoxic rats (Greenawalt *et al.*, 1962); (2) liver of rats after administration of ammonium carbonate (David and Kettler, 1961); (3) liver of rats poisoned with copper (Barka *et al.*, 1964); (4) brown adipose tissue of fetal rat (Suter, 1969; Barnard *et al.*, 1971); (5) adrenal cortex of rat, hamster and mouse (Lever, 1956; De Robertis and Sabatini, 1958; Zelander, 1959); (6) skeletal muscle of rat after thyroid hormone treatment (Gustafsson *et al.*, 1965); (7) thyroid of the partially metamorphosing derotreme (*Amphiuma means*) (Larsen, 1968); (8) neurons in the brain of the rat after delayed perfusion with fixative solution (Karlsson and Schultz, 1966); (9) reactive and regenerating axons in the spiral cord and medulla of rats (Lampert, 1967); (10) neurons in abdominal ganglia of the moth, *Galleria mellonella*, (Ashurst, 1965); (11) gills of the tropical fish popularly known as the 'Kissing gourami' (*Helostoma temmincki*) (Skobe *et al.*, 1970); (12) islet cell tumour of the golden hamster (Amherdt *et al.*, 1971); (13) renal cell carcinoma (Seljelid and Ericsson, 1965); (14) human ovarian carcinoma (Ghadially, unpublished observation); and (15) human acute leukaemic cells in peripheral blood (*Plate 91*).

In some of the above-mentioned examples only a small number of mitochondria showed longitudinally oriented cristae. In virtually all instances they were not enzymatically characterized so it is not possible to say whether they lacked cytochrome oxidase activity or not. However, in the case of the mitochondria in neonatal brown fat, Barnard *et al.* (1971) found that 30–40 per cent of the mitochondria contained longitudinal cristae but cytochemical studies showed that 'these had no observably different cytochrome oxidase activity compared to cristae oriented transversely'.

In the leukaemic cells studied by us (Ghadially and Skinnider, unpublished observations, *Plates 90* and *91*) and also in some of the examples mentioned above, mitochondria with longitudinally orientated cristae, showed C-shaped or ring-shaped configuration in ultrathin sections. It has been suggested that the ring form may be produced either by the approximation and fusion of the tips of a C-shaped mitochondrion, or that C-shaped and ring-shaped mitochondrial profiles represent sections through cup-shaped mitochondria. (For further comments on 'ring-shaped mitochondria', *see* page 278). Transitions from 'ring' forms to electron-dense membranous whorls have also been noted by us and others (*Plate 91, Figs. 2 and 3*). It is worth noting that the ring-shaped mitochondrial profile is not invariably associated with longitudinally orientated cristae, and that ring-shaped mitochondrial profiles with transversely orientated cristae also occur.

Plate 91

From human acute leukaemic cells.

Fig. 1. A partially transformed mitochondrion presenting a ring-shaped profile. × 74 000

Figs. 2 and 3. These illustrations probably depict the sequential stages of membranous whorl formation from mitochondria showing ring-shaped profiles. × 58 000; × 66 000

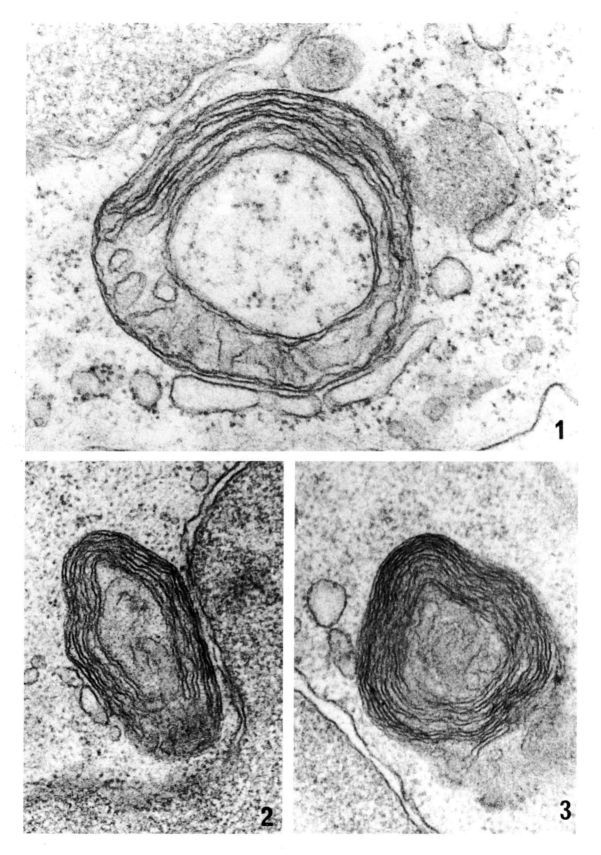

209

Prismatic cristae

The term 'prismatic cristae' is applied to cristae (*Plate 92*) which in transverse section present triangular or rhomboidal profiles and in longitudinal section appear as a pattern of parallel stripes. The fascicles of prismatic cristae may bend abruptly so that cross-cut triangular profiles and the longitudinal pattern of stripes may be seen adjacent to each other. Some lamellar cristae are usually also present in mitochondria with prismatic cristae.

Mitochondria with prismatic cristae have been found in: (1) mucus secreting cells of the salivary gland of the snail, *Limnae stagnalis* L. (Fain-Maurel, 1968); (2) sphincter muscle of the vas deferens of crayfish, *Astacus leptodaxtylus* Eschscholz and A. *astacus* L. (Murdock *et al.*, 1977); (3) kidneys of ammocetes (larvae of lampreys) of *Petromyzon marinus* L. (Youson, 1971); (4) cricothyroid muscle of bats (*Myotis lucifugus* and *Eptesicus fuscus*), (Revel *et al.*, 1963); (5) ischaemic skeletal muscle of rat (Hanzlíková and Schiaffino, 1977); (6) astrocytes from the brain and spinal cord of hamsters and cats (Blinzinger *et al.*, 1964, 1965; Korman *et al.*, 1970; Morales and Duncan, 1971); (7) kidney tubules of rats after subcutaneous injection of glycerin (Suzuki and Mostofi, 1967); (8) hepatocytes of the South African clawed toad (*Xenopus laevis*) after exposure to cold (Spornitz, 1975); and (9) myocardial cells of the oyster (*Crassostrea virginica* Gmelin) (Hawkins *et al.*, 1980).

Hexagonal arrays of filaments have been found between the prismatic cristae and it has been suggested (Korman *et al.*, 1970; Morales and Duncan, 1971) that an ordered packing of filaments transforms tubular cristae into prismatic cristae. Morales and Duncan (1971) point out that 'work with simple non-living models such as applicator sticks and plastic tubing of appropriate sizes results in the tubing assuming triangular outlines in cross sections when compression is applied to such an assembly'. However, it is evident that the filaments as such are not closely packed, and that there is a lucent interval between them. Therefore, Murdock *et al.* (1977) have postulated that these structures are rodlets with an electron-dense core and a less dense shell. Based on serial section studies they propose that 'close packing of these rodlets results in the regular hexagonal dot array. Deletion of three or four rodlets results in spaces with triangular or rectangular cross section. Lining of these spaces with membranes results in cristae with triangular or rectangular cross sections'.

Little however is known about the function or significance of prismatic cristae. Morphometric analysis by Murdock *et al.* (1977) has shown that the average size of a mitochondrion containing prismatic cristae does not differ significantly from that of normal mitochondria, but there is a significantly greater (75 per cent) surface area of cristal membranes in such mitochondria compared with the normal. Therefore one might argue that mitochondria containing prismatic cristae are metabolically more active than normal mitochondria. But it would be difficult to reconcile this with the diverse cell types in which such mitochondria have been found. Further such a hypothesis leaves unexplained the significance of the rodlets, or filaments.

It is well known that besides 'non-specific' ATP production for intracellular energy needs mitochondria in certain sites engage also in 'quite specific' intracellular metabolic processes (e.g. in steroid secreting cells). It is therefore tempting to suggest that mitochondria with so distinctive and highly organized a system of prismatic cristae and rodlets subserve some quite specific but as yet obscure metabolic activity in certain cells.

Plate 92

Mitochondria from the sphincter muscle of the crayfish vas deferens. (*From Murdock, Cahill and Reith, 1977*)

Fig. 1. Cross section of a mitochondrion showing dot array of filaments and triangular profiles of transversely cut prismatic cristae. × 152 000

Fig. 2. Mitochondrion showing dot array of filaments and rhomboidal profiles of transversely cut prismatic cristae. × 100 000

Fig. 3. Both transverse (T) and longitudinal (L) sections through the prismatic cristae are evident in this mitochondrion. A few lamellar cristae (arrowhead) are also present. × 43 000

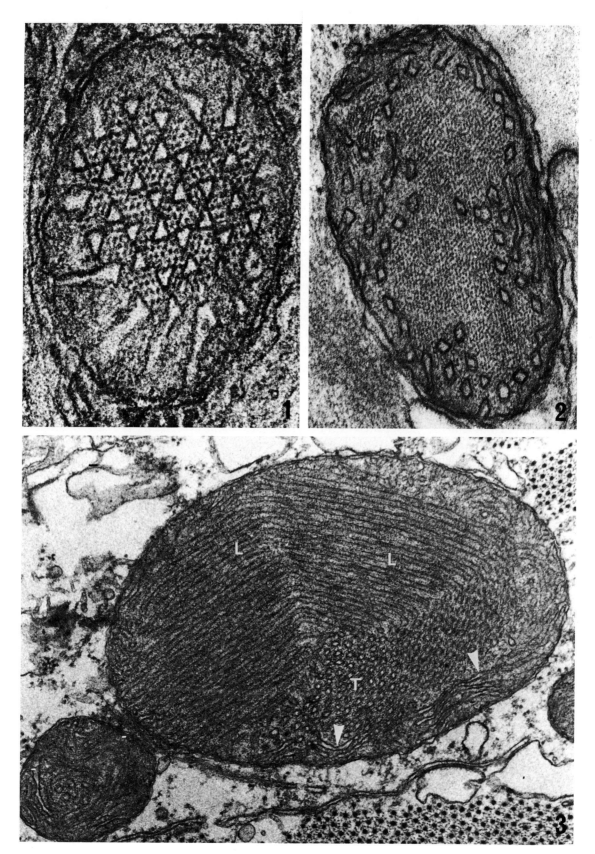

Sinuous undulating and reticular cristae

Depicted in *Plate 93, Figs. 1 and 2* are two unusual mitochondria, the like of which do not appear to have been described in the literature, and I might add that these two are the only such mitochondria I have ever encountered in the various tissues I have examined. The other mitochondria in the specimens in which these mitochondria occurred were unremarkable organelles with the usual lamellar cristae. The mitochondrion in *Fig. 1* was found in an example of the controversial tumour which is regarded by some to be a carcinoid of the breast. Others deny the existence of such an entity while yet others consider it to be an amphicrine tumour (Ghadially, 1985).

In this mitochondrion, the cristae create a reticular pattern. The reticulated appearance seems to be derived from irregularly deployed or sinuous or undulating cristae which have probably fused in places (or contact or overlay each other) enclosing islands or channels of mitochondrial matrix. In the absence of circular profiles suggesting the presence of tubules, one may surmise that the pattern seen here is produced by paired membranous lamellae derived from lamellar cristae. Similar in type but different in overall appearance are the giant mitochondria found in a pleomorphic adenoma by Tandler and Erlandson (1983). The cristae in these mitochondria are sparse and the undulations irregular. The pattern produced is more 'open' because of the abundance of matrix in these giant mitochondria. They call the pattern produced 'reticular pattern' and the cristae 'sinuous cristae', and they state that they are not aware (neither am I) of any other mammalian cell normal or neoplastic in which such mitochondria are found, but that comparable mitochondria occur in the *corpora allata* of locust during sexual maturation (Fain–Maurel and Cassier, 1969).

The mitochondrion in *Plate 93, Fig.2* was found in a metastatic melanoma. The pattern seen here is reminiscent of that thought to be produced by undulating or pouched paired membranous lamellae (i.e. a paired membrane complex) in the cytoplasm (*see Plates 84, 228 and 229*) and nucleus (*Plate 48*). In the case of this mitochondrion the undulating or pouched★ membranous lamellae appear to be derived from the usual or conventional lamellar cristae with which they appear to be continuous in places. The mode of formation and significance of these extremely rare transformations of mitochondrial morphology are totally obscure.

★The differences between undulating and pouched membranes are explained in a footnote on page 94.

Plate 93

Fig. 1. From a tumour diagnosed as a 'carcinoid of the breast'. This mitochondrion found in a tumour cell contains lamellar cristae forming a reticulum. × 64 000

Fig. 2. Metastatic melanoma. This mitochondrion found in a tumour cell contains a membrane complex composed of undulating or pouched lamellar cristae. Note the continuity of this membrane complex with conventional lamellar cristae (arrowheads). × 106 000

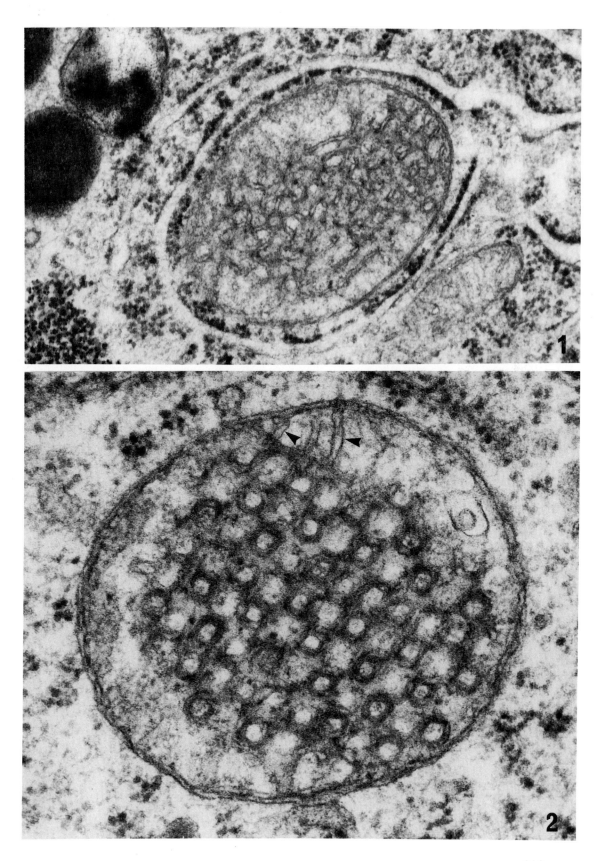

213

Mitochondriogenesis

Theories regarding the genesis of mitochondria may be divided into three not mutually exclusive groups: (1) *de novo* synthesis; (2) origin from non-mitochondrial structures such as nuclear envelope (Hoffman and Grigg, 1958; Brandt and Pappas, 1959), intracytoplasmic vacuoles or membranes (Linnane *et al.*, 1962; Berger, 1964; Threadgold and Lasker, 1967), cell membrane (Geren and Schmitt, 1954; De Robertis and Bleichmar, 1962), pinocytotic vesicles (Gey, 1956), and microbodies (Rouiller and Bernhard, 1956; Engfeldt *et al.*, 1958); (3) origin from pre-existing mitochondria with or without the prior formation of a partition (Fawcett, 1955; Campiche, 1960; André, 1962; Laguens and Bianchi, 1963; Svoboda and Higginson, 1963; Lafontaine and Allard, 1964; Arhelger *et al.*, 1965; Hübner, 1965; Schaffner and Felig, 1965; Glinsmann and Ericsson, 1966; Coupland and MacDougall, 1968; Flaks, 1968; Tandler *et al.*, 1969, 1970; Rifkin and Gahagan-Chase, 1970; Rohr *et al.*, 1970, 1971; Koch *et al.*, 1978).

The term '*de novo*' synthesis was used in earlier times to indicate a non-mitochondrial origin of mitochondria from structures not resolvable by light microscopy. Since the disclosure of numerous organelles by the electron microscope, this term is now restricted to mean origin from the cytoplasmic matrix. There is, however, little evidence that this in fact happens. Similarly, most of the claims regarding the origin of mitochondria from other organelles are also singularly tenuous. (*See* reviews by Novikoff, 1961 and Lehninger, 1965.) For instance the once-popular theory regarding the origin of mitochondria from microbodies (and vice versa) has lost favour as these structures have come to be recognized as organelles in their own right.

However, the idea that mitochondria may arise from some membrane systems, particularly the cell membrane, is at least theoretically admissible (Lehninger, 1965). Although unequivocal proof of origin of mitochondria from various cytomembranes is still lacking, some quite persuasive electron micrographs depicting the possible sequence of events leading to the production of mitochondria in this fashion have been published. For instance, from the morphological standpoint, there are quite interesting reports of origin of mitochondria from: (1) the axolemma of the nerve fibres of the infrared receptors in pit vipers (*Crotalus duvissus*) (De Robertis and Bleichmar, 1962); (2) reticular membranes of yeast (*Torulopsis utilis*) grown anaerobically and subsequently aerated (Linnane *et al.*, 1962); and (3) cytoplasmic vacuoles in certain cells in the skin of the larval sardine (*Sardinops carulae*) (Threadgold and Lasker, 1967) (*Plate 94*).

The view that mitochondria arise by a process of division from pre-existing mitochondria (*Plate 95*) is well substantiated by light microscopic studies of living and fixed cells (for references, *see* De Robertis and Bleichmar, 1962), and by studies which show that mitochondria contain DNA and RNA and that they are capable of synthesizing proteins and lipoproteins. It is

---

Plate 94

From the integumentary cells of the larval sardine. A possible mode of mitochondriogenesis from cytoplasmic vacuoles is depicted in these electron micrographs. (*Figs. 1–3, from Threadgold and Lasker, 1967; Fig. 4, Threadgold and Lasker, unpublished electron micrograph*)

Fig. 1. This electron micrograph shows a large vacuole into which has invaginated a short cytoplasmic process (arrow) containing some vesicles or tubules. × 30 000

Fig. 2. A further stage of evolution is depicted here. The invaginating cytoplasmic process (P) is now quite large, but still probably continuous with surrounding cytoplasm (arrow). The presumptive parts of the future mitochondrion can now be envisaged as follows: matrix chamber (M), outer chamber or intermembranous space (S) and cristae (C). × 36 000

Fig. 3. The invaginating process has almost completely filled the vacuole and nearly formed a normal mitochondrion. Only in one zone the intermembranous space (S) is still quite large. × 32 000

Fig. 4. A transversely cut normal mitochondrion (A) is seen here, as also is part of another (B) which is in a formative stage similar to that in *Fig. 2.* × 48 000

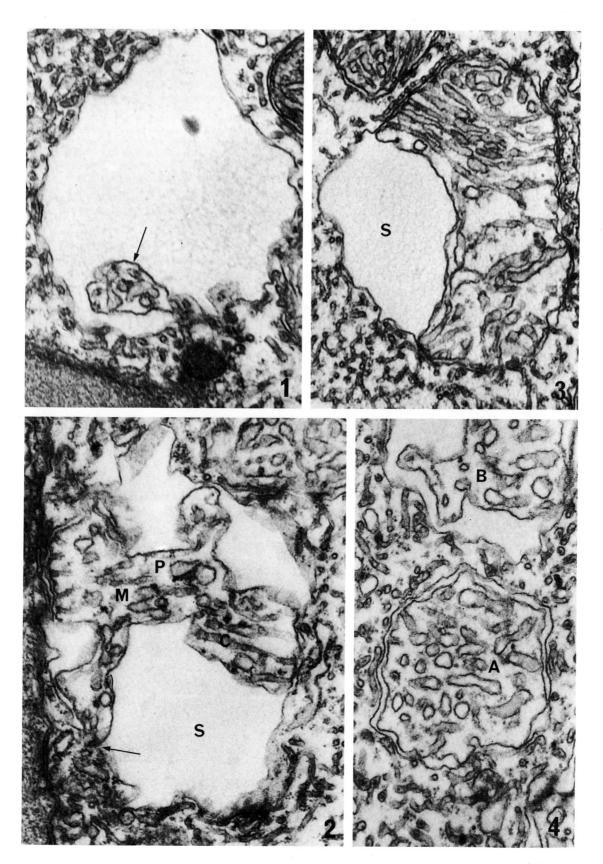

215

thought that mitochondrial protein synthesis independent of nuclear control, is almost exclusively directed to the production of the cristae and the inner membrane of the mitochondrial envelope★, but the synthesis of the outer membrane of the mitochondrial envelope is controlled by nuclear DNA-dependent RNA synthesis. (For references and support of these statements see Nass and Nass, 1963; Nass et al., 1965; Leduc et al., 1966; Anderson, 1969; Bergeron and Droz, 1969; Nussdorfer and Mazzochi, 1971.)

In ultrathin sections, mitochondrial profiles with deep indentations or constrictions suggesting fission or budding are sometimes seen (Plate 95, Figs. 3–6), but this could be the result of sectioning through an irregular or Y-shaped organelle. Even when a narrow connecting piece is demonstrated by serial sectioning, one cannot be certain whether one is witnessing fusion or fission. Nevertheless such considerations do not preclude the possibility that mitochondria may divide by a process of constriction or medial attenuation and indeed there is some experimental evidence to support such a contention (Tandler and Hoppel, 1974).

There is, however, one image which can confidently be interpreted as a dividing mitochondrion, and this process may be called partition and division (Plate 95, Figs. 1 and 2).

This observation, first made by Fawcett (1955), has now been confirmed by many studies. It would appear that in this process a partition forms from the inner mitochondrial membrane which divides the matrix chamber into two distinct compartments. A process of pinching off at the level of the partition then separates the two daughter mitochondria. Here again one may contend that this could be either fusion or fission, for a series of static pictures cannot on their own indicate the direction in which a process is moving. However, such arguments are silenced by the fact that partitioned mitochondria are seen in situations where we know an increase in mitochondrial population is occurring. For example, Tandler et al. (1968, 1969) have shown that in riboflavin-deficient mice the mitochondria are greatly enlarged but reduced in numbers. If riboflavin is administered to such mice the normal mitochondrial size and number are restored, and during this stage many partitioned mitochondria are seen. Similarly, morphometric analysis of perinatal rat livers has shown (Rohr et al., 1971) that the newly formed post-mitotic hepatocyte has only half the normal number of mitochondria. This is followed by a stage of mitochondrial enlargement (volume doubled) and, later, partition and division so that the hepatocyte eventually contains a mitochondrial population of normal size and number. I have observed partitioned mitochondria quite frequently in the regenerating post-hepatectomy liver of the rat but they are rarely seen in normal rat liver. Thus it would appear that one of the ways in which a mitochondrion divides is by first laying down a partition.

★Mitochondrial cristae are absent in certain petite mutant strains of yeast which completely lack mitochondrial DNA. However, the inner and outer membranes of the mitochondrion are not altered (Montisano and James, 1979). This suggests that the inner membrane can be produced under the control of nuclear DNA, but not the cristae.

Plate 95

Figs. 1 and 2. Partitioned mitochondria found in regenerating rat liver. × 45 000; × 43 000

Figs. 3–6. These electron micrographs show various mitochondrial profiles suggesting impending division, but such appearances could be due to sections through irregularly shaped mitochondria. From rat liver (*Figs. 3–5*) and human bone marrow (*Fig. 6*). × 43 000; × 50 000; × 42 000; × 45 000

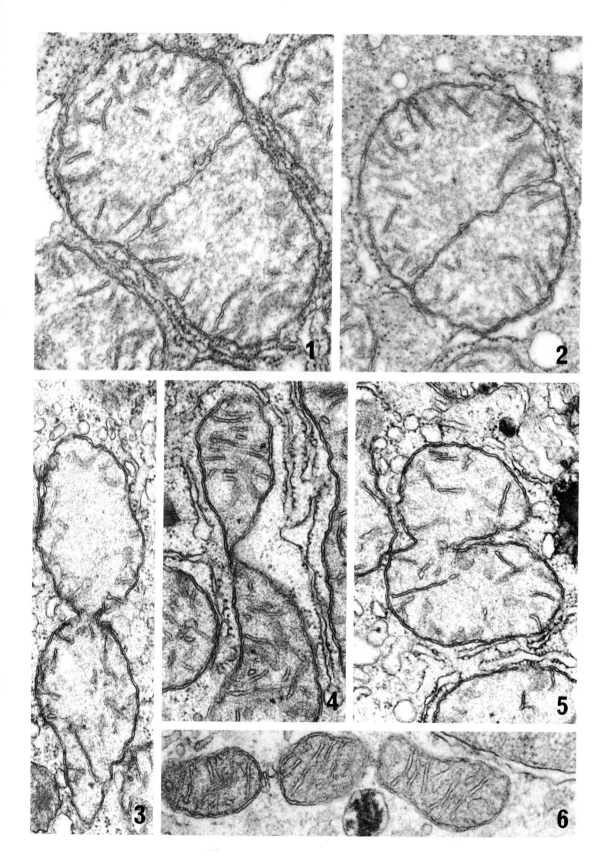

217

Mitochondrial involution and elimination

Numerous biochemical and autoradiographic studies indicate that there is a turnover of mitochondrial components (e.g. proteins, lipids and cytochrome C) and/or entire mitochondria★ in cells (Fletcher and Sanadi, 1961; Wilson and Dove, 1965; Bailey *et al.*, 1967; Beattie *et al.*, 1967; Gold and Menzies, 1968; Swick *et al.*, 1968; Bergeron and Droz, 1969; Mazzocchi *et al.*, 1976, 1977). Morphological evidence supporting the idea of a molecular or piecemeal repair and replacement of mitochondrial components is lacking but there is evidence that mitochondria can divide and multiply (page 216) and it would appear that old, effete or damaged mitochondria can suffer regressive changes and be removed in various ways in the cell. Images which may be interpreted as mitochondrial involution or dissolution are occasionally encountered in normal tissues, but many more are seen in pathological situations. The greater frequency of such changes in pathological states may be looked upon as an activation of normal mechanisms geared to the removal of organelles damaged by noxious influences. The various ways in which it is alleged that mitochondria are got rid of by the cell include: (1) mitochondrial pyknosis; (2) mitochondrial swelling (balloon degeneration); (3) cytolysosome formation; and (4) intracisternal sequestration.

Mitochondrial swelling which is part and parcel of cloudy swelling is a widely recognized and much studied phenomenon (*see* page 240). The converse change, mitochondrial pyknosis†, is not too well recognized and is only occasionally mentioned in the literature. Here a striking increase in the density of the matrix and a reduction of mitochondrial size occurs (*Plate 95*). The term 'mitochondrial pyknosis', which so succinctly describes this change was first employed by Wachstein and Besen (1964). These authors demonstrated mitochondrial pyknosis in coagulative necrosis produced in renal tissue with DL-serine. Both mitochondrial swelling and mitochondrial pyknosis were witnessed in adjacent cells and the contrast between these is beautifully illustrated in their paper.

Similar changes which can be interpreted as mitochondrial pyknosis have been observed in: (1) the liver of rats after (a) starvation (Rouiller, 1957), (b) carcinogenic diets (Rouiller and Simon, 1962), (c) necrogenic diets (Svoboda and Higginson, 1963); (2) human liver from cases of viral hepatitis (Pavel *et al.*, 1971); (3) hepatomas (Gansler and Rouiller, 1956); (4) experimentally induced renal tumours in hamsters (Mannweiler and Bernhard, 1957); and (5) human ovarian adenocarcinoma (*Plate 96*).

Pyknotic mitochondrial forms bear some resemblance to microbodies and indeed it has been suggested (e.g. Pavel *et al.*, 1971) that such dense mitochondria may represent an intermediate step leading to the formation of microbodies. In view of what is now known about microbodies, this does not seem a likely possibility.

★Estimates of the half-life of rat mitochondria are: (1) liver, 9.6–10.3 days; (2) kidney, 12.4 days; (3) adrenal cortex, 8.2–11.5 days (Fletcher and Sanadi, 1961; Wilson and Dove, 1965; Mazzocchi *et al.*, 1976).
†Mitochondrial pyknosis must not be confused with mitochondria showing a condensed configuration. Compare *Plate 96* with *Plates 108, 109* and *111*.

Plate 96

Fig. 1. A cell from adenocarcinoma of the human ovary showing mitochondrial pyknosis. In some instances where the matrix is not too dense, disorientated and fused cristae are discernible. × 7000

Fig. 2. High-power view of two mitochondria from *Fig. 1*, showing altered cristae and a dense matrix containing some intramatricial granules. × 13 500

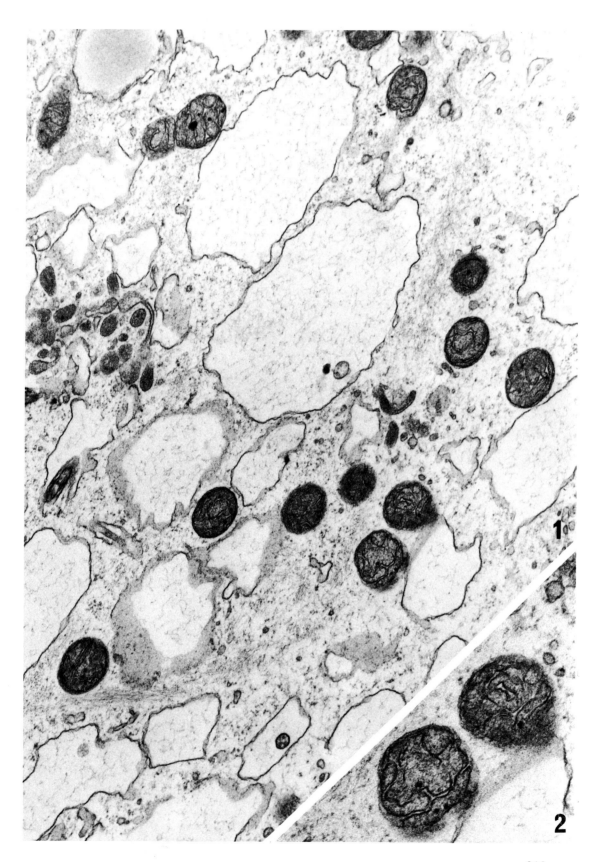

Mitochondrial swelling has at times been regarded as another possible fate that might befall effete mitochondria (Gansler and Rouiller, 1956; Rouiller, 1960). This must be distinguished from the well-known variety of mitochondrial swelling which affects virtually every mitochondrion in the cell and is the equivalent of the cloudy swelling and post-mortem change known to light microscopists (*see* page 240). This is not relevant here. What I wish to demonstrate (*Plate 97, Fig. 1*) is that one may occasionally find one or two grossly swollen mitochondria in company with other perfectly normal-looking mitochondria in a variety of experimental and other situations. Here, there is clearly no general derangement of osmotic forces within the cell. The primary defect obviously lies in the swollen mitochondrion itself, and this could well be regarded as an effete or damaged organelle about to suffer dissolution.

The transformation or incorporation of mitochondria into autolysosomes is perhaps the most common method by which these organelles are eliminated. Such methods of mitochondrial elimination include: (1) development of dense osmiophilic laminated or whorled membranes in mitochondria and conversion of such organelles into lysosomal bodies containing myelin figures; (2) incorporation of mitochondria into pre-existing lysosomes; and (3) sequestration of mitochondria with or without other organelles to form autolysosomes (*Plate 97, Figs. 2–5*).

Yet another ingenious method of involution is suggested by Pavel *et al.* (1971), which they describe as 'dissolution of mitochondria into the distended cisternae or vesicles of granular or agranular endoplasmic reticulum'. According to this concept the mitochondrion either fuses with the wall of a rough endoplasmic reticulum cisterna and discharges its contents, or herniates and falls into it and suffers subsequent dissolution.

This concept is reminiscent of the concept of intracisternal sequestration evoked by Blackburn and Vinijchaikul (1969) to explain the involution of the rough endoplasmic reticulum. Here it is postulated that invaginations of the rough endoplasmic reticulum into the cisternae occur, and portions of the papillary processes thus formed are detached and suffer dissolution (*see* page 544). One could also look upon intracisternal sequestration as one of the ways in which an autophagic vacuole or autolysosome commences.

Plate 97

Fig. 1. A solitary grossly swollen mitochondrion (M) with lucent matrix and disorganized cristae is seen among numerous normal-looking mitochondria. From the liver of a rat that had been treated with Atromid S. (*See also Plate 110, Fig. 2,* which shows a similar phenomenon in anoxic dog myocardium.) × 33 000

Fig. 2. Whorled membranous bodies (B), probably derived from involuting mitochondria. From cultured monkey kidney cells. × 28 000

Fig. 3. An autolysosome containing two mitochondria. From the same specimen as *Fig. 1.* × 40 000

Fig. 4. An autolysosome containing disintegrating mitochondrial remnants and other structures. From the liver of a tumour-bearing rat. × 40 000. (*Ghadially and Parry, unpublished electron micrograph*)

Fig. 5. Autolysosome containing mitochondrial remnants. From the kidney of a rat poisoned with lead acetate. × 42 000

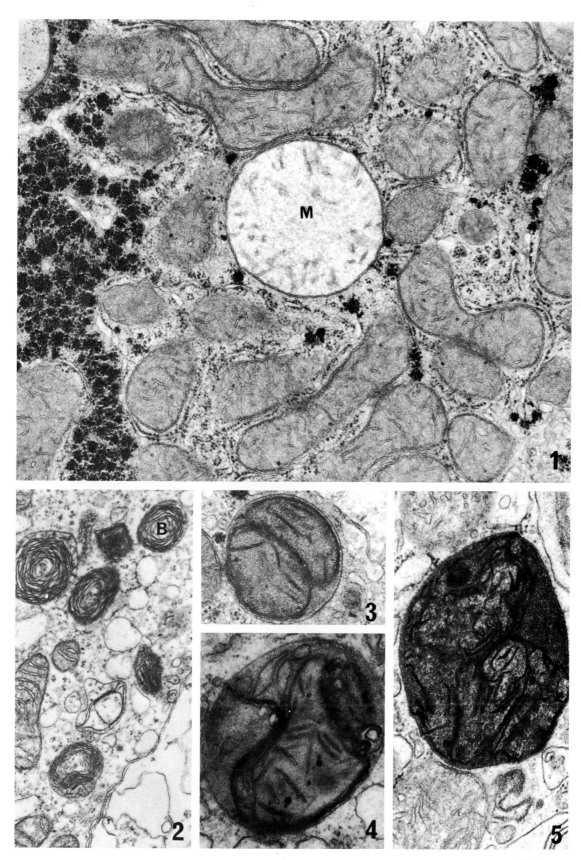

Mitochondrial associations

Although in most cells mitochondria appear to be randomly scattered in the cytoplasm, there are many instances where a close association occurs between mitochondria and other organelles and inclusions. Such associations seem to be quite meaningful and provide satisfying examples of correlation between structure and function. Various observations indicate that mitochondria are often located near a supply of substrate, or at sites in the cell known to require the ATP generated by the mitochondrion (Lehninger, 1965).

One of the frequently observed associations is between mitochondria and lipid droplets. Occasional examples of this may be found in a variety of tissues, but this association is of common occurrence in the myocardium, liver, pancreas and brown adipose tissue. A variety of appearances is seen. A single mitochondrion may appear close to, spread out over, or fused to the surface of a small lipid droplet, or several mitochondria may be seen surrounding a larger lipid droplet. In other instances the lipid droplet may lie in a deep invagination of the mitochondrial envelope and it is clear that in another plane of sectioning such a droplet could easily be mistaken for a lipid inclusion in the mitochondrion (*Plate 98, Figs. 1 and 2*), particularly if the invaginating membranes are not visualized (*see below*).

Often, when such close contact has occurred, it is impossible to resolve the mitochondrial membranes adjacent to the lipid droplet. Such an appearance could be explained on the basis of oblique sectioning through this area, and it has been debated whether a true continuity between the lipid and the mitochondrial matrix ever occurs (*see* the discussion in Napolitano and Fawcett, 1958, and in Novikoff, 1961). Some workers have adopted an intermediate view that only the outer membrane of the mitochondrion suffers dissolution but the inner membrane remains intact.

Since mitochondria are known to contain many of the enzymes (*see also* page 192) necessary for the metabolism of triglycerides (fatty acid oxidases), it has been suggested (Palade and Schidlowsky, 1958; Palade, 1959) that this is a meaningful juxtaposition which brings the mitochondrial enzymes into close association with the lipidic substrate. Close association between mitochondria and lipid is much more frequent and obvious in the liver and pancreas of fasted, rather than fully fed animals. This is in keeping with the idea that in the fasted animal the cells, having depleted much of the glycogen reserves, have shifted to the utilization of lipid to a greater extent than before for their metabolic needs.

However, when mitochondria have been seen in close association with lipid droplets in situations where lipid is accumulating as in brown adipose tissue, it has been suggested that the

---

Plate 98
Fig. 1. Rat hepatocyte mitochondria, showing close association with a lipid droplet (L). × 21 000
Fig. 2. A human myocardial mitochondrion, showing a deep invagination occupied by a lipid droplet (L). × 51 000
Fig. 3. Liver of day-old rat, showing close association of mitochondria with loops of rough endoplasmic reticulum. × 32 000

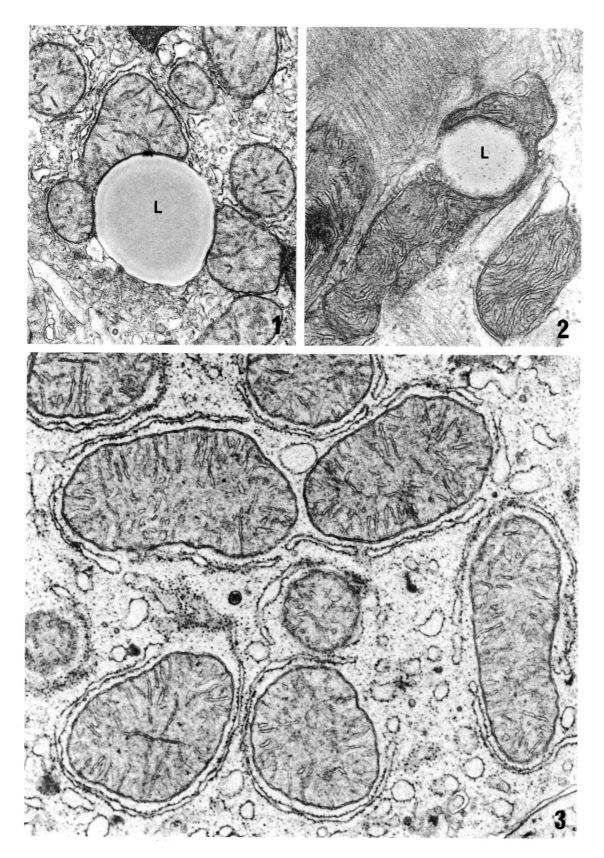

223

organelle may be involved in active synthesis of lipid (Napolitano and Fawcett, 1958). Apparently, most, but perhaps not all, of the enzymes necessary for this are present in the mitochondrion (*see* page 192). For instance, beef heart mitochondria and also mitochondria from some other sites are capable of quite rapid long-chain fatty acid synthesis (Hulsmann, 1962).

Another example of close association is that seen between the rough endoplasmic reticulum and the mitochondrion. The common pattern seen in such instances consist of curved profiles of rough endoplasmic reticulum, partially or almost completely encircling mitochondria but with a narrow zone of cytoplasm persisting between them (*Plate 98, Fig. 3*). Instances of continuity or apparent continuity have, however, been reported to occur between the mitochondrial membranes and the rough endoplasmic reticulum in the irradiated Rhesus hepatocyte (Ghidoni and Thomas, 1969) and between the mitochondrion and sarcoplasmic reticulum in skeletal and cardiac myocytes (Walker *et al.*, 1965; Walker and Schrodt, 1966; Bowman, 1967).

Even if the vagaries of sectioning geometry are accounted for and one concedes that true contact or continuity has in fact been demonstrated beyond reasonable doubt, one still wonders whether such rare examples of contact are fortuitous or artefactual rather than meaningful. On the other hand, one cannot exclude the possibility that the rarity of such images may indicate a transient but meaningful episode, which does occur in the living cell.

Profiles of rough endoplasmic reticulum wrapping around mitochondria are not so rare, however, particularly in cells engaged in active protein synthesis (e.g. the pancreas), and here is one of many examples where juxtaposition of this organelle to a site of energy utilization occurs. Bernhard and Rouiller (1956) reported that in fasted rats the rough endoplasmic reticulum regresses, but some is still seen around mitochondria. On re-feeding, the reticulum is

Plate 99

An oblique section through a portion of the distal tubule of mouse kidney. Note the close association of mitochondria with the highly folded basal part of the plasma membrane of the tubular epithelial cells. Basal lamina lining the circumference of the tubule is indicated by arrows. × 21 000

224

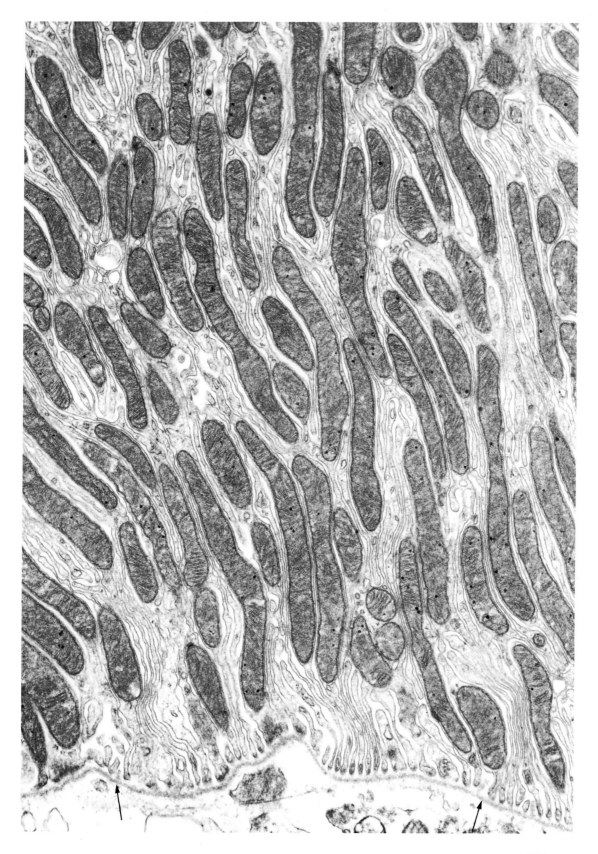

225

re-formed and, according to these authors, the mitochondria provide energy for its regrowth. Similarly in the liver of the newborn rat, where an active growth and proliferation of cells and organelles is in progress, a close association between mitochondria and developing rough endoplasmic reticulum is clearly evident (*Plate 98, Fig. 3*). A close association has also been noted between smooth endoplasmic reticulum and mitochondria (*Plate 84, Fig. 2*), as for example in dragonfly flight muscle (Smith, 1961) and in the pseudobranch gland of *Fundulus heteroclitus*. In the latter instance this is considered to be related to the high rate of carbonic anhydrase synthesis (Copeland and Dalton, 1959).

One of the most striking associations is that seen between mitochondria and myofilaments. In longitudinal sections of cardiac and skeletal muscle, rows of mitochondria are seen lying closely apposed to such filaments (*Plate 110, Fig. 2*) while in transverse sections through the I-band region, rings or girdles of mitochondria may be seen surrounding groups of myofilaments. It would appear that such an arrangement ensures that the ATP produced by the mitochondria is readily available via short diffusion paths to the myofilaments which need ATP for contraction.

Another frequently noted example of mitochondrial associations is the juxtaposition of mitochondria to cell membranes engaged in active transport of ions or other tasks involving high expenditure of energy. Thus in the distal convoluted tubule of the kidney (*Plate 99*), the basal plasma membrane is deeply infolded, and in the cleft-like spaces thus created lodge long slender mitochondria. A similar but not quite so elaborate arrangement is seen in the cells of the proximal tubule of the kidney, striated duct cells of the salivary gland, vestibular cells of cristae ampullaris, and marginal cells of the stria vascularis (for details, *see* Lentz, 1971). In all these instances a close association occurs over an extensive area between the mitochondrion and the cell membrane, and a topographical situation is created whereby the energy producer is brought into close apposition to the site of energy utilization.

Other examples of proximity of mitochondria to sites of energy utilization may be summarized briefly as follows: (1) in the Schwann cell for energy needed for the synthesis of large expanses of cell membrane to form the myelin sheath (Geren and Schmitt, 1954); (2) in synaptic junctions of axons for energy exchanges during impulse transmission (Palay, 1956); (3) in rat and guinea-pig spermatids for energy needed for the synthesis of the acrosome (Palade, 1952; Watson, 1952; Fawcett, 1959); and (4) in ciliated cells (*Plate 100*) for energy needed for ciliary motion (Lehninger, 1965).

Plate 100
Human bronchial mucosa, showing mitochondrial aggregates in the apical cytoplasm adjacent to the ciliary border. × 8000

226

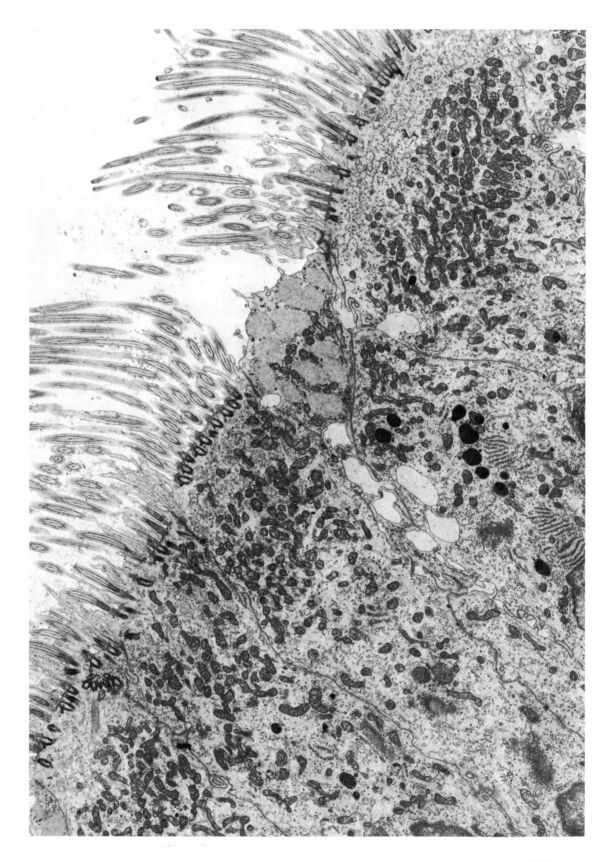

227

Intermitochondrial herniations, whorls and bridges

The principal alteration here appears to be the protrusion of a knob or finger-like projection (evagination) from one mitochondrion into an invagination in a neighbouring mitochondrion (*Plates 101* and *102*). The term 'herniation' has been used to describe this phenomenon although it is not strictly correct to do so. The term 'bridge' is also not a very appropriate description of the changes seen. Yet the lack of a better term forces us to continue their use. If membranous structures such as rough endoplasmic reticulum lie between the mitochondria they are dragged into these herniations. Depending upon the plane of section, and further structural modifications, such herniations present as intermitochondrial membranous whorls or bridges or as myelin figures apparently lying free in the mitochondrial matrix.

Such alterations of mitochondrial morphology have been noted in: (1) hepatocytes of vitamin E deficient rats (Sulkin and Sulkin, 1962); (2) hepatocytes of rats on a necrogenic diet (Svoboda and Higginson, 1963); (3) hepatocytes of rats after a single large dose of diethanolamine (Hruban *et al.*, 1965); (4) hepatocytes of rats after ligation of the portal vein (Kumano, 1973); (5) hepatocytes of rats bearing carcinogen-induced sarcomas in their flanks during the terminal stages of their life (Parry and Ghadially, 1966); (6) hepatocytes of rats breathing pure oxygen (Schaffner and Felig, 1965); (7) hepatocytes of riboflavin deficient mice (Tandler *et al.*, 1968); (8) hepatocytes of mice on galactoflavin-supplemented riboflavin-free diet (Tandler and Hoppel, 1974); (9) hepatocytes of dogs after *E. coli* endotoxin administration (Boler and Bibighaus, 1967); (10) human hepatoma (Ghadially and Parry, 1966); (11) autonomic ganglion cells of scorbutic guinea-pigs (Sulkin and Sulkin, 1967); and (12) adrenocortical cells of rats following hypophysectomy (Volk and Scarpelli, 1966).

Plate 101

From the liver of a tumour-bearing rat collected during the terminal stage of life. Herniation of one mitochondrion into another (arrows). The rough endoplasmic reticulum (R) is dragged into the herniation. × 53 000 (*From Parry and Ghadially, 1966*)

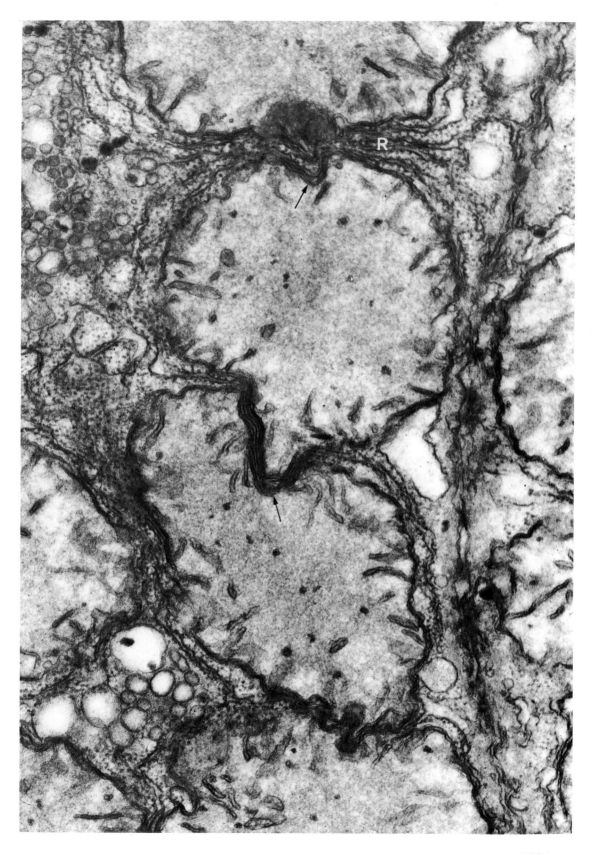

229

The notion that this phenomenon may be dependent on close packing and crenation of mitochondria, due perhaps to the use of hypertonic fixatives or to fluid loss due to other reasons, does not stand up to critical examination, for mitochondrial herniations may affect grossly hydropic mitochondria and can be seen even when only a few mitochondria are present. Sulkin and Sulkin (1962) found that the most striking alteration after prolonged vitamin E deficiency was the occurrence of mitochondrial protrusions projecting into adjacent mitochondria, and this occurs in mitochondria which are markedly swollen. Since during the later phases of the experiment such herniations disappeared and enlarged mitochondria occurred, they suggest that coalescence of mitochondria may have been achieved in this fashion. Similarly, mitochondrial hernias have been implicated in the formation of enlarged or giant mitochondria by other workers (Svoboda and Higginson, 1963; Volk and Scarpelli, 1966; Tandler et al., 1968). In our material such a correlation was not noted, for markedly enlarged or giant mitochondria were not evident, either in the tumour-bearing rat liver or the human hepatoma.

It is also worth noting that, although the union between the mitochondria resembles a joint of the peg-and-socket type rather than a dovetail joint, it is nevertheless quite firm, for such coupled mitochondria can be found also in pellets of isolated mitochondria (Tandler et al., 1968). In view of this, and the subsequent development of myelin figures at this site, it would appear that these junctions represent sites of focal damage and rearrangement of the membrane of the mitochondrial envelope.

Plate 102

From the same block of tissue as *Plate 101*. Intermitochondrial bridges (A) of electron-dense whorled membranes or myelin figures are seen connecting adjacent mitochondria. Some (B) appear to lie free in the mitochondrial matrix but they could be continuous with a mitochondrial envelope in another plane. Most of the appearances seen here can be interpreted as transverse or oblique sections through herniations of the type shown in *Plate 101*. × 48 000 (*From Parry and Ghadially, 1966*)

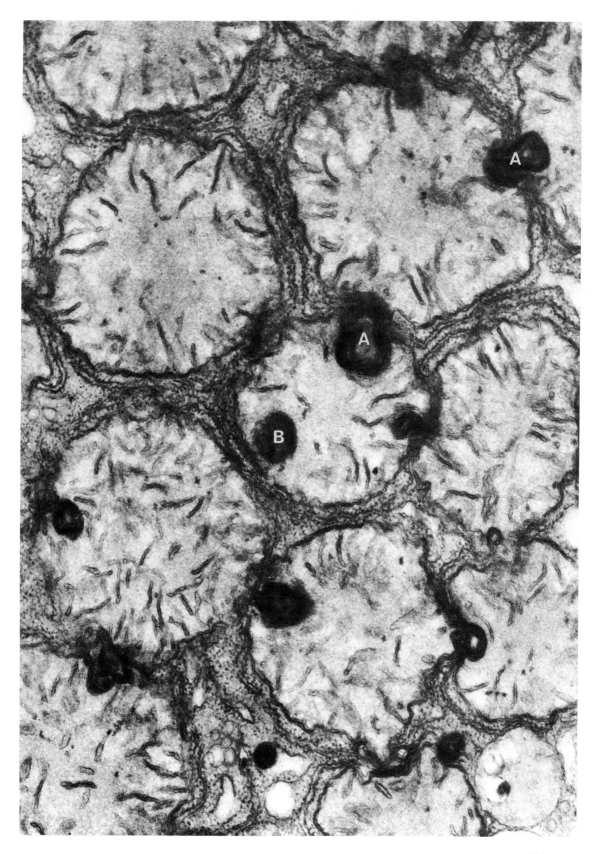

231

Variations in dense granules and calcification

It has already been noted (page 192) that the matrices of mitochondria contain electron-dense granules, and that they are more prominent and encountered more frequently in the mitochondria of tissues which transport large quantities of water and ions. Such dense granules measure 20–50 nm in diameter and at times it can be demonstrated that they are composed of subunits 5–7 nm in diameter. Studies on isolated dense granules indicate that they contain calcium, magnesium, phosphorus and inorganic material, which is mainly lipid (Matthews *et al.*, 1971). In keeping with this is the fact that these granules are osmiophilic (Barnard and Afzelius, 1972), but considerable doubt now exists as to whether *in vivo* the 20–50 nm dense granules in normal mitochondria contain divalent cations such as calcium (*see below*).

It has long been known from studies on isolated cell fractions that mitochondria contain relatively large amounts of calcium and magnesium, and it has also been shown that they can accumulate these and other ions, such as strontium and manganese, *in vitro*. Further *in vivo* experimental studies and histochemical studies also implicate mitochondria as sites of divalent cation localization (for references *see* Peachey, 1964).

The elegant studies of Peachey (1964), carried out with the excised toad bladder and isolated kidney mitochondria of the rat, show that when the incubating medium contains calcium, strontium or barium, these ions are concentrated in the pre-existing dense granules of the mitochondrial matrix, as evidenced by their increased size and density. This is particularly well demonstrated with barium because of its high atomic number (Ba 56, Sr 38, Ca 20) and, hence, marked electron density as visualized in electron micrographs. Often such deposits assumed the shape of hollow spheres, suggesting that barium had been deposited around a pre-existing matrical granule probably in exchange for other ions at that site. Similarly, in cultures from the heart tissue of day-old rats, Porter and Hogeboom (1964) observed an increase in the size but not the number of matrical-dense granules in the mitochondria of cells exposed to an excess of calcium, strontium or barium ions.

Large electron-opaque granules, often attaining a diameter of 100 nm, were observed by Lehninger *et al.* (1963) in the matrix of rat liver mitochondria incubated in a medium containing both calcium and inorganic phosphate, and it has been debated whether such large deposits represent enlarged dense granules or fresh deposits in the matrix.

Peachey (1964) has proposed that divalent cations may be retained in the mitochondrion in two possible forms: (1) bound to organic phosphate in the form of granules pre-existing in the matrix; and (2) as an inorganic precipitate. The concept here is that if modest amounts of calcium ions are presented to the mitochondrion, they will be deposited on the dense granules, but if large amounts of calcium ions, preferably with inorganic phosphate, are offered, they are likely to form *de novo* precipitates of calcium phosphate in the mitochondrial matrix.

Plate 103

Fig. 1. A modest increase in size of matrical dense-granules is seen in this group of mitochondria from the kidney tubule of a mouse treated with parathyroid hormone. × 26 000 (*Ghadially and Ailsby, unpublished electron micrograph*)

Fig. 2. Small calcareous deposits (C) are seen in the thickened basal lamina of a kidney tubule. From a mouse treated with calcium gluconate. × 24 000 (*Ghadially and Ailsby, unpublished electron micrograph*)

Fig. 3. Numerous calcified laminated bodies (B) are seen at the periphery of the kidney tubules of a mouse treated with calcium gluconate. The dense granules in the mitochondria appear normal in size and number. × 26 000 (*Ghadially and Ailsby, unpublished electron micrograph*)

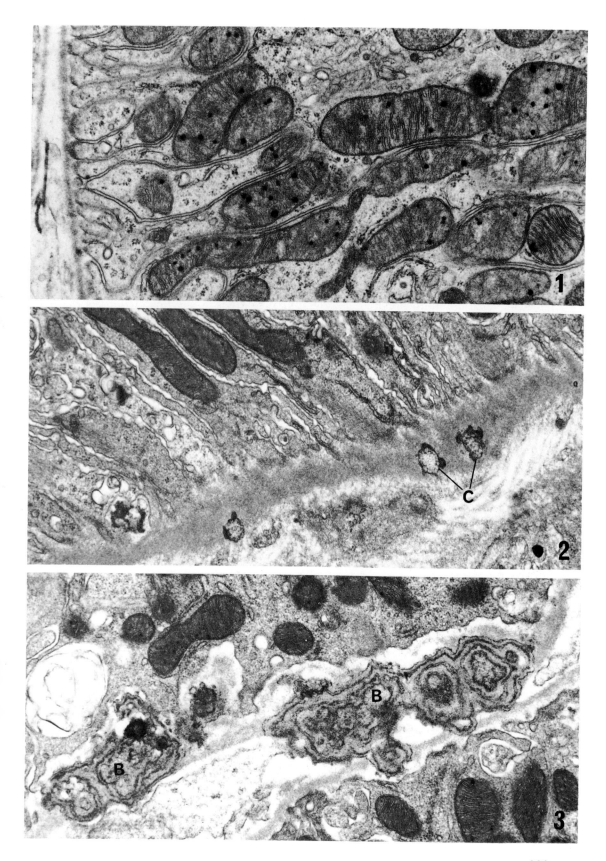

233

With the advent of electron-probe x-ray analysis* attempts have been made to determine the elemental composition of intramitochondrial dense granules with this technique. A few studies deal with the composition of these granules as found in sections of plastic embedded tissues prepared by conventional methods or minor modifications of such methods (Sutfin *et al.*, 1971; Ashraf and Bloor, 1976; Buja *et al.*, 1976). Calcium and at times also phosphorus† have been demonstrated in the granules by this method.

However, when tissues are exposed to aqueous solution‡, one wonders whether the elements found in the granules: (1) accurately reflect the *in vivo* situation; (2) derive from redistribution (translocation) of calcium in the tissue during preparative procedures; or (3) result from an uptake of calcium from preparative solutions§. To circumvent some of these possibilities electron-probe x-ray analysis has been carried out on intramitochondrial granules found in freeze-dried cryosections of unfixed frozen tissues and calcium and phosphorus has been demonstrated in such preparations also (Christensen, 1971; Somlyo *et al.*, 1975; Barnard and Seveus, 1976: Landis *et al.*, 1977; Mergner *et al.*, 1977; Saetersdal *et al.*, 1977).

However, an examination of published electron micrographs of 'intramitochondrial granules' in cryosectioned tissues shows that these granules are more dense and much larger and more numerous (often the entire mitochondrion is packed with such granules) than the relatively small intramitochondrial dense granules one finds in ultrathin sections of routinely prepared tissues. Indeed, the granules in most cryosectioned material more resemble the granules found in mitochondria incubated in media containing phosphorus and calcium. One may argue that the small size and paucity of granules in routine preparations reflect a loss of calcium during preparative procedures; or one can argue that the very large granules are artefactually produced by the cryotechniques employed, probably as a result of damage to the cell membrane and an influx of calcium into the cell and mitochondrion or as a result of local concentration and precipitation of calcium and phosphorus due to extraction of water (particularly if ice crystals form or if thawing and regelation occurs).

---

*This is a relatively non-destructive form of analysis by which elements from Na upwards (i.e. above Z number 10) can be simultaneously detected and displayed as a spectrum. The best spatial resolution that can be obtained is of the order of 20 nm. The sensitivity of detection varies with the elements but is of the order of 10^{-18}g. It is the only way of analysing minute inclusions *in situ* within the cell and so correlate morphology with atomic composition. (For a review *see* Ghadially, 1979a.)

†With energy dispersive spectrometry it is difficult to convincingly demonstrate small amounts of phosphorus in osmicated tissue because of the proximity of the M peak of osmium (1.914 ke V) and the Kα peak of phosphorus (2.012 ke V). The resolution of the x-ray detector is usually only about 150 eV so peaks separated by an interval of only 99 eV are not well resolved.

‡*See* Chandler (1977) and Morgan (1979) for succinct accounts on how conventional wet chemical preparative techniques disturb the *in vivo* chemical integrity of biological tissues.

§For example commercial glutaraldehyde contains calcium (Oschman and Wall, 1972). Distilled glutaraldehyde is free from this defect.

Plate 104

From the proximal tubule of the kidney of mouse treated with parathyroid hormone (*Ghadially and Ailsby, unpublished electron micrographs*)

Fig. 1. Large electron-opaque spherules, presumed to be enlarged matrical granules (G), are seen within the mitochondria. One mitochondrion however, contains normal-sized matrical granules (arrow). × 46 000

Fig. 2. In contrast to *Fig. 1,* most of the calcareous deposits here present as hollow spheres. Note also the tendency of fragmented and disorientated cristae (arrow) to wrap around these highly electron-opaque deposits. × 40 000

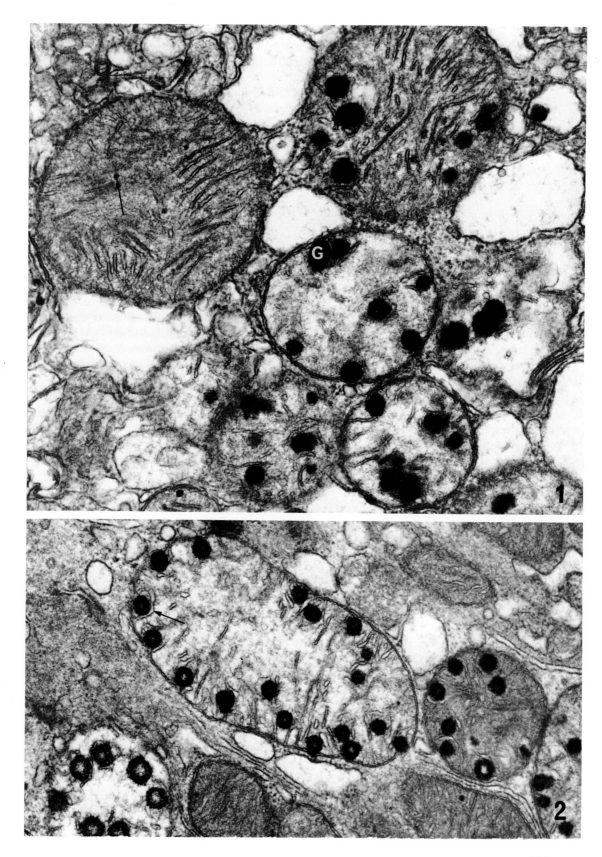

In this respect the work of Sevéus *et al.* (1978) is most revealing for these authors have found that these large granules are not formed if sections are cut at − 110°C, but they are seen in sections cut at about − 80°C. Therefore these authors quite rightly point out that these large granules are 'formed by electrolyte diffusion in the section and therefore cannot be considered as representing the *in vivo* pool of mitochondrial calcium'. Regarding the much smaller granule seen in routine preparations some doubt must remain as to their true composition *in vivo*. As we have seen they contain much lipid hence, to a large extent at least, their electron density is due to osmiophilia (Barnard and Afzelius, 1972; Barnard and Ruusa, 1979)★.

Be that as it may, it is important to realize that the 'new' findings with crytotechniques do not disprove the 'old' idea (Peachey, 1964; Lehninger, 1970b) that cation sequestration can occur *in vivo* either at *de novo* sites in the mitochondrial matrix or on pre-existing mitochondrial dense granules. In the text that follows we deal with changes in dense granules (pre-existing or *de novo*) observed in routinely prepared tissues.

An increase in density, size and number of dense granules has been reported to occur in diverse pathological and experimental states. In extreme examples the mitochondrion may be filled with calcium deposits, and fusion of such calcified mitochondria may result in irregular calcified masses within and/or outside the cell.

The more dramatic examples of this kind have been observed following some procedures which produce focal necrosis. It is worth noting that one is not witnessing calcification of necrotic tissue, for intramitochondrial calcification precedes the necrosis and indeed appears to be a factor in its production. Such examples of intramitochondrial calcification include: (1) the rat myocardium in magnesium deficiency (Heggtveit *et al.*, 1964); and (2) the kidney tubules of mice after the administration of parathyroid extract (Caulfield and Schrag, 1964).

The effect of experimentally produced hypercalcaemia on renal tissues has been the subject of many studies, quite a few at the ultrastructural level (for references *see* Duffy *et al.*, 1971). Such studies have revealed essentially three types of lesions in the proximal tubules: (1) changes in dense granules and intramitochondrial calcification; (2) amorphous or crystalline calcium deposits in the cytoplasm; and (3) calcium deposits and calcified laminated bodies in the basal lamina (*Plates 103–106*).

A clear relationship between the lesion produced and the agent used to produce the hypercalcaemia does not seem to exist, but there are probably species differences. Our observations (Ghadially and Ailsby, unpublished) and those of Caulfield and Schrag (1964) show that in mice, parathyroid extract leads to mitochondrial calcification while calcium gluconate does not produce such mitochondrial changes but leads to laminated calcium deposits in the basal lamina (*Plate 103, Figs. 2 and 3*). In the rat, however, calcium gluconate produces both calcified mitochondria and laminated calcium deposits in the basal lamina (Duffy *et al.*, 1971).

★The controversy about the composition and function of matrical dense granules seems to be unending. Biochemical analysis of isolated granules by Brdiczka and Barnard (1980) suggest that they are composed of phospholipoprotein and that under some *in vitro* conditions this lipoprotein can bind calcium. Regarding the function of these granules *in vivo*, Fawcett (1981) feels that in most sites they are probably not involved in calcium sequestration but they may be involved in this activity in mineralized tissues. Further he suggests that since these granules are closely associated with the cristae they may be 'involved in assembly of the mitochondrial inner membrane'. In epiphysial growth plate cartilage, the matrical dense granules of mitochondria in the hypertrophic zone accumulate calcium and phosphorus. In the degenerating zone the calcium and phosphorus are liberated into the matrix where calcification ensues.

Plate 105

From the proximal tubule of the kidney of mouse treated with parathyroid hormone.

Fig. 1. Mitochondria containing 'hollow' calcified spheres (arrows) and electron-dense calcified masses which at higher magnification are seen to be composed of needle-shaped crystals. × 24 000

Fig. 2. High-power view of calcified mitochondria demonstrating crystalline calcium (C) deposits. × 46 000

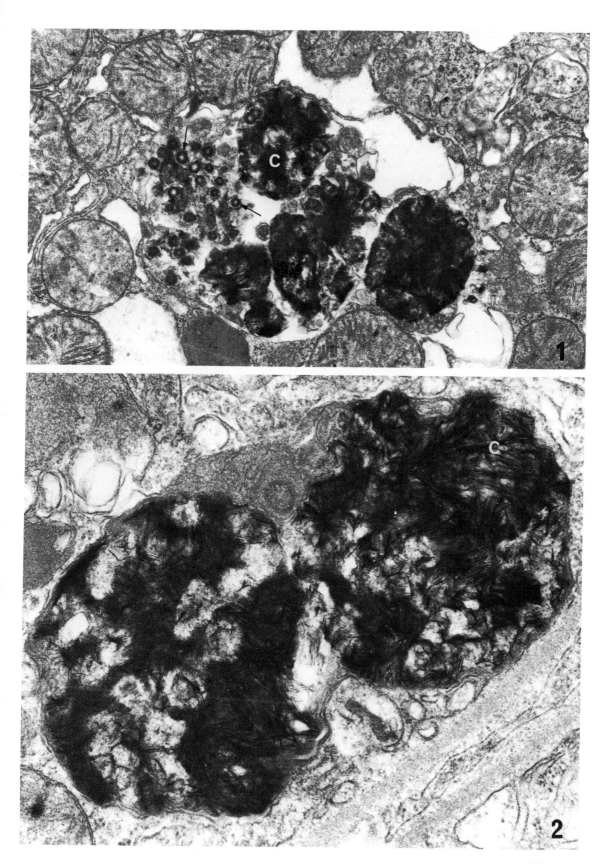

237

The sequence of events occurring in the proximal tubule of the mouse after parathyroid hormone treatment is depicted in *Plate 103, Fig. 1* and *Plates 104–106*. The earliest change is a modest increase in size of intramitochondrial dense granules. Not all proximal tubules nor all the cells in a proximal tubule show this alteration. Later, cells containing mitochondria with huge dense granules are seen. They may present either as solid or hollow electron-dense spheres (*Plate 104*). Some mitochondria also come to contain crystalline calcium deposits (*Plate 105*).

In some instances the dense granules appear to be enveloped in a membrane, probably derived from disintegrating cristae (*Plate 106*). There is no evidence that calcium deposits occur in the intracristal space. It is interesting to note that not all mitochondria within a given cell show such changes, and that normal-looking mitochondria with normal-sized dense granules may occur in the same cell. Finally, fusion of calcified mitochondria and/or enlarged dense granules liberated from ruptured mitochondria produce calcareous masses in the cytoplasm and lumen of the kidney tubule.

Numerous other instances of increase in number and size of intramitochondrial dense granules have been reported in the literature. They vary from quite modest changes to changes almost, but not quite, as severe as those discussed earlier. Such examples include: (1) ischaemic dog myocardium (Herdson *et al.*, 1965); (2) rat myocardium after administration of steroids and sodium phosphate (D'Agostino, 1964; Horvath *et al.*, 1970); (3) rat heart poisoned with plasmocid (D'Agostino, 1963); (4) cardiomyopathy associated with a phaeochromocytoma (Alpert *et al.*, 1972); (5) a variety of megamitochondria (*see* page 266); (6) liver of tumour-bearing rats (Ghadially and Parry, 1965); (7) liver of rats poisoned with carbon tetrachloride (Reynolds, 1963); (8) liver cell necrosis due to heliotrine (Kerr, 1969); (9) chilled dog kidneys used for transplantation (Fisher *et al.*, 1967); (10) tetanus-intoxicated mouse and human muscles (Zacks and Sheff, 1964; Zacks *et al.*, 1966); and (11) osteoclasts, osteoblasts and enterocytes following the administration of parathormone (Matthews *et al.*, 1971).

A decrease or disappearance of matrical dense granules has also at times been noted to occur. Particularly interesting is the observation by Trump *et al.* (1965a) that the earliest change (15 minutes) which occurs in mouse liver after excision is a disappearance of intramitochondrial dense granules. Similarly, within ten minutes after occluding the superior mesenteric artery, Brown *et al.* (1970) found a loss of intramitochondrial dense granules in ileal mucosal cells of the dog, and under similar experimental conditions Aho *et al.* (1970) reported a loss of matrical granules in the jejunal mucosal cells. In excised rat and dog kidneys an early disappearance of intramitochondrial dense granules has been noted (MacKay *et al.*, 1968). A decrease in dense granules has also been reported to occur after histamine stimulation of gastric parietal cells and pancreozymin stimulation of pancreas, (Fawcett, 1966). Dense granules in hepatocyte mitochondria disappear in normal and tumour-bearing rats two hours after partial hepatectomy, but return in both cases six hours after the operation (Parry, personal communication).

Plate 106

From kidney of mouse treated with parathyroid hormone. Necrotic cells containing numerous mitochondria with calcareous deposits are seen in the top half of this electron micrograph. Many of the intramitochondrial dense deposits seem to be surrounded by a membrane (arrow). In the lower half of the picture a portion of a kidney tubule containing much necrotic debris, calcified mitochondria (M), and a large calcareous deposit (D) is seen. × 28 000 (*Ghadially and Ailsby, unpublished electron micrograph*)

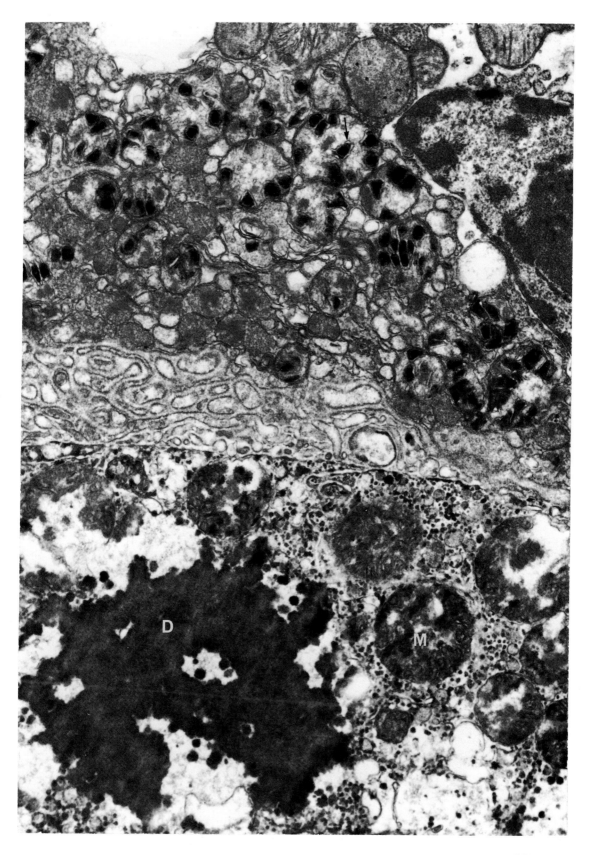

239

Swollen or hydropic mitochondria

A common and easily recognized variety of mitochondrial enlargement, a swollen or hydropic mitochondrion is due to the entry of water (and solutes) into the organelle, and can be engendered by numerous agents which produce cell damage. Mitochondrial swelling, together with swelling and vesiculation of the rough endoplasmic reticulum, constitutes the change called cloudy swelling by pathologists (*see also* page 430).

Various alterations of mitochondrial morphology are seen, depending upon the stage reached by the process and also upon which of the two mitochondrial chambers is primarily involved. As pointed out earlier (page 192), there are two compartments in a mitochondrion: (1) the outer or intermembranous chamber lying between the two membranes of the mitochondrial envelope and extending either as a potential space or as a cleft-like or tubular space within the cristae; and (2) the inner chamber which contains the mitochondrial matrix. Since the permeability of the inner and outer mitochondrial membranes is known to be different, it follows that flooding of one or other, or both, chambers may occur.

By far the commonest variety of swelling seen is that due to the involvement of the matrix or inner chamber (*Plate 107*). In the early stages or in mild degrees of swelling there is only a modest increase in the size of the mitochondrion, and dilution of the matrix, as evidenced by a decreased density, is barely discernible. The cristae, however, appear displaced to the periphery and may show varying degrees of disorientation, shortening and reduction in numbers.

In this early stage, the matrix, although somewhat paler, retains its homogeneous character; but with advancing hydration it shows a patchy appearance due to development of multiple electron-lucent foci, and in time frank cavitation of the mitochondrial matrix occurs. Loss of matrix density is due at first to dilution but later there is a loss of matrix substance. Breaks in the mitochondrial-limiting membranes are also encountered, particularly in grossly swollen mitochondria. The intramitochondrial dense granules tend to disappear at an early stage of swelling, but this is not invariably the case.

Plate 107

Mitochondria from the liver of a rat bearing a carcinogen-induced subcutaneous sarcoma, showing varying degrees (increasing from *Figs. 1 to 3*) of swelling of the matrical chamber (*Ghadially and Parry, unpublished electron micrographs*)

Fig. 1. A slightly swollen mitochondrion (M) showing peripherally placed cristae and a fairly homogeneous, medium-density matrix. Intramitochondrial dense granules are absent. × 32 000

Fig. 2. Markedly swollen mitochondria with peripherally placed, disorientated, and disintegrating cristae. The matrix has a patchy appearance and a break (arrow) is evident in the wall of a mitochondrion. Dense granules are abundant. Note also the vesiculation (V) of the rough endoplasmic reticulum. In pathological terms, this cell is showing cloudy swelling. × 46 000

Fig. 3. This grossly swollen mitochondrion shows frank cavitation of the mitochondrial matrix (M) and loss of cristae. The lower half of the mitochondrial wall is attenuated and probably ruptured (arrow). × 46 000

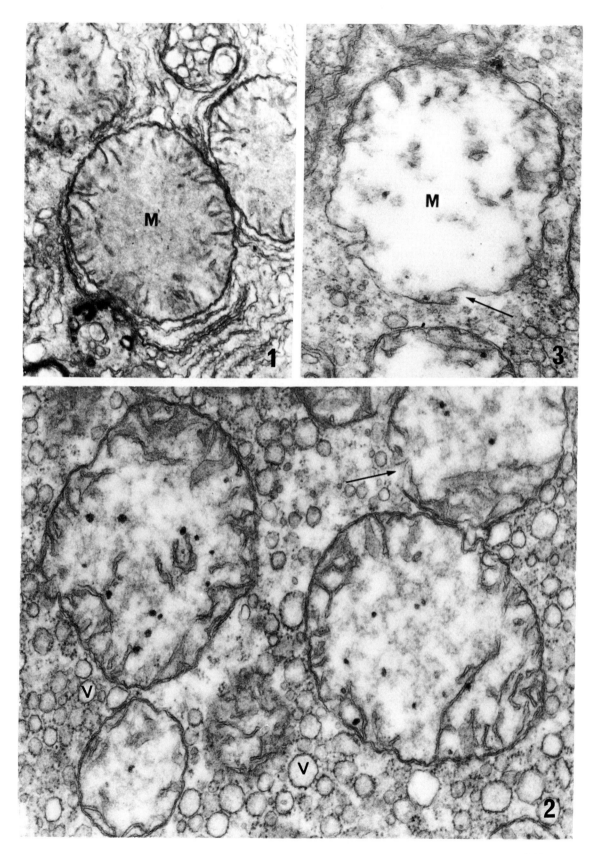

241

Mitochondrial swelling due to influx of water into the outer chamber is usually of a modest degree and is frequently limited to a ballooning of the cristae (intracristal swelling). It is only occasionally accompanied by separation of the inner and outer membranes of the envelope, and even then often only a segment of the wall is affected, forming a 'blister' on the wall of the mitochondrion (*Plate 108*). In instances where only intracristal swelling is present, there may be no obvious increase in the over-all size of the mitochondrion, and the matrix may appear quite dense★. However, with advanced swelling of the intermembranous space, an overall increase in size of the mitochondrion becomes evident (*Plates 108* and *109*). These remarks apply to mitochondria seen in ultrathin sections of tissues.

Studies with isolated mitochondria and cells or tissues *in vitro* show that similar changes can be produced in mitochondria by various experimental procedures (Trump and Ginn, 1968; Butler and Judha, 1970; Gordon and Bernstein, 1970; Laiho *et al.*, 1971). In such *in vitro* studies normal mitochondria are often referred to as showing an orthodox configuration, and those with dense matrix and swollen cristae as showing a condensed configuration. In Ehrlich ascites tumour cells taken directly from the animal, the mitochondria display a normal configuration, but when such cells are repeatedly washed, transformation of mitochondria to condensed configuration occurs (Gordon and Bernstein, 1970). The mechanism by which this change is produced is not understood. It is thought that such changes are accompanied by conformational changes of the inner membrane protein (Wrigglesworth and Packer, 1968) and that the condensed configuration indicates a 'low energy state' and the orthodox form a 'high energy state' (Hackenbrock, 1968a, b).

In Ehrlich ascites tumour cells transformation from orthodox to condensed configuration can be induced in all mitochondria in less than 6 seconds by the addition of 2-deoxyglucose which rapidly generates adenosine diphosphate from adenosine triphosphate in the cell and this in turn induces oxidative phosphorylation in mitochondria (Hackenbrock *et al.*, 1971). This supports the idea that the transformation from orthodox to condensed configuration is linked to oxidative phosphorylation.

Mitochondria with expanded matrical chambers have been produced by the addition of valinomycin to the medium, which produces a rapid potassium ion influx. This has been demonstrated with isolated rat liver mitochondria (Butler and Judha, 1970) and also with the washed Ehrlich ascites cells mentioned earlier. The addition of calcium chloride or phosphate ions also induces swelling of the matrix chamber but there is also much loss of matrix material.

★The densification of the matrix is probably due to movement of water from the matrix to the intracristal space.

Plate 108

Fig. 1. A monkey kidney cell from a culture infected with herpesvirus. Mitochondria cut in various planes clearly show markedly ballooned cristae (C) and a moderately dense matrix (M), but there is no separation of the outer and inner mitochondrial membranes. This (and also *Fig. 2*) is the appearance which is sometimes referred to as a 'condensed configuration'. Several matrical dense granules are present. × 41 000

Fig. 2. Two mitochondria, which no doubt escaped while the tissue (frog kidney) was being minced in osmium, are now seen lying free in the embedding medium. Both show markedly ballooned cristae (C), a dense matrix and some intramitochondrial dense granules. There is focal separation of inner and outer membranes (arrow) in one mitochondrion, while in the other the separation is much more extensive. These mitochondria are grossly swollen compared to the mitochondria (M) within the kidney tubule. × 32 000

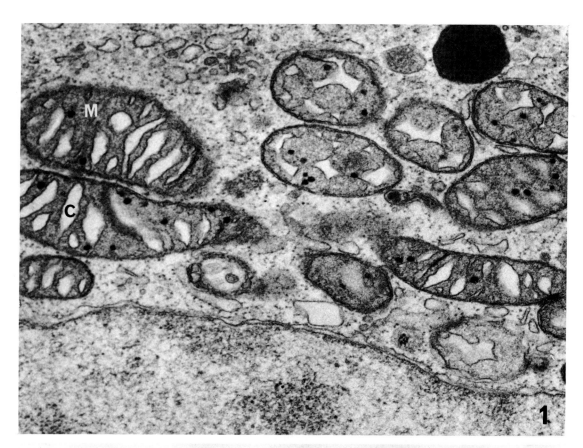

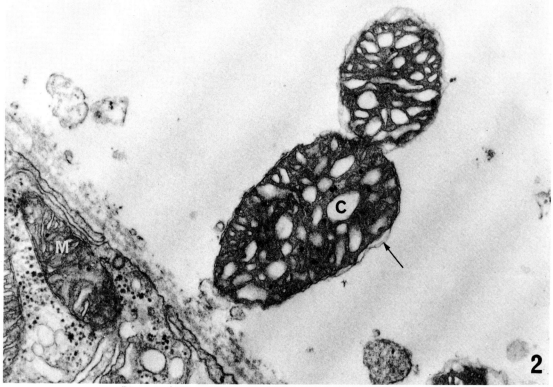

Trump and Bulger (1967, 1968) and Trump and Ginn (1968) have noted, in isolated flounder kidney tubules injured in various ways, that there is first an expansion of the intracristal space and only later is this followed by a swelling of the matrix compartment. Similar sequential swelling of the two chambers has often been observed by us in cultures of herpesvirus-infected cells harvested at different time intervals (*Plates 108* and *110*). Indeed, on occasions, both varieties of swollen mitochondria may be seen in the same cell, or adjacent cells and, as Trump and Ginn (1968) point out, at times one portion of the mitochondrion may show intracristal swelling and dense matrix, while the remainder may show marked swelling of the matrix chamber (*Plate 111*)★.

Only a few of the studies on volume changes in isolated mitochondria have been mentioned above, but a voluminous literature on this subject exists (*see* reviews by Lehninger, 1962, 1965). These studies, although of great interest, do not directly concern us here, because correlated ultrastructural studies were performed only occasionally, and often artefacts due to the separation procedure and different methods of fixation employed make correlations between these results and what one finds in ultrathin tissue sections difficult. However, these studies have demonstrated that mitochondria can show two types of swelling: (1) a passive swelling, which can be produced by altering the osmolarity of the medium; and (2) an active swelling, which is dependent on electron transport, and can be brought about in isotonic solutions by adding minute amounts of various swelling-inducer agents, such as phosphorus, calcium and mercury ions, fatty acids, thyroxine, oxytocin, vasopressin, insulin and hydrocortisone. It would appear that in many pathological situations the initial mitochondrial swelling is of the active type, but that later, when the cell becomes flooded with water, a passive enlargement also occurs.

★It is thought that this phenomenon is possible because in some mitochondria the matrix chamber occurs as two separate compartments divided by a crista. It seems to me that a more plausible explanation would be that this is a dividing mitochondrion at a stage when the partition has cleaved the matrix chamber into two as explained on page 216.

Plate 109

Fig. 1. Synovial intimal cell from a case of haemachromatosis. The mitochondria show a severe degree of intracristal swelling. The matrix chamber presents as electron-dense bands or ribbons. × 48 000

Fig. 2. HeLa cell exposed to 200 µg/ml of *cis*-dichlorodiammine-platinum (II) for five hours. At this concentration this drug is quite toxic and kills cells in a few hours. In this electron micrograph we are witnessing one of the terminal stages of intracristal swelling. The matrix now forms an electron-dense band at the periphery of the mitochondrion. × 46 000 (*Ghadially and Yang-Steppuhn, unpublished electron micrograph*)

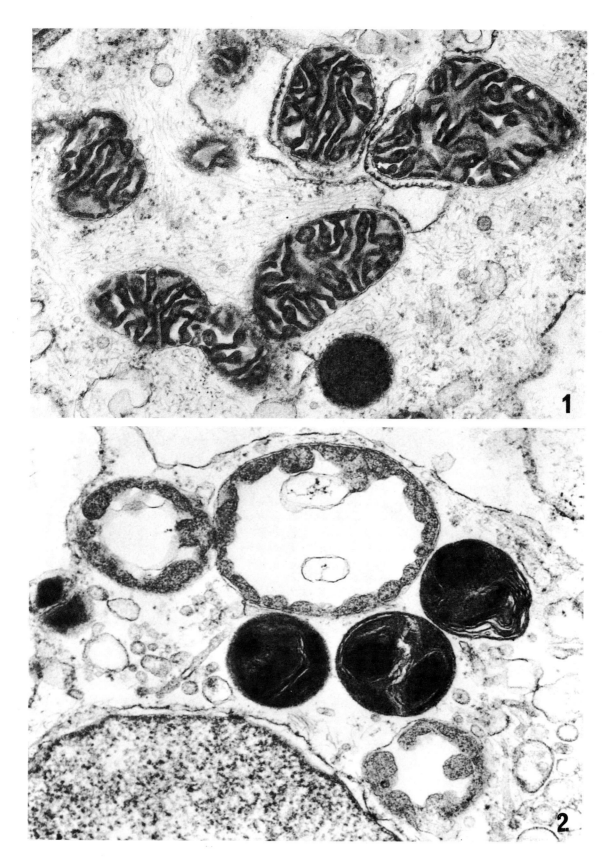

The equivalent of passive swelling is also clearly seen as an artefact in tissues which are fixed in hypotonic solutions (Ogura and Furuta, 1957). Other procedures where mitochondrial swelling might be artefactually introduced in the specimen include hypoxia due to the use of a tourniquet prior to surgical biopsy, delay in collecting tissues, and using blocks of tissues too large to permit rapid penetration of fixative solution (David, 1964; Trump *et al.*, 1965a, b; Ericsson and Biberfeld, 1967; Petersen, 1977). Distinction between this kind of artefactual swelling and that produced by pathological processes which one might be investigating can be difficult or impossible.

Multiple factors appear to be involved in the production of mitochondrial hydrops. Osmotic changes in the external environment of mitochondria are clearly a factor in some cases but, since hydropic and normal mitochondria can at times be found in the same cell (*Plate 110, Fig. 2; Plate 97, Fig. 1*), it has been suggested (Rouiller, 1960; David, 1964) that the primary chemical derangement can also occur in the organelle itself, and that alterations in membrane permeability may be involved.

Plate 110

Fig. 1. Monkey kidney cell from a culture infected with herpesvirus. During the early stages mitochondria with ballooned cristae, as shown in *Plate 108, Fig. 1*, are found. At a later stage such mitochondria suffer swelling of the inner chamber also, producing the appearance shown in this electron micrograph. Note the swollen cristae (C), focal separation of the outer and inner mitochondrial membranes (F), cavitation of the matrix (M), and breaks in the wall of the mitochondrion (arrow). × 49 000

Fig. 2. Dog myocardium subjected to anoxia. Only a few of the mitochondria show matrical lucency and some swelling. The others are not markedly altered. × 23 000

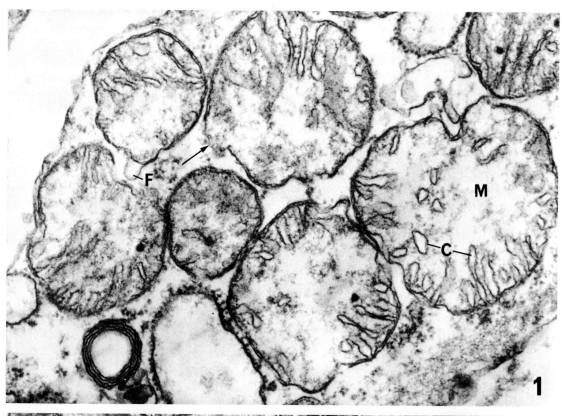

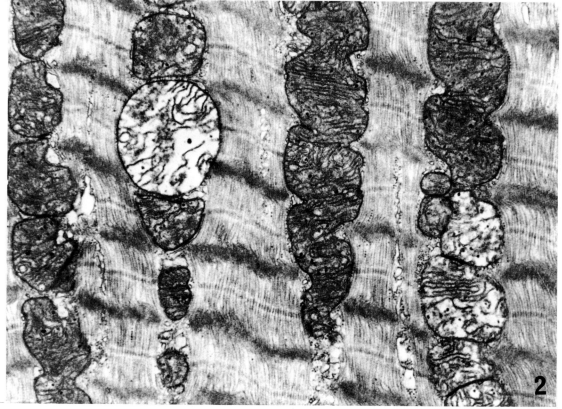

247

Swollen mitochondria (like cloudy swelling) have been observed in almost every type of tissue subjected to a variety of pathological influences. It is so protean a manifestation of cell injury that it would be impossible to list every situation in which this change has been noted. David (1964) lists the following conditions in which mitochondrial swelling has been seen in the liver: starvation, kwashiorkor, choline deficiency, vitamin B_1 deficiency, enteromelia of mouse, hepatitis, yellow fever, x-rays, ethionine intoxication, dimethylaminoazobenzene-feeding, hepatoma, diphtheria toxin, cirrhosis, bile duct obstruction, phosphorus poisoning, hormone action and shock.

The term 'cloudy swelling' was coined by Virchow to describe intracellular water accumulation in cells subject to toxic stress. He believed it to be a primary cause of cell death. (A detailed historical review of this subject has been presented by Cameron, 1952.) The pathogenesis of cloudy swelling is still not fully understood, but it is now believed that it involves a failure of cellular osmotic control mechanisms. It would appear that damage and swelling of mitochondria lead to a suppression of ATP production, which in turn leads to a failure of the ATP-dependent sodium pump at the cell membrane, resulting in the cellular compartments becoming flooded with water.

Plate 111

Fig. 1. Oncocytic adenoma of parathyroid gland. Two cells are seen in this electron micrograph. The one on the left contains swollen mitochondria with cavitation of the matrix and a variable loss of cristae, while the one on the right contains mitochondria showing a condensed configuration. × 30 000

Fig. 2. Same specimen as *Fig. 1.* In one and the same cell we find a mitochondrion (A) with a swollen matrix chamber, another (B) where the matrix is dense and yet another where one part of the mitochondrion (a) resembles mitochondrion (A) and another part (b) resembles mitochondrion (B). × 59 000

248

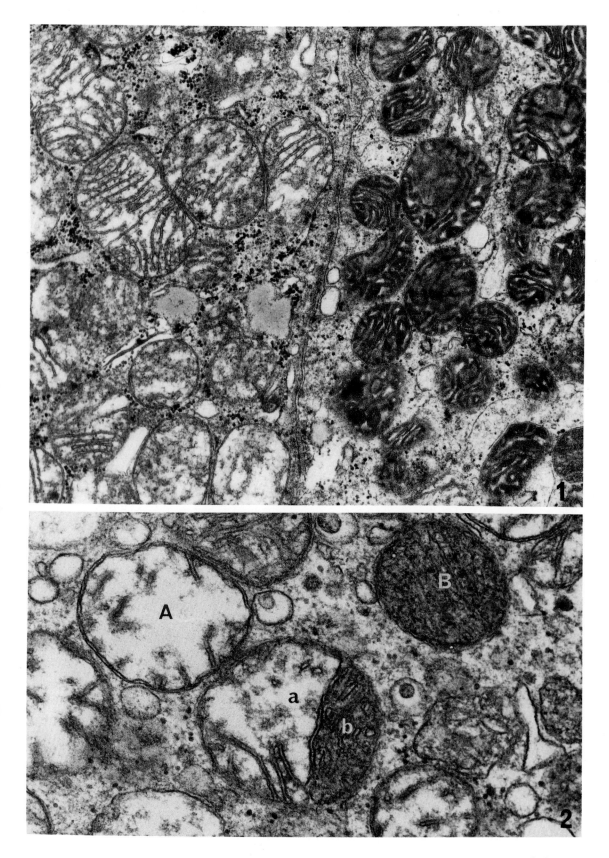

Flocculent or woolly densities in mitochondria

A much studied intramitochondrial inclusion is the matrical flocculent density or woolly density (*Plates 112* and *113*), which is at times also called 'dense matrical deposit' and 'amorphous matrical deposit'. These densities present as irregular medium-density deposits with a woolly filamentous border. However, at times these densities can be quite electron-dense and the woolly nature hard to discern.

Among the many ultrastructural alterations that occur in the lethally injured cell, the development of woolly densities is thought to be the most reliable early manifestation of irreversible cell injury, cell death and ensuing necrosis (*Plate 112*). However, if such densities are seen only in one or two mitochondria in an otherwise normal-looking cell then that is not an indicator of cell death but of a damaged or effete organelle(s) (*see* page 296).

Woolly densities were noted by Trump *et al.* (1965a, b) during their studies on *in vitro* ischaemia. This phenomenon is studied by sampling at various time intervals excised tissue (usually mouse or rat liver, but sometimes kidney, pancreas or myocardium) maintained in a moist environment at normothermic (37°C) or hypothermic (4°C) temperature (Trump *et al.*, 1965a, b; Glaumann *et al.*, 1977; Jennings *et al.*, 1975; Jones and Trump, 1975; Penttila and Ahonen, 1976; Nevalainen and Anttinen, 1977; Kahng *et al.*, 1978; Trump *et al.*, 1982; Myagkaya *et al.*, 1984, 1985).

Intramitochondrial woolly densities have also been seen: (1) after *in vivo* ischaemia, e.g. myocardial infarcts (Jennings and Ganote, 1974, 1976; Buja *et al.*, 1976); (2) after several types of cell injury including heavy metal and other types of poisoning and immune cytolysis (Greene *et al.*, 1979); (3) in cardiac and central nervous system mitochondria after hyperbaric oxygen (Balentine, 1974; Hughson and Balentine, 1974); (4) in surgically removed tissues where there has been a substantial delay between cutting off the blood supply and fixation (personal observations); and (5) in tissues obtained at autopsy (personal observations).

Flocculent or woolly densities are believed to be precipitates of denatured mitochondrial matrix proteins and/or proteins and lipids liberated from disintegrating cristae (Collan *et al.*, 1981; Itkonen and Collan, 1983) when a cell is irreversibly damaged and mitochondrial function becomes disorganized. Woolly densities are moderately electron-dense in unstained sections which suggests that they contain some osmiophilic lipid. They are negative for calcium and phosphorus by electron-probe x-ray analysis (Hughson and Balentine, 1974), which shows that they (i.e woolly densities) are different from the calcified granules (*Plates 104–106*) found in mitochondria in certain pathological states.

A quantitative study of woolly densities which develop in the mitochondria of rat hepatocytes during *in vitro* ischaemia (Myagkaya *et al.*, 1985) shows that the frequency and size (mean diameter given in brackets) of woolly densities produced at various time intervals in tissue maintained at 37°C★ are: (1) 30 minutes, 0 per cent; (2) 1 hour, 8 per cent (170 nm); (3) 1.5 hours, 37 per cent (207 nm); (4) 2 hours, 48 per cent (235 nm); (5) 4 hours, 57 per cent (337 nm).

Myagkawa *et al.* (1985) attempt to correlate their findings with the work on *in vivo* ischaemia (Bassi and Bernelli-Zazzera, 1964; James, 1968; Yamauchi *et al.*, 1982; Frederiks *et al.*, 1984) which indicates that after 1 hour of ischaemia 10 per cent of rat hepatocytes become necrotic while after 2 hours 50–90 per cent become necrotic. They conclude from this and their own *in*

★The corresponding figures for liver tissue kept at 4°C are: (1) 2 days, 3.4 per cent; (2) 4 days, 8.4 per cent (i.e. comparable to 1 hour ischaemia at 37°C); (3) 7 days, 25 per cent; (4) 9 days, 31 per cent; (5) 11 days, 34 per cent; (6) 14 days, 43 per cent.

Plate 112

Fig. 1. Rat liver collected 1 hour after the animal was killed and placed in an incubator at 37°C. Seen here are hepatocellular mitochondria with woolly densities (arrows) which abut the mitochondrial envelope. × 41 000

Fig. 2. Human liver tissue obtained at an autopsy which was performed 8 hours after death. The swollen extracted mitochondria contain quite large electron-dense woolly densities (arrows). Their woolly nature is evident only when the periphery of the densities is closely examined. × 16 000

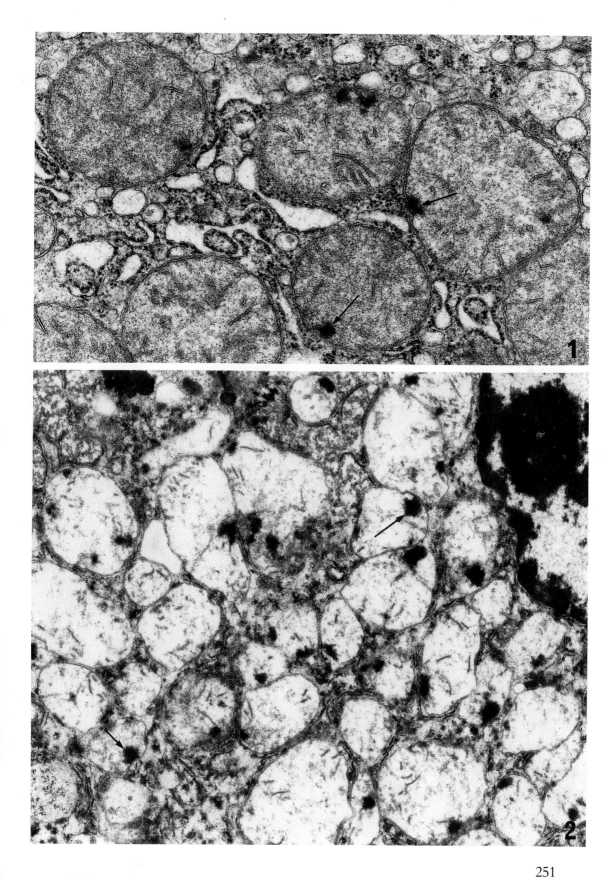

251

vitro study that '1.5 hour incubation may be the decisive cut-off time following which irreversible damage to the majority of hepatocytes occurs'. However, the logical basis for comparing these *in vivo* and *in vitro* figures is rather tenuous because: (1) in sectioned material which shows only a minute slice of a mitochondrion there will be a gross underestimation of the number of woolly densities and number of mitochondria bearing woolly densities; and (2) the real figure needed for comparison is not the percentage of mitochondria containing woolly densities, but the percentage of hepatocytes containing mitochondria with woolly densities, for only then one can see if the percentage of hepatocytes containing mitochondria with woolly densities after *in vitro* ischaemia is similar to the percentage of necrotic cells seen after *in vivo* ischaemia.

Be that as it may, the results of this study are in keeping with the long-held view that the presence of a few intramitochondrial woolly densities is no firm indicator of cell death, and that only when substantial numbers of mitochondria contain woolly densities can one entertain such a notion.

As is to be expected at 4°C, necrotic or autolytic changes in the cell and its mitochondria are markedly decelerated because protein denaturation is retarded by cooling (Majno *et al.*, 1960). Myagkaya *et al.*, (1985) found that in liver pieces kept for 2 days at this temperature only 3.4 per cent of the mitochondria contained woolly densities and they state that: 'after 14 days incubation at 4°C the general morphological appearance, the size of woolly densities and the percentage of mitochondria containing them, were comparable with those observed after 2 hours of normothermal ischaemia'. They (Myagkaya *et al.*, 1985) therefore conclude that for cells maintained at 4°C woolly densities are a poor criterion for assessing cell death.

Until now we have discussed studies on woolly densities in the mitochondria of experimental animals. Corresponding studies on human tissues obtained at biopsy or autopsy do not appear to have been executed but I will report several observations that I have made. As is to be expected in promptly collected and fixed biopsy material (neoplastic or non-neoplastic), woolly densities are not seen except in the odd degenerate or necrotic cell, but when there is a prolonged delay between collection and fixation intramitochondrial woolly densities are frequently encountered. In autopsy material woolly densities abound.

I have seen woolly densities in many tissues and tumours, but oncocytomas with their numerous mitochondria best demonstrate this phenomenon (*Plate 113*). Woolly densities vary much in size and electron density. Small woolly densities are at times mistaken for matrical dense granules, while large ones for intramitochondrial lipid inclusions. Yet such errors can be avoided by careful inspection, because woolly densities have a fuzzy border and they often abut the mitochondrial envelope. Neither lipid droplets nor matrical granules show these features. The former (matrical granules) have a compact granular appearance and they lie in association with the cristae. Since they are as a rule lost during the early phases of ischaemia (i.e. in about 15 minutes), they are hardly likely to be present at the late phase when woolly densities occur. Osmiophilic lipid droplets are homogeneously electron-dense and as a rule have a sharp border (*see also* footnote on page 260).

Plate 113

Renal oncocytoma. Incidental finding in an autopsy performed approximately 12 hours after death. (*Ghadially and Lew, unpublished electron micrographs*)

Fig. 1. Several mitochondria containing woolly densities (arrows) are seen in the tumour cells. × 12 500

Fig. 2. A higher-power view of woolly densities (arrowheads). The woolly nature is demonstrated at the periphery of these densities. × 81 000

252

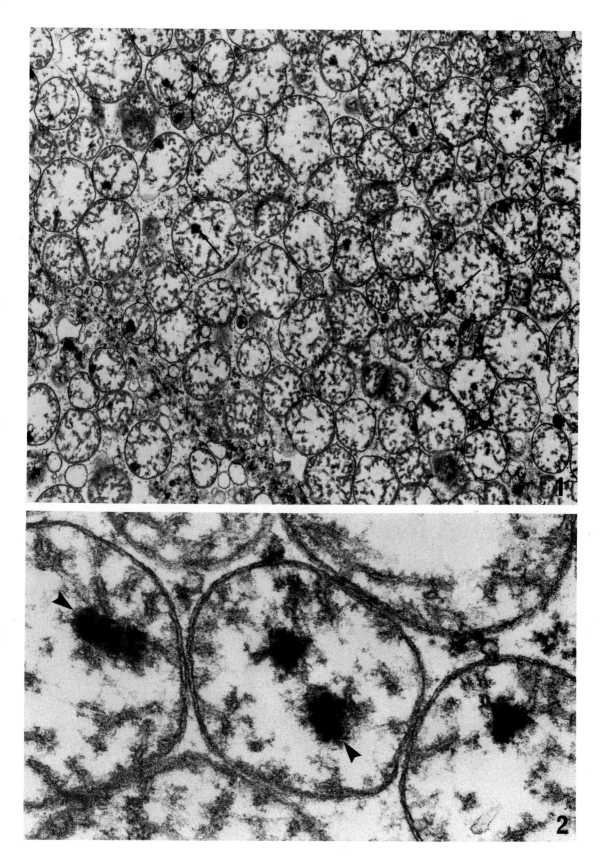

Mitochondrial hypertrophy and hyperplasia

Mitochondrial enlargement due to hypertrophy is distinguishable from swelling or hydrops, because in the former there is no dilution of the matrix, and hence no reduction of matrix density. Also, in hypertrophied mitochondria the concentration of cristae is normal or increased, but in swollen mitochondria the cristae are lost or displaced to the periphery.

Examples of increase in the size (hypertrophy) and/or number (hyperplasia) of mitochondria have been observed in cardiac, uterine and skeletal muscle subject to various pathological and experimental states where an increased functional demand is made on the tissue. Thus the marked hypertrophy of the myometrium during pregnancy is matched not only by a great increase in the number and size of mitochondria but also by an increase in the number of cristae (Dessouky, 1968). Similar mitochondrial changes have also been observed in the myocardium after acute and exhaustive exercise (Laguens *et al.*, 1966; Pelosi and Agliati, 1968) and in cardiac hypertrophy produced by natural disease or experimental situations (Meerson *et al.*, 1964; McCallister and Brown, 1965; Bishop and Cole, 1969; Zak and Rabinowitz, 1973). Such studies show that mitochondrial hypertrophy commences during the early stages of cardiac hypertrophy, before the hypertrophy of myofibrils. During the final stage of exhaustion and cardiac failure there is a decrease in the mitochondrial mass, and also swelling of mitochondria.

A single non-lethal but toxic dose of digoxin has also been shown to produce a significant increase in the quantity of mitochondria and enhanced energy production by rat myocardial cells (Arcasoy and Smuckler, 1969). In the rat gastrocnemius muscle, Gustafsson *et al.* (1965) noted an increase in the size and number of mitochondria and an increase in the number and length of cristae after the administration of L-thyroxine under anabolic conditions. In these hypermetabolic rats, the enlargement of the mitochondrial apparatus amounted to an increase two and a half times normal. No simple correlation, however, exists between the enhanced metabolic activity produced by thyroxine and mitochondrial hypertrophy and hyperplasia, for even three weeks after cessation of thyroxine treatment, mitochondrial hypertrophy and hyperplasia persist although their elevated respiratory activity has returned to normal. Strangely enough thyroidectomy also produces a small but definite enlargement of the mitochondrial apparatus.

Plate 114
An oncocyte from a bronchial mucosal gland of man, showing cytoplasm packed with mitochondria. × 24 000

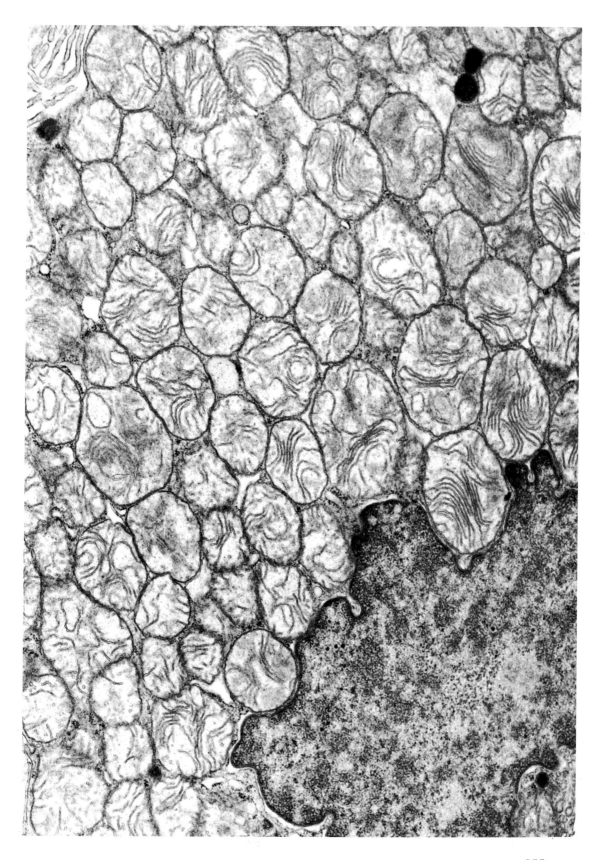

255

Cortisone treatment on the other hand produces a fourfold increase in the volume of hepatocellular mitochondria in the rat but there is a decrease in the number of mitochondria per cell such that the total mitochondrial volume per cell remains approximately unchanged, as does the total amount of cristae surface per cell (Wiener et al., 1968). This is accompanied by an uncoupling of oxidative phosphorylation, a lowering of the P : O ratios and a 14–40 per cent decrease in the amount of oxygen consumed per mg of mitochondrial protein.

Perhaps the largest concentration of mitochondria (see footnote on page 264) known to occur is seen in the cells called 'oncocytes'. As is well known, these acidophilic cells with a markedly granular cytoplasm arise in tissues that have already attained histological maturity. For instance, in salivary glands, transition from normal epithelial cells to oncocytes is known to occur (Tandler, 1966a). During such transformation a remarkable hyperplasia of mitochondria occurs. Oncocytes from various sites show certain common features, the most important being the abundance of mitochondria (Plate 114) which usually lack matrical dense granules similar to those so commonly seen in normal mitochondria (see footnote on page 260). Indeed, often the cytoplasm contains little besides mitochondria, but it is difficult to see what energy requirement so remarkable a collection of mitochondria is supposed to meet. A plausible explanation that has been offered is that these mitochondria are probably biochemically defective and that this is an example of compensatory hyperplasia occurring at the organelle level (Tandler and Shipkey, 1964; Tandler et al., 1970).

In normal brown adipose tissue exceedingly numerous mitochondria are found (Plate 115)

Plate 115

Brown adipose cell of golden mantled squirrel (*Citellus lateralis*) showing a few lipid droplets (L) and numerous mitochondria well endowed with cristae but lacking in dense granules. × 19 500. (*From a block of tissue, supplied by Dr I. Grodums*)

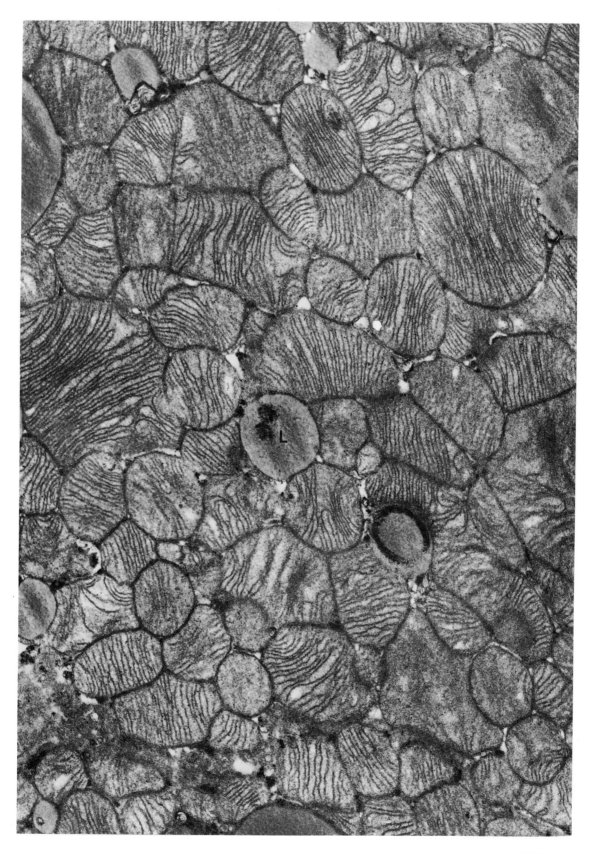

257

and they undergo a hypertrophy during hibernation (Grodums, 1977). They provide the energy required for the degradation of fat to yield the heat necessary to raise the body temperature during arousal from hibernation in hibernating animals (Smallely and Dryer, 1963; Smith and Hock, 1963; Smith and Horwitz, 1969; Suter, 1969; Grodums, 1977) and for non-shivering thermogenesis in human neonates and other non-hibernating animals (Aherne and Hull, 1966; Brück, 1970). In keeping with this is the observation that numerous mitochondria occur also in hibernomas (Levine, 1972; Seemayer *et al.*, 1975; Fleishman and Schwartz, 1983). Here (*Plate 116*) a variety of cells are seen, including: (1) cells containing several large lipid droplets with a few mitochondria between them; (2) cells with medium-sized lipid droplets with collections of many mitochondria; and (3) cells resembling oncocytes which are packed with innumerable mitochondria with only a rare small lipid droplet between them.

All the above-mentioned cells also contain a few lysosomal bodies containing electron-dense granules and lipid droplets (i.e. lipofuscin granules). Intramatrical dense granules are difficult to find in the mitochondria of hibernoma but then they are rare or inconspicuous in mitochondria of brown adipose tissue also★. There is no reason to suppose that mitochondria in hibernoma are biochemically defective and no reason whatsoever to classify a hibernoma as an oncocytoma, even though it contains cells that morphologically resemble oncocytes. Further, the cells in brown fat and hibernoma do not derive by transformation of cells that have reached histological maturity as do oncocytes. Thus the large number of mitochondria in hibernoma are no more than a counterpart of that found in brown fat, its parent tissue of origin.

★In the brown adipose tissue of the rat, intramitochondrial granules are quite prominent in the perinatal period, but they vanish within a day or two after birth.

Plate 116

Fig. 1. Hibernoma. The cell on the left contains several lipid droplets (L), some mitochondria (M) and a few lysosomes (arrows). The cell on the right resembles an oncocyte in that it is packed with numerous mitochondria (M). A few lipid droplets (L) and lysosomes (arrows) are also present. × 4800 (*From a block of tissue supplied by Dr T. A. Seemayer*)

Fig. 2. Hibernoma. A higher-power view showing mitochondria (M) and lysosomes (L) in the cell shown in the right part of *Fig. 1.* × 16 500 (*From a block of tissue supplied by Dr T. A. Seemayer*)

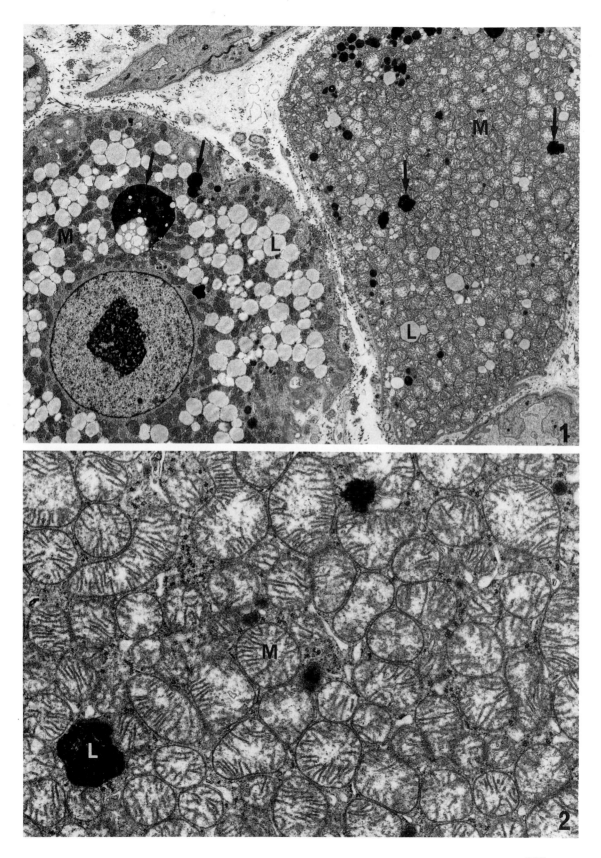

259

Mitochondria in oncocytes and oncocytomas

The term 'oncocyte' was coined by Hamperl (1950) to describe the large eosinophilic (acidophilic) cells of Hürthle cell tumours of the thyroid gland. He suggested that this was a special class of cell and that tumours of these cells should be called 'oncocytomas'.

It is now well known that these acidophilic (oxyphil) cells with a granular cytoplasm★ are found in a variety of normal and pathological tissues (e.g. normal salivary gland, parathyroid gland, pancreas, liver, Graves disease and Hashimoto's thyroiditis) and that they arise from normal epithelial cells that have already reached histological maturity. In salivary glands, transition from normal epithelial cells to oncocytes has been demonstrated by Tandler (1966a), and there is ultrastructural evidence that Hürthle cells derive from the thyroid epithelium (Feldman *et al.*, 1972). Light and electron microscopic studies (Hamperl, 1936, 1937; *Plate 113*) have shown oncocytes in the ducts and acini of bronchial mucosal glands, particularly in older individuals. It is said (Matsuba *et al.*, 1972) that normally oncocytes are not found in the bronchi of persons less than 33 years old. Bonikos *et al.* (1977) have shown that oncocytic change can be induced in the conducting airways by high oxygen tension.

Ultrastructurally, oncocytes (*Plate 114*) and cells of oncocytomas (*Plates 117* and *118*) are characterized by a cytoplasm packed with innumerable mitochondria which usually lack intramitochondrial dense granules†. In some instances such mitochondria may contain glycogen or lipid or filamentous inclusions (*Plates 133, 134* and *139*). Tumours deserving to be called oncocytomas include: (1) Warthin's tumour (adenolymphoma of parotid gland) (Tandler and Shipkey, 1964; McGavran, 1965; Tandler, 1966b; Hubner *et al.*, 1971; Allegra, 1971; Sun *et al.*, 1976); (2) oxyphil cell adenoma of the major salivary glands (Tandler *et al.*, 1970; Kay and Still, 1973; Sun *et al.*, 1975; Lee and Roth, 1976; Carlsöö *et al.*, 1979); (3) oxyphil cell adenomas of parathyroid gland (Marshall *et al.*, 1967; Heinmann *et al.*, 1971; Arnold *et al.*, 1974; McGregor *et al.*, 1978); (4) oncocytic adenoma of pituitary gland (Kovacs and Horvath, 1973; Landolt and Oswald, 1973; Kovacs *et al.*, 1974; Scanarini and Mingrino, 1974; Bauserman *et al.*, 1978; Roy, 1978; Goebel *et al.*, 1980; Kalyanaraman *et al.*, 1980); (5) Hürthle cell tumours (also called 'Askanazy cell tumours' or 'oxyphil tumours') of the thyroid (Tonietti *et al.*, 1967; Michel-Bechet *et al.*, 1971; Feldman *et al.*, 1972; Valenta *et al.*, 1974; Ghadially, 1985; Sobrinho-Simões *et al.*, 1985; Nesland *et al.*, 1985); (6) bronchial oncocytoma (Fechner and Bentinck, 1973); (7) fibrolamellar oncocytic hepatoma (a variety of hepatocellular carcinoma, usually not associated with cirrhosis. They appear to have a better prognosis than other varieties of hepatocellular carcinomas) (Farhi *et al.*, 1982; Baithun and Pollock, 1983); (8) intracystic oncocytic papilloma of the breast (Nielsen, 1981); (9) renal oncocytoma, which has been

---

★An eosinophilic granular cytoplasm usually indicates the presence of either numerous mitochondria or numerous lysosomes. Tumours in which large numbers of mitochondria occur (i.e. oncocytomas) are dealt with here. Tumours in which large numbers of lysosomes are found are dealt with on page 684.

†By this I mean that the ubiquitous matrical dense granules (20–50 nm in diameter in which subunits 5–7 nm in diameter may at times be discerned) which are seen in most normal mitochondria are rarely, if ever, seen in mitochondria of normal or neoplastic oncocytes. Confusion and controversy has developed in the literature on this point, which I think stems from problems of interpretation and nomenclature. Woolly densities (*Plates 112* and *113*) are at times confused with matrical dense granules (*Plate 83*) and the much larger electron-dense lipidic inclusions (*Plate 134*) are also at times referred to as 'dense bodies' or 'dense granules' by some. Yet others talk about 'dense core granules' which is truly bewildering. It is possible that some of the 'dense bodies' may represent calcium deposits like the ones shown in *Plate 104, Fig. 1* but this is pure speculation on my part. I have not found indubitable 'normal' matrical dense granules in any of the numerous oncocytomas I have studied, but woolly densities are all too common (because of anoxia produced during surgery and/or delays in collecting and processing) and intramitochondrial lipidic inclusions are uncommon but not rare.

Plate 117
Oxyphil adenoma of parathyroid gland. The cells are packed with numerous mitochondria. × 8300 (*From a block of tissue supplied by Dr S. Cinti*)

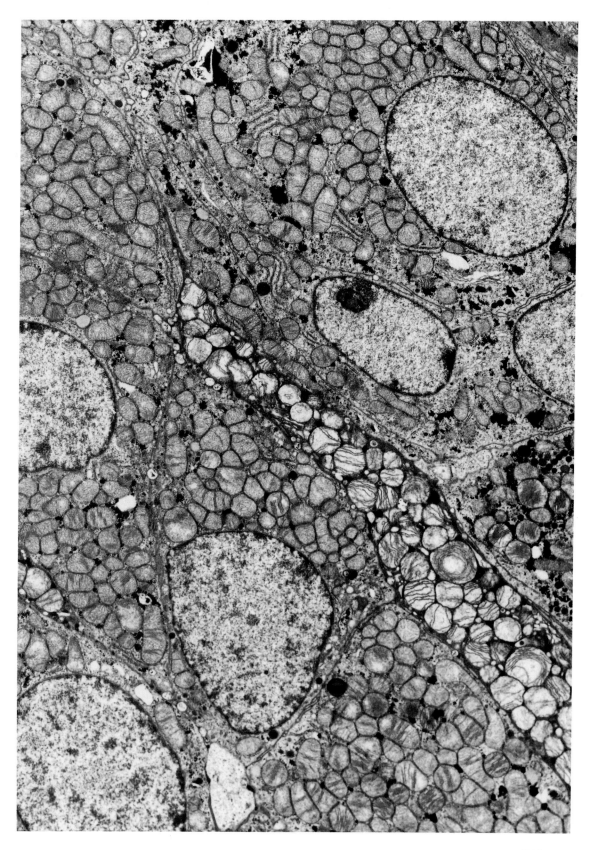

261

wrongly diagnosed as carcinoma in the past (Murphy and Ghadially, 1983; Ghadially, 1985); (10) cycasin-induced oncocytic adenomas of rat kidney (Gusek, 1975); and (11) ovarian oncocytoma (Yoshida et al., 1984).

It is important to note that when a tumour seems to consist only of oncocytes (apart of course, from stromal cells) and the term 'oncocytoma' suggests itself, great care must be taken to exclude the possible presence of other elements in the tumour. Sections from several blocks of tumour tissue must be examined to exclude the possible presence of non-oncocytic areas, lest an error in diagnosis is made and a malignant tumour containing oncocytic areas, is mistaken for a benign oncocytoma. However, oncocytic transformation of a lesser degree (i.e. few, several or many neoplastic oncocytes or mitochondria-rich cells resembling oncocytes admixed with other tumour cells) is also known to occur. Such examples include: (1) carcinoma of the kidney (Seljelid and Ericsson, 1965; Keyhani, 1969. See also Chapter 11 in Ghadially, 1985); (2) fibroadenoma of breast (Archer and Omar, 1969); (3) oxyphil adenoma of the lacrimal caruncle (Radnot and Lapis, 1970); (4) oncocytic adenocarcinoma of the ovary (Takeda et al., 1983); (5) oxyphil cell carcinoma* of parathyroid gland (Obara et al., 1985); (6) oncocytic carcinoid of bronchus† (Ghadially and Block, 1985); and (7) plasmacytoma with oncocytic change† (Posalaky and McGinley, 1985).

Plate 119 illustrates an oncocytic carcinoid of the bronchus. Grossly, the tumour presented as an oval pale yellowish mass (3 × 2 × 2 cm) projecting into the lumen of a medial lobe segmental bronchus as a polypoid structure and extending into the adjacent lung parenchyma from which it was separated by a fibrous capsule. The tumour was composed principally of closely-packed small clusters of cells, but in some areas the cells were arranged in columns. Some of the cells had a granular cytoplasm. The histopathological diagnosis was 'bronchial carcinoid-lung (right lower lobe)'. Ultrastructural appearances suggest that the tumour was basically a neuroendocrine tumour (i.e. a carcinoid) with oncocytic transformation of some neuroendocrine cells. A spectrum of appearances was seen, ranging from cells with many neuroendocrine granules and few mitochondria (neuroendocrine cells) to cells containing more mitochondria and few granules (intermediate cells) to cells which contained numerous mitochondria and virtually no neuroendocrine granules (oncocytes). A few enlarged mitochondria containing

---

*Parathyroid carcinoma is a rare tumour. The reported cases have been of the chief cell type, indubitable cases of oxyphil cell carcinoma are hard to find. The two tumours reported by Obara et al. (1985) were composed almost entirely of quite typical oncocytes, but cells containing other organelles such as rough endoplasmic reticulum, Golgi complex and secretory granules were also present. The tumours were functionally active.

†One generally associates oncocytic transformation with epithelial cells such as those found in kidney, thyroid and bronchus. The occurrence of oncocytic bronchial carcinoids (only seven cases recorded so far) shows that this change can occur in a neuroendocrine cell. Even more intriguing is the report by Posalaky and McGinley (1985) which shows that oncocytic change can occur in plasma cells. The cells in laryngeal rhabdomyoma of the dog contain numerous mitochondria, and such tumours have been misdiagnosed as laryngeal oncocytomas with the light microscope but electron microscopy shows that besides many mitochondria these cells also contain myofibrils (Meuten et al., 1985). A priori one can argue that an enzymic defect in the mitochondria of any cell type may lead to a compensatory proliferation of mitochondria and the emergence of an oncocyte. Finally, it is worth noting that oncocytic transformation is not exclusively associated with ageing or neoplasia. For example, several cases of oncocytic cardiomyopathy have been described (myocytes are loaded with mitochondria), the most interesting case being that described by Silver et al. (1980) where an 11-week-old female showed extensive oncocytic transformation of cardiac myocytes and oncocytes were found also in endocrine (pituitary, thyroid) and exocrine (submandibular, sublingual, minor salivary) glands.

Plate 118
Warthin's tumour (adenolymphoma of parotid gland). The cytoplasm of the tumour cells is packed with innumerable mitochondria. × 3700 (*Tandler, unpublished electron micrograph*)

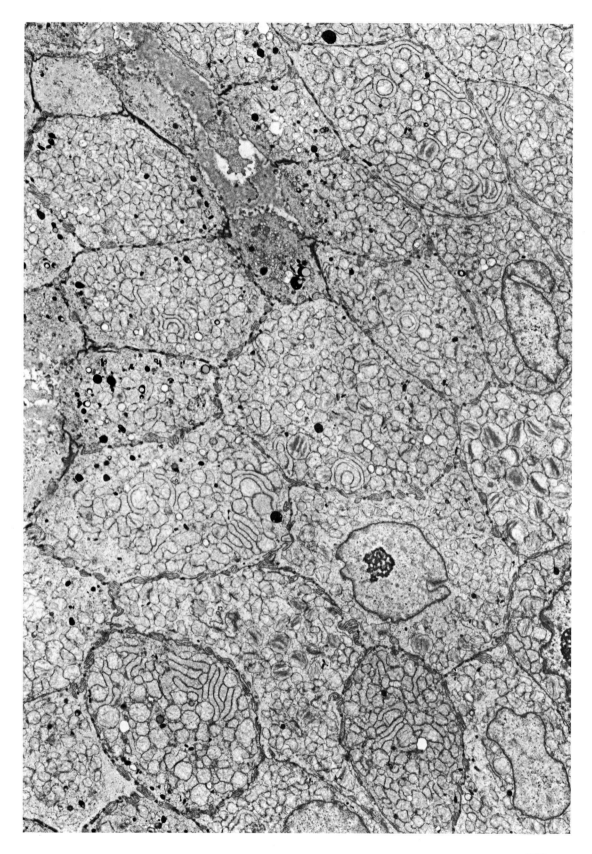

263

filamentous or paracrystalline inclusions were seen in the tumour cells (*Plate 139*). Several varieties of mitochondrial anomalies (e.g. concentric cristae, centrally stacked cristae and chondriospheres) and inclusions (*Plate 133* and *Plate 134, Fig. 5*) are associated with oncocytic transformation so the occurrence of these filamentous inclusions may be regarded as a part and parcel of this phenomenon.

Oncocytomas are essentially benign tumours, but rare malignant variants are also known to occur (Gray *et al.*, 1976; Lee and Roth, 1976; Ghadially, 1985). Perhaps the best known is the malignant oncocytoma of the thyroid gland (Hürthle cell carcinoma). Bondeson *et al.* (1981) reviewed 42 cases of Hürthle cell tumours, two of which had produced distant metastasis. Several cases of malignant oncocytomas of the salivary glands have been described but Gray *et al.* (1976) could only accept ten cases in the literature as being indubitably malignant. Leiber *et al.* (1981) studied 90 cases of renal oncocytoma, four of whom died from metastatic disease.★

There is, of course, no specific ultrastructural feature which distinguishes benign from malignant oncocytoma, but as one would expect they usually show the well known features one associates with malignancy, namely enlarged and irregular nuclei and nucleoli, abundant polyribosomes lying free in the cytoplasm, poorly developed or absent basal lamina, and sparse poorly differentiated cell junctions.

One may well ask what energy requirement so remarkable a collection of mitochondria† is supposed to meet in the oncocyte? Conflicting results have been obtained by histochemical studies and studies on isolated mitochondria. Some studies suggest that there is a high level of oxidative activity, while others have found that the mitochondria are deficient in various ways and have a low level of succinoxidase activity. Tandler *et al.* (1970) give an excellent critique on this subject and conclude that these mitochondria are biochemically defective and that this is an example of compensatory hyperplasia occurring at the organelle level; on the other hand Feldmann *et al.* (1968) discuss the possibility that the increase in mitochondrial mass may be due to a prolonged life-span (i.e. a diminished rate of elimination) of mitochondria in these cells.

The idea of organelle atrophy, hypertrophy or hyperplasia is not too difficult to accept, but it takes somewhat more imagination to accept a concept of organelle neoplasia. Since mitochondria have their own DNA one can envisage a mutation but this could hardly lead to an increased proliferation of mitochondria because mitochondrial DNA codes for only a fraction of mitochondrial proteins (*see* page 216). However, such a theory has been proposed by Sun *et al.* (1975) who suggest that an oncocytoma may represent 'an intracellular "neoplasm" of the mitochondria proliferating at the expense of the cell's own economy'. Be that as it may, ultrastructural studies have clearly defined a group of tumours which can be confidently identified by their characteristic mitochondrial population.

★Light microscopic study. I am not aware of an ultrastructurally confirmed renal oncocytoma which has metastasized.
†Carlsöö *et al.* (1979) found that the volume fraction occupied by mitochondria in a parotid oncocytoma was close to 60 per cent of the cytoplasm. This is higher than for any other cell type so far investigated. Comparative figures for other cells are: rat parietal cells 35 per cent; human hepatocytes 19 per cent; guinea-pig pancreatic acinar cells 8 per cent.

Plate 119

Fig. 1. Oncocytic carcinoid of bronchus. Neuroendocrine cells containing numerous characteristic neuroendocrine granules (arrows). × 7500

Fig. 2. Oncocytic carcinoid of bronchus. Same case as *Fig. 1*. Two cells are portrayed here. The one on the left shows incomplete oncocytic transformation in that besides many mitochondria (M), it contains some neuroendocrine granules (thin arrows) and short strands of rough endoplasmic reticulum (arrowheads). The one on the right shows complete oncocytic transformation in that it contains little besides mitochondria (M). × 12 500 (*From Ghadially and Block, 1985*)

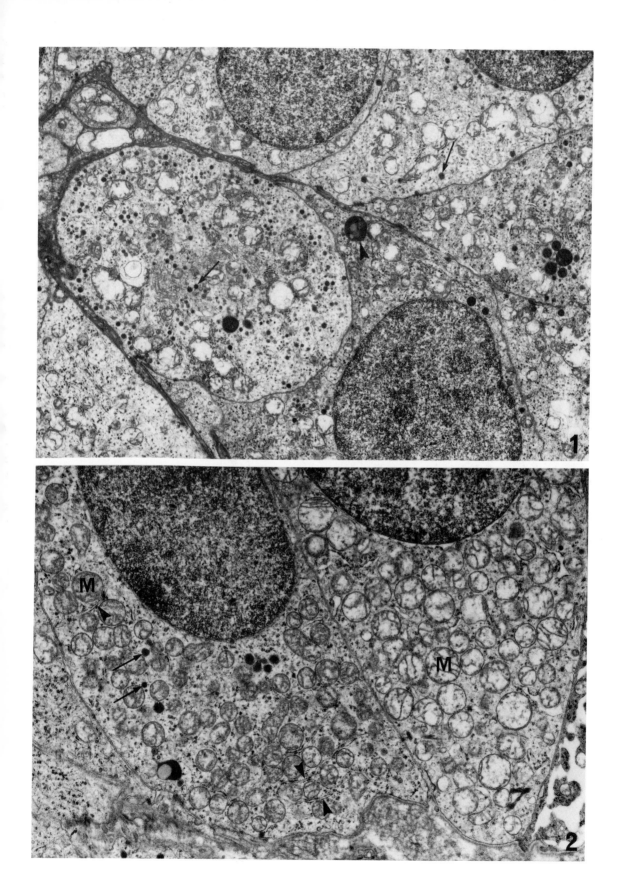

Giant mitochondria

Grossly enlarged mitochondria have been observed in a variety of tissues under diverse situations, and terms such as 'megamitochondria' and 'giant mitochondria' have been employed to describe them. Such organelles may evolve either by fusion of a number of mitochondria or by growth of a single mitochondrion, or both. Often such enlargement affects only one or two mitochondria in a cell, the size and number of the remainder being normal or even diminished. Giant mitochondria frequently show highly interesting alterations of internal structure (*Plates 120–124*), such as an increase in the number of cristae (often showing novel arrangements), myelin figures, prominent dense granules, and crystalline and lipidic inclusions. Some of these alterations, such as crystalline inclusions, are at times also seen in some of the remaining normal-sized mitochondria in the cell containing the giant forms.

A study of published electron micrographs and tissues containing giant mitochondria leads one to believe that in the evolution of these organelles there is a phase of enlargement followed by a phase of degeneration and disintegration of internal architecture. The former phase is characterized by an abundance of well preserved cristae, matrix and, at times, large, numerous matrical dense granules. The formation of myelin figures, granular amorphous debris and osmiophilic lipidic material may be regarded as regressive changes due to degeneration and disintegration within the enlarged organelle. Later, segmental or total dissolution of the inner mitochondrial membrane may occur, and a single-membrane-bound body containing membrane remnants and electron-dense material, morphologically acceptable as a autolysosome, may develop (*Plate 122, Fig. 2*).

Plate 120

From non-neoplastic human liver adjacent to a hepatoma.

Fig. 1. A giant mitochondrion containing tubular cristae (C), crystalline inclusions (arrow) and large matrical dense granules (D) is seen in this liver cell. The remarkable increase in size of this organelle is well demonstrated by comparison with normal-sized mitochondria in the bottom right corner of the picture. × 43 000 (*From Ghadially and Parry, 1966*)

Fig. 2. A small part of a giant golf-club-shaped mitochondrion is illustrated here. Several intramitochondrial crystalline inclusions are present. They present profiles suggesting longitudinally (L) and transversely (T) cut filaments, but actually (as explained on page 298) these crystals are composed of globular, not filamentous subunits. × 75 000 (*Ghadially and Parry, unpublished electron micrograph*)

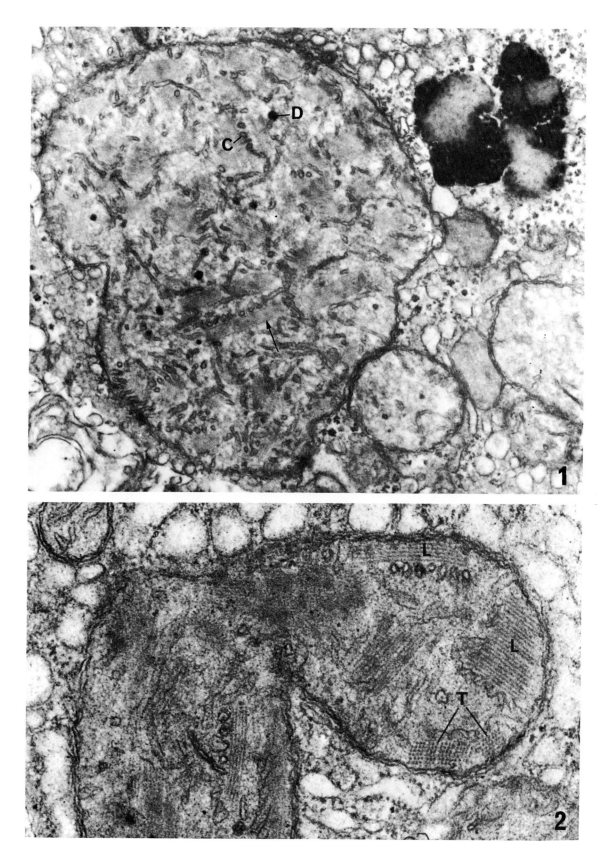

267

Mitochondrial abnormalities of the sort described above have been seen in various tissues under apparently unrelated conditions, and different theories regarding their genesis have been suggested.

Hormonal mechanisms have been held responsible for the giant mitochondria produced in some situations, as in: (1) rat adrenal (seen with greater frequency in female rats) after hypophysectomy (Sabatini et al., 1962; Volk and Scarpelli, 1966); (2) the fetal zone of the human adrenal cortex during the sixth and twelfth weeks of gestation (Luse, 1961; Ross, 1962); (3) rats given ACTH, and also in rats given aminoglutethimide which blocks steroid synthesis (Racela et al., 1969); (4) endometrium of mink during the phase of delayed implantation of early pregnancy (Enders et al., 1963); (5) liver of healthy women on oral contraceptives (Pihl et al., 1968; Perez et al., 1969; Martinez-Manautou et al., 1970; Reid et al., 1978); and (6) liver of castrated sheep treated with the synthetic anabolic steroid, trenbolone acetate (Reid et al., 1978).

Protein, vitamin and related nutritional deficiencies seem to be associated with another group of cases (seen mainly in the liver) where giant mitochondria and moderately enlarged mitochondria are found, although in some of these cases hormonal imbalance and toxic factors may also be involved. Thus, such mitochondria have been seen in: (1) the pancreas in kwashiorkor (Blackburn and Vinijchaikul, 1969); (2) the liver and adrenals of protein-deficient rats (Svoboda and Higginson, 1964; Svoboda et al., 1966); (3) the liver of riboflavin-deficient mice (Tandler et al., 1968); (4) liver of morbidly obese patients (open liver biopsy obtained during jejuno-ileal bypass operation) (Friedman et al., 1977); (5) human liver surrounding a large but well differentiated hepatoma (*Plates 120–122*) (Ghadially and Parry, 1966); and (6) biopsy specimens of livers containing metastatic carcinoma (Albukerk and Duffy, 1976). The association of tumours and giant mitochondria is interesting, for profound disturbances of protein metabolism also occur in the neoplastic state, and the cachexia and anaemia which occur in the tumour-bearing host are well recognized (Greenstein, 1954; Wiseman and Ghadially, 1958).

Chronic alcoholism in which complex nutritional deficiencies may also be operative provides another interesting situation where megamitochondria occur in the liver. At one time it was thought that the hyaline eosinophilic Mallory's bodies were megamitochondria and their degenerate remains (Porta et al., 1965). Later it was contended that they were areas of focal cytoplasmic degradation (i.e. autolysosomes) involving various organelles besides mitochondria (Flax and Tisdale, 1964). We now know that these concepts are erroneous and that Mallory's bodies are in fact accumulations of cytokeratin filaments in the cytoplasm of hepatocytes (*see* page 902 for more details).

Plate 121

From non-neoplastic human liver adjacent to a hepatoma. Same case as *Plates 120* and *122*. A bipartite (fusion?) giant mitochondrion is seen in this hepatocyte. Abundant cristae and crystals are seen in the upper part of the organelle while the lower part is filled with granular matrix. × 50 000 (*Ghadially and Parry, unpublished electron micrograph*)

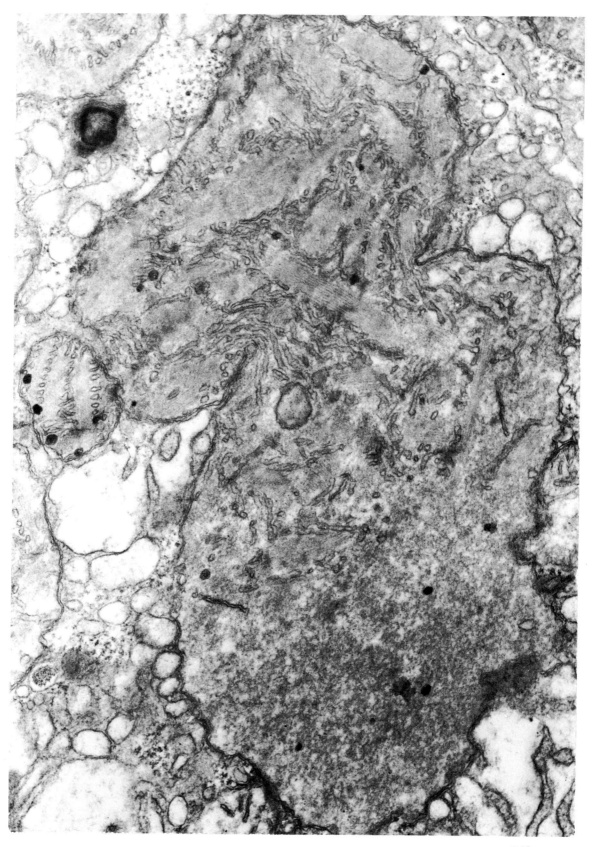

269

Rats given special diets and alcohol also develop megamitochondria in their hepatocytes (Porta *et al.*, 1969). In passing one may note that rat liver is not quite as susceptible to the formation of megamitochondria as is the human liver and bizarre giant mitochondria as found in human liver are not seen in the rat. That there are species differences in the production of megamitochondria is attested also by the fact that cuprisone produces megamitochondria in the mouse liver but not in the rat liver (Hoppel and Tandler, 1973). That there are organ-specific or cell-specific differences is attested by the fact that administration of isonicotinic acid derivatives (nialamide, iproniazid, isoniazid) to mice produces giant mitochondria in hepatocytes but not in Kupffer cells, cardiocytes and renal tubular epithelial cells (Wakabayashi *et al.*, 1979).

The list of diseases and conditions in which megamitochondria (with or without crystalline inclusions) have been seen in the human hepatocyte is indeed quite formidable and the final common pathway by which this change is produced is not understood. Besides the examples already mentioned above, megamitochondria in human hepatocytes have been seen in: (1) viral hepatitis (Jézéquel, 1959; Wills, 1968; Spycher and Rüttner, 1968); (2) amyloidosis (Thiery and Caroli, 1962); (3) carcinoma of bile duct (Jézéquel, 1959); (4) alcoholic hepatitis (Svoboda and Manning, 1964; Feldmann *et al.*, 1970a); (5) porphyria (Jean *et al.*, 1968); (6) leptospirosis (Sandborn *et al.*, 1966); (7) recurrent jaundice in pregnancy (Adlercreutz *et al.*, 1967; Van Haelst and Bergstein, 1970); (8) Dubin-Johnson syndrome (Minio and Gautier, 1967; Feldmann *et al.*, 1970b); (9) Gilbert's disease (Minio and Gautier, 1967; Feldmann *et al.*, 1968); (10) Sanfilippo's disease (Haust, 1968); (11) Wilson's disease (Sternlieb, 1968); and (12) systemic scleroderma (Feldmann *et al.*, 1977).

A moderate degree of mitochondrial enlargement with crystalline inclusions or normal-sized mitochondria with crystals have often been reported to occur in apparently normal human liver (Reppart *et al.*, 1963; Mugnaini, 1964a; Svoboda and Manning, 1964; Wills, 1965; Lynn *et al.*, 1969), and regarding giant mitochondria in the liver, David (1964) states, 'We have been able to notice it in various non-characteristic diseases without any pathological-histological findings on the liver'. The view that mitochondria with crystalline inclusions can occur in normal human liver has been challenged by Bhagwat and his co-workers (Bhagwat and Ross, 1971; Bhagwat *et al.*, 1972), who point out that in such studies the normality of the livers can be seriously questioned and that, when stricter criteria are employed in selecting normal human liver, mitochondria with crystalline inclusions are not seen. (*See also* pages 298 and 306.)

Plate 122

From non-neoplastic human liver adjacent to a hepatoma. Same case as *Plates 120* and *121* (*Ghadially and Parry, unpublished electron micrographs*)

Fig. 1. The giant mitochondrion in the centre of this illustration shows early degenerative changes as evidenced by the presence of osmiophilic lipidic material (L) and disintegration of internal architecture. Compare with *Plates 120* and *121.* × 32 000

Fig. 2. A large, single-membrane-bound body, presumably derived from a giant mitochondrion, is seen in this electron micrograph. It contains amorphous material similar to that found in giant mitochondria, and paired membranous structures which could be derived from disintegrating cristae (arrows). A lipid droplet (L) is also present. × 40 000

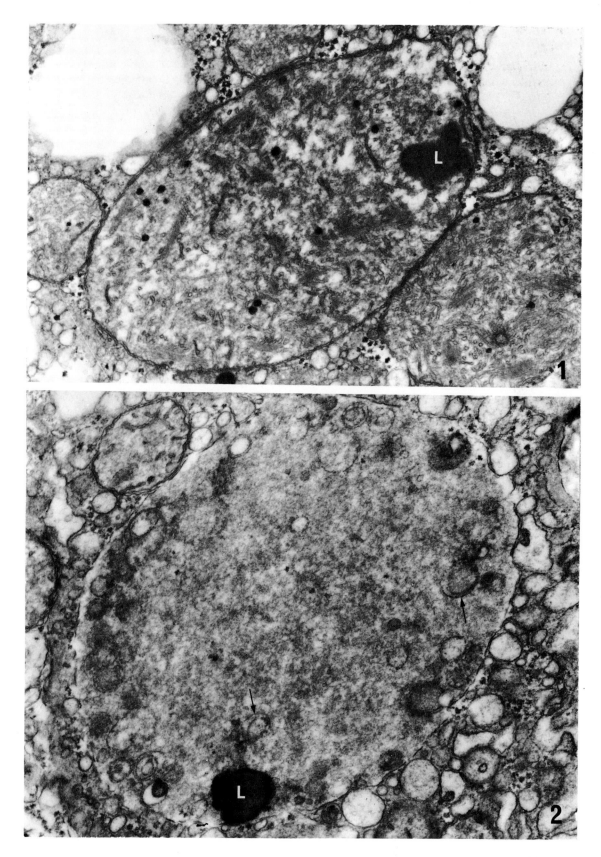

In *Plate 123* are illustrated two giant mitochondria found in the liver of an apparently normal dog; but, as can be seen, the internal architecture of these organelles is different from the giant mitochondria illustrated in the previous plates (*Plates 120* and *121*). Such mitochondria with an abundant matrix but sparse cristae★ are readily produced in the liver of mice fed cuprizone (Suzuki, 1969). Giant mitochondria with crystalline inclusions have been seen in dogs two and three-quarter hours after reversible hypovolaemic shock (Blair *et al.*, 1968), but these resembled more the giant mitochondria of human liver described earlier.

Giant mitochondria have not often been reported to occur in haemopoietic tissues but they have been seen in: (1) bone marrow macrophages from a case of myeloid leukaemia (Bessis and Breton-Gorius, 1969); (2) bone marrow macrophages from a case of erythroleukaemia (Ghadially and Skinnider, 1974) (*Plate 124, Fig. 2* and *Plate 125*); and (3) plasma cells from a case of myeloma in which an acute leukaemia had developed (Skinnider and Ghadially, 1975).

The mitochondria of striated muscle appear to be singularly prone to fusion and formation of giant mitochondria. Even in apparently normal muscle, long mitochondria extending over several sarcomere lengths are encountered at times, and these are almost certainly due to end-to-end fusion of pre-existing mitochondria. This is in keeping with Fawcett's (1966) statement that 'the majority of mitochondria in muscle are 2 to 3 μm long but it is not uncommon to find a few 8 or even 10 μm in length'. Giant mitochondria, presumably produced by end-to-end fusion and also lateral fusion, can develop within a few minutes of myocardial hypoxia (*Plate 124, Fig. 1*). Giant mitochondria in muscle tissue have been seen also in various pathological and experimental states, but in some instances they could equally well have been formed by the enlargement of solitary mitochondria.

Thus giant mitochondria (including long end-to-end fused mitochondria) have been seen in: (1) hypoxic myocardium of dogs (Lozada and Laguens, 1966); (2) myocardium of dogs with aortic stenosis (Wollenberger and Schulze, 1961); (3) hypoxic isolated perfused rat hearts (Sun *et al.*, 1969); (4) myocardium of rats maintained for long periods on small doses of thyroxine (Zaimis *et al.*, 1969); (5) myocardium of dogs treated with quinidine (Hiott and Howell, 1971); (6) myocardium of mouse, bat and dog after the administration of reserpine (Wilcken *et al.*, 1967; Sun *et al.*, 1968; Hagopian *et al.*, 1972); (7) myocardium of a patient on digitalis therapy assumed to have a primary cardiomyopathy (Kraus and Cain, 1980); and (8) in various myopathies of man (Luft *et al.*, 1962; Gruner, 1963; Shy *et al.*, 1966; Shafiq *et al.*, 1967). Particularly interesting are the enlarged mitochondria found in some myopathies, for crystalline inclusions occur in the intracristal compartment and not as they usually do (e.g. liver) in the matrix compartment (*see Plates 137* and *140*).

★Such mitochondria, however, are viable and functional as attested by their ability to accumulate calcium and phosphate under loading conditions (thought to be a test of energy coupling from either electron transport or the hydrolysis of ATP) and to produce ATP (Maloff *et al.*, 1978).

Plate 123

Figs. 1 and 2. Two giant mitochondria from the liver of an apparently normal dog. The remarkable increase in size is demonstrated by comparison with a normal-sized mitochondrion (M) in *Fig. 1*. These giant mitochondria show a paucity of cristae (arrow) but an abundance of granular matrix and intramatrical dense granules (G) of a similar size to that seen in the normal-sized mitochondrion. × 35 000; × 37 000

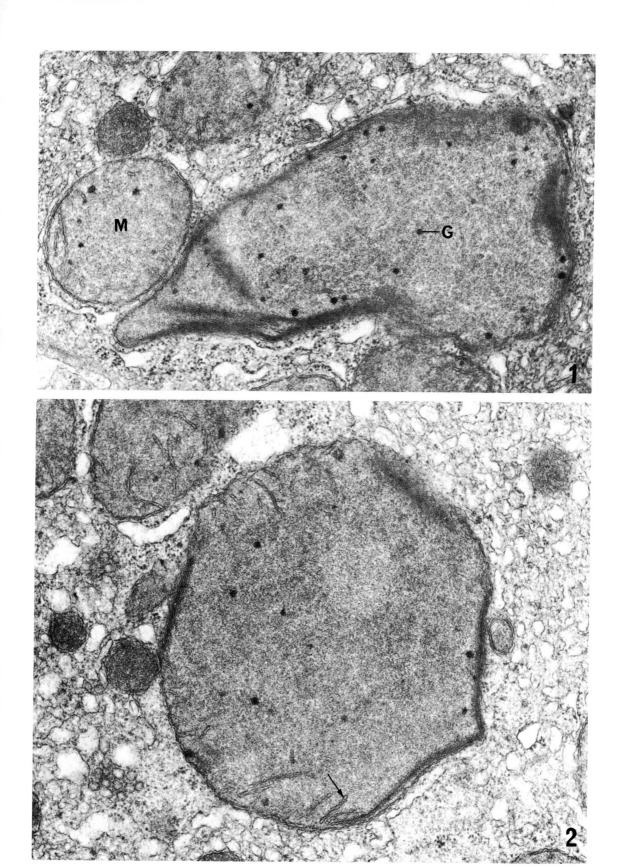

273

The occurrence of various mitochondrial abnormalities, particularly giant or enlarged mitochondria with or without crystalline and/or other inclusions, has led to the idea that such defects may be primarily responsible for the production of certain diseases of muscle in man. The idea of a mitochondrial disease was first put forward by Luft *et al.* (1962) and later developed by Gonatas and Shy (1966) and by Shy *et al.* (1966), who found mitochondrial abnormalities in two cases of slowly progressive muscular dystrophy. In one case there were enlarged and giant mitochondria; this condition they named 'megaconial myopathy'. In the other case the mitochondria were small but very numerous; this they described as 'pleoconial myopathy'. The term 'mitochondrial myopathy' has been employed by Spiro *et al.* (1970) and other workers to describe muscular disorders where abnormal mitochondria are found.

However, some 40 cases or more of a great variety of muscular disorders with mitochondrial alterations have now been described (for references, *see* Mair and Tomé, 1972) and it would appear that such changes are neither primary nor specific for a particular disease or group of diseases. The mitochondrial changes seen no doubt reflect deranged mitochondrial metabolism, but this is more likely to be a secondary change engendered by various disease processes and noxious influences. Thus, little aetiological significance can be attached to the finding of abnormal mitochondria in pathological muscle tissue of man (Peter *et al.*, 1970).

A quite unusual variety of giant mitochondria was found by Tandler and Erlandson (1983) in a pleomorphic adenoma of the parotid gland (*see also* page 212). These mitochondria contained abundant matrix in which lay sparse sinuous or irregularly undulating cristae. They call the pattern produced 'reticular pattern' and the cristae 'sinuous cristae'. Apparently such mitochondria have not been found in any other mammalian cell, normal or neoplastic, but somewhat comparable mitochondria have been seen in the *corpora allata* of the locust during sexual maturation (Fain-Maurel and Cassier, 1969).

The precise manner in which giant mitochondria (in all sites) are born is debatable, but as suggested earlier this can be by enlargement of pre-existing mitochondria or by fusion of smaller organelles to form large ones. It is also conceivable that both these processes (which are not mutually exclusive) may be involved in any given instance.

Plate 124

Fig. 1. Giant mitochondrion found in dog myocardium. Mitochondria from adjacent rows are seen in the process of fusing with the main mass forming the giant mitochondrion. × 20 000

Fig. 2. Giant mitochondrion found in a bone marrow macrophage from a case of erythroleukaemia. × 17 500 (*Ghadially and Skinnider, unpublished electron micrograph*)

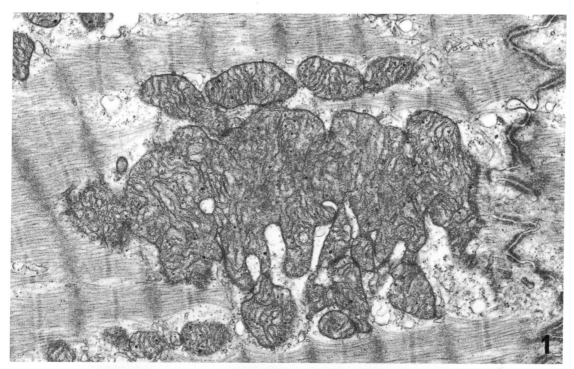

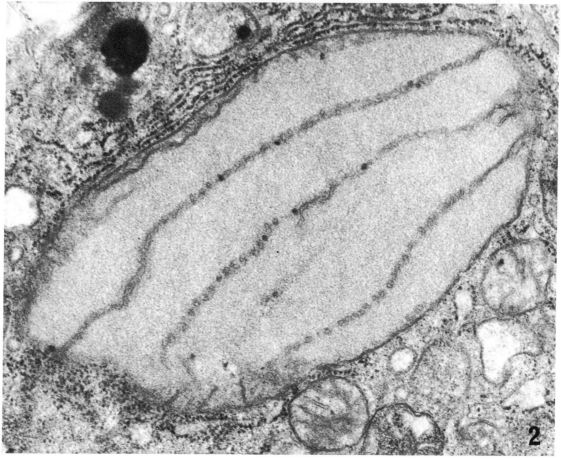

Some giant mitochondria have a fairly regular margin and a round or ovoid shape. They also contain a fairly regular pattern of cristae within them and there is little need to postulate that anything more than an enlargement of a single organelle has occurred. More frequently, however, giant mitochondria have irregular contours, and show bipartite or lobular forms. This, taken in conjunction with the reduction in the number of mitochondria so often seen in their neighbourhood, suggests that a fusion process may also be involved. This seems clearly to be the case at least in some of the giant mitochondria found in the myocardium (Kraus and Cain, 1980) and is also probably the case in some of the giant mitochondria seen in hepatocytes (Ghadially and Parry, 1966). On the other hand, in giant mitochondria in the epithelium of the renal tubules of rats with spontaneous nephropathy (Kraus and Cain, 1975) and in the case of erythroleukaemia studied by us (Ghadially and Skinnider, 1974) the morphological evidence indicates that these giant mitochondria are derived by enlargement of individual mitochondria rather than fusion of pre-existing mitochondria (*Plate 125*). Barastegui and Ruano-Gil (1984) found giant mitochondria, five to ten times longer than normal mitochondria in the epithelium of the ureter of senile rats. Their paper deals largely with the rod-like crystals (similar to those shown in *Plate 138*) that were present in the mitochondria, rather than the genesis of these mitochondria. However, the electron micrographs and line drawings in the paper support the idea that here too giant mitochondria were derived by enlargement of individual mitochondria rather than fusion of pre-existing normal-sized mitochondria.

Crystalline inclusions are a common feature of giant mitochondria in various tissues, but particularly so in the liver. They are generally considered to be protein or lipoprotein in nature. Such crystals often bear a close relationship to the cristae and may at times appear to overlie them or even arise from them. Svoboda and Manning (1964) have interpreted this as a degenerative change in the cristae, leading to a release and subsequent crystallization of lipoproteins derived from the membranes of the cristae.

Plate 125

Bone marrow macrophage from a case of erythroleukaemia. Appearances seen here suggest that giant mitochondria in this site and situation develop by enlargement of solitary mitochondria. The probable stages of evolution from normal to giant mitochondria are depicted by letters A, B, C, D, and E. × 25 000 (*From Ghadially and Skinnider, 1974*)

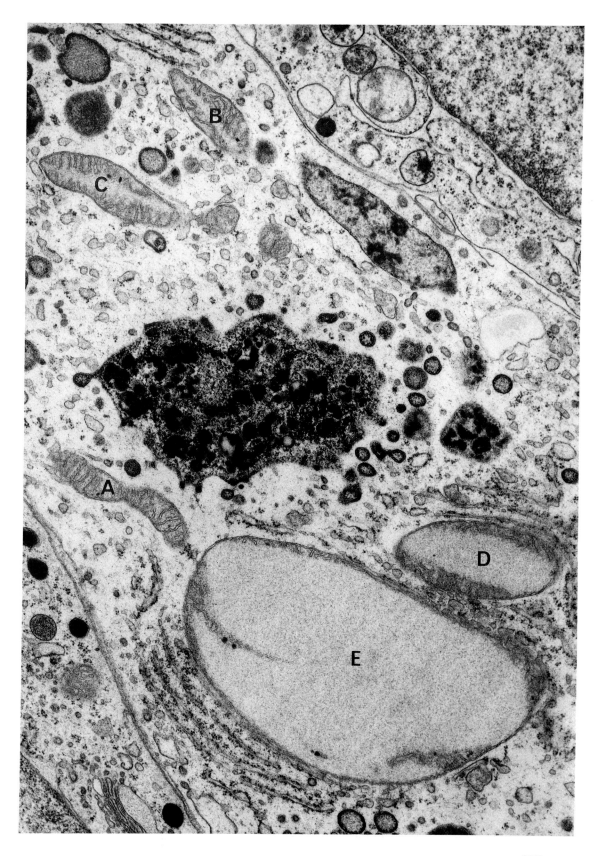

Ring-shaped and cup-shaped mitochondria

In ultrathin sections, mitochondria showing C-, U- and O-shaped profiles have at times been seen in normal and pathological tissues (*Plate 126*). It is now believed that in most instances such mitochondrial profiles represent sections in various planes through cup-shaped organelles.

Mitochondria with the O-shaped configuration in section are often referred to loosely as 'doughnut mitochondria' or 'ring-shaped mitochondria'. The 'hole' within such forms may be placed centrally or eccentrically, and usually contains cytoplasmic matrix and various structures such as ribosomes, rough endoplasmic reticulum or glycogen (*see Plate 131*). The material, however, is clearly demarcated from the mitochondrion by the double membrane of the mitochondrial envelope and is akin in some ways to a pseudoinclusion. If, due to obliquity of sectioning, the membranes are not visualized, an erroneous impression of a true intramitochondrial inclusion could be created. Usually the 'hole' is quite small, but at times it can be quite large so that a long slender, ring-shaped mitochondrial profile is seen surrounding a large volume of cytoplasm. At times two or more cup-shaped mitochondria may be stacked within one another so that in section they appear as concentric rings of mitochondria. Such an appearance is at times referred to as a chondriosphere (page 282).

It is conceivable that ring-shaped mitochondrial profiles could represent a section through a genuine doughnut-shaped organelle produced perhaps by the fusion of the tips of a curved mitochondrion, and indeed such an interpretation has at times been favoured in the earlier literature. However, the chances of cutting a three-dimensionally doughnut-shaped structure so that it presents as a ring are small, and since such 'ring-shaped mitochondria' are almost invariably seen in company with C-shaped and U-shaped forms, it is now generally conceded that these forms (C, U and O) represent sections through mitochondria which are in fact, cup-shaped. It is also clear that at times the ring form represents sections through mitochondria with complex irregular forms such as the one shown in *Plate 126, Fig. 2*. Yet another possibility is that a ring-shaped appearance may be created by a circularly arranged crista near the central part of the mitochondrion. We (Ghadially and Ailsby, unpublished observations) have seen this in an apparently normal cow adrenal (*Plate 127*) where such mitochondria were abundant but C- or U-shaped mitochondrial profiles were absent. At times a single modified crista lined the central 'hole'; in other instances two or more cristae encircled this region. Also, at times mitochondria with two 'holes' were noted.

'Ring-shaped mitochondria' or mitochondria judged to be cup-shaped by the above-mentioned criteria have been seen in a variety of normal tissues, such as: (1) interstitial cells of rat testis; (2) opossum Leydig cells; (3) nurse cells of *Drosophila* testis; (4) grasshopper and

---

Plate 126

Fig. 1. A mitochondrion showing a U-shaped profile. × 32 000

Fig. 2. An irregular shaped mitochondrion: one end of the mitochondrion presents as a C-shaped profile, the other end an O-shaped profile. × 25 000

Fig. 3. A C-shaped mitochondrial profile. Note the narrow opening through which continuity of cytoplasmic structures is maintained. × 29 000

Figs. 4 and 5. 'Ring forms' with centrally placed 'holes'. × 34 000; × 48 000

Figs. 6 and 7. 'Ring forms' with eccentrically placed 'holes'. × 29 000 × 40 000

278

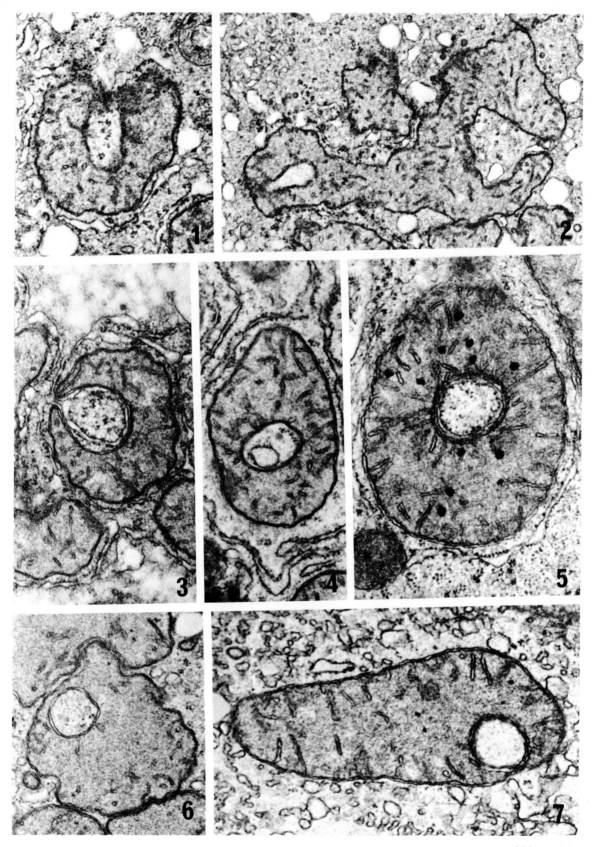

279

scorpion testes during spermatogenesis; (5) adrenal cortex of hamsters; (6) beta cells of the islets of embryonic mouse pancreas; (7) occasional hepatocytes in apparently normal rat liver (for references to the above-mentioned examples, *see* Stephens and Bils, 1965); (8) brown fat in rats (Suter, 1969); and (9) livers of four apparently normal dogs (*Plate 126, Fig. 5*).

The rat liver seems to be quite prone to the formation of such mitochondria, and this kind of mitochondrial transformation has been seen after the administration of various drugs, such as: (1) carbon tetrachloride (Reynolds, 1960) (*Plate 126, Figs. 1–4, 6* and *7*); (2) ammonium carbonate (David and Kettler, 1961); and (3) alcohol (Kiessling and Tobe, 1964; Porta *et al.*, 1965; Koch *et al.*, 1968). Such mitochondria have also been seen in the liver of fetal rats when the mothers received prednisolone during pregnancy (Hill and Blackburn, 1967).

Other situations in which these mitochondria have been seen include: (1) the great alveolar cells of oxygen-adapted rats exposed to 100 per cent oxygen (Rosenbaum *et al.*, 1969; Yamamoto *et al.*, 1970); (2) kidney of winter-starved frogs (Karnovsky, 1962, 1963); (3) rat brain tissue fixed by glutaraldehyde perfusion after a delay of one hour (Karlsson and Schultz, 1966); (4) clear cell carcinoma of kidney (Seljelid and Ericsson, 1965); (5) oncocytoma (Askew *et al.*, 1971); (6) Fortner hamster melanoma (Wolff *et al.*, 1971); and (7) human leukaemia (*Plate 91*).

The significance of such transformation of mitochondrial morphology is obscure. Since cup-shaped mitochondria have been seen in the liver after administration of various toxic agents, and at times these organelles proceed to the formation of membranous whorls and myelin figures, one could argue that this is a degenerative phenomenon. On the other hand, such mitochondria were considered by Rosenbaum *et al.* (1969) to represent an adaptive change in the lungs of rats treated with various concentrations of oxygen, and evidence was presented that this change may be reversible. Others (Stephens and Bils, 1965) have seen an analogy between the cup-shaped mitochondrion and the mitochondria associated with lipid droplets. In the latter instance the mitochondrion spreads out over a lipid droplet and assumes a cup-shaped form, and this, as we have noted, seems to be a functionally meaningful relationship (*see* page 222). Hence, one can argue that, since in the cup-shaped mitochondrion there is an increase in the mitochondrial surface and a more extensive or close relationship between the mitochondrion and cytoplasmic structures, this may facilitate exchanges between the cytoplasm and the mitochondrion.

Plate 127

From the adrenal cortex of a normal cow (*Ghadially and Ailsby, unpublished electron micrographs*).

Fig. 1. Numerous mitochondria with crescentric or concentric cristae, demarcating a circular area of mitochondrial matrix, are evident. × 23 000

Fig. 2. Two 'doughnut' mitochondria (A and B) and a mitochondrion (C) with a crescentric crista are present. It is evident that in certain planes of sectioning C would present an image similar to that seen at A or B. × 35 000

Figs. 3 and 4. Another 'ring-shaped mitochondrion' with a large central 'hole', and a mitochondrion with two 'holes'. × 53 000; × 46 000

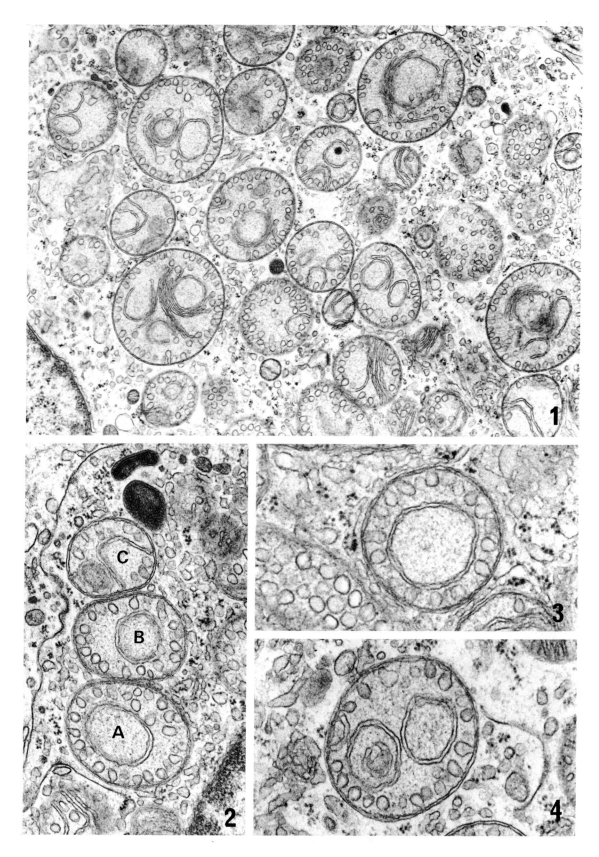

Chondriospheres

As pointed out in the previous section (page 278), when a ring-shaped mitochondrial profile is seen in sectioned material it usually represents a horizontal or transverse section through a cup-shaped mitochondrion (i.e. plane of section parallel to the mouth of the cup) while a vertical section through the base of the cup-shaped mitochondrion presents a C-shaped or U-shaped profile. Usually the hollow of the 'cup' contains cytoplasmic material but sometimes it may contain one or more spherical mitochondria. At times two or more cup-shaped mitochondria may be stacked within one another so that in transverse section they appear as 'concentric rings of mitochondria'. Such spherical aggregates of mitochondria of the type described above (*Plate 128*) are called 'chondriospheres' (De Robertis and Sabatini, 1958). Sometimes the cristae of mitochondria comprising a chondriosphere show the normal transverse orientation but more frequently a partial or total transformation to longitudinal cristae is evident. The mid-portion of such mitochondrial profiles appears attenuated and the ends often appear club-shaped.

Chondriospheres have been found in: (1) steroid secreting cells of the adrenal cortex and testis (De Robertis and Sabatini, 1958; Christensen and Chapman, 1959; Bhattacharyya and Butler, 1979; (2) Warthin's tumour (Tandler and Hoppel, 1972); (3) oncocytic adenoma of the parathyroid gland (Ghadially, 1985) (*Plate 128, Fig. 1*); (4) cycasin-induced oncocytic adenoma of the kidney of the rat (Gusek, 1975); (5) a plasma cell from a case of multiple myeloma (Ghadially, unpublished observation) (*Plate 128, Fig. 2*); (6) hepatocytes of the rat after ammonium carbonate administration (David and Kettler, 1961); (7) great alveolar cells (type II pneumocytes) of oxygen-adapted rats exposed to 100 per cent oxygen (Rosenbaum *et al.*, 1969); (8) prothoracic glands of insects (Beaulaton, 1968; Cassier and Fain-Maurel, 1971); and (9) corpora allata of insects (Cassier, 1979).

The significance of chondriospheres is obscure. These structures are usually seen in situations where cup-shaped mitochondria occur, hence common theories regarding their biological significance have been propounded (page 280). Since transitions between chondriospheres and osmiophilic membranous whorls (myelin figures) have frequently been observed, most authors regard the formation of chondriospheres as a preliminary stage of a degenerative phenomenon. On the other hand, some authors like Rosenbaum *et al.* (1969) have argued that it is an adaptive change which is reversible, and does not always proceed to degeneration and myelin figure formation.

Plate 128

Fig. 1. Oxyphil adenoma of parathyroid gland. Horizontal (H) and vertical (V) sections through quite large or giant cup-shaped mitochondria are evident. Compare with the normal sized mitochondria (M) which are also present. Note also the chondriosphere (arrowhead) composed of one mitochondrion enveloping another. × 31 000 (*From Ghadially, 1985*)

Fig. 2. Plasma cell from a case of multiple myeloma, showing a chondriosphere composed of two cup-shaped mitochondria surrounding a centrally placed mitochondrion. × 56 000

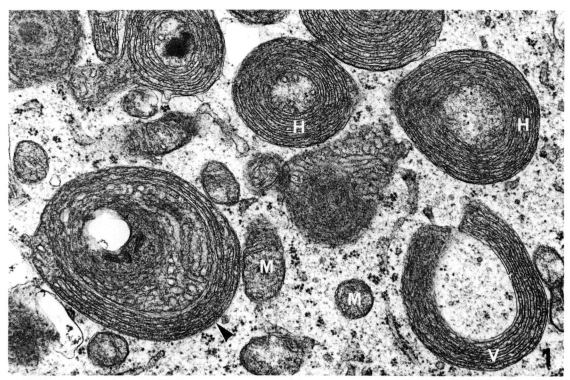

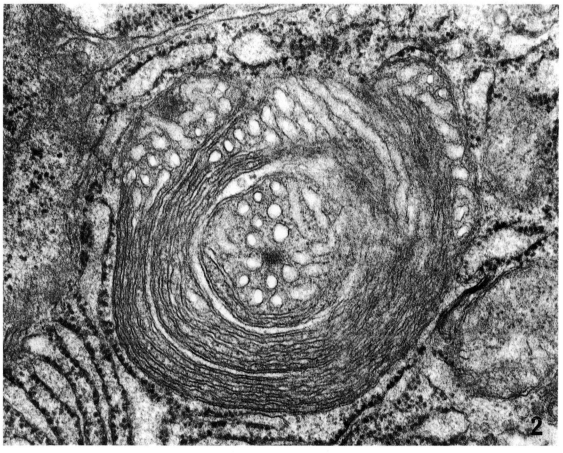

Mitochondrial changes in neoplasia

Although no constant or specific alteration of mitochondrial morphology characterizes the neoplastic state, one does find a host of changes which have interesting implications and certain aspects of mitochondrial morphology are of value in the differential diagnosis of tumours. Numerous studies have long established the fact that there is a positive correlation between the metabolic activity of a tissue and the number and size of mitochondria and also the size, surface area and concentration of cristae (for examples attesting this generalization *see* pages 194 and 254).

In malignant tumours we find an exception or an apparent exception to this rule, for here we have a metabolically active fast-growing tissue where the mitochondria are often too few (compared with the cell of origin). Further they are more fragile than normal and quite pleomorphic, in the sense that in a given tumour or even a single tumour cell one may find large and small mitochondria with sparse or numerous cristae. One or more of these features is quite prominent in fast-growing malignant tumours but less apparent or absent in well-differentiated tumours and benign tumours.

The idea that mitochondria in tumours are defective is also supported by many biochemical studies. Thus, for example, it has been shown that mitochondria isolated from hepatomas exhibit a lower respiratory capacity than mitochondria from normal liver (Kielley, 1952; Emmelot *et al.*, 1959; Devlin and Pruss, 1962; Fiala and Fiala, 1967; Arcos *et al.*, 1969; Sordahl *et al.*, 1969; Pedersen *et al.*, 1970).

The paradox of a fast-growing tissue with a paucity of mitochondria and/or defective mitochondria may be explained by recalling the historical work of Warburg (1956, 1962), which showed the predominance of glycolysis over respiration in the energy metabolism of tumours. Since the enzymes of anaerobic glycolysis* occur in the cytoplasmic matrix, and not in the mitochondria, one may argue that a paucity of a functioning mitochondrial mass would hardly embarrass the metabolic activity of a malignant tumour. Thus, in fact, there seems to be a good correlation between what is seen with the electron microscope and the respiratory biochemistry of neoplastic tissue.

It is worth noting that many alterations of mitochondrial morphology are encountered in tumours and that normal-looking well-preserved mitochondria are infrequently seen in malignant neoplasms (*Plate 129*). The mitochondria are frequently swollen and at times disrupted owing to a flooding of the matrix chamber with water. Less frequently it is the intracristal space which is flooded. This produces mitochondria with a dense matrix (i.e. condensed configuration).

---

*In passing it is worth noting that cells with an anaerobic mode of life (e.g. *Entamoeba histolytica*) lack mitochondria (Griffin and Juniper, 1971).

Plate 129

Seminoma. The swollen mitochondria (S) in the neoplastic cell are well contrasted from the normal-looking mitochondria (M) in the non-neoplastic lymphocyte. × 18 000 (*From Ghadially, 1985*)

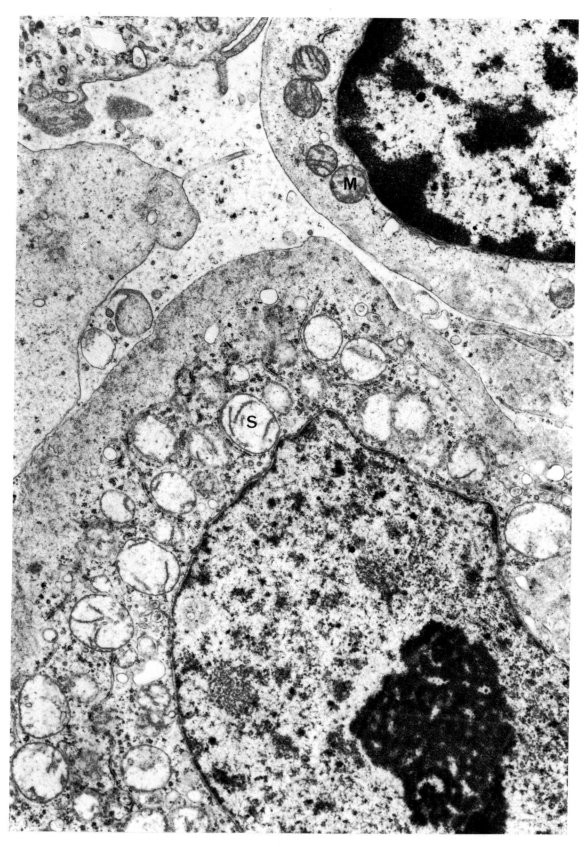

Changes of the type described above are probably multifactorial. They may be due to factors such as: (1) hypoxia produced during surgery (e.g. application of a tourniquet or clamping of blood vessels before the tumour is removed); (2) cell injury and cloudy swelling due to vascular and/or metabolic disturbances (naturally occurring or produced by therapy) in the tumour; and (3) delayed or improper fixation.

That this is not the whole story is attested by the fact that while the mitochondria in the tumour cells may be grossly swollen, those in accompanying non-neoplastic cells may be fairly well-preserved (*Plate 129*). Thus, once again we have to fall back on the idea that mitochondria in tumours are abnormal and unusually fragile.

Various other less common alterations of mitochondrial morphology are also found in tumours. These include: (1) pyknotic mitochondria (*Plate 96*) which are thought to indicate a regressive or involutionary mitochondrial change; and (2) mitochondria which present rod-shaped, C-shaped or ring-shaped profiles with longitudinal instead of the usual transverse cristae (*Plates 90* and *91*). This transformation (i.e. transverse to longitudinal cristae) may denote a deficiency of cytochrome oxidase in the mitochondrion. However, it should be remembered that the above-mentioned mitochondrial changes are seen in non-neoplastic states also.

Finally, it is worth noting that certain aspects of mitochondrial morphology are of value in the electron microscopic diagnosis of tumours. As noted before (page 198) in most cells mitochondria with lamellar cristae are found, but in steroid-secreting cells mitochondria have tubular and vesicular cristae. This difference is carried over into tumours (*Plate 130*), hence this is of diagnostic value in identifying tumours of steroid secreting cells (for references and review *see* Ghadially, 1985). Similarly, the differential diagnosis of tumours whose cells show a granular eosinophilic cytoplasm at light microscopy is facilitated by electron microscopic examination, for in the case of oncocytomas (page 260 and Ghadially, 1985) the cytoplasm is packed with mitochondria (which are biochemically defective) while in the case of tumours such as granular cell myoblastoma (page 684 and Ghadially, 1985) the cells contain numerous lysosomes.

Plate 130

Fig. 1. Aldosteronoma (Conn's syndrome). A variety of cristal profiles are seen in the mitochondria; some acceptable as sections through lamellar cristae and others as sections through tubular and vesicular cristae. × 46 000. (*From a block of tissue supplied by Dr T. K. Shnitka*)

Fig. 2. An ovarian tumour produced by grafting a piece of ovary into the spleen of an ovarectomized rat. The mitochondria show tubulovesicular cristae. Note also the lipid droplets (L) in the cytoplasmic matrix and similar lipidic inclusions (arrows) in the mitochondria. × 21 000

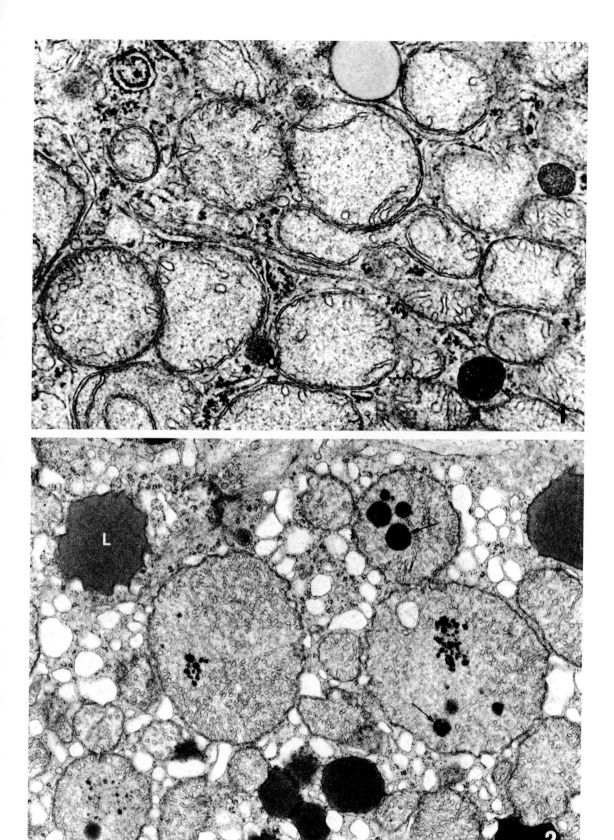

287

Intramitochondrial glycogen inclusions

Glycogen inclusions in mitochondria appear morphologically similar to the common glycogen deposits that occur in the cytoplasm (*see Plates 406–408*). Usually such inclusions consist of monoparticulate glycogen (β-glycogen, 15–35 nm diameter), but glycogen rosettes (α-glycogen, 60–90 nm) are also at times seen. Both true and false inclusions (i.e. pseudoinclusions) occur. The latter are distinguishable by the double membranes of the mitochondrial envelope demarcating them from the mitochondrial matrix (*Plate 131*).

True intramitochondrial glycogen inclusions (*Plates 132* and *133*) present as: (1) small deposits of glycogen particles lying within expanded cristae; (2) larger deposits lying in a compartment enclosed by a single membrane; or (3) a collection of glycogen particles apparently lying in the mitochondrial matrix.

Numerous studies attest to the fact that glycogen is deposited in the intracristal space (i.e. the outer mitochondrial compartment). It seems that the single-membrane-limited type of deposit is a further stage of development of this process whereby the intracristal compartment is dilated to form a vacuole which accommodates the growing glycogen deposit. When the vacuole is further distended the limiting membrane comes to lie against the wall of the mitochondrion and becomes difficult to discern. At this stage an erroneous impression may be created that the glycogen is lying in the matrix, but the electron lucency of the region in which the glycogen lies should prevent one from making such an error. However, the possibility that true matrical deposits (i.e. in the inner mitochondrial compartment) also sometimes occur cannot be completely ruled out*.

*My view based on a study of the published illustrations is that in all but perhaps one instance (*Plate 2, Fig. 3* from Fain-Maurel, 1966) glycogen deposits have been found only in the outer compartment of the mitochondrion.

Plate 131
Pleomorphic adenoma of parotid gland. A tumour cell containing double-membrane-bound (arrows) intramitochondrial pseudoinclusions. Three of the four inclusions contain cytoplasmic matrix and glycogen (small arrowheads), the remaining one contains a vacuole (large arrowhead) also. The profiles seen here could be produced by a section through an invagination of the double-membraned mitochondrial envelope like that seen in *Plate 98, Fig. 2* or it could be due to a section through cup-shaped mitochondria like the ones shown on *Plate 126*. × 64 000

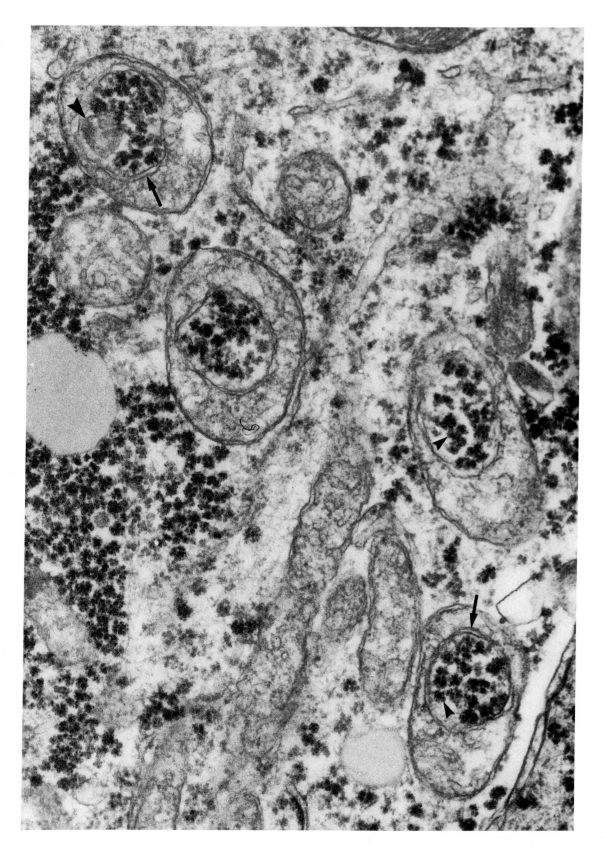

289

Intramitochondrial glycogen has been seen in: (1) spermatozoa of pulmonates and sea-urchin (Personne and André, 1964; André, 1965; Anderson, 1968; Personne and Anderson, 1970); (2) prothoracic gland of silkworm (Beaulaton, 1964); (3) hypobranchial gland of molluscs (Fain-Maurel, 1966); (4) digestive cells of *Hydra* (Lentz, 1966); (5) inter-renal (adrenocortical) cells of the spotted salamander (Picheral, 1968; Berchtold, 1969); (6) *Drosophila* heart (Burch *et al.*, 1970); (7) rat pinealocytes (Lin, 1965); (8) retinal receptor cells of the rat, toad and giant salamander (Ishikawa and Pei, 1965; Ishikawa and Yamada, 1969); (9) lumbar spinal ganglia of frog (Berthold, 1966); (10) axons in prelaminar optic nerve of normal monkeys (Schutta *et al.*, 1970); (11) neurons of rats with bilirubin encephalopathy (Schutta *et al.*, 1970); (12) dystrophic axoplasm in brain of vitamin E deficient rats (Lampert, 1967); (13) brown adipose tissue of 19-day rat fetus (Suter, 1969); (14) mouse hepatocytes in riboflavin deficiency (Tandler *et al.*, 1968, 1969); (15) myocardium of swine fed rapeseed diets (Vodovar *et al.*, 1977); (16) myopathy and cardiomyopathy in man (Hulsmann *et al.*, 1967; D'Agostino *et al.*, 1968; Schellens and Ossentjuk, 1969; Hug and Schubert, 1970); (17) Quebec beer-drinkers' cardiomyopathy (Auger and Chenard, 1967; Bulloch *et al.*, 1970; Alexander, 1972); (18) myocardium of a patient on digitalis therapy assumed to have a primary cardiomyopathy (these were giant mitochondria) (Kraus and Cain, 1980); (19) canine myocardium as a delayed response to prolonged periods (30–45 minutes) of anoxic cardiac arrest (Buja *et al.*, 1972); (20) Fallot's tetralogy (Roberts and Ferrans, 1975); (21) cardiac hypertrophy due to aortic valvular disease (Maron and Ferrans, 1978); (22) human adenolymphoma (Warthin's tumour) and oncocytoma (Tandler and Shipkey, 1964; Tandler, 1966; Hübner *et al.*, 1967; Tandler *et al.*, 1970; Carlsöö *et al.*, 1979; Ghadially, 1985); and (23) canine plasmacytoma (Ghadially *et al.*, 1977).

Plate 132

Glycogen deposits in mitochondria from visual receptor cells of normal rat retina. Such deposits are not seen in newborn rats; they are first detectable at three months and are quite common in rats over one year old. (*From Ishikawa and Pei, 1965*)

Fig. 1. A mitochondrion in a synaptic spherule, showing a few glycogen particles lying in the intracristal space (arrow). × 41 000

Figs.2 and 3. Intramitochondrial single-membrane-bound glycogen deposits are seen in these electron micrographs. × 41 000; × 41 000

Fig. 4. A large glycogen deposit is seen in a mitochondrion. The cristae are pushed to the periphery. × 38 000

Fig. 5. Mitochondrion from the inner segment of rat retina incubated with saliva. The clear area represents a zone from which glycogen was removed by this procedure. × 33 000

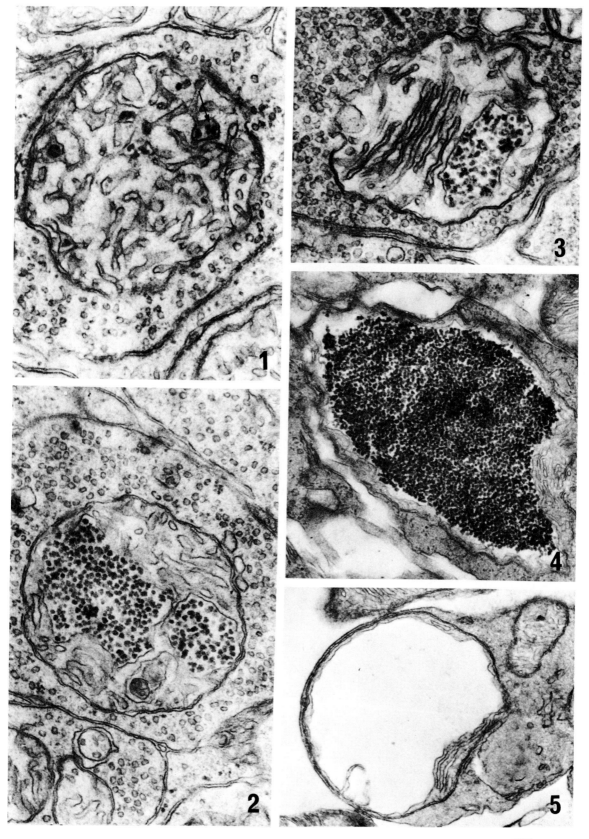

The manner in which glycogen appears in the mitochondrion and the significance of this phenomenon is difficult to evaluate. In the case of the giant mitochondria Kraus and Cain (1980) suggest that glycogen could have been trapped (i.e. accidentally included) during fusion of normal-sized mitochondria to form giant mitochondria. However, for glycogen in normal-sized mitochondria, one may argue that glycogen particles are taken in by some process akin to 'phagocytosis', or that glycogen is synthesized or polymerized from morphologically undetectable units (monomers or dimers) taken up via the external membrane of the mitochondrial envelope. For the former hypothesis there is no support, and against the latter hypothesis (synthesis of glycogen in mitochondria) there is the widely accepted idea, based mainly on studies in isolated liver and muscle mitochondria that the enzymes necessary for glycogenesis and glycogenolysis reside outside these organelles.

Nevertheless, differences may exist between mitochondria in different sites, and there may also be differences engendered by altered physiological and pathological states. Certainly the notion that synthesis or polymerization of glycogen can occur in some mitochondria is compatible with morphological appearances. An observation made by Tandler *et al.* (1970) seems pertinent here (*Plate 133*). They found α-glycogen-containing mitochondria in oncocytes whose cytoplasm contained only β-glycogen, and they state 'at a minimum oncocytoma mitochondria possess the enzymes necessary to convert β-glycogen to α-glycogen'.

In the plasmacytoma we (Ghadially *et al.*, 1977) studied, mainly monoparticulate glycogen was found in the mitochondria but no glycogen could be detected in the cytoplasm. This virtually rules out the possibility that preformed glycogen was taken up by the mitochondrion from the cytoplasm and one is left with the possibility that most, perhaps all, the stages of glycogen synthesis were accomplished within the mitochondrion and that the enzymes necessary to do this were present at this site.

Regarding the occurrence of glycogen in hypertrophied myocardium, Maron and Ferrans (1978) state that 'Intramitochondrial glycogen probably occurs due to increased permeability (a consequence of hypoxia or other metabolic changes) of the outer mitochondrial membranes, which permits diffusion of solubilized enzymes of glycogen synthesis from the cytoplasm into the outer mitochondrial compartment where they eventually proceed to synthesize glycogen'. This is an attractive hypothesis which also explains why glycogen deposits occur in the outer mitochondrial compartment and not in the inner mitochondrial compartment which is limited by a membrane known to have a different permeability (*see* page 192). In the case of the spermatocyte mitochondria mentioned earlier (Anderson, 1968; Personne and Anderson, 1970) there is evidence that enzymes for synthesis and degradation of glycogen exist in these organelles and that such deposits provide energy for metabolism and motility.

Plate 133

Glycogen-containing mitochondria from an oncocytoma (*From Tandler, Hutter and Erlandson, 1970*)

Fig. 1. Three glycogen-containing mitochondria. × 23 000

Fig. 2. A mitochondrion containing glycogen rosettes (α-glycogen). × 44 000

Fig. 3. A dividing mitochondrion. A single-membrane-bound glycogen deposit is present. × 52 000

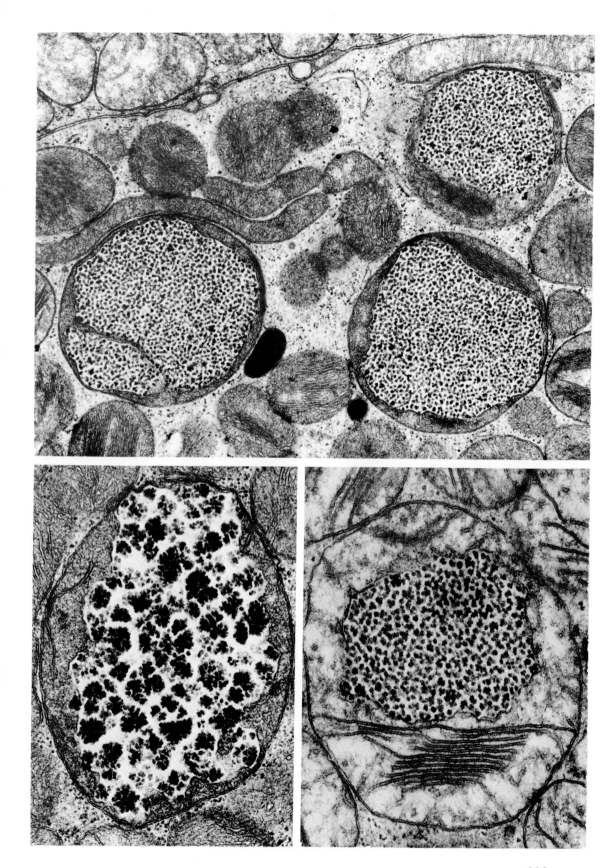

293

Intramitochondrial lipidic inclusions

As noted in an earlier section (page 232) the normally occurring ubiquitous intramitochondrial dense granules measuring 2–5 nm in diameter are composed largely of lipid. These lipidic inclusions do not concern us here. In this section we deal with much larger lipidic inclusions which are at times found in mitochondria (*see Plates 412 and 413*).

Intramitochondrial lipidic inclusions are characterized by the lack of a limiting membrane, an amorphous appearance, a medium to high electron density, and a rounded or irregular form (*Plate 134; see also Plate 130, Fig. 2*). Either solitary or multiple inclusions can occur in a single mitochondrion. Morphologically then, these inclusions are similar to the lipid inclusions found in the cytoplasm of various cells.

Nevertheless, confident diagnosis of lipid inclusions in mitochondria is beset by many difficulties. When a medium or high density inclusion, morphologically similar to a cytoplasmic lipid droplet, is sighted in a mitochondrion, it is difficult to rule out the possibility that it could be some entirely different material or that it may contain other constituents besides lipid★.

Therefore in the electron microscopic literature, many examples of presumably lipidic inclusions have been referred to by the non-committal term 'dense inclusions'. Since such inclusions are smaller than mitochondria, histochemical analysis with the light microscope is hardly feasible, and unless numerous mitochondria in a sample of tissue contain such inclusions the effect of lipid solvents cannot be confidently assessed with the aid of the electron microscope.

Yet another source of difficulty stems from the close association which develops between mitochondria and cytoplasmic lipid droplets. It has already been noted (page 222) that in such an instance a lipid droplet may lie in a deep invagination of the mitochondrial envelope and that in certain planes of sectioning it may appear to lie within the mitochondrion. The situation here is analogous to pseudoinclusions of the nucleus, and one could contend that the lipid droplet is still in fact outside the mitochondrion. However, contact between the mitochondrion and lipid droplet is said at times to lead to the dissolution of the mitochondrial envelope, so one might also contend that a true intramitochondrial lipid inclusion could be derived in this fashion.

Besides the above-mentioned situation, intramitochondrial inclusions acceptable as lipidic in nature on morphological grounds have been seen in a variety of tissues. Occasional mitochondria of the suprarenal cortex of normal man and other animals contain one or two small osmiophilic lipidic droplets (*Plate 134*). Many mitochondria in the brown adipose tissue of neonatal rats also contain one or two electron-dense lipidic droplets morphologically similar to those illustrated in the suprarenal cortex of the cow, and Suter and Staubli (1970) have shown

★For example, dense granules containing calcium such as those shown in *Plate 104, Fig. 1* could be confused with osmiophilic lipid droplets shown in *Plate 134*.

Plate 134

Figs. 1 and 2. Mitochondria from the brown fat of a squirrel, showing lipid droplets (L) apparently lying in the mitochondrion. Many examples of close association of lipid and mitochondria were present in this tissue. This, combined with the fact that there is a dense halo around the droplets, suggests the presence of obliquely sectioned membranes in this region. It is therefore difficult to accept these as examples of true intramitochondrial lipid inclusions. × 39 000; × 26 000 (*Grodums, unpublished electron micrographs*)

Figs. 3 and 4. Mitochondria from the suprarenal cortex of a cow showing small and large electron-dense lipidic (L) inclusions. × 39 000; × 41 000

Fig. 5. Mitochondria from an oxyphil adenoma of the parathyroid gland showing quite large lipidic (L) inclusions. × 55 000 (*From Ghadially, 1980*)

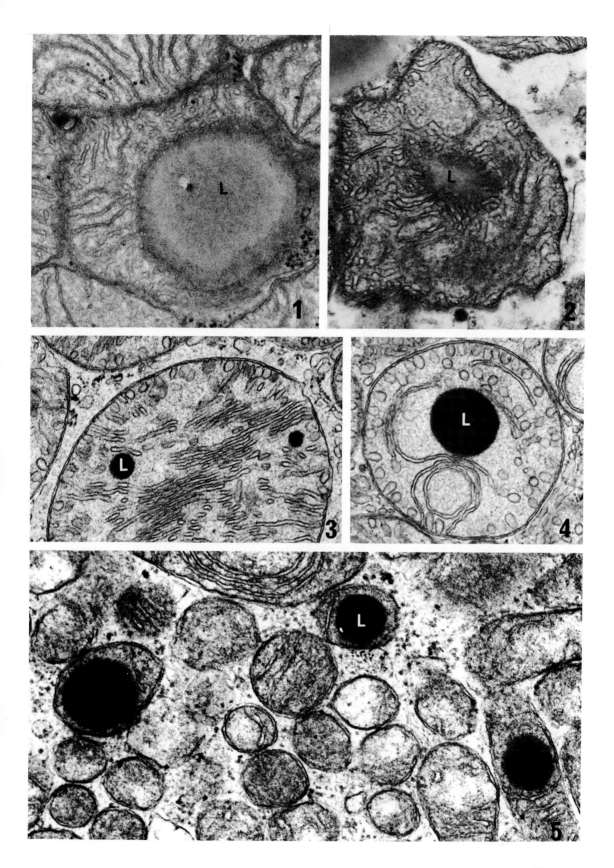

that such inclusions are absent in isolated mitochondria treated with lipid solvents. Prolonged treatment with pronase did not affect the inclusions, so they probably do not contain much protein. Since these intramitochondrial lipidic inclusions disappear during early post-natal life, at a stage when the mitochondria in the brown fat enlarge in size, it has been suggested by these authors that the lipid is probably used for the synthesis of the lipoprotein membranes of the cristae. Quite large presumably lipidic inclusions were seen (Ghadially, 1985) (*Plate 134, Fig. 5*) in the abundant mitochondria of an oxyphil adenoma of the parathyroid gland but their significance is obscure.

In most of the above-mentioned examples, lipidic inclusions were noted in normal-looking mitochondria with well formed cristae, where presumably the lipid has a physiological role. But there are other examples where lipidic inclusions have been seen in pathologically altered mitochondria with sparse cristae, and it would appear that such lipid or lipoprotein or lipid and protein containing inclusions are derived by a breakdown or disintegration of the cristae (*Plate 135*).

Such inclusions have been noted in degenerating giant mitochondria (*see Plate 122*) and we (Ghadially and Parry, unpublished observations) have seen similar intramitochondrial inclusions in the liver of rats bearing carcinogen-induced subcutaneous sarcomas, and also in a human hepatoma. Rat hepatocyte mitochondria with numerous irregular-shaped inclusions acceptable as containing lipid or lipoprotein or lipid and protein were found by Parry (personal communication), when an RD_3 sarcoma was transplanted into the livers of these animals (*Plate 135, Fig. 2*). Deposits of a similar morphology have also been noted in the mitochondria of stimulated rat adrenals (for references, *see* Giacomelli *et al.*, 1965) and other steroid-secreting cells in various experimental or pathological situations, and several workers have regarded them as intramitochondrial lipid accumulations (Lever, 1956; Gordon *et al.*, 1964).

Irregular-shaped electron-dense intramitochondrial inclusions were found in a great number of hepatocyte mitochondria of ethionine-fed rats by Minick *et al.* (1965), so they were able to trace the stages of development of these inclusions. Numerous mitochondria with centrally placed stacked cristae similar to those shown in *Plate 135, Fig. 1*, were seen, and they concluded that the inclusions were derived by breakdown of cristae of such altered mitochondria.

Thus it would appear that these inclusions derived from disintegrating cristae are an indicator of a noxious influence operating on the mitochondrion. These inclusions are in fact similar to the flocculent densities found in the mitochondria of lethally injured cells (*see* page 26) and which are now widely regarded as the hallmark of a dead cell, but in this instance many mitochondria are affected (*see* pages 250–253). It follows then that if only an occasional mitochondrion shows such inclusions in an otherwise intact cell it would not be wise to pronounce the cell as dead.

Plate 135

Fig. 1. Mitochondria from liver of a rat bearing a transplanted tumour in its flank. Note the centrally placed cristae (C) and irregular electron-dense deposit, presumably lipid, lipoprotein or lipid and protein (L). × 50 000

Fig. 2. A mitochondrion from a rat liver in which an RD3 sarcoma was transplanted. Note the irregular masses of electron-dense material, presumed to contain lipid, lipoprotein or lipid and protein (L). × 80 000 (*Parry, unpublished electron micrograph*)

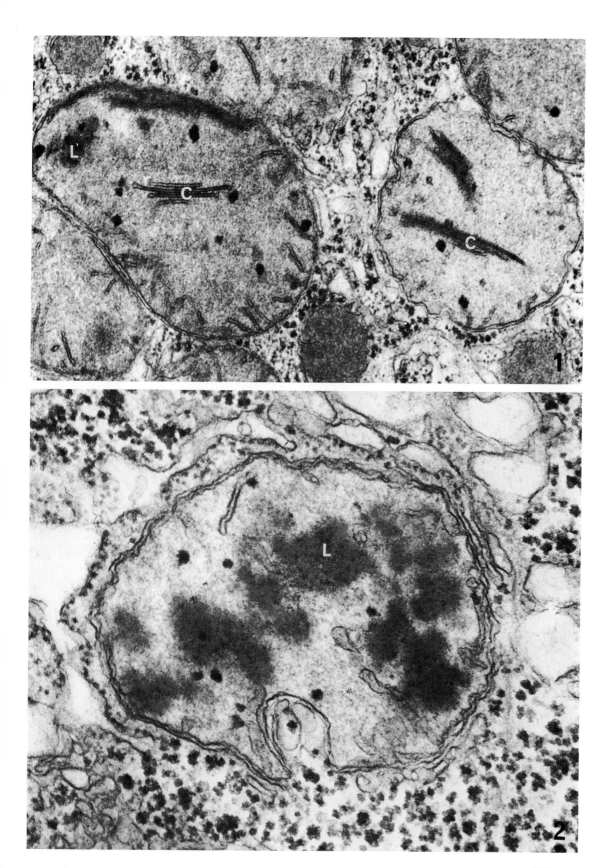

Intramitochondrial crystalline, paracrystalline and filamentous inclusions

Crystalline inclusions generally assumed to be protein have been noted in various cell compartments such as the nucleus (*see Plates 58* and *59*), cytoplasm (*see Plates 414–417*) and mitochondria. Details of structure vary, but the characteristic feature of crystals in all sites is that they have a highly ordered pattern of internal organization. Terms such as 'crystalloid' or 'paracrystalline' inclusions are employed when the ordered arrangement is less than the expected ideal. Obviously, many differences in fine structure exist between crystals found in various situations. However, certain general considerations about the appearance of crystals in electron micrographs are worth noting before dealing with intramitochondrial crystals.

The appearance of crystals in ultrathin sections depends, among other things, on the plane of sectioning with respect to the plane of the crystal lattice (*Plates 136* and *137*). Thus, in longitudinal sections a crystal may present as a system of closely spaced parallel 'lines', in transverse section as an ordered array of 'dots' and in oblique sections as a lattice, honeycomb pattern or reticular pattern. The 'parallel line' pattern has been interpreted in some instances as representing longitudinal sections through filaments, rods or microtubules; in other instances it is quite clear that this 'parallel line' image is produced by an off-register superimposition of rows of spherical or short cylindrical units. Similarly the 'dot' pattern may be interpreted either as transverse sections through rods or filaments, or as representing macromolecular units of globular, granular or short cylindrical form. The lattice pattern could be produced by interlacing filaments, or again by off-register superimposed images of closely packed but highly ordered arrays of 'dots'. The true three-dimensional structure of most crystals still awaits clarification.

Nevertheless, it is clear now that a variety of crystals and crystalloid inclusions occur in mitochondria; some that are composed of globular units, other composed of filaments, and yet others of microtubules. The arrangement and packing of these substructures also varies, for example, the filaments may be arranged in parallel arrays forming sheaves or the filaments may be coiled to form helical structures.

Although good examples of each variety of intramitochondrial crystal and paracrystal exist, it is not possible to sort out and classify all the published reports in such strictly defined categories, because in several instances inadequate or insufficient illustrations are provided and in a few instances the description and/or interpretations are suspect or erroneous. Therefore, I shall list the sites and situations where various types of crystalline and paracrystalline inclusions have been seen and then comment upon some that are of particular interest.

Plate 136

Intramitochondrial crystals from the liver of a patient with hepatitis.
Fig. 1. Longitudinally sectioned crystal, presenting as a series of evenly spaced parallel lines. × 89 000
Fig. 2. Transversely sectioned crystal, showing discrete dot pattern. × 200 000
Fig. 3. Obliquely sectioned crystal, showing a reticular pattern. × 220 000

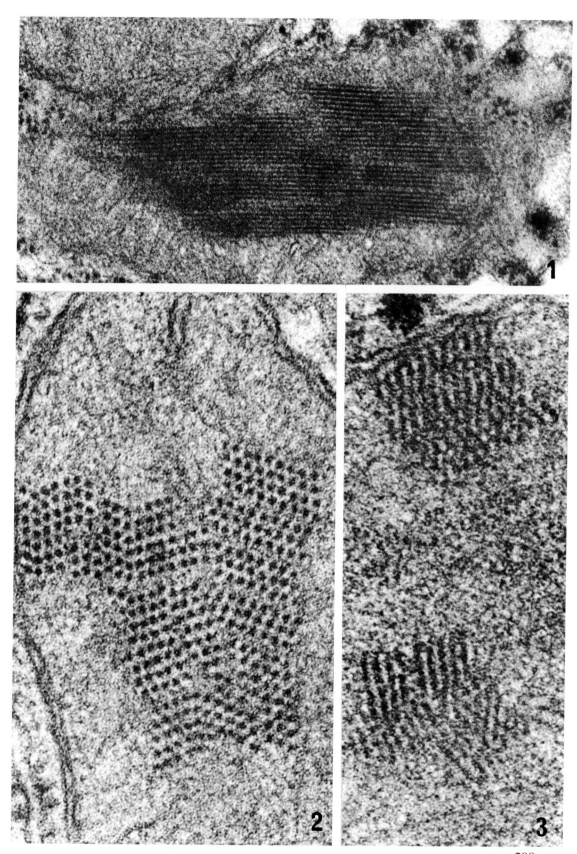

299

Intramitochondrial crystalline, paracrystalline or filamentous inclusions have been noted in various normal and pathological cells and tissues such as: (1) brown fat (Napolitano and Fawcett, 1958); (2) oocytes of amphibians and certain cells in early embryogenesis (Lanzavecchia and Le Coultre, 1958; Ward, 1962; Karasaki, 1963; Lanzavecchia, 1965; Massover, 1971); (3) bean root (Newcomb *et al.*, 1968); (4) ameloblasts of enamel organ (Jessen, 1968); (5) various cell types of the striped snake (*Elaphae quadrivirgata*) (Kurosumi *et al.*, 1966; Yamamoto *et al.*, 1969); (6) renal tubules of frogs collected in winter (*Plate 137, Fig. 3*); (7) renal tubules of rat (Osvaldo and Latta, 1966); (8) rat kidney after nickel subsulphide injection (Jasmin, 1978); (9) cat kidney (Bargmann *et al.*, 1977); (10) epithelial cells of rat ureter (Barastegui and Ruano-Gil, 1984); (11) kidney of ammocoetes (Youson, 1971); (12) epitheliomuscular cells of *Hydra* (Davis, 1967); (13) astrocytes in *Corpus striatum* in the rat (Mugnaini, 1964b); (14) retinal rods of the frog's eye (Yamada, 1959); (15) pinealocytes (Lin, 1965); (16) chorioallantoic placenta of the rat (Ollerich, 1968); (17) rat and domestic fowl adrenals fixed by perfusion with glutaraldehyde (Kjaerheim, 1967); (18) adrenal glands of normal rats (Saito and Fleischer, 1971); (19) adrenal glands of rats on a sodium–deficient diet (Giacomelli *et al.*, 1965); (20) thyroid follicular cells of rats treated with propylthiouracil and potassium iodide (Fujita and Machino, 1964); (21) thyroid follicular cells of the bat during the euthyroid state which follows the period of arousal (Nunez *et al.*, 1975); (22) normal rabbit thyroid gland (incidence of paracrystalline inclusions decreased when the thyroid gland was repressed by castration) (Nathaniel, 1976, 1978, 1980); (23) insect sperm (crystals shown to contain proline-rich proteins) (Baccetti *et al.*, 1977); (24) pancreatic acinar cells of starved Japanese newts (*Triturus pyrogaster*) (Taira, 1979); (25) myocardial cells of oyster (*Crassostrea virginica* Gmelin) (Hawkins *et al.*, 1980); (26) hypotrichous ciliates (*Pseudourostyla cristata* and *P. levis*) incubated in various media (Suganuma and Yamamoto, 1980); (27) neurons in cerebral cortex and spinal cord after delayed fixation (Pena, 1980) (*Plate 138*); (28) cortical dendrites in Alzheimer's disease (Saraiva *et al.*, 1985); (29) cortical dendrites from patients with early forms of sclerosing panencephalitis (Paula-Barbosa *et al.*, 1984); (30) stored skeletal muscle of ox and pig (Cheah *et al.*, 1973); (31) beef heart (Hall and Crane, 1971; Wakabayashi *et al.*, 1971); (32) liver of slender salamander *Batrachoseps attenuatus* (Hamilton *et al.*, 1966); (33) liver of human and dog (references given below) (*Plates 136* and *137, Fig. 2*); (34) sphincter muscle of crayfish vas deferens (Murdock *et al.*, 1977); (35) various myopathies in man (references given later) (*Plate 137, Fig. 1* and *Plate 140*); (36) giant mitochondria in some tissues (pages 266–277); (37) glioblastoma (Tani *et al.*, 1971); (38) neuroblastoma (Brawn and Mackay, 1980); (39) rhabdomyoma (Marquart, 1978); (40) breast tumours (benign and malignant) (Seman and Gallagher, 1979); and (41) oncocytic carcinoid of lung (Ghadially and Block, 1985) (*Plate 139*).

Plate 137

Fig. 1. A mitochondrion from an atrophic deltoid muscle showing rectangular crystalline inclusions lying in the intracristal space. Each crystal is surrounded by a membrane, derived from a crista. × 71 000 (*Ghadially and Ailsby, unpublished electron micrograph*)

Fig. 2. Most of the crystals in this hepatocyte mitochondrion from a case of hepatitis present as a highly ordered array of electron–dense dots. In one instance, however (arrow), the plane of sectioning is such that the dots are partially superimposed to form a pattern of dotted parallel lines. × 72 000

Fig. 3. A mitochondrion containing a crystalline inclusion, from a renal tubular cell of a winter-starved frog. × 107 000

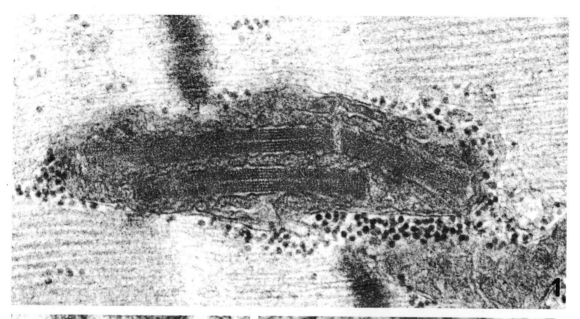

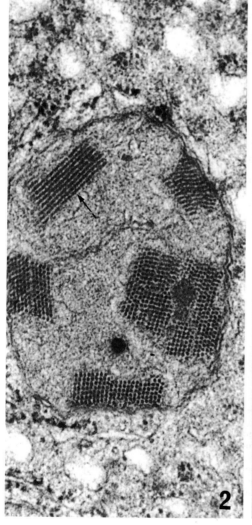

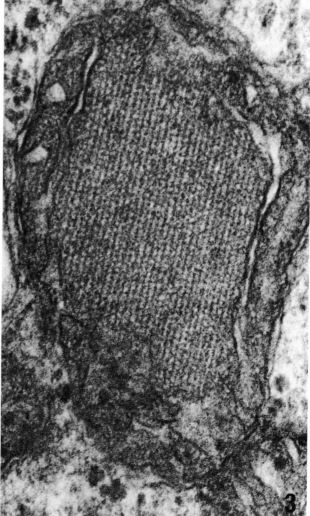

A review of the literature cited above shows that while some of these are 'true' structures presumably produced *in vivo* (e.g. those encountered in hepatocytes), others are artefacts of delayed tissue fixation. Such artefactually produced crystalline or paracrystalline structures appear to be formed by crystallization of proteins and lipids released from degenerating and disintegrating cristae during tissue autolysis. These inclusions, often described as 'rod-like' or 'plate-like' inclusions, have been found in several types of normal cells and some neoplastic cells (Cheah *et al.*, 1973; Pena, 1980; Jaworski, 1984; Barastegui and Ruano-Gil, 1984).

The artefactual nature of most, if not all, these rod-like inclusions is suggested by the work of Pena (1980) who studied neuronal mitochondria in surgical biopsies and autopsy material. The rod-like crystals were not found in surgical material, but were sometimes seen in autopsy material obtained 2–4 hours after death and constantly seen in autopsy material obtained 4–15 hours after death.

These crystalline inclusions, which show a rod-like profile, occur in the intracristal space or its continuation, the outer chamber of the mitochondrion, which lies between the inner and outer membranes of the mitochondrial envelope. The segment of the crista or envelope where crystallization occurs usually appears thicker and more electron-dense. The three-dimensional morphology of these crystals is not clearly established and there may well be variations in these inclusions found in various sites and situations. In sectioned material these crystals usually present as a periodic array of 'dots' (*Plate 138*), which could represent transverse sections through parallel straight filaments or a longitudinal mid-section through a helical filament. Sometimes a ladder-like pattern is seen (*Plate 138, Fig. 2*) which could be attributed to oblique sectioning through straight filaments or a tangential cut such that the coils of the helix are visualized. However, the failure to visualize 'straight parallel lines' representing longitudinal sections of filaments argues against the idea that these crystals are composed of straight filaments. The possibility that these crystals are composed of globular units is also feasible for any section normal to the flat surface of this presumably plate-like structure would yield an image with 'dots' lying in a rod-like profile.

As mentioned earlier (page 298), crystals composed of globular units can in some planes of sectioning look as if they were composed of filaments, hence such inclusions are at times erroneously described as filamentous inclusions or paracrystalline inclusions composed of filaments. *Plate 139* shows paracrystalline inclusions★ which are indubitably composed of

★Only truly crystalline inclusions where the globular units are arranged in a highly ordered fashion can give images suggesting that parallel filaments or a lattice of filaments is present (*Plates 136* and *137*). In the case of paracrystalline inclusions like the ones shown in *Plate 138*, the real question that arises is whether they are composed of filaments or lamellae. Continual failure to demonstrate circular profiles acceptable as transverse sections through filaments in several such structures would support the idea that lamellae are present. The presence of such profiles (*Plate 139, Fig. 3*) would confirm that the paracrystal is composed of filaments.

Plate 138

Fig. 1. From a specimen of human cerebral cortex collected at an autopsy performed 8 hours after death. A paracrystalline inclusion (arrowhead) with a rod-like profile has developed in the mitochondrion in a neurite. It presents here as a row of regularly spaced electron-dense dot-like profiles, lying between rigid-looking electron-dense segments of the outer and inner membranes of the mitochondrial envelope. × 131 000

Fig. 2. From rat cerebral cortex maintained at 37°C in a moist environment for 4 hours. A paracrystalline inclusion (arrowhead) is seen in the intracristal space of a mitochondrion in a neuron. It appears to be somewhat obliquely cut so that its details are not too well revealed and instead of 'dots' we see a periodic structure which resembles the rungs of a ladder. × 121 000

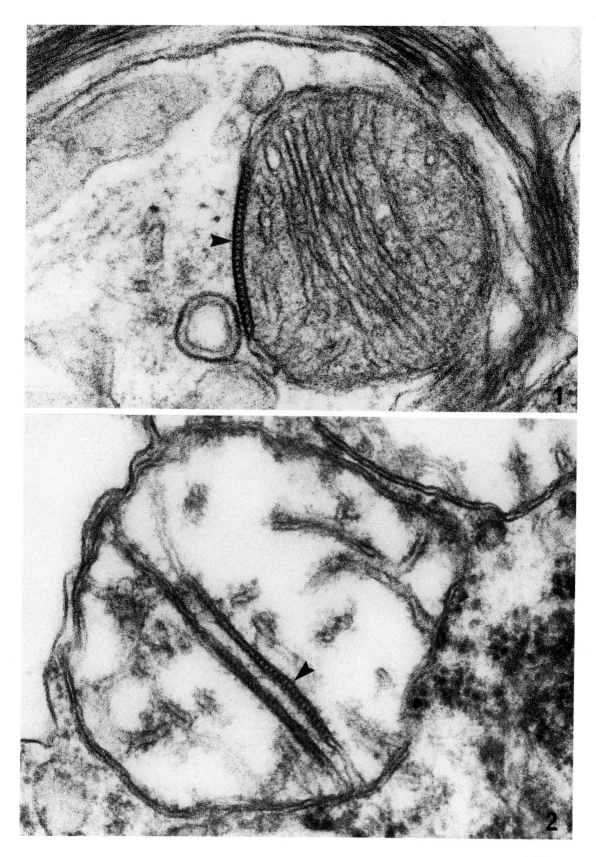

303

sheaves of straight and whorled filaments. These paracrystalline inclusions were found in a few mitochondria in an oncocytic carcinoid of the lung (Ghadially and Block, 1985). The intramitochondrial inclusion described by Saraiva *et al.*, (1985) in dendrites of patients with Alzheimer's disease looks somewhat similar, and the authors talk about filaments and lamellae; but in one of their illustrations the appearance suggests that transversely-sectioned microtubules rather than filaments may be present. Convincing examples of paracrystalline inclusions composed of helical filaments are shown by Mugnaini (1964b) and good examples of paracrystalline inclusions composed of microtubules are presented by Kjaerheim (1967).

In the liver of man, intramitochondrial crystals have been seen in giant mitochondria, and also at times in normal-sized mitochondria in various pathological states, such as carcinoma of the bile duct, obstructive jaundice, viral hepatitis, alcoholism, diabetes mellitus, Weil's disease, Waldenström's disease, bacterial infections, amyloidosis, congenital defects of bilirubin metabolism, hepatitis, mucopolysaccharidosis, type I hyperlipoproteinaemia, Wilson's disease, mushroom poisoning and after prolonged use of oral contraceptives. Such crystalline inclusions are also said to occur occasionally in the mitochondria of normal human liver, but this view has been challenged (for references, *see* David, 1964; Shiraki and Neustein, 1971; Bhagwat and Ross, 1971; Bhagwat *et al.*, 1972).

Plate 139

Oncocytic carcinoid of bronchus. Same case as *Plate 119* (*From Ghadially and Block, 1985*)

Fig. 1. An enlarged or giant mitochondrion (about 2.5 times greater in diameter than the average mitochondrion in this tumour) containing sheaves of filaments producing a paracrystalline inclusion. × 47 000

Fig. 2. Higher-power view of an intramitochondrial paracrystalline inclusion composed of sheaves of filaments cut longitudinally or obliquely. The two membranes comprising the mitochondrial envelope (arrowheads) are clearly visualized. × 54 000

Fig. 3. Another high-power view of an intramitochondrial filamentous or paracrystalline inclusion. Rounded profiles (arrows) of transversely cut filaments (about 10 nm in diameter) can be detected here. The two membranes of the mitochondrial envelope (arrowheads) are clearly visualized. × 95 000

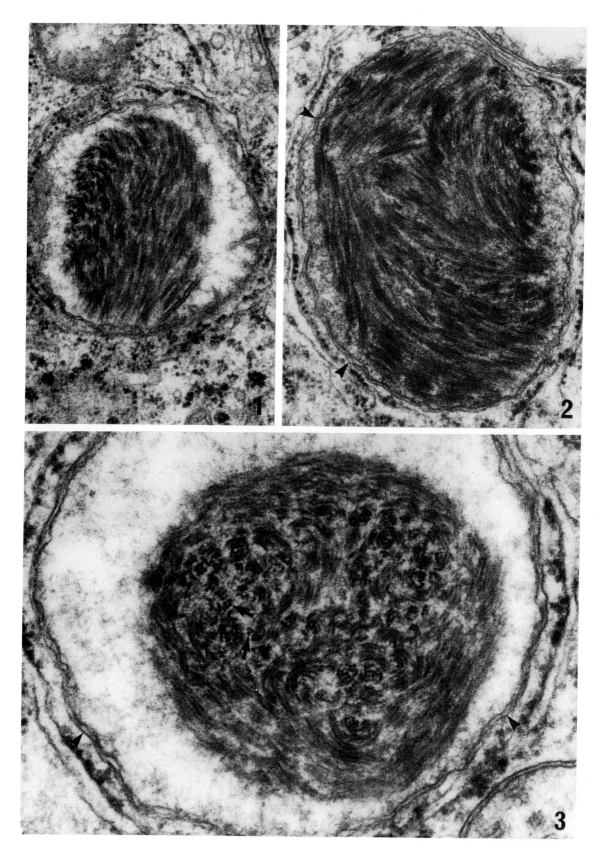

305

The mitochondria of human liver seem to be singularly prone to crystal formation. Reports dealing with such crystals in the liver of other animals are few except for the dog, where they have been reported to occur in: (1) protein deficiency (Ericsson *et al.*, 1966); (2) sulphamethoxypyrazine administration (Stein *et al.*, 1966); (3) *in vivo* ischaemia (Swenson *et al.*, 1967); (4) hypovolaemic shock (Blair *et al.*, 1968); and (5) three apparently normal dogs (Shiraki and Neustein, 1971). Intramitochondrial crystals have also been noted in the liver of monkeys receiving alcohol (Voelz, 1968) and in the liver of pigs poisoned with lead (Watrach, 1964).

Intramitochondrial crystals, usually rectangular in shape have been found in a variety of myopathies (Norris and Panner, 1966; Shy *et al.*, 1966; Price *et al.*, 1967; Shafiq *et al.*, 1967; D'Agostino *et al.*, 1968; Chou, 1969; Fisher and Danowski, 1969; Schellens and Ossentjuk, 1969; Spalke *et al.*, 1975). These crystals seem to develop in the intracristal or intermembranous compartment (*Plate 137, Fig. 1* and *Plate 140*), in contrast to the crystals in hepatocyte mitochondria mentioned above, which develop in the matrix compartment (*Plate 136*). Some workers consider that the crystals in muscular tissue are composed of spherical subunits 5–10 nm in diameter, but Chou (1969) considers that the subunits are filamentous structures arranged in a double helix.

A perusal of this section of the text devoted to intramitochondrial crystals and crystalloids will show the reader how difficult, if not near impossible, it is to assess the true three-dimensional morphology of many of these structures from a few random images. Little wonder then, that one finds conflicting interpretations in the literature. Only meticulous study of several images, combined with studies using the tilting stage and serial sections can resolve such problems. Such studies have rarely been executed, hence the true morphology of many crystals remains an enigma.

Little is known about the chemistry or significance of intramitochondrial crystals. Such crystals in hibernating animals and oocytes may well represent a form of protein storage, but those seen in human hepatocytes are generally regarded as a product of degenerative changes in the mitochondrion. Another possibility is that they might represent crystallized mitochondrial enzymic proteins. There is as yet little to support or refute such assumptions.

Plate 140

Biopsy from a case of ocular muscular dystrophy (*Specimen supplied by Dr T. M. Mukherjee*)

Fig. 1. In a pocket between the myofibrils and the bulging cell membrane lie numerous mitochondria containing crystalline inclusions which are cut more or less transversely and show a quadrilateral or rectangular shape. × 21 000

Fig. 2. Longitudinal and oblique sections through these intramitochondrial crystals reveal a fine somewhat difficult to discern lamellar pattern. × 53 000

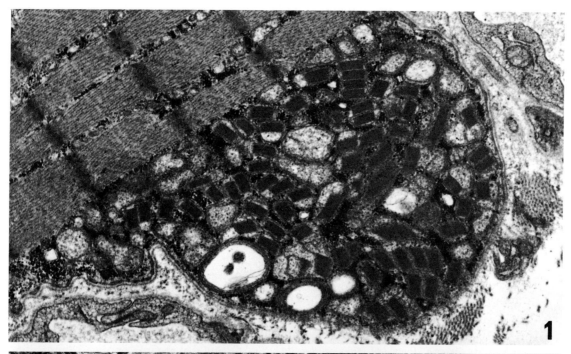

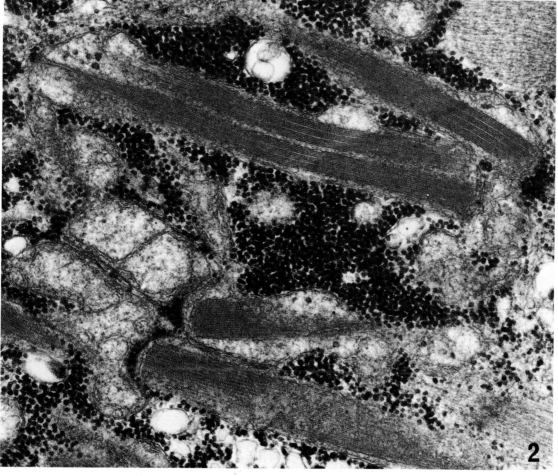

Intramitochondrial iron inclusions

Small deposits of intracellular electron-dense iron-containing particles (ferritin and/or haemosiderin) may normally be found in the reticuloendothelial system. Larger deposits occur locally in tissues after a haemorrhage (*see* page 636) or in the reticuloendothelial system, liver and other sites in conditions of iron overload produced by a variety of diseases and experimental procedures. Such deposits take the form of fine electron-dense particles scattered diffusely in the cytoplasmic matrix and/or collections of particles in single-membrane-bound lysosomal bodies called sidersomes (Richter, 1957). In the early literature, before the lysosome concept had evolved, iron deposits were at times erroneously thought to be localized in mitochondria. However, it is now clear that as a rule intramitochondrial iron deposits do not occur in such conditions (Kuff and Dalton, 1957; Bessis and Caroli, 1959; Ghadially, 1979b, c).

Substantial deposits of intramitochondrial iron are, however, frequently observed in erythroblasts and reticulocytes in sideroblastic anaemia (Bessis and Breton-Gorius, 1961; Sorenson, 1962; Heilmeyer *et al.*, 1962; Larizza and Orlandi, 1964; Tanaka, 1967).

Mollin and Hoffbrand (1968) defined sideroblastic anaemia as 'a dyshaemopoietic anaemia in which there is defective synthesis of haemoglobin associated with an abnormal accumulation of ionizable iron granules in the erythroblasts, some of which show a 'ring' or 'collar' of iron granules around the nucleus'. Electron microscopy shows that the ring sideroblast owes its appearance to a perinuclear distribution of iron-containing mitochondria (*Plate 141, Fig. 1*). At higher magnifications it is abundantly clear that the iron deposits lie in the mitochondrial matrix between the cristae (*Plate 141, Fig. 2; Plate 142, Fig. 1*), and that the iron occurs in a much finer form than the occasional aggregates of ferritin or haemosiderin* found in these cells (*Plate 142, Fig. 2*).

Tanaka (1967) has claimed that intramitochondrial iron is also seen in reticulum cells of the bone marrow in sideroblastic anaemia, but other workers (including myself) have not observed this in their material. Intramitochondrial iron has also been reported to occur in erythroid cells of apparently normal guinea-pigs and in thalassaemia (Bessis and Breton-Gorius, 1961), but this has not been reported by other workers. I can, however, confirm that the guinea-pig marrow does at times contain mitochondria with iron inclusions.

Sideroblastic anaemia is a chronic anaemia which is usually refractory to treatment and occurs despite the presence of adequate or large iron stores and high serum iron values. Two main varieties of this anaemia are known to occur. A primary or idiopathic variety which is sometimes hereditary, and a secondary variety associated with various disorders (for details, *see* Mollin and Hoffbrand, 1968) including malignancies such as Hodgkin's disease (*Plates 141 and 142*).

---

*Contrary to past belief it is not possible to confidently identify ferritin in electron micrographs. (The reasons for this are discussed on page 640.) However, evenly spaced particles of the type marked 'B' in *Plate 142, Fig. 2*, are more likely to be ferritin than haemosiderin. One may envisage that the even spacing is produced by close-packing of ferritin molecules which consist of an electron-lucent protein (apoferritin) shell (which blends with the cytoplasmic matrix and is hence not visualized) and a centrally placed electron-dense core.

Plate 141

From bone marrow of a case of sideroblastic anaemia secondary to Hodgkin's disease.

Fig. 1. Normoblast, showing perinuclear distribution of mitochondria containing iron deposits. × 19 000

Fig. 2. A group of iron-containing mitochondria found in the cytoplasm of a reticulocyte. × 78 000

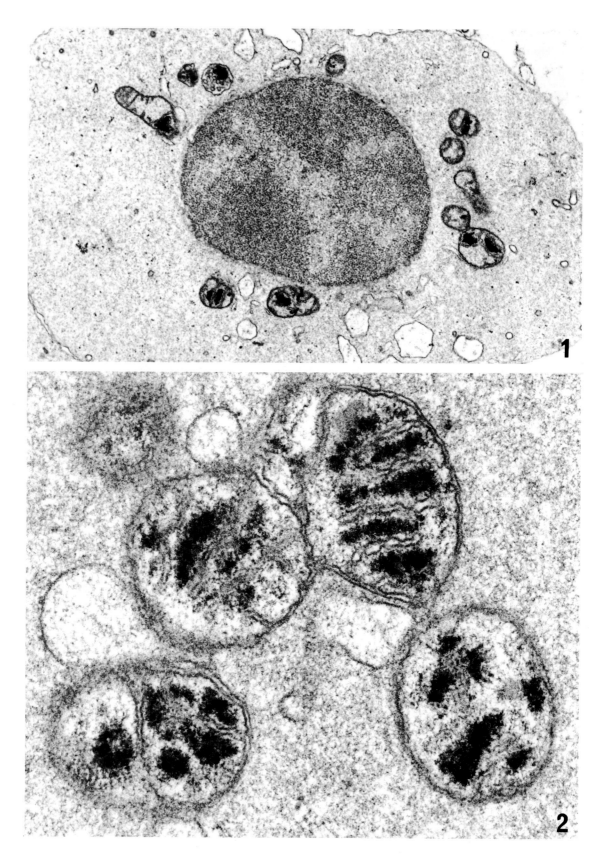

It would appear that the accumulation of iron in mitochondria is provoked by deficient porphyrin or haem synthesis. Mitochondria are known to be involved in the synthesis of porphyrin and the incorporation of iron into porphyrin to produce haem (Remington, 1957; Sano *et al.*, 1959). It is conceivable, therefore, that enzymatic defects in mitochondria may hinder such a synthesis and the iron destined for incorporation into haemoglobin would then accumulate in the mitochondrion. In some cases of acquired or hereditary forms of the disease, there is haem deficiency in the erythroid cells and also an unbalanced globin-chain synthesis with decreased β-chain formation (Grasso and Hines, 1969; Hines and Grasso, 1970; Cartwright and Deiss, 1975).

Thus it would appear that more than one biochemical defect can lead to the formation of iron-loaded mitochondria, and that sideroblastic anaemia may be a heterogeneous group of disorders. Such an idea is supported also by studies (Chui *et al.*, 1977) on mice carrying two mutant genes at the flexed-tail locus (*ff*) on chromosome 13 which develop severe anaemia during fetal development. The reticulocytes contain mitochondrial iron deposits similar to those seen in patients with sideroblastic anaemia. The intracellular free haem pool is elevated but there is diminished globin-chain production (Chui *et al.*, 1977).

Little is known about the chemical composition of the intramitochondrial inclusions seen in cases of sideroblastic anaemia except that they contain iron. It would be difficult to obtain enough human material for cell fractionation and chemical analysis and there would also be the problem of separating iron-laden mitochondria from iron-laden lysosomes (siderosomes) in the bone marrow macrophages. The only hope lies in *in situ* analysis of these inclusions by electron probe x-ray analysis. In one such study (Trump *et al.*, 1978), it is claimed that besides iron these deposits contain potassium. However, this was in tissue stained *en bloc* with uranium where the analysis is complicated by peak overlap problems between uranium and potassium.

Our (Ghadially *et al.*, 1979) electron-probe x-ray analytical studies carried out on unosmicated unstained preparations showed no potassium. Iron was demonstrated in every inclusion analysed, but a few also contained some phosphorus and/or sulphur. A consideration of the atomic ratios of the elements present led us to conclude that the iron in these inclusions probably occurs as a hydrated ferric oxide or ferric hydroxide oxide [FeO (OH). n H$_2$O] and that the phosphorus and sulphur detected in some of these inclusions indicates the presence of some organic compounds.

Plate 142

From the same tissue as *Plate 141*.

Fig. 1. High-power view of an iron-containing mitochondrion. The fine particulate nature of the deposit and the high electron density are clearly seen. The iron deposits lie in the matrix between the cristae. × 110 000

Fig. 2. The difference between the fine powdery intramitochondrial deposits of iron (A) and ferritin or haemosiderin (B) in the cytoplasm is demonstrated in this electron micrograph. × 100 000

310

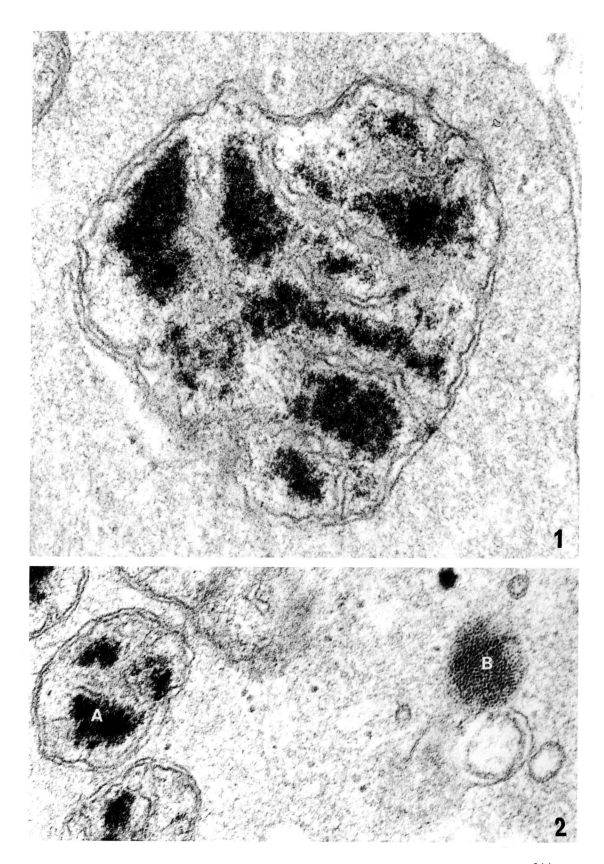

311

References

Aldercreutz, H., Svanborg, A. and Ånberg, Å. (1967). Recurrent jaundice in pregnancy. I. A clinical and ultrastructural study. *Am. J. Med.* **42**, 335

Aherne, W. and Hull, D. (1966). Brown adipose tissue and heat production in the newborn infant. *J. Path. Bact.* **91**, 223

Aho, A. J., Arstila, A. U., Ahonen, J. and Scheinin, T. M. (1970). The fine structural changes in intestinal epithelium cells in acute experimental mesenteric vascular occlusion. *Scand. J. clin. Lab. Invest.* **25**, Suppl. 113, 58

Albukerk, J. and Duffy, J. L. (1976). Ultrastructural alterations in livers with metastasis. *Arch. Path. Lab. Med.* **100**, 168

Alexander, C. S. (1972). Cobalt-Beer Cardiomyopathy. *Am. J. Med.* **53**, 395

Allegra, S. R. (1971). Warthin's tumour: A hypersensitivity disease? *Human Path.* **2**, 403

Alpert, L., Pai, S. H., Zak, F. G. and Werthamer, S. (1972). Cardiomyopathy associated with a pheochromocytoma. *Archs Path.* **93**, 544

Amherdt, M., Orci, L., Track, N. S., Lambert, A. E., Kanazawa, Y. and Stauffacher, W. (1971). An ultrastructural study of the islet cell tumor of the golden hamster. *Hormone Metab. Res.* **3**, 252

Anderson, W. A. (1968). Cytochemistry of sea urchin gametes. I. Intramitochondrial localisation of glycogen, glucose-6-phosphatase, and adenosine triphosphatase activity in spermatozoa of *Paracentrotus lividus. J. Ultrastruct. Res.* **24**, 398

Anderson, W. A. (1969). Nuclear and cytoplasmic DNA synthesis during early embryogenesis of *Paracentrotus lividus. J. Ultrastruct. Res.* **26**, 95

André, J. (1962). Contribution à la connaissance due chondriome; étude de ses modifications ultrastructurales pendant la spermatogénèse. *J. Ultrastruct. Res.* Suppl. 3

André, J. (1965). Quelques données recentes sur la structure et la physiologie des mitochondries: glycogène, particules elementaires, acides nucleiques. *Archs Biol., Liege,* **76**, 277

Arcasoy, M. M. and Smuckler, E. A. (1969). Acute effects of digoxin intoxication on rat hepatic and cardiac cells. *Lab. Invest.* **20**, 190

Archer, F. and Omar, M. (1969). Pink cell (oncocytic) metaplasia in a fibro-adenoma of the human breast. Electron microscopic observations. *J. Path.* **99**, 119

Arcos, J. C., Mathison, J. B., Tison, M. J. and Mouledoux, A. M. (1969). Effect of feeding amino azo dyes on mitochondrial swelling and contraction. Kinetic evidence for deletion of membrane regulatory sites. *Cancer Res.* **29**, 1288

Arhelger, R. B., Broom, J. S. and Boler, R. K. (1965). Ultrastructural hepatic alterations following tannic acid administration to rabbits. *Am. J. Path.* **46**, 409

Arnold, B. M., Kovacs, K., Horvath, E., Murray, T. M. and Higgins, H. P. (1974). Functioning oxyphil cell adenoma of the parathyroid gland: evidence for parathyroid secretory activity of oxyphil cells. *J. Clin. Endocr.* **38**, 459

Ashhurst, D. E. (1965). Mitochondrial particles seen in sections. *J. Cell Biol.* **24**, 497

Ashraf, M. and Bloor, C. M. (1976). X-ray microanalysis of mitochondrial deposits in ischemic myocardium. *Virchows Arch. B Cell Path.* **22**, 287–297

Askew, J. B., Fechner, R. E., Bentinck, D. C. and Jenson, A. B. (1971). Epithelial and myoepithelial oncocytes. Ultrastructural study of a salivary gland oncocytoma. *Archs Otolar.* **93**, 46

Auger, C. and Chenard, J. (1967). Quebec beer-drinkers' cardiomyopathy: ultrastructural changes in one case. *Can. Med. Ass. J.* **97**, 916

Baccetti, A., Dallai, R., Pallini, V., Rosati, F. and Afzelius, B. A. (1977). Protein of insect sperm mitochondrial crystals. Crystallomitin. *J. Cell Biol.* **73**, 594

Bailey, E., Taylor, C. B. and Bartley, W. (1967). Turnover of mitochondrial components of normal and essential fatty acid-deficient rats. *Biochem. J.* **104**, 1026

Baithun, S. I. and Pollock, D. J. (1983). Oncocytic hepatocellular tumour. *Histopathology* **7**, 107

Ballentine, J. D. (1974). Ultrastructural pathology of hyperbaric oxygenation in the central nervous system. *Lab. Invest.* **31**, 580

Barastegui, C. A. and Ruano-Gil, D. (1984). Atypical cristae (paracrystalline inclusions) in mitochondria of epithelial cells of the rat ureter. 1. Ultrastructural features. *J. Submicrosc. Cytol.* **16**, 299

Bargmann, W., Krish, B. and Leonhardt, H. (1977). Lipids in the proximal convoluted tubule of the cat kidney and the reabsorption of cholesterol. *Cell and Tiss. Res.* **177**, 523

Barka, T., Scheuer, P. J., Schaffner, F. and Popper, H. (1964). Structural changes of liver cells in copper intoxication. *Archs Path.* **78**, 331

Barnard, T. and Afzelius, B. A. (1972). The matrix granules of mitochondria. A Review. *Sub-Cell. Biochem.* **1**, 375

Barnard, T. and Ruusa, J. (1979). Mitochondrial matrix granules in soft tissues. 1. Elemental composition by x-ray microanalysis. *Exp. Cell Res.* **124,** 339

Barnard, T. and Seveus, L. (1976). Distinction between matrix granules and Ca stores in mitochondria of brown adipose tissue. *J. Cell Biol.* **70,** p. 142a (Abstract 425)

Barnard, T., Afzelius, B. A. and Lindberg, O. (1971). A cytochemical investigation into the distribution of cytochrome oxidase activity within the mitochondria of brown adipose tissue from the prenatal rat. *J. Ultrastruct. Res.* **34,** 544

Bassi, M. and Bernelli-Zazzera, A. (1964). Ultrastructural cytoplasmic changes of liver cells after reversible and irreversible ischemia. *Exp. Mol. Path.* **3,** 332

Bauserman, S. C., Hardman, J. M., Schochet, S. S. and Earle, K. M. (1978). Pituitary oncocytomas. *Archs Path. Lab. Med.* **102,** 456

Beams, H. W. and Tahmisian, T. N. (1954). Structure of the mitochondria in the male germ cells of Helix as revealed by the electron microscope. *Exp. Cell Res.* **6,** 87

Beattie, D. S., Basford, R. E. and Koritz, S. B. (1967). The turnover of the protein components of mitochondria from rat liver, kidney, and brain. *J. Biol. Chem.* **242,** 4584

Beaulaton, J. (1964). Sur l'accumulation intramitochondriale de glycogène dans la gland prothoracigne du ver à soie du chêne *Antheraea peruyi* (Guér) pendant les quatrième et cinquième stades larvaires. *C. R. Acad. Sci. (D),* Paris **258,** 4139

Beaulaton, J. A. (1968). Modifications ultrastructurales des cellules sécrétrices de la glande prothoracique de vers à soie au cours des deux derniers âges larvaires. 1. Le chondriome, et ses relations avec le reticulum agranulaire. *J. Cell Biol.* **39,** 501

Benda, C. (1902). Die mitochondria, *Ergebn. Anat. Entw. Gesch.* **12,** 743

Berchtold, J. P. (1969). Contribution à l'étude ultrastructurale des cellules interrénales de *Salamandra salamandra L* (Amphibien urodèle). 1. Conditions normales. *Z. Zellforsch. Mikrosk. Anat.* **102,** 357

Berger, E. R. (1964). Mitochondria genesis in the retinal photoreceptor inner segment. *J. Ultrastruct. Res.* **11,** 90

Bergeron, M. and Droz, B. (1969). Protein renewal in mitochondria as revealed by electron microscope radioautography. *J. Ultrastruct. Res.* **26,** 17

Bernhard, W. and Rouiller, C. (1956). Close topographical relationship between mitochondria and ergastoplasm of liver cells in a definite phase of cellular activity. *J. biophys. biochem. Cytol.* **2,** Suppl., 73

Berthold, C. H. (1966). Ultrastructural appearance of glycogen in the β-neurons of the lumbar spinal ganglia of the frog. *J. Ultrastruct. Res.* **14,** 254

Bessis, M. and Breton-Gorius. J. (1961). Presence de fer dans les mitochondries des erythroblastes chez le cobaye normal. *Nouv. Rev. franc. Hemat.* **1,** 356

Bessis, M. and Breton-Gorius, J. (1969). Pathologie et asynchronisme de developpmente des organelles cellulaires au cours des leucemies aigues granulocytaires. *Nouv. Rev. franc. Hemat.* **9,** 245

Bessis, M. and Caroli, J. (1959). A comparative study of hemachromatosis by electron microscopy. *Gastroenterology* **37,** 538

Bhagwat, A. G. and Ross, R. C. (1971). Hepatic intramitochondrial crystalloids. *Archs Path.* **91,** 70

Bhagwat, A. G., Ross, R. C. and Currie, D. J. (1972). Ultrastructure of normal human liver. *Archs Path.* **93** 227

Bhattacharyya, T. K. and Butler, D. G. (1979). Fine structure of the adrenocortical homologue in the North American eel and modifications following seawater adaptation. *Anat. Rec.* **193** 213

Bishop, S. P. and Cole, C. R. (1969). Ultrastructural changes in the canine myocardium with right ventricular hypertrophy and congestive heart failure. *Lab. Invest.* **20,** 219

Blackburn, W. R. and Vinijchaikul, K. (1969). The pancreas in kwashiorkor. An electron microscopic study. *Lab. Invest.* **20,** 305

Blair, O. M., Stenger, R. J., Hopkins, R. W. and Simeone, F. A. (1968). Hepatocellular ultrastructure in dogs with hypovolemic shock. *Lab. Invest.* **18,** 172

Blinzinger, K., Rewcastle, N. B. and Hager, H. (1964). Beobachtungen uber Mitochondrien mit eigenartiger Innenstruktur (Prisma-Typ) in Astrozyten des Goldhamstergehirns. *Z. Naturforschg.* **19,** 514

Blinzinger, K., Rewcastle, N. B. and Hager, H. (1965). Observations on prismatic type mitochondria within astrocytes of the Syrian hamster brain. *J. Cell Biol.* **25,** 293

Boler, R. K. and Bibighaus, A. J. (1967). Ultrastructural alterations of dog livers during endotoxin shock. *Lab. Invest.* **17,** 537

Bondeson, L., Bondeson, A-G., Ljungberg, O. and Tibblin, S. (1981). Oxyphil tumours of the thyroid. *Ann. Surg.* **194,** 677

Bonikos, D. S., Bensch, K. G., Watt, T. and Northway, W. H. Jr. (1977). Pulmonary oncocytes in prolonged hyperoxia. *Exp. Mol. Path.* **26,** 92

Bowman, R. W. (1967). Mitochondrial connections in canine myocardium. *Tex. Rep. Biol. Med.* **25,** 517

Brandt, P. W. and Pappas, G. D. (1959). The nuclear-mitochondrial relationship in *Pelomyxa carolinensis*. *J. biophys. biochem. Cytol.* **6,** 91

Brawn, P. N. and Mackay, B. (1980). Intracristal crystalline inclusions in mitochondria of a neuroblastoma. *Ultrastruct. Path.* **1,** 495

Brdiczka, D. and Barnard, T. (1980). Mitochondrial matrix granules in soft tissues. II. Isolation and initial characterization of a calcium-precipitable, soluble lipoprotein subfraction from brown fat and liver mitochondria. *Exp. Cell Res.* **126,** 127

Brown, R. A., Chiu, C., Scott, H. J. and Gurd, F. N. (1970). Ultrastructural changes in the canine ileal mucosal cell after mesenteric arterial occlusion. *Archs. Surg., Chicago* **101,** 290

Brück, K. (1970). Nonshivering thermogenesis and brown adipose tissue in relation to age, and their integration in the thermoregulatory system. *Brown Adipose Tissue.* Ed. by O. Lindberg, Ch. 5, p. 117. New York: Elsevier Publishing Co.

Buja, L. M., Ferrans, V. J. and Levitsky, S. (1972). Occurrence of intramitochondrial glycogen in canine myocardium after prolonged anoxia cardiac arrest. *J. Mol. Cell. Cardiol.* **4,** 237

Buja, L. M., Dees, J. H., Harling, D. F. and Willerson, J. T. (1976). Analytical electron microscopic study of mitochondrial inclusions in canine myocardial infarcts. *J. Histochem. Cytochem.* **24,** 508

Bulloch, R. T., Murphy, M. L. and Pearce, M. B. (1970). Fine structural lesions in the myocardium of a beer drinker with reversible heart failure. *Am. Heart J.* **80,** 629

Burch, G. E., Sohal, R. and Fairbanks, L. D. (1970). Ultrastructural changes in Drosophila heart with age. *Archs Path., Chicago* **89,** 128

Butler, W. H. and Judha, J. D. (1970). Ultrastructural studies on mitochondrial swelling. *Biochem. J.* **118,** 883

Cameron, G. R. (1952). *Pathology of the Cell.* Edinburgh: Oliver and Boyd

Campiche, M. (1960). Les inclusions lamellaires des cellules alvéolaires dans le poumon du raton. Relations entre l'ultrastructure et la fixation. *J. Ultrastruct. Res.* **3,** 302

Carlsöö, B., Domeij, S. and Helander, H. F. (1979). A quantitative ultrastructural study of a parotoid oncocytoma. *Arch. Path. Lab. Med.* **103,** 471

Cartwright, G. E. and Deiss, A. (1975). Sideroblasts, siderocytes, and sideroblastic anemia. *N. Engl. J. Med.* **292,** 185

Cassier, P. (1979). The corpora allata of insects. In *Int. Rev. Cytol.* **57,** 1-73. Ed. by G. H. Bourne & J. F. Danielli. New York: Academic Press.

Cassier, P. and Fain-Maurel, M. A. (1971). Modalités de l'évolution et du renouvellement du chondriome au cours des cycles d'activité des glandes de mue de *Petrobius maritimus* leach (*Insecte aptérygote*). *Arch. Zool. Exp. Gen.* **112,** 457

Caulfield, J. B. and Schrag, P. E. (1964). Electron microscopic study of renal calcification. *Am. J. Path.* **44,** 365

Chandler, J. A. (1977). *X-ray Microanalysis in the Electron Microscope.* Amsterdam, New York: North Holland Publishing

Cheah, K. S., Cheah, A. M. and Voyle, C. A. (1973). Paracrystalline arrays in mitochondria following ageing of mitochondria *in situ. Bioenergetics* **4,** 383

Chou, S. M. (1969). 'Megaconial' mitochondria observed in a case of chronic polymyositis. *Acta neuropath.* **12,** 68

Christensen, A. K. (1971). Frozen thin sections of fresh tissue for electron microscopy with a description of pancreas and liver. *J. Cell Biol.* **51,** 772

Christensen, A. K. and Chapman, G. B. (1959). Cup-shaped mitochondria in interstitial cells of the albino rat testis. *Exp. Cell Res.* **18,** 576

Chui, D. H. K., Sweeney, G. D., Patterson, M. and Russell, E. S. (1977). Hemoglobin synthesis in siderocytes of flexed-tailed mutant (*f/f*) mice. *Blood,* **50,** 165

Collan, Y., McDowell, E. and Trump, B. F. (1981). Studies on the pathogenesis of ischemic cell injury. VI. Mitochondrial flocculent densities in autolysis. *Virchows Arch. B Cell Pathol.* **35,** 189

Copeland, D. E. and Dalton, A. J. (1959). An association between mitochondria and the endoplasmic reticulum in cells of the pseudobranch gland of a Teleost. *J. biophys. biochem. Cytol.* **5,** 393

Coupland, R. E. and MacDougall, J. D. B. (1968). The effect of hyperbaric oxygen on rat liver cells in organ culture: a light- and electron-microscope study. *J. Path. Bact.* **96,** 149

Daems, W. Th. and Wisse, E. (1966). Shape and attachment of the cristae mitochondriales in mouse hepatic cell mitochondria. *J. Ultrastruct. Res.* **16,** 123

D'Agostino, A. N. (1963). An electron microscope study of skeletal and cardiac muscle of the rat poisoned by plasmocid. *Lab. Invest.* **12,** 1060

D'Agostino, A. N. (1964). An electron microscopic study of cardiac necrosis produced by 9-α-fluorocortisol and sodium phosphate. *Am. J. Path.* **45,** 633

314

D'Agostino, A. N., Ziter, F. A., Rallison, M. L. and Bray, P.F. (1968). Familial myopathy with abnormal muscle mitochondria. *Archs Neurol., Chicago* **18**, 388

Dalton, A. J. and Felix, M. D. (1957). Electron microscopy of mitochondria and the Golgi complex. *Symp. Soc. exp. Biol.* **10**, 148

David, H. (1964). *Submicroscopic Ortho and Pathomorphology of the Liver.* Translated by H. G. Epstein. Berlin: Akademie-Verlag. Oxford: Pergamon Press; New York: Macmillan

David, H. and Kettler, L. H. (1961). Degeneration von Lebermitochondrien nach ammonium-intoxikation. *Z. Zellforsch. mikrosk. Anat.* **53**, 857

Davis, L. E. (1967). Intramitochondrial crystals in Hydra. *J. Ultrastruct. Res.* **21**, 125

De Robertis, E. and Bleichmar, H. (1962). Mitochondriogensis in nerve fibers of the infrared receptor membrane of pit vipers. *Z. Zellforsch. mikrosk. Anat.* **57**, 572

De Robertis, E. and Sabatini, D. (1958). Mitochondrial changes in the adrenocortex of normal hamsters. *J. biophys. biochem. Cytol.* **4**, 667

Dessouky, D. A. (1968). Electron microscopic studies of the myometrium of the guinea pig. *Am. J. Obstet. Gynec.* **100**, 30

Devlin, T. M. and Pruss, M. P. (1962). Oxidative phosphorylation and ATPase activity of mitochondria from rat hepatomas. *Proc. Am. Assoc. Cancer Res.* **3**, 315

Duffy, J. L., Suzuki, Y. and Churg, J. (1971). Acute calcium nephropathy. Early proximal tubular changes in the rat kidney. *Archs Path.* **91**, 340

Emmelot, P., Bos, C. J., Brombacher, P. J. and Hampe, J. F. (1959). Studies on isolated tumour mitochondria: biochemical properties of mitochondria from hepatomas with special reference to a transplanted rat hepatoma of the solid type. *Br. J. Cancer* **13**, 348

Enders, A. C., Enders, R. K. and Schlafke, S. (1963). An electron microscope study of the gland cells of the mink endometrium. *J. Cell Biol.* **18**, 405

Engfeldt. B., Gardell, S., Hellstrom, J., Ivemark, B., Rhodin, J. and Strandh, J. (1958). Effect of experimentally induced hyperparathyroidism on renal function and structure. *Acta endocr.* **29**, 15

Ephrussi, B. (1953). *Nucleocytoplasmic Relations in Microorganisms*, p. 124. London: Oxford University Press

Ericsson, J. L. E. and Biberfeld, P. (1967). Studies on aldehyde fixation. Fixation rates and their relation to fine structure and some histochemical reactions in liver. *Lab. Invest.* **17**, 281

Ericsson, J. L.E., Orrenius, S. and Holm, I. (1966). Alterations in canine liver cells induced by protein deficiency: ultrastructural and biochemical observations. *Expl. Molec. Path.* **5**, 329

Ernster, L. and Luft, R. (1963). Further studies on a population of human skeletal muscle mitochondria lacking respiratory control. *Exp. Cell Res.* **32**, 26

Fain-Maurel, M.-A. (1966). Localisations intramitochondriale et intracisternale de glycogene monoparti-culaire. *C. R. Acad. Sci. (D) Paris* **263**, 1107

Fain-Maurel, M.-A. (1968). Variabilité de la structure mitochondriale dans les mucocytes des glands salivaires de Limnaea stagnalis L. (Gastéropode Pulmoné). *C. R. Acad. Sci.* **267**, 1614

Fain-Maurel, M.-A. and Cassier, P. (1969). Pléomorphisme mitochondrial dans les corpora allata de *Locusta migratoria migratorioides* (R et F.) au cours de la vie imaginale. *Z. Zellforsch.* **102**, 543

Farhi, D. C., Shikes, R. H. and Silverberg, S.G. (1982). Ultrastructure of fibrolamellar oncocytic hepatoma. *Cancer* **50**, 702

Fawcett, D. W. (1955). Observations on the cytology and electron microscopy of hepatic cells. *J. natn. Cancer Inst.* **15**, (Suppl.), 1475

Fawcett, D. W. (1959). In *Developmental Cytology*. Chapter 8. Ed. by D. Rudnick. New York: Ronald Press

Fawcett, D. W. (1966). *The Cell: Its Organelles and Inclusions.* Philadelphia and London: Saunders

Fawcett, D. W. (1981). *The Cell.* Philadelphia: W. B. Saunders Co.

Fawcett, D. W. and McNutt, N. S. (1969). The ultrastructure of the cat myocardium I. Ventricular papillary muscle. *J. Cell Biol.* **42**, 1

Fechner, R. E. and Bentinck, B. R. (1973). Ultrastructure of bronchial oncocytoma. *Cancer* **31**, 1451

Feldman, P. S., Horvath, E. and Kovacs, K. (1972). Ultrastructure of three Hürthle cell tumours of the thyroid. *Cancer* **30**, 1279

Feldmann, G., Oudea, P., Domart-Oudéa, M.-C., Molas, G. and Fauvert, R. (1968). L'ultrastructure hepatique au cours de la maladie de Gilbert. *Path. Biol.* **16**, 943

Feldmann, G., Oudea, P., Molas, G., Domart-Oudea, M. -C. and Fauvert, R. avec la collaboration technique de Mme J. Penaud (1970a). L'ultrastructure des hepatocytes au cors des cirrhoses alcooliques. *Presse Med.* **78**, 409

Feldmann, G., Molas, G., Groussard, O. and Domart-Oudéa, M. C. (1970b). Die Ultrastruktur der Leber bei chronischem idiopathischem Ikterus. *Münch. med Wschr.* **39**, 1725

Feldmann, G., Maurice, M., Husson, J. M., Fiessinger, J.N., Camilleri, J. P., Benhamou, J. P. and Housset, E. (1977). Hepatocyte giant mitochondria: An almost constant lesion in systemic scleroderma. *Virchows Arch. A Path. Anat Histol.* **374**, 215

Ferrans, V. J., Hibbs, R. G., Weily, H. S., Weilbaecher, D. G., Walsh, J. J. and Burch, G. E. (1970). A histochemical and electron microscopic study of epinephrine-induced myocardial necrosis. *J. Molec. Cell. Cardiol.* **1**, 11

Ferrans, V. J., Buja, L. M., Levitsky, S. and Roberts W. C. (1971). Effects of hyperosmotic perfusate on ultrastructure and function of the isolated canine heart. *Lab. Invest.* **24**, 265

Fiala, S. and Fiala, A. E. (1967). Structural and metabolic distinction between Morris hepatoma 5123A and normal rat liver. *Int. J. Cancer* **2**, 344

Fisher, E. R. and Danowski, T. S. (1969). Mitochondrial myopathy. *Am. J. clin. Path.* **51**, 619

Fisher, E. R. and Horvat, B. (1971). Experimental production of so-called spironolactone bodies. *Archs Path.* **91**, 471

Fisher, E. R., Copeland, C. and Fisher, B. (1967). Correlation of ultrastructure and function following hypothermic preservation of canine kidneys. *Lab. Invest.* **17**, 99

Flaks, B. (1968). Unusual aspects of ultrastructural differentiation in rat heptoma cells. *J. Cell Biol.* **38**, 230

Flax, M. H. and Tidale, W. A. (1964). An electron microscopic study of alcoholic hyalin. *Am. J. Path.* **44**, 441

Fleishman, J. S. and Schwartz, R. A. (1983). Hibernoma: Ultrastructural observations. *J. Surg. Oncol.* **23**, 285

Fletcher, M. J. and Sanadi, D. R. (1961). Turnover of rat-liver mitochondria. *Biochem. Biophys. Acta* **51**, 356

Frederiks, W. M., Fronik, G. M. and Hessling, J. G. M. (1984). A method for quantitative analysis of the extent of necrosis in ischemic rat liver. *Exp. Mol. Path.* **41**, 119

Friedman, H. I., Chandler, J. G. and Nemeth, T. J. (1977). Hepatic intramitochondrial filaments in morbidly obese patients undergoing intestinal bypass. *Gastroenterology* **73**, 1353

Fujita, H. and Machino, M. (1964). Fine structure of intramitochondrial crystals in rat thyroid follicular cell. *J. Cell Biol.* **23**, 383

Gansler, H. and Rouiller, C. (1956). Modifications physiologiques et pathologiques du chondriome. Étude au microscope életronique. *Schweiz. Z. Path. Bact.* **19**, 217

Geren, B. B. and Schmitt, F. O. (1954). The structure of the Schwann cell and its relation to the axon in certain invertebrate nerve fibers. *Nat. Acad. Sci. Proc.* **40**, 863

Gey, G. O. (1956). Some aspects of the constitution and behaviour of normal and malignant cells maintained in continuous culture. *Harvey Lect.* **50**, 154

Ghadially, F. N. (1979a). Invited review: the technique and scope of electron-probe x-ray analysis in pathology. *Pathology* **11**, 95

Ghadially, F. N. (1979b). Ultrastructural localization and *in situ* analysis of iron, bismuth and gold inclusions. *CRC Critical Reviews in Toxicology*, November 1979 **6**, 303

Ghadially, F. N. (1979c). Haemorrhage and Haemosiderin. *J. Submicr. Cytol.* **11**, 271

Ghadially, F. N. (1980). *Diagnostic Electron Microscopy of Tumours*. London: Butterworths

Ghadially, F. N. (1985). *Diagnostic Electron Microscopy of Tumours*, 2nd Edition. London: Butterworths

Ghadially, F. N. and Block, H. J. (1985). Oncocytic carcinoid of the lung. *J. Submicrosc. Cytol.* **17**, 435

Ghadially, F. N. and Parry, E. W. (1965). Ultrastructure of the liver of the tumor-bearing host. *Cancer* **18**, 485

Ghadially, F. N. and Parry, E. W. (1966). Ultrastructure of a human hepatocellular carcinoma and surrounding non-neoplastic liver. *Cancer* **19**, 1989

Ghadially, F. N. and Skinnider, L. F. (1974). Giant mitochondria in erythroleukaemia. *J. Path.* **114**, 113

Ghadially, F. N., Lalonde, J-M. A. and Mukherjee, T. M. (1979). Electron-probe x-ray analysis of intramitochondrial iron deposits in sideroblastic anaemia. *J. Submicrosc. Cytol.* **11**, 503

Ghadially, F. N., Lowes, N. R. and Mesfin, G. M. (1977). Atypical glycogen deposits in a plasmacytoma: An ultrastructural study. *J. Path.* **122**, 157

Ghidoni, J. J. and Thomas, H. (1969). Connection between a mitochondrion and endoplasmic reticulum in liver. *Experientia* **25**, 632

Giacomelli, F., Weiner, J. and Spiro, D. (1965). Cytological alterations related to stimulation of the zona glomerulosa of the adrenal gland. *J. Cell Biol.* **26**, 499

Glaumann, B., Glaumann, H., Berezesky, I K. and Trump, B. F. (1977). Studies on cellular recovery from injury. II. Ultrastructural studies on the recovery of the pars convoluta of the proximal tubule of the rat kidney from temporary ischemia. *Virchows Arch. B Cell Path* **24**, 1

Glinsmann, W. H. and Ericsson, J. L. E. (1966). Observations on the subcellular organization of hepatic parenchymal cells. II. Evolution of reversible alterations induced by hypoxia. *Lab. Invest.* **15**, 762

316

Goebel, H. H., Schulz, F. and Rama, B. (1980). Ultrastructurally abnormal mitochondria in the pituitary oncocytoma. *Acta Neurochirurg.* **51**, 195

Gold, P. H. and Menzies, R. A. (1968). Mitochondrial turnover in several tissues of the rat. *Fed. Proc.* **27**, p. 832 (Abstract 3483)

Gonatas, N. K. and Shy, G. M. (1966). Childhood myopathies with abnormal mitochondria. *Proc. 5th Int. Congr. Neuropath.*, Zurich, 1965. Int. Congr. Ser. No. 100, p. 606. Amsterdam: Excerpta Medica

Gordon, E. E. and Bernstein, J. (1970). Effect of valinomycin on mitochondrial ultrastructure and function of intact Ehrlich ascites tumor cells. *Biochem. biophys. Acta* **205**, 464

Gordon, G. B., Miller, L. R. and Bensch, K. G. (1964). Electron microscopic observations of the gonad in the testicular feminization syndrome. *Lab. Invest.* **13**, 152

Grasse, P. P., Carasso, N. and Favard, P. (1956). Les ultrastructures cellulaires au cours de la spermiogenese de l'escargot (*Helix pomatia L.*). *Annls sci. nat. Zool. (11)* **18**, 339

Grasso, J. A. and Hines, J. D. (1969). A comparative electron microscopic study of refractory and alcoholic sideroblastic anaemia. *Br. J. Haematol.* **17**, 35

Gray, S. R., Cornog, J. L. and Seo, I. S. (1976). Oncocytic neoplasms of salivary glands—a report of 15 cases including two malignant oncocytomas. *Cancer* **38**, 1306

Greenawalt, J. W., Foster, G. V. and Lehninger, A. L. (1962). The observation of unusual membranous structures associated with liver mitochondria in thyrotoxic rats. In *Electron Microscopy*, Vol. 2, p. 00-5. Ed. by S. S. Breese, Jr. New York: Academic Press

Greene, W.B., Balentine, J. D. and Hennigar, G. R. (1979). Selective mitochondrial degeneration in renal tubules following hyperbaric oxygen exposure. *Am. J. Path* **96**, 737

Greenstein, J. P. (1954). *Biochemistry of Cancer*. New York: Academic Press

Griffin, J. L. and Juniper, K. Jr. (1971). Ultrastructure of *Entamoeba histolytica* from human amebic dysentery. *Arch. Path.* **21**, 271

Grodums, E. I. (1977). Ultrastructural changes in mitochondria of brown adipose cells during the hibernation cycle of *Citellus lateralis*. *Cell Tiss. Res.* **185**, 231

Gruner, J. E. (1963). Sur quelques anomalies mitochondriales observées au cours d'affections musculaires variées. *C.r. Soc. Biol. Paris, Strasbourg* **157**, 181

Gusek, W. (1975). Die Ultrastruktur Cycasin-induzierter Nierenadenome. *Virchows Arch. A. Path. Anat. Histol.* **365**, 221

Gustafsson, R., Tata, J. R., Lindberg, O. and Ernster, L. (1965). The relationship between the structure and activity of rat skeletal muscle mitochondria after thyroidectomy and thyroid hormone treatment. *J. Cell Biol.* **26**, 555

Hackenbrock, C. R. (1968a). Ultrastructural bases for metabolically linked mechanical activity in mitochondria. II. Electron transport linked ultrastructural transformations in mitochondria. *J. Cell. Biol.* **37**, 345

Hackenbrock, C. R. (1968b). Chemical and physical fixation of isolated mitochondria in low-energy and high-energy states. *Proc. natn. Acad. Sci., USA* **61**, 598

Hackenbrock, C. R., Rehn, T. G., Weinbach, E. C. and Lemasters, J. J. (1971). Oxidative phosphorylation and ultrastructural transformation in mitochondria in the intact ascites tumor cell. *J. Cell Biol.* **51**, 123

Hagopian, M., Gershon, M. D. and Nunez, E. A. (1972). An ultrastructural study of the effect of reserpine on ventricular cardiac muscle of active and hibernating bats (*Myotis lucifugus*). *Lab. Invest.* **27**, 99

Hall, J. D. and Crane, F. L. (1971). Intracristal rods. A new structure in beef heart mitochondria. *J. Cell Biol.* **48**, 420

Hamilton, D. W., Fawcett, D. W. and Christensen, A. K. (1966). The liver of the slender salamander *Batrachoseps attenuatus*. *Z. Zellforsch.* **70**, 347

Hamperl, H. (1936). Über das Vorkommen von Oncocyten in verschiedenen Organen und ihren Geschwulsten (Mundspeicheldrüsen, Bauchspeichrüse, Epithelkörperchen, Hypophyse, Schilddrüse, Eileiter). *Virchows Arch. Pathol. Anat.* **298**, 327

Hamperl, H. (1937). Über gutartige Bronchialtumoren (Cylindrome und Carcinoide). *Virchows Arch. Path. Anat.* **300**, 46

Hamperl, H. (1950). Onkocytes and so-called Hürthle cell tumor. *Arch. Path.* **49**, 563

Hanzlíková, V. and Schiaffino, S. (1977). Mitochondrial changes in ischemic skeletal muscle. *J. Ultrastruct. Res.* **60**, 121

Haust, D. M. (1968). Crystalloid structure of hepatic mitochondria in children with heparitin sulfate mucopolysaccharidosis (Sanfilippo type). *Exp. mol. Path.* **8**, 123

Hawkins, W. E., Howse, H. D. and Foster, C. A. (1980). Prismatic cristae and paracrystalline inclusions in mitochondria of myocardial cells of the oyster *Crassostrea virginica* Gmelin. *Cell Tissue Res.* **209**, 87

Heggtveit, H. A., Herman, L. and Mishra, R. K. (1964). Cardiac necrosis and calcification in experimental magnesium deficiency. *Am. J. Path.* **45**, 757

Heilmeyer, V. L., Merker, H., Molbert, E. and Neidhardt, M. (1962). Zur Mikromorphologie der hereditaren hypochromen sideroachrestischen Anamie. *Acta Haemat.* **27**, 78

Heinmann, P., Hansson, G. and Nilsson, O. (1971). Primary hyperparathyroidism in a case of oxyphilic adenoma. *Acta Path. microbiol Scand. Sect. A* **79**, 10

Herdson, P. B., Sommers, H. M. and Jennings, R. B. (1965). A comparative study of the fine structure of normal and ischemic dog myocardium with special reference to early changes following temporary occlusion of a coronary artery. *Am. J. Path.* **46**, 367

Hill, R. B. and Blackburn, W. R. (1967). Effect of prednisolone treatment of pregnant rats on fetal liver structure and metabolism. *Lab. Invest.* **17**, 146

Himmelhoch, S. R. and Karnovsky, M. J. (1961). Oxidative and hydrolytic enzymes in the nephron of *Necturus maculosus. J. biophys. biochem. Cytol.* **9**, 893

Hines, J. D. and Grasso, J. A. (1970). The sideroblastic anemias. *Semin. Hematol.* **7**, 86

Hiott, D. W. and Howell, R. D. (1971). Acute electron microscopic changes in myocardial cells induced by high doses of quinidine. *Toxic. appl. Pharmac.* **18**, 964

Hoffman, H. and Grigg, G. W. (1958). An electronmicroscopic study of mitochondria formation. *Exp. Cell Res.* **15**, 118

Hoppel, C. L. and Tandler, B. (1973). Biochemical effects of cuprizone on mouse liver and heart mitochondria. *Biochem. Pharmacol.* **22**, 2311

Horvath, E., Somogyi, A. and Kovacs, K. (1970). Histochemical study of the electrolyte-steroid-cardiopathy with necrosis (ESCN) in rats. *Cardiovasc. Res.* **4**, 355

Howatson, A. F. and Ham, A. W. (1957). The fine structure of cells. *Can. J. Biochem. Physiol.* **35**, 549

Hruban, Z., Swift, H. and Slesers, A. (1965). Effect of triparanol and diethanolamine on the fine structure of hepatocytes and pancreatic acinar cells. *Lab. Invest.* **14**, 1652

Hübner, G. (1965). Elektronenmikrokopische Untersuchungen zur Allylalkoholvergiftung der Mäuseleber. *Verh. deutsch. Ges. Path.* **49**, 256

Hübner, G., Paulussen, F. and Kleinsasser, O. (1967). Zur Feinstruktur und Genese der Onkocyten. *Virchows Arch. path. Anat. Physiol.* **343**, 34

Hübner, G., Klein, H. J., Kleinsasser, O. and Schiefer, H. G. (1971). Role of myoepithelial cells in the development of salivary gland tumors. *Cancer* **27**, 1255

Hug, G. and Schubert, W. K. (1970). Idiopathic cardiomyopathy. Mitochondrial and cytoplasmic alterations in heart and liver. *Lab. Invest.* **22**, 541

Hughson, M. and Balentine, J. D. (1974). Focal myocardial lesions in rats exposed to hyperbaric oxygen: light and ultrastructural observations. In *Fifth International Hyperbaric Conference*. Eds. by W. G. Trapp, E. Banister, A. Davison and P. Trapp, p. 685. British Columbia, Canada: Simson Fraser University

Hulsmann, W. C. (1962). Fatty acid synthesis in heart sarcosomes. *Biochim. biophys. Acta* **58**, 417

Hulsmann, W. C., Bethlem, J., Meijer, A. E. F. H., Fleury, P. and Schellens, J. P. M. (1967). Myopathy with abnormal structure and function of muscle mitochondria. *J. Neurol. Neurosurg. Psychiat.* **30**, 519

Ishikawa, T. and Pei, Y. F. (1965). Intramitochondrial glycogen particles in rat retinal receptor cells. *J. Cell Biol.* **25**, 402

Ishikawa, T. and Yamada, E. (1969). Atypical mitochondria in the ellipsoid of the photoreceptor cells of vertebrate retinas. *Invest. Ophthal.* **8**, 302

Itkonen, P. and Collan, Y. (1983). Mitochondrial flocculent densities in ischemia. Digestion experiments. *Acta Path. Microbiol. Immunol. (Scand). Sect. A.* **91**, 463

James, J. (1968). Feulgen-DNA changes in rat liver cell nuclei during the early phase of ischaemic necrosis. *Histochemie* **13**, 312

Jasmin, G. (1978). Ultrastructural patterns of Ni-induced crystalline inclusions in mitochondria of renal tubules. *Exp. Mol. Path.* **29**, 199

Jaworski R. C. (1984). Intramitochondrial paracrystalline inclusions in chondrosarcoma. *Pathology* **16**, 172

Jean, G., Lambertenghi, G. and Ranzi, T. (1968). Ultrastructural study of the liver in hepatic porphyria. *J. clin. Path.* **21**, 501

Jennings, R. B. and Ganote, C. E. (1974). Structural changes in myocardium during acute ischemia. *Circulation Res.* Suppl. III to **34** and **35**, 111–156

Jennings, R. B. and Ganote, C. E. (1976). Mitochondrial structure and function in acute myocardial ischemic injury. *Circulation Res.* Suppl. 1, **38**, 1–80

Jennings, R. B., Ganote, C. E. and Reimer, K. A. (1975). Ischemic tissue injury. *Am. J. Path.* **81**, 179

Jessen, H. (1968). The morphology and distribution of mitochondria in ameloblasts with special reference to a helix-containing type. *J. Ultrastruct. Res.* **22**, 120

Jézéquel, A. M. (1959). Dégénérescence myélinique des mitochondries de foie humain dans un épithélioma du cholédoque et un ictère viral. *J. Ultrastruct. Res.* **3**, 210

Jones, R. T. and Trump, B. F. (1975). Cellular and subcellular effects of ischemia on the pancreatic acinar cell. *Virchows Arch. B Cell Path.* **19**, 325

Kagawa, Y., Racker, E. and Hauser, R. E. (1966). Partial resolution of the enzymes catalyzing oxidative phosphorylation X: Correlation of morphology and function in submitochondrial particles. *J. Biol. Chem.* **241**, 2475

Kahng, M. W., Berezesky, I. K. and Trump, B. F. (1978). Metabolic and ultrastructural response of rat kidney cortex to *in vitro* ischemia. *Exp. Mol. Path.* **29**, 183

Kalyanaraman, U. P., Halmi, N. S. and Elwood, P. W. (1980). Prolactin-secreting pituitary oncocytoma with galactorrhea-amenorrhea syndrome. *Cancer* **46**, 1584

Karasaki, S. (1963). Studies on amphibian yolk. I. The ultrastructure of the yolk platelet. *J. Cell Biol.* **18**, 135

Karlsson, U. and Schultz, R. L. (1966). Fixation of the central nervous system for electron microscopy by aldehyde perfusion. III. Structural changes after exsanguination and delayed perfusion. *J. Ultrastruct. Res.* **14**, 47

Karnovsky, M. J. (1962). Mitochondrial changes and cytochrome oxidase in the frog nephron. In *Electron Microscopy*, Vol. 2, p. Q 9. Ed. by S. S. Breese, Jr. New York: Academic Press

Karnovsky, M. J. (1963). The fine structure of mitochondria in the frog nephron correlated with cytochrome oxidase activity. *Exp. Mol. Path.* **2**, 347

Kay, S. and Still, W. J. S. (1973). Electron microscopic observations on a parotid oncocytoma. *Arch. Path.* **96**, 186

Kerr, J. F. R. (1969). An electron-microscope study of liver cell necrosis due to heliotrine. *J. Path.* **97**, 557

Keyhani, E. (1969). Anomalies de structure de mitochondries dans un adénocarcinome rénal spontané de la souris. *Arch. Biol. (Liege)* **80**, 153

Kielley, R. K. (1952). Oxidative phosphorylation by mitochondria of transplantable mouse hepatoma and mouse liver. *Cancer Res.* **12**, 124

Kiessling, K. H. and Tobe, U. (1964). Degeneration of liver mitochondria in rats after prolonged alcohol consumption. *Exp. Cell Res.* **33**, 350

Kimberg, D. V., Loud, A. V. and Wiener, J. (1968). Cortisone-induced alterations in mitochondrial function and structure. *J. Cell Biol.* **37**, 63

Kjaerheim, A. (1967). Crystallized tubules in the mitochondrial matrix of adrenal cortical cells. *Exp. Cell Res.* **45**, 236

Koch, O. R., Porta, E. A. and Hartroft, W. S. (1968). A new experimental approach in the study of chronic alcoholism. III. Role of alcohol versus sucrose or fat-derived calories in hepatic damage. *Lab. Invest.* **18**, 379

Koch, O. R., Roatta de Conti, L. L., Bolanos, L. P. and Stoppani, A. O. M. (1978). Ultrastructural and biochemical aspects of liver mitochondria during recovery from ethanol-induced alterations. *Am. J. Path.* **90**, 325

Korman, E. F., Harris, R. A., Williams, C. H., Wakabayashi, T., Green, D. E. and Valdivia, E. (1970). Paracrystalline arrays in mitochondria. *Bioenergetics* **1**, 387

Kovacs, K. and Horvath, E. (1973). Pituitary 'Chromophobe' adenoma composed of oncocytes. *Arch. Path.* **95**, 235

Kovacs, K., Horvath, E. and Bilbao, J. M. (1974). Oncocytes in the anterior lobe of the human pituitary gland. A light and electron microscopic study. *Acta neuropath. (Berl.)* **27**, 43

Kraus, B. and Cain, H. (1975). Mitochondrienveränderungen des Tubulusepithels bei Wistarratten mit spontaner Nephropathie. *Virchows Arch. B Cell Path.* **19**, 179

Kraus, B. and Cain, H. (1980). Giant mitochondria in the human myocardium – morphogenesis and fate. *Virchows Arch. B Cell Path.* **33**, 77

Kuff, E. L. and Dalton, A. J. (1957). Identification of molecular ferritin in homogenates and sections of rat liver. *J. Ultrastruct. Res.* **1**, 62

Kumano, H. (1973). Light and electron microscopic observations on the liver cells after the ligation of the portal vein. *Hiroshima J. med. Sci.* **22**, 103

Kurosumi, K., Matsuzawa, T. and Watari, N. (1966). Mitochondrial inclusions in the snake renal tubules. *J. Ultrastruct. Res.* **16**, 269

Lafontaine, J. G. and Allard, C. (1964). A light and electron microscope study of the morphological changes induced in rat liver cells by the azo dye 2-ME-DAB. *J. Cell. Biol.* **22**, 143

Laguens, R. P. and Bianchi, N. (1963). Fine structure of the liver in human idiopathic diabetes mellitus. 1. Parenchymal cell mitochondria. *Exp. Mol. Path.* **2**, 203

Laguens, R. P., Lozada, B. B., Gomez-Dumm, C. L. and Beramendi, A. R. (1966). Effect of acute and exhaustive exercise upon the fine structure of heart mitochondria. *Experientia* **22**, 244

Laiho, K. U., Shelburne, J. D. and Trump, B. F. (1971). Observations on cell volume, ultrastructure, mitochondrial conformation and vital dye uptake in Ehrlich ascites tumor cells: effects of inhibiting energy production and function of the plasma membrane. *Am. J. Path.* **65**, 203

Lampert, P. W. (1967). A comparative electron microscopic study of reactive, degenerating, regenerating and dystrophic axons. *J. Neuropath. Exp. Neurol.* **26**, 345

Landis, W. J., Hauschka, B. T., Rogerson, C. A. and Glimcher, M. J. (1977). Electron microscopic observations of bone tissue prepared by ultracryomicrotomy. *J. Ultrastruct. Res.* **59**, 185

Landolt, A. M. and Oswald, U. W. (1973). Histology and ultrastructure of an oncocytic adenoma of the human pituitary. *Cancer* **31**, 1099–1105

Lanzavecchia, G. (1965). Structure and demolition of yolk in *Rana esculenta* L. *J. Ultrastruct. Res.* **12**, 147

Lanzavecchia, G. and Le Coultre, A. (1958). Origine dei mitocondri durante lo sviluppo embrionale di *Rana esculenta*. Studio al microscopio elettronico. *Arch. Ital. Anat. Embriol.* **63**, 447

Larizza, P. and Orlandi, F. (1964). Electron microscopic observations on bone marrow and liver tissue in non-hereditary refractory sideroblastic anemia. *Acta haemat.* **31**, 9

Larsen, J. H. (1968). Ultrastructure of thyroid follicle cells of three salamanders (*Amblystoma, Amphiuma and Necturus*) exhibiting varying degrees of neoteny. *J. Ultrastruct. Res.* **24**, 190

Leduc, E. H., Bernhard, W. and Tournier, P. (1966). Cyclic appearance of atypical mitochondria containing DNA fibers in cultures of an adenovirus-12-induced hamster tumor. *Exp. Cell Res.* **42**, 597

Lee, S. C. and Roth, L. M. (1976). Malignant oncocytoma of the parotid gland. *Cancer,* **37**, 1607

Leeson, C. R. and Leeson, T. S. (1969). Mitochondrial organization in skeletal muscle of the rat soft palate. *J. Anat.* **105**, 363

Lehninger, A. (1960). *Energy transformation in the cell.* Reprinted from Scientific American No. 69 (Published May 1960) San Francisco: W. H. Freeman & Co.

Lehninger, A. L. (1961). *How cells transform energy.* Reprinted from Scientific American No. 91 (Published September 1961, reprint 91) San Francisco: W. H. Freeman & Col.

Lehninger, A. L. (1962). Water uptake and extrusion by mitochondria in relation to oxidative phosphorylation. *Physiol. Rev.* **42**, 467

Lehninger, A. L. (1965). *The mitochondrion. Molecular basis of structure and function.* New York, Amsterdam: W. A. Benjamin Inc.

Lehninger, A. L. (1970a). *Biochemistry. The molecular basis of cell structure and function.* New York: Worth

Lehninger, A. L. (1970b). Mitochondria and calcium ion transport. *Biochem. J.* **119**, 129

Lehninger, A. L., Rossi, C. S. and Greenawalt, J. W. (1963). Respiration-dependent accumulation of inorganic phosphate and Ca^{++} by rat liver mitochondria. *Biochem. Biophys. Res. Comm.* **10**, 444

Lentz, T. L. (1966). Intramitochondrial glycogen granules in digestive cells of hydra. *J. Cell Biol.* **29**, 162

Lentz, T. L. (1971). *Cell Fine Structure.* Philadelphia, London and Toronto: Saunders

Lever, J. D. (1956). Physiologically induced changes in adrenocortical mitochondria. *J. biophys. biochem. Cytol.* **2**, Suppl. 313

Levine, G. D. (1972). Hibernoma. An electron microscopic study. *Human Path.* **3**, 351

Lieber, M. M., Tomera, K. M. and Farrow, G. M. (1981). Renal oncocytoma. *J. Urol* **125**, 481

Lin, H. S. (1965). Microcylinders within mitochondrial cristae in the rat pinealocyte. *J. Cell Biol.* **25**, 435

Linnane, A. W., Vitols, E. and Nowland, P. G. (1962). Studies on the origin of yeast mitochondria. *J. Cell Biol.* **13**, 345

Lozada, B. B. and Laguens, R. P. (1966). Hypoxia and the heart ultrastructure with special reference to the protective action of the coronary drug Persantin. *Cardiologia* **49**, Suppl., 1, 33

Luft, R., Ikkos, D., Palmieri, G., Ernster, L. and Afzelius, B. (1962). A case of severe hypermetabolism of non-thyroid origin with a defect in the maintenance of mitochondrial respiratory control: a correlated clinical, biochemical and morphological study. *J. clin. Invest.* **41**, 1776

Luse, S. (1961). Electron microscopic observations on the adrenal gland. In *The Adrenal Cortex,* Ed. by H. D. Moon, p. 46, New York: Hoeber

Lynn, J. A., Bailey, J. J., Willis, J. M. and Race, G. J. (1969). Hepatic ultrastructural variations in apparently 'normal' humans. *Lab. Invest.* Abstr. **20**, 594

McCallister, B. D. and Brown, A. L. (1965). A quantitative study of myocardial mitochondria in experimental cardiac hypertrophy. *Lab. Invest.* **14**, 692

McGavran, M. H. (1965). The ultrastructure of papillary cystadenoma lymphomatosum of the parotid gland. *Virchows Arch. Pathol. Anat.* **338**, 195

McGregor, D. H., Lotuaco, L. G. and Chu, L. L. H. (1978). Functioning oxyphil adenoma of parathyroid gland. An ultrastructural and biochemical study. *Am. J. Path.* **92**, 691

MacKay, B., Moloney, P. J. and Rix, D. B. (1968). The use of electron microscopy in renal preservation and perfusion. In *Organ Perfusion and Preservation,* p. 697. Ed. by J. C. Norman, J. Folkman, W. G. Hardison, L. E. Rudolf and F. J. Veith. New York: Appleton-Century-Crofts

McNutt, N. S. and Fawcett, D. W. (1969). The ultrastructure of the cat myocardium. II. Atrial muscle. *J. Cell Biol.* **42**, 46

Mair, W. G. P. and Tomé, F. M. S. (1972). *Atlas of the Ultrastructure of Diseased Human Muscle.* Edinburgh and London: Churchill Livingstone

Majno, G., La Gattuta, M. and Thompson, T. E. (1960). Cellular death and necrosis: chemical, physical and morphologic changes in rat liver. *Virchows Arch. Path. Anat.* **333**, 421

Maloff, B. L., Scordilis, S. P. and Tedeschi, H. (1978). Assays of the metabolic viability of single giant mitochondria. *J. Cell Biol.* **78**, 214

Mannweiler, K. L. and Bernhard, W. (1957). Recherches ultrastructurales sur une tumeur rénale experimentale du hamster. *J. Ultrastruct. Res.* **1**, 158

Maron, B. J. and Ferrans, V. J. (1978). Ultrastructural features of hypertrophied human ventricular myocardium. *Progress Cardiovasc. Dis.* **21**, 207

Marquart, K-H. (1978). Intracristale lineare Einschlusse in Mitochondrien menschlicher Rhabdomyom-zellen. *Virchows Archiv A.* **378**, 133

Marshall, R. B., Roberts, D. K. and Turner, R. A. (1967). Adenomas of the human parathyroid. Light and electron microscopic study following selenium 75 methionine scan. *Cancer* **20**, 512

Martinez-Manautou, J., Aznar-Ramos, R., Bautista-O'Farrill, J. and González-Angulo. A. (1970). The ultrastructure of liver cells in women under steroid therapy. II. Contraceptive therapy. *Acta Endocrinol.* **65**, 207

Massover, W. H. (1971). Intramitochondrial yolk-crystals of frog oocytes. II. Expulsion of intramitochondrial yolk-crystals to form single-membrane bound hexagonal crystalloids. *J. Ultrastruct. Res.* **36**, 603

Matsuba, K., Takizawa, T. and Thurlbeck, W. M. (1972). Oncocytes in human bronchial mucous glands. *Thorax* **27**, 181

Matthews, J. L., Martin, J. H., Arsenis, C., Eisenstein, R. and Kuettner, K. (1971). The role of the mitochondria in intracellular calcium regulation. In *Cellular Mechanisms for Calcium Transfer and Homeostasis,* p. 239. Ed. by G. Nichols and R. H. Wasserman. New York and London: Academic Press

Mazzocchi, G., Neri, G., Belloni, A. S., Robba, C. and Nussdorfer, G. G. (1977). Investigations on the turnover of adrenocortical mitochondria. XI. Effects of dexamethasone on the half-life of mitochondria from the rat zona fasciculata. *Beitr. Path.* **161**, 221

Mazzocchi, G., Robba, C., Neri, G., Gottardo, G. and Nussdorfer, G. G. (1976). Investigations on the turnover of adrenocortical mitochondria. V. An autoradiographic study of the radioactivity decay in the mitochondrial compartment from the adrenal cortex of 3H-Thymidine-injected rats. *Cell Tiss. Res.* **172**, 149

Meerson, F. Z., Zaletayeva, T. A., Lagutchev, S. S. and Pshennikova, M. G. (1964). Structure and mass of mitochondria in the process of compensatory hyperfunction and hypertrophy of the heart. *Exp. Cell Res.* **36**, 568

Mergner, W. J., Chang, S. H., Jones, R. T. and Trump, B. F. (1977). Microprobe analysis and fine structure of mitochondrial granules in ultrathin frozen sections of rat pancreas. *Exp. Cell Res.* **108**, 429

Meuten, D. J., Calderwood Mays, M. B., Dillman, R. C., Cooper, B. J., Valentine, B. A., Kuhajda, F. P. and Pass, D. A. (1985). Canine laryngeal rhabdomyoma. *Vet. Pathol.* **22**, 533

Michel-Bechet, M., Valenta, L. J. and Athouel-Haon, A. M. (1971). In *Further advances in thyroid research.* Ed. by K. Fellinger and R. Hofer. Wien: Vrlg. Wiener Med. Acad.

Minick, O. T., Kent, G., Orfei, E. and Volini, F. I. (1965). Non-membrane enclosed intramitochondrial dense bodies. *Expl. Molec. Path.* **4**, 311

Minio, F. and Gautier, A. (1967). L'ultrastructure du foie humain lors d'icteres idiopathiques chroniques. *Zeitschrift fur Zellforschung* **78**, 267

Mollin, D. L. and Hoffbrand, A. V. (1968). Sideroblastic anaemia. In *Recent Advances in Clinical Pathology,* p. 273. Ed. by S. C. Dyke. Edinburgh and London: Churchill Livingstone

Montisano, D. F. and James T. W. (1979). Mitochondrial morphology in yeast with and without mitochondrial DNA. *J. Ultrastruct. Res.* **67**, 288

Moore, D. H. and Ruska, H. (1957). Electron microscope study of mammalian cardiac muscle cells. *J. biophys. biochem. Cytol.* **3**, 261

Morales, R. and Duncan, D. (1971). Prismatic and other unusual arrays of mitochondrial cristae in astrocytes of cats and hamsters. *Anat. Rec.* **171**, 545

Morgan, A. J. (1979). Non-freezing techniques of preparing biological specimens for electron microprobe x-ray microanalysis. *Scan. Electron Microsc.* **11**, 635

Mugnaini, E. (1964a). Filamentous inclusions in the matrix of mitochondria from human livers. *J. Ultrastruct. Res.* **11**, 525

Mugnaini, E. (1964b). Helical filaments in astrocytic mitochondria of the *Corpus striatum* in the rat. *J. Cell Biol.* **23**, 173

Murdock, L. L., Cahill, M. A. and Reith, A. (1977). Morphometry and ultrastructure of prismatic cristae in mitochondria of a crayfish muscle. *J. Cell Biol.* **74**, 326

Murphy, Fergus and Ghadially, F. N. (1983). Case 3: Renal oncocytoma. *Ultrastruct. Path.* **5**, 285

Myagkaya, G., van Veen, H. and James, J. (1984). Ultrastructural changes in rat liver sinusoids during prolonged normothermic and hypothermic ischaemia *in vitro*. *Virchows Arch. B Cell Path.* **47**, 361

Myagkaya, G. L., van Veen, H. and James, J. (1985). Quantitative analysis of mitochondrial flocculent densities in rat hepatocytes during normothermic and hypothermic ischemia *in vitro*. *Virchows Arch. B Cell Path.* **49**, 61

Napolitano, L. and Fawcett, D. (1958). The fine structure of brown adipose tissue in the newborn mouse and rat. *J. biophys. biochem. Cytol.* **4**, 685

Nass, M. M. K. and Nass, S. (1963). Intramitochondrial fibers with DNA characteristics. I. Fixation and electron staining reactions. II. Enzymatic and other hydrolytic treatments. *J. Cell Biol.* **19**, 593

Nass, M. M. K., Nass, S. and Afzelius, B. A. (1965). The general occurrence of mitochondrial DNA. *Exp. Cell Res.* **37**, 516

Nathaniel, D. R. (1976). Helical inclusions and atypical cristae in the mitochondria of the rabbit thyroid gland. *J. Ultrastruct. Res.* **57**, 194

Nathaniel, D. R. (1978). Effect of gonadectomy on the follicular cell and inclusions in mitochondria of rabbit thyroid gland. *Am. J. Path.* **91**, 137

Nathaniel, D. R. (1980). Paracrystalline arrays in atypical cristae and mitochondrial division. *J. Cell Sci.* **42**, 23

Nesland, J. M., Sobrinho-Simões, M. A., Holm, R., Sambade, M. C. and Johannessen, J. V. (1985). Hurthle cell lesions of the thyroid: a combined study using transmission electron microscopy, scanning electron microscopy, and immunocytochemistry. *Ultrastruct. Path.* **8**, 269

Nevalainen, T. J. and Anttinen, J. (1977). Ultrastructural and functional changes in pancreatic acinar cells during autolysis. *Virchows Arch. B Cell Path.* **24**, 197

Newcomb, E. H., Steer, M. W., Hepler, P. K. and Wergin, W. P. (1968). An atypical crista resembling a 'tight junction' in bean root mitochondria. *J. Cell Biol.* **39**, 35

Nielsen, B. B. (1981). Oncocytic breast papilloma. *Virchows Arch. A (Path. Anat.)* **393**, 345

Norris, F. H. and Panner, B. J. (1966). Hypothyroid myopathy. *Arch. Neurol.* **14**, 574

Novikoff, A. B. (1961). Mitochondria (Chondriosomes). In *The Cell*, Vol. 2, p. 299. Ed. by J. Brachet and A. E. Mirsky. New York and London: Academic Press

Nunez, E. A., Greif, R. L. and Gershon, M. D. (1975). Paracrystalloids from mitochondria in thyroid follicular cells. Normal occurrence and experimental induction. *Lab. Invest.* **33**, 352

Nussdorfer, G. G. and Mazzochi, G. (1971). Effect of ACTH on mitochondrial RNA synthesis of rat adrenocortical cells. *Z. Zellforsch.* **118**, 35

Obara, T., Fujimoto, Y., Yamaguchi, K., Takanashi, R., Kino, I. and Sasaki, Y. (1985). Parathyroid carcinoma of the oxyphil cell type. *Cancer* **55**, 1482

Ogura, M. and Furuta, Y. (1957). A study of fixation for electron microscopy (on the effect of osmotic pressure). *Electron Microscopy* **5**, 15

Ollerich, D. A. (1968). An intramitochondrial crystalloid in element III of rat chorioallantoic placenta. *J. Cell Biol.* **37**, 188

Oschman, J. L. and Wall, B. J. (1972). Calcium binding to intestinal membranes. *J. Cell Biol.* **55**, 58

Osvaldo, L. and Latta, H. (1966). Interstitial cells of the renal medulla. *J. Ultrastruct. Rest.* **15**, 589

Palade, G. E. (1952). The fine structure of mitochondria. *Anat. Rec.* **114**, 427

Palade, G. E. (1953). An electron microscope study of the mitochondrial structure. *J. Histochem. Cytochem.* **1**, 188

Palade, G. E. (1959). In *Subcellular Particles*, p. 64. Ed. by T. Hagashi. New York: Roland Press

Palade, G. E. and Schidlowsky, G. (1958). Functional association of mitochondria and lipide inclusions. *Anat. Rec.* **130**, 352

Palay, S. L. (1956). Synapses in the central nervous system. *J. biophys. biochem. Cytol.* **2**, Suppl., 193

Pappas, G. D. and Brandt, P. W. (1959). Mitochondria. I. Fine structure of the complex patterns in the mitochondria of *Pelomyxa carolinensis* Wilson (*Chaos chaos* L.). *J. biophys. biochem. Cytol.* **6**, 85

Parry, E. W. and Ghadially, F. N. (1966). Ultrastructural changes in the liver of tumour-bearing rats during the terminal stages of life. *Cancer* **19**, 821

Paula-Barbosa, M. M., Tavares, M. A. and Borges, M. M. (1984). Mitochondrial abnormalities in cortical dendrites from patients with early forms of subacute sclerosing panencephalitis (SSPE). *Acta Neuropathol. (Berl.)* **63**, 117

Pavel, I., Bonaparte, H. and Petrovici, A. (1971). Involution of liver mitochondria in viral hepatitis. *Archs Path.* **91**, 294

Peachey, L. D. (1964). Electron microscopic observations on the accumulation of divalent cations in intramitochondrial granules. *J. Cell Biol.* **20**, 95

Pedersen, P. L., Greenawalt, J. W., Chan, T. L. and Morris, H., P. (1970). A comparison of some ultrastructural and biochemical properties of mitochondria from Morris hepatomas 9618A, 7800 and 3924A. *Cancer Res.* **30**, 2620

Pelosi, G. and Agliati, G. (1968). The heart muscle in functional overload and hypoxia. A biochemical and ultrastructural study. *Lab. Invest.* **18**, 86

Pena, C. E. (1980). Periodic units in the intracristal and envelope spaces of neuronal mitochondria. An artifact due to delayed fixation. *Acta Neuropathol. (Berl.)* **51,** 249

Penttila, A. and Ahonen, A. (1976). Electron microscopical and enzyme histochemical changes in the rat myocardium during prolonged autolysis. *Beitr. Path.* **157,** 126

Perez, V., Gorodisch, S., De Martire, J., Nicholson, R. and Dipaola, G. (1969). Oral contraceptives: Long-term use produces fine structural changes in liver mitochondria. *Science* **165,** 805

Personne, P. and Anderson, W. (1970). Localisation mitochondriale d'enzymes liées au metabolisme du glycogéne dans le spermatozoide de l'escargot. *J. Cell Biol.* **44,** 20

Personne, P. and André, J. (1964). Existence de glycogene mitochondrial dans le spermatozoide de la testacelle. *J. Microscopie* **3,** 643

Peter, J. B., Stempel, K. and Armstrong, J. (1970). Biochemistry and electron microscopy of mitochondria in muscular and neuromuscular diseases. In *Proceedings of the International Congress on Muscle Diseases.* Int. Congr. Ser. No. 199, p. 228. Ed. by J. N. Walton, N. Canal and G. Scarlato. Amsterdam: Excerpta Medica

Petersen. P. (1977). Glutaraldehyde fixation for electron microscopy of needle biopsies from human livers. *Acta path. microbiol. scand. Sect. A.* **85,** 373

Picheral, B. (1968). Les tissues elaborateurs d'hormones steroides chez les amphibiens urodeles. II. Aspects ultrastructuraux de la glande interrenale de *Salamandra salamandra* (L). Etude particuliére du glycogéne. *J. Microscopie* **7,** 907

Pihl, E., Rais, O. and Zeuchner, E. (1968). Functional and morphological liver changes in women taking oral contraceptives. *Acta Chir. Scand.* **134,** 639

Polack, F. M., Kanai, A. and Hood, C. I. (1971). Light and electron microscopic studies of orbital rhabdomyosarcoma. *Am. J. Ophthal.* **71,** 75

Porta, E. A., Hartroft, W. S. and de la Iglesia, F. A. (1965). Hepatic changes associated with chronic alcoholism in rats. *Lab. Invest.* **14,** 1437

Porta, E. A., Koch, O.R. and Hartroft, W. S. (1969). A new experimental approach in the study of chronic alcoholism. IV. Reproduction of alcoholic cirrhosis in rats and the role of lipotropes versus vitamins. *Lab. Invest.* **20,** 562

Porter, K. R. and Hogeboom, G. (1964). Addendum to paper by Peachey, L. D. (1964). Electron microscopic observations on the accumulation of divalent cations in intramitochondrial granules. *J. Cell Biol.* **20,** 109

Posalaky, Z. and McGinley, D. (1985). Plasmacytoma with oncocytic changes. *J. Submicrosc. Cytol.* **17,** 263

Price, H. M., Gordon, G. B., Munsat, T. L. and Pearson, C. M. (1967). Myopathy with atypical mitochondria in Type I skeletal muscle fibers. *J. Neuropath. exp. Neurol.* **26,** 475

Racela, A., Azarnoff, D. and Svoboda, D. (1969). Mitochondrial cavitation and hypertrophy in rat adrenal cortex due to aminoglutethimide. *Lab. Invest.* **21,** 52

Racker, E. (1968). The membrane of the mitochondrion. *Scientific American* **218,** 32 (Reprint 1101)

Racker, E. (Ed.) (1969). *Structure and Function of Membranes of Mitochondria and Chloroplasts.* New York: Reinhold

Radnot, M. and Lapis, K. (1970). Ultrastructure of the caruncular oncocytoma. *Ophthalmologica* **161,** 63

Reid, I. M., Donaldson, I. A. and Heitzman, R. J. (1978). Effects of anabolic steroids on liver cell ultrastructure in sheep. *Vet. Pathol.* **15,** 753

Remington, C. (1957). Connaissances recentes sur la biosynthese des porphyrines et de l'heme. *Revue Hémat.* **12,** 591

Reppart, J. T., Peters, R. L., Edmondson, H. A. and Baker, R. F. (1963). Electron and light microscopy of sclerosing hyaline necrosis of the liver. *Lab. Invest.* **12,** 1138

Revel, J. P., Fawcett, D. W. and Philpott, C. W. (1963). Observations on mitochondrial structure. Angular configurations of the cristae. *J. Cell Biol.* **16,** 187

Reynolds, E. S. (1960). Cellular localization of calcium deposition in liver of rat poisoned with carbon tetrachloride. *J. Histochem. Cytochem.* **8,** 331

Reynolds, E. S. (1963). The nature of calcium-associated electron-opaque masses in mitochondria of livers of carbon tetrachloride poisoned rats. *J. Cell Biol.* **19,** 58A

Rhodin, J. A. G. (1963). *An Atlas of Ultrastructure.* Philadelphia and London: Saunders

Richter, G. W. (1957). A study of hemosiderosis with the aid of electron microscopy. *J. Exp. Med.* **106,** 203

Rifkin, R. J. and Gahagan-Chase, P. A. (1970). Morphologic and biochemical effects of a chelating agent, α,α'-dipyridyl, on kidney and liver in rats. *Lab. Invest.* **23,** 480

Roberts, W. C. and Ferrans, V. J. (1975). Pathologic anatomy of the cardiomyopathies. Idiopathic dilated and hypertrophic types, infiltrative types and endomyocardial disease with and without eosinophilia. *Human Path.* **6,** 287

Rohr, H. P., Strebel, H., Henning, L. and Bianchi, L. (1970). Ultrastrukturell-morphometrische Untersuchungen, an der Rattenleberparenchymzelle in der Frühphase der Regeneration nach partieller Hepatektomie. *Beitr. path. Anat.* **141,** 52

Rohr, H. P., Wirz, A., Henning, L. C., Riede, U. N. and Bianchi, L. (1971). Morphometric analysis of the rat liver cell in the perinatal period. *Lab. Invest.* **24,** 128

Rosenbaum, R. M., Wittner, M. and Lenger, M. (1969). Mitochondrial and other ultrastructural changes in great alveolar cells of oxygen adapted and poisoned rats. *Lab. Invest.* **20,** 516

Ross, M. H. (1962). Electron microscopy of the human foetal adrenal cortex. In *The Human Adrenal Cortex*, p. 558. Ed. by A. R. Cumie, T. Symington and J. K. Grant. Edinburgh and London: Churchill Livingstone

Rouiller, C. (1957). Contribution de la microscopie électronique á l'étude du foie normal et pathologique. *Annls Anat. path.* **2,** 548

Rouiller, C. (1960). Physiological and pathological changes in mitochondrial morphology. *Int. Rev. Cytol.* **9,** 227

Rouiller, C. and Bernhard, W. (1956). Microbodies and the problem of mitochondrial regeneration in liver cells. *J. biophys. biochem. Cytol.* **2,** Suppl., 355

Rouiller, C. and Simon, G. (1962). Contribution de la microscopie electronique au progres de nos connaissances en cytologie et en histopathologie hepatique. *Revue int. Hépat.* **12,** 167

Roy, S. (1978). Ultrastructure of oncocytic adenoma of the human pituitary gland. *Acta neuropath. (Berl.)* **41,** 169

Sabatini, D. D., De Robertis, E. D. P. and Bleichmar, H. B. (1962). Submicroscopic study of the pituitary action on the adrenocortex of the rat. *Endocrinology* **70,** 390

Saetersdal, T. S., Myklebust, R., Berg Justesen, N. -P. and Engedal, H. (1977). Calcium containing particles in mitochondria of heart muscle cells as shown by cryo-ultramicrotomy and x-ray microanalysis. *Cell Tiss. Res.* **182,** 17

Saito, A. and Fleischer, S. (1971). Intramitochondrial tubules in adrenal glands of rat. *J. Ultrastruct. Res.* **35,** 642

Sandborn, E. B., Côté, M. G. and Viallet, A. (1966). Electron microscopy of a human liver in Weils' disease (*Leptospirosis icterohaemorrhagica*). *J. Path. Bact.* **92,** 369

Sano, S., Inoue, S., Tanabe, Y., Sumiya, C. and Koike, S. (1959). Significance of mitochondria for porphyrin and heme biosynthesis. *Science* **129,** 275

Saraiva, A. A., Borges, M. M., Madeira, M. D., Tavares, M. A. and Paula-Barbosa, M. M. (1985). Mitochondrial abnormalities in cortical dendrites from patients with Alzheimer's disease. *J. Submicrosc. Cytol.* **17,** 459

Scanarini, M. and Mingrino, S. (1974). Clinical, histological and ultrastructural observations upon the oncocytoma of the human pituitary gland. *J. Neurosurg. Sci* **18,** 263

Schaffner, F. and Felig, P. (1965). Changes in hepatic structure in rats produced by breathing pure oxygen. *J. Cell Biol.* **27,** 505

Schellens, J. P. M. and Ossentjuk, E. (1969). Mitochondrial ultrastructure with crystalloid inclusions in an unusual type of human myopathy. *Virchows Arch. B Zellpath.* **4,** 21

Schutta, H. S., Johnson, L. and Neville, H. E. (1970). Mitochondrial abnormalities in bilirubin-encephalopathy. *J. Neuropath. exp. Neurol.* **29,** 296

Seemayer, T. A., Knaack, J., Wang, N. -S. and Ahmed, M. N. (1975). On the ultrastructure of hibernoma. *Cancer* **36,** 1785

Seljelid, R. and Ericsson, J. L. E. (1965). An electronmicroscopic study of mitochondria in renal clear cell carcinoma. *J. Microscopie* **4,** 759

Seman, G. and Gallagher, H. S. (1979). Intramitochondrial rod-like inclusions in human breast tumors. *Anat Rec.* **194,** 267

Sevéus, L., Brdiczka, D. and Barnard, T. (1978). On the occurrence and composition of dense particles in mitochondria in ultrathin frozen dry sections. *Cell Biol. Int. Reports* **2,** 155

Shafiq, S. A., Milhorat, A. T. and Gorycki, M. A. (1967). Giant mitochondria in human muscle with inclusions. *Arch. Neurol.* **17,** 666

Shiraki, K. and Neustein, H. B. (1971). Intramitochondrial crystalloids and amorphous granules. Occurrence in experimental hepatic ischemia in dogs. *Archs Path.* **91,** 32

Shy, G. M., Gonatas, N. K. and Perez, M. (1966). Two childhood myopathies with abnormal mitochondria. I. Megaconial myopathy. II. Pleoconial myopathy. *Brain* **89,** 133

Siekevitz, P. (1957). *Powerhouse of the Cell.* Reprint from *Scientific American* (Reprint #36) July 1957. San Francisco: W. H. Freeman & Co.

Silver, M.M., Burns, J. E., Sethi, R. K. and Rowe, R. D. (1980). Oncocytic cardiomyopathy in an infant with oncocytosis in exocrine and endocrine glands. *Human Pathol.* **11,** 598

Sjostrand, F. S. (1956). The ultrastructure of cells as revealed by the electron microscope. *Int. Rev. Cytol.* **5,** 455

Skinnider, L. F. and Ghadially, F. N. (1975). Ultrastructure of acute myeloid leukaemia arising in multiple myeloma. *Human Path.* **6,** 379

Skobe, Z., Garant, P. R. and Albright, J. T. (1970). Ultrastructure of a new cell in the gills of the air-breathing fish *Helostoma temmincki. J. Ultrastruct. Res.* **31,** 312

Slautterback, D. B. (1961). The fine structure of shrew (*Blarina*) cardiac muscle. *Anat. Rec.* **139,** 274

Slautterback, D. B. (1965). Mitochondria in cardiac muscle cells of the canary and some other birds. *J. Cell Biol.* **24,** 1

Smallely, R. L. and Dryer, R. L. (1963). Brown fat: thermogenic effect during arousal from hibernation of the bat. *Science* **140,** 1333

Smith, D. S. (1961). The organization of the flight muscle in a dragonfly *Aeshna* Sp. *(Odonata). J. biophys. biochem. Cytol.* **11,** 119

Smith, D. S. (1963). The structure of flight muscle sarcosomes in the blowfly *Calliphora erythrocephala (Diptera). J. Cell Biol.* **19,** 115

Smith, R. E. and Hock, R. J. (1963). Brown fat: thermogenic effector of arousal in hibernators. *Science* **140,** 199

Smith, R. E. and Horwitz, B. A. (1969). Brown fat and thermogenesis. *Physiol. Rev.* **49,** 330

Sobrinho-Simões, M. A., Nesland, J. M., Holm, R., Sambade, M. C. and Johannessen, J. V. (1985). Hurthle cell and mitochondrion-rich papillary carcinomas of the thyroid gland: an ultrastructural and immunocytochemical study. *Ultrastruct. Path.* **8,** 131

Somlyo, A. V., Silcox, J. and Somlyo, A. P. (1975). Electron probe anaylsis and cryoultramicrotomy of cardiac muscle: Mitochondrial granules. *Proceedings of the Annual Meeting* — 33, p. 532. Electron Microscopy Society of America

Sordahl, L. A., Blailock, Z. R., Liebelt, A. G., Kraft, G. H. and Schwartz, A. (1969). Some ultrastructural and biochemical characteristics of tumor mitochondria isolated in albumin-containing media. *Cancer Res.* **29,** 2002

Sorenson, G. D. (1962). Electron microscopic observations of bone marrow from patients with sideroblastic anemia. *Am. J. Path.* **40,** 297

Spalke, G., Heene, R. and Herold, D. (1975). Mitochondrienveränderungen im Skeletmuskel bei neuraler Muskelatrophie (Charcot-Marie-Tooth). *J. Neurol.* **209,** 9

Spiro, A. J., Prineas, J. W. and Moore, C. L. (1970). A new mitochondrial myopathy in a patient with salt craving. *Archs Neurol., Chicago* **22,** 259

Spornitz, U. M. (1975). Studies of the liver of *Xenopus laevis.* 1. The ultrastructure of the parenchymal cell. *Anat. Embryol.* **146,** 245

Spycher, M. A. and Rüttner, J. R. (1968). Kristalloide Einschlüsse in menschilchen Lebermitochondrien. *Virchows Arch. Abt. B Zellpath.* **1,** 211

Stein, R. J., Ritcher, W. R. and Brynjolfsson, G. (1966). Ultrastructural pharmacopathology. I. Comparative morphology of the livers of the normal street dog and purebred beagle: a base-line study. *Expl Molec. Path.* **5,** 195

Stenger, R. J. and Spiro, D. (1961). The ultrastructure of mammalian cardiac muscle. *J. biophys. biochem. Cytol.* **9,** 325

Sternlieb, I. (1968). Mitochondrial and fatty changes in hepatocytes of patients with Wilson's disease. *Gastroenterology* **55,** 354

Stephens, R. J. and Bils, R.F. (1965). An atypical mitochondrial form in normal rat liver. *J. Cell Biol.* **24,** 500

Suganuma, Y. and Yamamoto, H. (1980). Occurrence, composition and structure of mitochondrial crystals in a hypotrichous ciliate. *J. Ultrastruct. Res.* **70,** 21

Sulkin, N. M. and Sulkin, D. (1962). Mitochondrial alterations in liver cells following vitamin E deficiency. In *Proceedings of the Fifth international Congress for Electron Microscopy*, Vol. 2, p. vv-8. Ed. by S. S. Breese. New York: Academic Press

Sulkin, D. F. and Sulkin, N. M. (1967). An electron microscopic study of autonomic ganglion of guinea pigs during ascorbic acid deficiency and partial inanition. *Lab. Invest.* **16,** 142

Sun, C. N., Dhalla, N. S. and Olson, R. E. (1969). Formation of gigantic mitochondria in hypoxic isolated perfused rat hearts. *Experientia* **25,** 763

Sun, C. N., White, H. J. and Thompson, B. W. (1975). Oncocytoma (mitochondrioma) of the parotid gland. An electron microscopical study. *Arch. Path.* **99,** 208

Sun, C. N., White, H. J. and Thompson, B. W. (1976). Warthin's tumor of the parotid gland. An electron microscopic study. *Exp. Path. Bd.* **12,** 269

Sun, S. C., Sohal, R. S., Colcolough, H. L. and Burch, G. E. (1968). Histochemical and electron microscopic studies of the effects of reserpine on the heart muscle of mice. *J. Pharmac. exp. Ther.* **161,** 210

Suter, E. R. (1969). The fine structure of brown adipose tissue. II. Perinatal development in the rat. *Lab. invest.* **21,** 246

Suter, E. R. (1969). The fine structure of brown adipose tissue. III. The effect of cold exposure and its mediation in newborn rats. *Lab. Invest.* **21,** 259

Suter, E. R. and Staubli, W. (1970). An ultrastructural histochemical study of brown adipose tissue from neonatal rats. *J. Histochem. Cytochem.* **18,** 100

Sutfin, L. V., Holtrop, M. E. and Ogilvie, R. E. (1971). Microanalysis of individual mitochondrial granules with diameters less than 1000 Angstroms. *Science* **174,** 947

Suzuki, K. (1969). Giant hepatic mitochondria: production in mice fed with cuprizone. *Science* **163,** 81

Suzuki. T. and Mostofi, F. K. (1967). Intramitochondrial filamentous bodies in the thick limb of Henle of the rat kidney. *J. Cell Biol.* **33,** 605

Svoboda, D. J. and Higginson, J. (1963). Ultrastructural hepatic changes in rats on a necrogenic diet. *Am. J. Path.* **43,** 477

Svoboda, D. J. and Higginson, J. (1964). Ultrastructural changes produced by protein and related deficiencies in the rat liver. *Am. J. Path.* **45,** 353

Svoboda, D. J. and Manning, R. T. (1964). Chronic alcoholism with fatty metamorphosis of the liver — mitochondrial alterations in hepatic cells. *Am. J. Path.* **44,** 645

Svoboda, D. J., Grady, H. and Higginson, J. (1966). The effect of chronic protein deficiency in rats. II. Biochemical and ultrastructural changes. *Lab. Invest.* **15,** 731

Swenson, O., Grana, L., Inouye, T. *et al.* (1967). Immediate and long-term effects of acute hepatic ischemia. *Archs Surg., Chicago* **95,** 451

Swick, R. W., Rexroth, A. K. and Stange, J. L. (1968). The dynamic state of rat liver mitochondria. *Fed. Proc.* **27,** p. 462 (Abstract No. 1379)

Taira, K. (1979). Studies on intramitochondrial inclusions on the pancreatic acinar cells of the Japanese newt, *Triturus pyrrogaster.* 1. Occurrence of intramitochondrial inclusions with long-term starvation. *J. Ultrastruct. Res.* **67,** 89

Takeda, A., Matsuyama, M., Sugimoto, Y., Suzumori, K., Ishiwata, T., Ishida, S. and Nakanishi, Y. (1983). Oncocytic adenocarcinoma of the ovary. *Virchows Arch. Path. Anat.* **399,** 345

Tanaka, Y. (1967). Iron-laden mitochondria in reticulum cells of hypersiderotic human bone marrows. *Blood* **29,** 747

Tandler, B. (1966a). Fine structure of oncocytes in human salivary glands. *Virchows Arch. A Path. Anat.* **341,** 317

Tandler, B. (1966b). Warthin's tumor. *Arch. Otolaryng.* **84,** 68

Tandler, B. and Hoppel, C. L. (1972). *Mitochondria.* New York, London: Academic Press

Tandler, B. and Hoppel, C. L. (1974). Ultrastructural effects of dietary galactoflavin on mouse hepatocytes. *Exp. Molec. Path.* **21,** 88

Tandler, B. and Shipkey, F. H. (1964). Ultrastructure of Warthin's Tumor. 1. Mitochondria. *J. Ultrastruct. Res.* **11,** 292

Tandler, B. and Erlandson, R. A. (1983). Giant mitochondria in a pleomorphic adenoma of the submandibular gland. *Ultrastruct. Path.* **4,** 85

Tandler, B., Erlandson, R. A. and Wynder, E. L. (1968). Riboflavin and mouse hepatic cell structure and function. 1. Ultrastructural alterations in simple deficiency. *Am. J. Clin. Path.* **52,** 69

Tandler, B. Erlandson, R. A., Smith, A. L. and Wynder, E. L. (1969). Riboflavin and mouse hepatic cell structure and function. II. Division of mitochondria during recovery from simple deficiency. *J. Cell Biol.* **41,** 477

Tandler, B., Hutter, R. V. P. and Erlandson, R. A. (1970). Ultrastructure of oncocytoma of the parotid gland. *Lab. Invest.* **23,** 567

Tani, E., Ametani, T., Higashi, N. and Fugihara, E. (1971). Atypical cristae in mitochondria of human glioblastoma multiforme cells. *J. Ultrastruct. Res.* **36,** 211

Thiery, J. P. and Caroli, J. (1962). Etude comparative en microscopie electronique de l'amylose hepatique primaire humaine et de l'amylose experimentale de la souris. *Revue int. Hépat.* **12,** 207

Threadgold, L. T. and Lasker, R. (1967). Mitochondrogenesis in integumentary cells of the larval sardine (*Sardinops caerulea*). *J. Ultrastruct. Res.* **19,** 238

Tonietti, G., Baschieri, L. and Salabe, G. (1967). Papillary and micro-follicular carcinoma of human thyroid. An ultrastructural study. *Archs Path.* **84,** 601

Trump, B. F. and Bulger, R. E. (1967). Studies of cellular injury in isolated flounder tubules. I. Correlation between morphology and function of control tubules and observations of autophagocytosis and mechanical cell damage. *Lab. Invest.* **16,** 453

Trump, B. F. and Bulger, R. E. (1968). Studies of cellular injury in isolated flounder tubules. III. Light microscopic and functional chnages due to cyanide. *Lab. Invest.* **18,** 721

Trump, B. F. and Ginn, F. L. (1968). Studies of cellular injury in isolated flounder tubules. II. Cellular swelling in high potassium media. *Lab. Invest.* **18,** 341

Trump, B. F., Berezesky, I. K. and Cowley, R. A. (1982). The cellular and subcellular characteristics of acute and chronic injury with emphasis on the role of calcium. In *Pathophysiology of Shock, Anoxia and Ischemia*, Chapter 1. Ed. by R. A. Cowley and B. F. Trump. Baltimore: Williams and Wilkins

Trump, B. F., Goldblatt, P. J. and Stowell, R. E. (1965a). Studies on necrosis of mouse liver *in vitro*: ultrastructural alterations in the mitochondria of hepatic parenchymal cells. *Lab. Invest.* **14,** 343

Trump, B. F., Goldblatt, P. J. and Stowell, R. E. (1965b). Studies on necrosis *in vitro* of mouse hepatic parenchymal cell. Ultrastructural alterations in endoplasmic reticulum Golgi apparatus, plasma membrane and lipid droplets. *Lab. Invest.* **14,** 2000

Trump, B. F., Berezesky, I. K., Jiji, R. M., Mergner, W. J. and Bulger, R. E. (1978). Energy dispersive x-ray microanalysis of mitochondrial deposits in sideroblastic anemia. *Lab. Invest.* **39,** 375

Valenta, L. J., Michel-Bechet, M., Warshaw, J. B. and Maloof, F. (1974). Human thyroid tumors composed of mitochondrion-rich cells: Electron microscopic and biochemical findings. *J. clin. endocrin. Metab.* **39,** 719

Van Haelst, U. and Bergstein, N. (1970). Electron microscopic study of the liver in so-called idiopathic jaundice of late pregnancy. *Path. europ.* **5,** 198

Vodovar, N., Desnoyers, F., Cluzan, R. and Levillain, R. (1977). Pathologie ultrastructurale des mitochondries des cellules myocardiques de Porc, induite par les lipides alimentaires. *Biologie Cellulaire* **29,** 37

Voelz, H. (1968). Structural comparison between intramitochondrial and bacterial crystalloids. *J. Ultrastruct. Res.* **25,** 29

Volk, T. L. and Scarpelli, D. G. (1966). Mitochondrial gigantism in the adrenal cortex following hypophysectomy. *Lab. Invest.* **15,** 707

Wachstein, M. and Besen, M. (1964). Electron microscopy of renal coagulative necrosis due to *dl*-serine, with special reference to mitochondrial pyknosis. *Am. J. Path.* **44,** 383

Wakabayashi, T., Smoly, J. M., Hatase, O. and Green, D. E. (1971). A lattice structure in beef heart mitochondria induced by phosphotungstic acid. *Bioenergetics* **2,** 167

Wakabayashi, T., Asano, M. and Kawamoto, S. (1979). Induction of megamitochondria in the mouse liver by isonicotinic acid derivatives. *Exp. Mol. Path.* **31,** 387

Walker, S. M. and Schrodt, G. R. (1966). Evidence for connections between mitochondria and the sarcoplasmic reticulum and evidence for glycogen granules within the sarcoplasmic reticulum. *Am. J. Phys. Med.* **45,** 25

Walker, S. M., Schrodt, G. R., Truong, X. T. and Wall, E. J. (1965). Evidence for structural connections between mitochondria and intermediate elements of triads. *Am. J. phys. Med.* **44,** 26

Warberg, O. (1956). The metabolism of tumors (English translation), London 1930. *Science* **123,** 309

Warberg, O. (1962). Uber die fakultative de anaerobiose de krebszellen und ihre amuedung auf die chemotherapie. In *On Cancer and Hormones. Essays in Experimental Biology*, p.29. Chicago: University of Chicago Press

Ward, R. T. (1962). The origin of protein and fatty yolk in *Rana pipiens*. II. Electron microscopical and cytochemical observations of young and mature oocytes. *J. Cell Biol.* **14,** 309

Watrach, A. M. (1964). Degeneration of mitochondria in lead poisoning. *J. Ultrastruct. Res.* **10,** 177

Watson, M. L. (1952). University of Rochester (New York) Atomic Energy Project, unclassified report. U. R. 185

Wendel, P. -O. and Barnard, T. (1974). A cytochemical approach to the lipid composition of mitochondrial matrix granules in brown adipose tissue and liver. *J. Histochem. Cytochem.* **22,** 1028

Wiener, J., Loud, A. V., Kimberg, D. V. and Spiro, D. (1968). A quantitative description of cortisone-induced alterations in the ultrastructure of rat liver parenchymal cells. *J. Cell Biol.* **37,** 47

Wilcken, D. E. L., Brender, D., Shorey, C. D. and MacDonald, G. J. (1967). Reserpine: effect on structure of heart muscle. *Science* **157,** 1332

Wills, E. J. (1965). Crystalline structures in the mitochondria of normal human liver parenchymal cells. *J. Cell Biol.* **24,** 511

Wills, E. J. (1968). Acute infective hepatitis. *Arch. Path.* **86,** 184

Wilson, J. E. and Dove, J. L. (1965). Turnover of mitochondria in rat liver, kidney and heart. *J. Elisha Mitchell Sci Soc.* **81,** 21

Wiseman, G. and Ghadially, F. N. (1958). A biochemical concept of tumour growth infiltration and cachexia. *Br. med. J.* **2,** 18

Wolff, H. H., Balda, B. R., Birkmayer, G. D. and Braun-Falco, O. (1971). Zur Ultrastruktur des Hamster-Melanoms A Mel 3 von Fortner. *Arch. Derm. Forsch.* **240,** 192

Wollenberger, A. and Schulze, W. (1961). Mitochondrial alterations in the myocardium of dogs with aortic stenosis. *J. biophys. biochem. Cytol.* **10,** 285

Wrigglesworth, J. M. and Packer, L. (1968). Optical rotary dispersion and circular dichroism studies on mitochondria: correlation of ultrastructure and metabolic state with molecular conformational changes. *Archs Biochem. Biophys.* **128,** 790

Yamada, E. (1959). A crystalline body found in the rod inner segment of the frog's eye. *J. biophys. biochem. Cytol.* **6**, 517

Yamamoto, T., Ebe, T. and Kobayashi, S. (1969). Intramitochondrial inclusions in various cells of a snake. *Elaphae quadrivirgata. Z. Zellforsch.* **99**, 252

Yamamoto, E., Wittner, M. and Rosenbaum, R. M. (1970). Resistance and susceptibility to oxygen toxicity by cell types of the gas-blood barrier of the rat lung. *Am. J. Path.* **59**, 409

Yamauchi, H., Mittmann, U., Geisen, H. P. and Salzer, M. (1982). Postischemic liver damage in rats: amino acid analysis and morphometric studies. *Tohoku J. Exp. Med.* **138**, 49

Yoshida, Y., Tenzaki, T., Ishiguro, T., Kawanami, D. and Ohshima, M. (1984). Oncocytoma of the ovary: Light and electron microscopic study. *Cynecologic Oncol.* **18**, 109

Yotsuyanagi, Y. (1959). Etude au microscope electronique des coupes ultra-fines de la levure. *Compt. Rend.* **248**, 274

Youson, J. H. (1971). Prismatic cristae and matrix granules in mitochondria of the kidneys of ammocoetes. *J. Cell Biol.* **48**, 189

Zacks, S. I. and Sheff, M. F. (1964). Studies on tetanus toxin. I. Formation of intramitochondrial dense granules in mice acutely poisoned with tetanus toxin. *J. Neuropath. exp. Neurol.* **23**, 306

Zacks, S. I., Hall, J. A. S. and Sheff, M. F. (1966). Studies on tetanus. IV. Intramitochondrial dense granules in skeletal muscle from human cases of tetanus intoxication. *Am. J. Path.* **48**, 811

Zaimis, E., Papadaki, I., Ash, A. S. F., Larbi, E., Kakari, S., Matthew, M. and Paradelis, A. (1969). Cardiovascular effects of thyroxine. *Cardiovasc. Res.* **3**, 118

Zak, R. and Rabinowitz, M. (1973). Metabolism of the ischemic heart. *Med. clins N. Am.* **57**, 93

Zelander, T. (1959). Ultrastructure of the mouse adrenal cortex. An electron microscopical study in intact and hydrocortisone-treated male adults. *J. Ultrastruct. Res.* Suppl. **2**, 1

Golgi complex and secretory granules

Introduction

In 1898 Golgi reported the occurrence of a new organelle in nerve cells. He called it 'appareil réticulaire interne' ('internal reticular apparatus'), but later workers dropped this appellation and adopted the term 'Golgi apparatus'. This term has also lost favour now; today the organelle is more frequently referred to as the 'Golgi complex'.

Heated controversy raged for many years regarding the existence of this organelle in living cells, for the chief way in which it could be convincingly demonstrated was in tissues fixed for prolonged periods in solutions containing silver or osmium. It became clear that most cells contained an area of cytoplasm which could reduce silver and osmium salts, but whether this indicated the presence of a specific organelle in the living cell was doubted. With ordinary light microscopy it is, as a rule, not demonstrable in the living cell, nor can it be unequivocally demonstrated in routine histological preparations in most cell types. (For a critique on this old controversy, *see* Bensley, 1951 and Dalton, 1961.) However, it should be noted that in cells with a well developed Golgi complex a 'negative image' of the Golgi complex is discernible as a clear area in the juxtanuclear position. A well-known example of this is the 'Hof', seen as a clear crescentric area adjacent to the nucleus of the plasma cell.

With the advent of phase-contrast microscopy, some of the doubts regarding the existence of this organelle in the living cell were removed, but the controversy was not truly settled until, with the electron microscope, Dalton and Felix (1954a, b) demonstrated that the silver or osmium deposits produced in the cell by the classic methods were associated with a membranous organelle of characteristic morphology.

In ultrathin sections the Golgi complex presents as stacks of flattened 'sacs' or 'saccules' (it is not customary to refer to these as 'cisternae' even though most of them are no doubt cisternae) and associated vacuoles and vesicles. Like the smooth endoplasmic reticulum, it is composed of smooth membrane, but as a rule it can be distinguished from the former because of the characteristic organization of its elements. Regions of specialization exist within this organelle, for with silver and osmium impregnation methods only the outer stacks (the forming face) show the characteristic 'staining'; no amount of prolonged fixation will stain all the elements of the Golgi complex. When thick sections through such preparations are examined with the high voltage electron microscope it is found that the outermost 'saccule' and some of the 'vesicles' of the forming face actually consist of a tubular polygonal network which is in keeping with Golgi's original description and the term he adopted 'appareil réticulaire interne' (Rambourg *et al.*, 1973).

Numerous studies have now shown that in many cells which produce a protein-rich secretion, the contents of the rough endoplasmic reticulum are transported to the Golgi where they are condensed, modified and packaged to form secretory granules (*Plate 143*). In cells that secrete glyoproteins, much of the carbohydrate component is added to the protein (derived from the rough endoplasmic reticulum) in the Golgi complex. Sulphation of glycosaminogly-cans (mucopolysaccharides) also occurs in this organelle. Other roles of the Golgi include packaging of hydrolytic enzymes to form primary lysosomes and the repair and replenishment of the cell membrane and the glycoprotein coat of cells. The latter process is believed to be achieved by vacuoles arising from the Golgi which fuse with the cell membrane and discharge their contents on to the cell surface. The Golgi complex is also believed to be involved in the production of melanosomes (Chapter 9) and rod-shaped microtubulated bodies (Chapter 10). It is also involved in lipid and lipoprotein transport and secretion in certain cell types.

Secretory granules of various endocrine and exocrine cells show many variations in size and fine structure which among other things reflect the chemical composition of the secretory product they contain. For example, the contents of mucous granules are usually flocculent and electron-lucent, while zymogen granules are as a rule homogeneously electron-dense. The insulin-containing secretory granule of the beta cell of the pancreatic islet is characterized by the presence of a crystal or crystals in its interior.

It follows then that one should be able to identify the type of secretory cell by the type of secretory granule it contains. This is a point of value in the differential diagnosis of adenomas and adenocarcinomas where quite often secretory granules of a morphology similar to the cell of origin occur (Ghadially, 1985).

It behoves us then to be cognizant of the morphology of various secretory granules and the variations engendered in them by pathological (including neoplastic) states. Much of the latter part of this chapter is devoted to such matters. The secretory granules selected for inclusion in this text are mainly those of value in the differential diagnosis of tumours.

Plate 143

Mucus-secreting cell from human bronchial mucosa, showing a large Golgi complex comprising stacks of flattened sacs (S) and numerous vacuoles and vesicles. Current concepts regarding the manner in which secretory granules containing mucin (a glycoprotein which with water forms mucus) are made is illustrated with the aid of this electron micrograph. The protein part of the glycoprotein is synthesized from the amino acids by the polyribosomes of the rough endoplasmic reticulum, and travel along its cisternae (A). Some sugars may be added to the protein at this stage. Intermediate or transport vesicles containing the newly synthesized material bud off (B) from the margins of the cisternae and coalesce with the saccules of the Golgi complex. The completion of synthesis is achieved in the Golgi complex by the addition of other sugars and the fully formed glycoprotein then emerges as single-membrane-bound granules (at times called droplets) by a process of budding from the Golgi stacks (C). In merocrine glands the secretory granules (D) then travel to the apex of the cell where the membrane bounding the granule fuses with the cell membrane prior to discharge of its contents. Thus at no stage is the cell cytoplasm exposed to the exterior during merocrine secretion. × 23 000

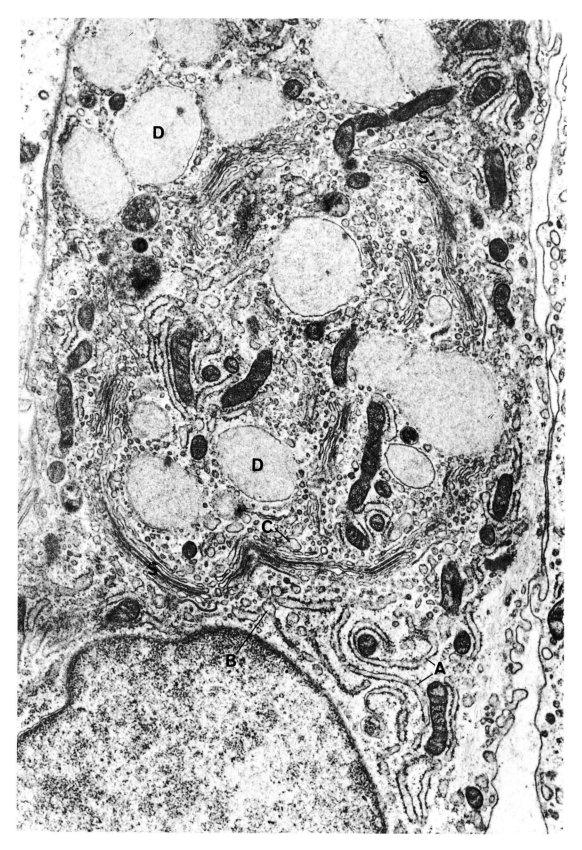

Structure and function

Although the Golgi complex is a pleomorphic organelle which shows some variations in morphology and distribution within various cell types, there is also a distinctiveness about its membranous formations which clearly allows its identification and establishes it as an organelle in its own right (*Plates 143–147*).

The Golgi complex is composed of three basic elements, the most characteristic part being a stack of flattened sacs the ends of which are often slightly dilated. The stack of sacs is occasionally straight but more often is slightly or markedly curved (*Plates 143* and *144*). On the convex or outer face of the stack (at times referred to also as the forming face or immature face) lie numerous vesicles. There is ample evidence now that these vesicles arise by a process of budding from the endoplasmic reticulum and bring with them not only products made in this organelle for processing and packing in the Golgi complex but also add to the pool of Golgi complex membranes. On the inner or concave face (at times referred to as the mature or maturing face) of the stack are vacuoles of various dimensions containing secretory material which has been condensed and packaged and is leaving the Golgi complex.

The packaging of material into vacuoles involves the utilization of membranes from the Golgi stacks. This, however, is continually replenished by the membranes derived from the small vesicles (called 'intermediate vesicles') migrating from the endoplasmic reticulum to the Golgi complex. The alternative idea that the secretory products from the endoplasmic reticulum flow via 'permanent' connections between this organelle and the Golgi sacs is difficult to support on available evidence. Since ribosomes are essential for protein synthesis and the Golgi complex is composed only of smooth membranes, the most logical site for new membrane formation must be the rough endoplasmic reticulum, and one can therefore argue that the ultimate source of the Golgi membranes is also likely to be derived from this structure.

The above description depicts the basic unit of the Golgi complex and the probable mode of turnover of its components. More often than not, several such Golgi units of curved packets of flattened sacs and associated vesicles and vacuoles are seen arranged in a circular, oval, crescentic or cup-shaped configuration within the cytoplasm of a variety of cells (*Plates 143* and *144*). It would appear that the system of peripherally placed stacks is the equivalent of the 'dictyosome' of light microscopists, while the centrally placed vacuoles with the secretory contents correspond to the 'archoplasm'. In keeping with general practice, I have avoided using the perfectly appropriate term 'cisternae' for the flattened sacs of the Golgi complex. The reason for such reluctance is not clear but perhaps this attitude stems from a desire to avoid confusion with the cisternae of the rough endoplasmic reticulum.

The circular or oval configuration of the Golgi complex mentioned above is characteristic of many but not all cell types. In others the stacks appear somewhat randomly distributed, and at times groups of stacks with their associated vacuoles and vesicles placed quite far apart in the cytoplasm may be found in a cell (*Plate 145*). In such cases (particularly in pathological tissues) one is left wondering whether there are two or more Golgi complexes present or whether continuity between the two systems would be demonstrable by serial sectioning.

The Golgi complex generally occupies a juxtanuclear position. In secretory epithelia the position of the complex is in the juxtanuclear cytoplasm facing the apical portion of the cell. In hepatocytes the Golgi complex is usually represented by only a few rather slightly curved stacks adjacent to the cell membrane. Occasionally, however, it is seen extending from the nucleus to

---

Plate 144

A zone 3 chondrocyte from articular cartilage of a nine-month-old rabbit showing characteristic glycogen deposits (G), intracytoplasmic filaments (F) and cell processes (P) extending into the matrix. The well developed Golgi complex shows many stacks and secretory vacuoles (V), the contents of which are remarkably similar in appearance to the cartilage matrix. × 31 000 (*From Ghadially and Roy, 1969*)

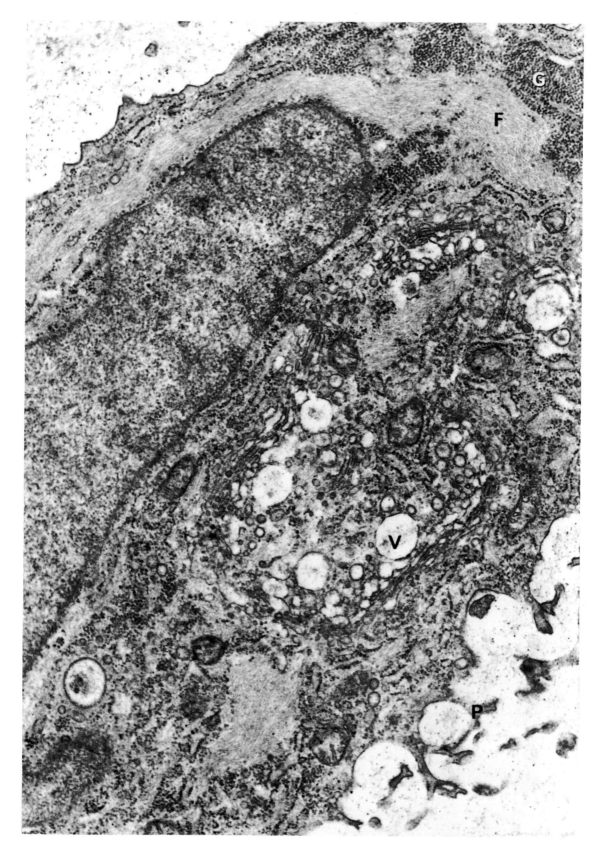

the cell membrane. In neurons the Golgi complex is quite diffuse and its components have a perinuclear distribution.

Although in most cells the Golgi complex is located in the apical portion of the cell (in the juxtanuclear zone), there are instances in which this organelle occupies the basal part of the cell (*see* the review by Kirkman and Severinghaus, 1938), and examples have also been cited where the Golgi shifts from one pole of the cell to the other. Thus in ameloblasts the Golgi complex migrates from the apical to the basal pole prior to the production of the enamel matrix (Jasswoin, 1924; Beams and King, 1933). Two similar shifts in the position of the Golgi have also been noted to occur during the development of the chick corneal epithelium. The first is related to the formation of the primary corneal stroma and the second shift occurs when Bowman's membrane is forming beneath the epithelium (Trelstad, 1970).

The functions of the Golgi complex are many and varied. Its involvement in secretory processes had long been suspected by light microscopists, because of the prominence of this organelle in such cells and the presence of secretory droplets in the Golgi region. Thus, on the basis of such observation, in 1914 Cajal had already envisaged that in the goblet cells of intestinal epithelium mucus was synthesized within the Golgi complex. The remarkable clarity with which some light microscopists saw the involvement of the Golgi complex in secretory activity is demonstrated in a review by Bowen (1929) who wrote, 'Secretion is in essence a phenomenon of "granule" or droplet formation. Starting with a single such secretory droplet about to be expelled from the cell, we find it possible to trace its origin step by step to a minute vacuole, which has thus from the beginning served as a segregation centre for a specific secretion material. The primordial vacuole is found to arise in that zone of the cell characterized by the presence of the Golgi apparatus, and the evidence indicates, if it does not demonstrate, that the primary vacuole arises through the activity of the Golgi substance and undergoes a part at least of its development in contact with, or embedded in, the Golgi apparatus'.

A series of studies employing electron microscopic, cytochemical and autoradiographic techniques have now established beyond doubt that the Golgi complex is involved in the production of virtually every exocrine and endocrine secretion. A few examples to illustrate this will now be considered, together with the techniques used in elucidating the function of the Golgi complex.

The first study of this kind was on the exocrine cells of the pancreas where, by using radioactive amino acids, it was shown that the newly formed labelled protein appears first in the rough endoplasmic reticulum and is then transported to the Golgi where it is packaged to form secretory granules. However, in most proteinaceous secretions the protein is combined with carbohydrate, to form glycoproteins. The question then arose as to where the carbohydrate component was added to the protein. The presence of glycoprotein in the Golgi complex had long been demonstrated by histochemical methods, but it was the work of Leblond and his colleagues (Peterson and Leblond, 1964; Neutra and Leblond, 1966a, b) which convincingly demonstrated that it is the Golgi saccule where certain carbohydrates are added to the protein to form glycoprotein. These authors injected glucose-^{3}H into rats and found that the Golgi

---

Plate 145

Fig. 1. Type A cell from human synovial membrane, showing Golgi stacks (G), vacuoles containing secretory material (V) and mitochondria (M). The scant rough endoplasmic reticulum and ribosomes lying free in the cytoplasm are barely discernible. × 25 000 (*From Ghadially and Roy, 1969*)

Fig. 2. Type A cell from rat synovial membrane, showing mitochondria (M) and sparse rough endoplasmic reticulum (R). A characteristic feature of the synovial cells of this species is the occurrence of numerous rather large secretory vacuoles which contain electron-lucent material surrounded by some medium–density material and a few electron-dense granules. A gradation in size of the vacuoles (A, B and C) is seen stemming from the Golgi region (G) to the cell surface which lay just beyond the top edge of the picture. × 26 000 (*From Roy and Ghadially, 1967a*)

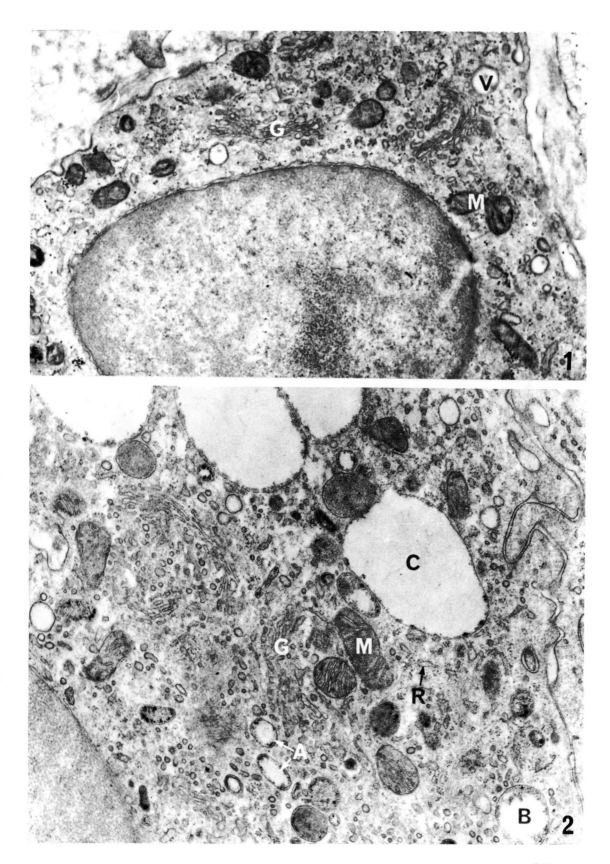

saccules of the goblet cells in the large intestine were labelled within 15 minutes. At 20 minutes the newly formed radioactive glycoprotein began to appear in the mucous droplets and by 40 minutes almost all the radioactive glycoprotein had migrated from the Golgi to the collection of mucous droplets in the goblet cells.

However, it is worth noting that the Golgi complex is not the sole site of uptake and coupling of sugars to protein (see review by Rambourg, 1971). For example, while tritiated mannose is taken up primarily by the Golgi complex of intestinal epithelial cells (Ito, 1969), in thyroid follicular cells its primary site of incorporation is the rough endoplasmic reticulum (Whur et al., 1969). Similarly, in plasma cells the autoradiographic reaction following the administration of tritiated glucosamine is first seen in the rough endoplasmic reticulum (Zagury et al., 1970).

Further interesting insights into the function of the Golgi complex spring from studies on cartilage and synovial membrane. The matrix of cartilage comprises a collagenous framework within which is entrapped the ground substance or interfibrillary matrix rich in water and proteoglycans (known previously as protein-polysaccharides or chondromucoproteins). These macromolecules are constructed of a protein core to which a large number of glycosaminoglycan chains (chondroitin sulphate and keratan sulphate previously referred to collectively as mucopolysaccharides or sulphated mucopolysaccharides) are attached laterally. It would appear that the core protein is first synthesized by the polyribosomes of the rough endoplasmic reticulum and that the linkage region sugars are also mainly added in this region of the cell. Elongation of the chains and sulphation of the molecule occurs mainly in the Golgi complex (Horwitz and Dorfman, 1968).

Chondroitin sulphate and keratan sulphate are the two main glycosaminoglycans found in cartilage (a small amount of hyaluronic acid is also present). In contrast to chondroitin sulphate synthesis, little is known about the synthesis of keratan sulphate which has a slow rate of turnover.

The uptake of ^{35}S-sulphate into chondroctyes either in vivo or in vitro (Plate 146) has been used as an indicator of the synthesis of chondroitin sulphate (and hence of proteoglycan synthesis) (Dziewiatkowski, 1951; Bostrom and Aquist, 1952; Adams and Rienits, 1961). Electron microscopic observations on the autoradiographic localization of ^{35}S-sulphate in chondrocytes has shown (Fewer et al., 1964; Godman and Lane, 1964) that the radiosulphate is first localized mainly in the Golgi complex. Later the radioactivity is seen over large Golgi-derived secretory vacuoles, which then seem to migrate to the surface and discharge their contents into the matrix (Plate 146). Such experiments indicate that sulphation occurs in the Golgi complex. This has been confirmed by later studies (Martinez et al., 1977) but it would appear that some sulphotransferase activity is present also in the rough endoplasmic reticulum where the process of sulphation probably commences.

Plate 146

Fig. 1. Electron micrograph of an autoradiogram of a pair of chondrocytes 20 minutes after presentation of radiosulphate, illustrating the concentration of the grains over the vacuolated Golgi regions. × 18 500 (*From Godman and Lane, 1964*)

Fig. 2. Electron micrograph of an autoradiogram of a chondrocyte 19 hours after presentation of radiosulphate. The grains now overlie the large smooth-walled vacuoles, some of which (arrows) seem to be in the process of discharging their contents into the matrix. Many other grains, presumably discharged at an earlier stage, are also seen in the matrix. × 21 000 (*From Godman and Lane, 1964*)

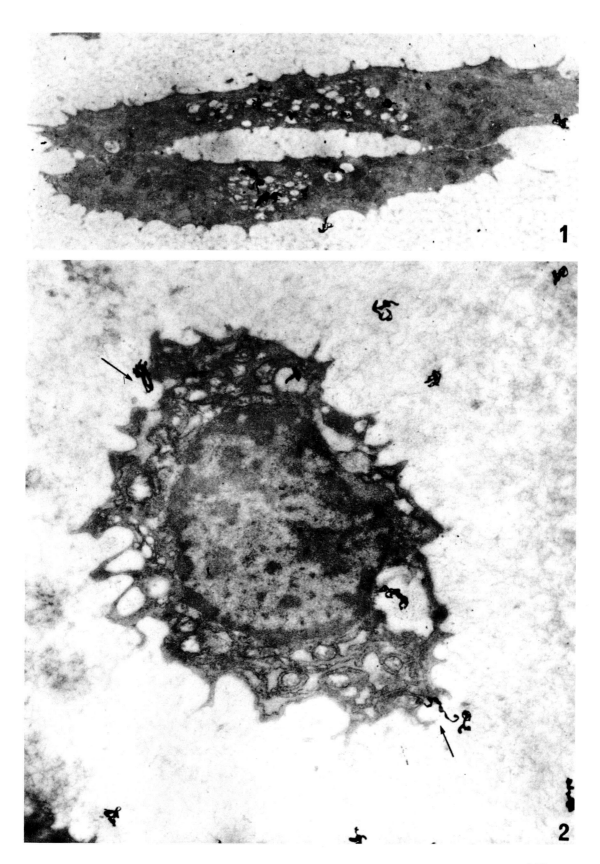

In the synovial membrane there is a somewhat different situation, for the glycosaminoglycan produced by the synovial intimal cells (i.e. hyaluronic acid) and poured into the joint cavity as a part of the synovial fluid is not sulphated. Virtually all of it occurs free (that is to say, not bound to protein) but a minute amount may be bound to protein (Hamerman and Sandson, 1963).

Thus here we have a tissue which produces much free glycosaminoglycan and the morphology of the synovial intima seems to reflect how this is accomplished. In the synovial intima of all species studied to date two main cell types have been found: one called type A cell, which contains abundant Golgi elements and numerous vacuoles and vesicles but little rough endoplasmic reticulum (*Plate 145*) and another called the type B cell, which contains abundant rough endoplasmic reticulum but in which the Golgi complex by comparison is poorly represented, and vacuoles and vesicles are scanty (*Plate 181* in Chapter 6). Intermediate forms also occur, clearly indicating that type A and B cells are not distinct cell lines but variants whose morphology reflects the kind of functional activity they are engaged in at a given moment.

In view of what is known about the functions of the rough endoplasmic reticulum and Golgi complex, one may surmise that type A cells which have little or no rough endoplasmic reticulum for export protein synthesis but well developed Golgi complexes for polysaccharide synthesis, produce the hyaluronic acid of the synovial fluid; indeed this material has been demonstrated within the Golgi complex and secretory vacuoles by colloidal iron staining and enzyme digestion (Roy and Ghadially, 1967b) (*Plate 147*). Much has been made of the role of type A cells in the removal of material from joints, while its role in the production of hyaluronic acid seems to have been largely overlooked; yet phagocytosed material is found in both cell types (at times more in type B than type A cells) and there is no reason to suppose that the type A cells of the synovial intima are devoted solely to scavenging activity (Ghadially, 1978, 1980, 1983).

There are very few anatomic sites where a substantial pool of free hyaluronic acid is found. One such site is the joint cavity and another the vitreus of the eye. In the cortical layer of the vitreus is found a homogeneous population of cells called 'hyalocytes' which are thought to produce the ground substances (hyaluronic acid) of the vitreus and to have macrophage-like properties (Hogan *et al.*, 1971; Grabner *et al.*, 1980). The hyalocytes bear a remarkable resemblance to type A synovial cells, in that they have virtually no rough endoplasmic reticulum, a well-developed Golgi complex and some vesicles, vacuoles and lysosomes. One may therefore, with some justification speculate that a cell type of characteristic morphology (e.g. hyalocyte and type A cell) adapted to produce large amounts of hyaluronic acid occur in these sites. On the other hand, in sites where smaller amounts of hyaluronic acid occur, such as various connective tissues, it is the fibroblast (well endowed with rough endoplasmic reticulum and Golgi complex) which produces hyaluronic acid.

Plate 147

The illustrations on this plate show the results obtained with the colloidal iron technique for localizing glycosaminoglycans (hyaluronic acid) in synovial cells. Osmium-fixed tissue was treated with colloidal iron and embedded in araldite. Sections were not stained. The black granular iron deposit is located at sites where glycosaminoglycan is present. In tissues pre-treated with hyaluronidase such deposits were not seen (*From Roy and Ghadially, 1967b*)

Fig. 1. Normal rabbit synovial membrane, showing deposits of electron-dense iron particles on the surface of the synovial cell (S) facing the joint cavity (J). A large number of electron-dense particles can be seen localized in a large smooth-walled vacuole (V). A less intense but still fairly distinct localization of dense particles is seen in smaller vacuoles and vesicles (v). Dense particles can also been seen localized in the matrix (M) between the synovial cells. × 37 000

Fig. 2. Normal rabbit type A synovial cell, showing iron particles localized in Golgi vesicles (G) and a large smooth-walled vacuole (V). × 61 000

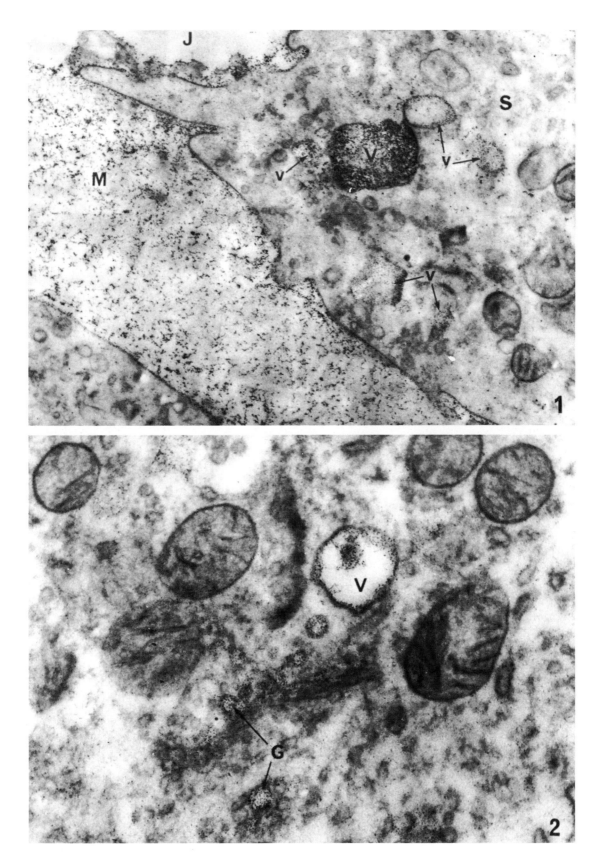

Golgi complex in cell differentiation and neoplasia

The Golgi complex is a specialized structure which performs many functions. Its activity may therefore be looked upon as an expression of cellular differentiation and fuctional maturity of the cell. In keeping with this is the oft-made observation that immature cells or undifferentiated cells (i.e. stem cells or blast cells) have a poorly developed Golgi complex as compared to their normal mature counterparts. Similarly, fast-growing cells such as cells in tissue culture and anaplastic tumour cells, where the accent is on growth and multiplication rather than on differentiation and function, also tend to have a poorly developed Golgi complex.

Exceptions or apparent exceptions to such generalization are also easily found. Thus, in the erythroid series of cells, all organelles including the Golgi complex (which is not too prominent to begin with) are lost in the mature red blood cell. Similarly, in the mature granulocytes the Golgi complex is small or hard to find because once the various granules are formed, the Golgi complex disappears or becomes markedly atrophic.

Light microscopic studies on tumours (Ludford, 1929, 1952; Severinghaus, 1937; Dalton and Edwards, 1942; Bothe et al., 1950) have shown many variations in size and distribution of the Golgi complex but none that can be considered specific for the neoplastic state. Electron microscopic studies have done little besides confirm and clarify these findings (Haguenau and Lacour, 1955; Haguenau and Bernhard, 1955; Howatson and Ham, 1955, 1957; Dalton and Felix, 1956; Selby et al., 1956; Suzuki, 1957; Epstein, 1957a, b; Dalton, 1959, 1961; Oberling and Bernhard, 1961; Bernhard, 1969).

From a review of the literature and personal observations on human tumours and tumours of experimental animals, the following tentative conclusions are drawn: (1) in fast-growing anaplastic tumours the Golgi complex is almost invariably poorly developed or difficult to identify; (2) there is a rough correlation between the degree of differentiation and the size of the Golgi complex in a given tumour type, the less differentiated tumours having poorer Golgi complexes; (3) relatively well differentiated malignant tumours and benign tumours usually have a well developed Golgi complex if the parent tissue of origin is also well endowed in this respect; and (4) marked hypertrophy, dilatation and distortion of the Golgi complex are, at times, found in some tumours.

We (Ghadially and Parry, 1966) have seen hypertrophy, dilatation and distortion of Golgi complexes in a human hepatoma (*Plate 148*) and such changes have also been reported by other workers in some examples of: (1) mouse and rat hepatomas (Dalton and Edwards, 1942; Bothe et al., 1950; Dalton, 1961, 1964); (2) Rous sarcoma (Bernhard, 1969); and (3) experimentally produced pituitary adenomas (Severinghaus, 1937). It must, however, be stressed that as a general rule tumours are poorly endowed with Golgi complexes as compared to their cell of origin.

Most of the above-mentioned variations are easily reconciled with our concepts of cell differentiation and function on the one hand and the anaplasia and loss or impairment of functional ability in the tumour cell on the other. The marked hypertrophy of Golgi complexes seen in some tumours is also not particularly surprising because excessive production of secretory materials is, at times, a feature of some tumours.

Plate 148

Figs. 1–3. Examples of hypertrophy, dilatation and distortion of Golgi complexes found in a singularly well differentiated human hepatoma. × 38 000; × 17 000; × 25 000 (*Fig. 1, from Ghadially and Parry, 1966; Figs. 2 and 3, Ghadially and Parry, unpublished electron micrographs*)

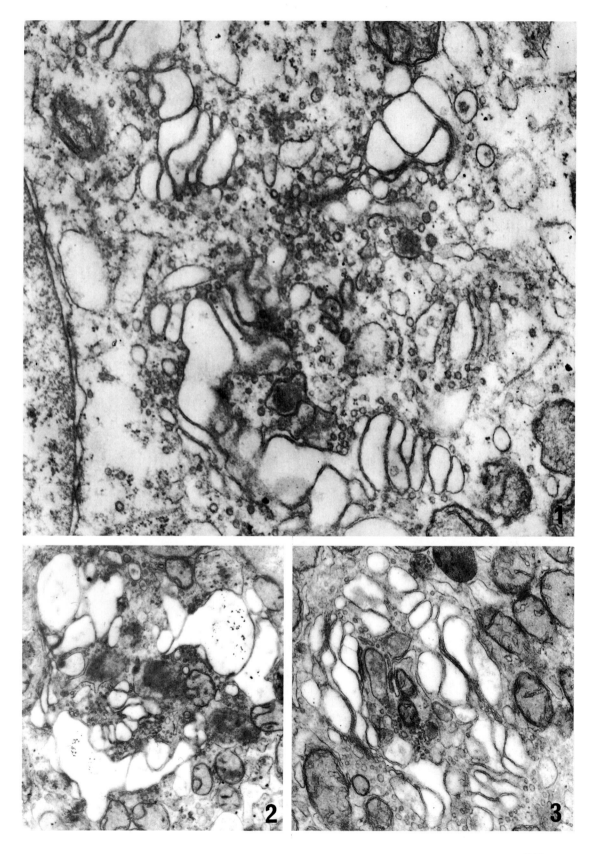

Hypertrophy and atrophy of Golgi complex

A variety of changes have been reported to occur in the Golgi complex in normal and pathological tissues. Such differences can be accounted for in terms of cell differentiation (already dealt with on page 340), physiological activity and pathological or toxic influences. The changes themselves comprise: (1) hypertrophy or atrophy of the Golgi complex; (2) dilatation or collapse of the Golgi elements; (3) changes in intracellular positions of the Golgi complex (page 334); and (4) quantitative and/or qualitative differences in the contents of the Golgi complex (page 344). So frequent are reports of slight alterations of Golgi complex morphology and contents that they cannot all be cited here; however, a few examples will be quoted which illustrate the significance of such changes.

Hypertrophy of the Golgi elements (i.e. stacks, vesicles and vacuoles), evidenced by an increase in the number of Golgi units (i.e. a set of stacks and associated vacuoles and vesicles) or by multiple Golgi complexes occupying larger areas of the cell cytoplasm, can usually be correlated with an increased secretory activity (i.e work hypertrophy) or a compensatory hypertrophy (i.e. secondary to atrophy or malfunction in adjacent cells). Thus, during experimentally induced adrenal cortical regeneration in the rat there is a remarkable hypertrophy of the Golgi complexes in the ACTH-secreting cells of the adenohypophysis, presumably reflecting the increased synthesis of ACTH which ensues. When adrenal regeneration is nearing completion and the ACTH level falls, the Golgi complex is restored to normal size (Nakayama *et al.*, 1969). After the injection of papain there is a depletion of matrix from the rabbit ear cartilage and the ears become floppy. During the subsequent phase of restoration of the matrix and recovery of the ears to an erect position the activity synthesizing chondrocytes show a remarkable Golgi hypertrophy (Sheldon and Robinson, 1960; Sheldon and Kimball, 1962).

Marked atrophy or destruction and the disappearance of recognizable Golgi elements have been noted to occur in various situations; for example, in enucleate *Amoeba proteus* (Flickinger, 1970) where a suppression of lipoprotein synthesis necessary for the formation and maintenance of membranes may be responsible. In cases of osteoarthritis (Roy, 1967; Ghadially and Roy, 1969) marked atrophy of Golgi complexes is seen in many synovial intimal cells. This is evidenced by a smaller cell area being occupied by the organelle and by the small size and number of stacks and vesicles (*Plate 149*). In some neighbouring cells, however, there were a large number of Golgi units and a singularly large number of associated vesicles which occupied quite large areas of the cytoplasm. Nevertheless, in both instances, vacuoles containing secretory material were hard to find (*Plate 149*). Thus the appearance seen here suggests an attempt at compensatory hypertrophy in response to atrophy of this organelle in adjacent cells. Such changes are in keeping with the reduced amount of hyaluronic acid known to occur in the synovial fluid from osteoarthritic joints (Decker *et al.*, 1959; Castor *et al.*, 1966).

Atrophic changes and destruction and the disappearance of Golgi elements have also been noted in hepatocytes subject to a variety of toxic influences. In such instances the disturbance of lipoprotein synthesis and secretion which occurs is reflected also by alterations of the Golgi complex and endoplasmic reticulum contents (pages 344 and 526).

Plate 149

Synovial cells from an osteoarthritic human joint.
Fig. 1. A synovial cell showing a markedly atrophic Golgi complex. × 42 000 (*From Roy, 1967*)
Fig. 2. A synovial cell showing Golgi stacks and an unusually large number of associated vesicles. × 39 000 (*From Ghadially and Roy, 1969*)

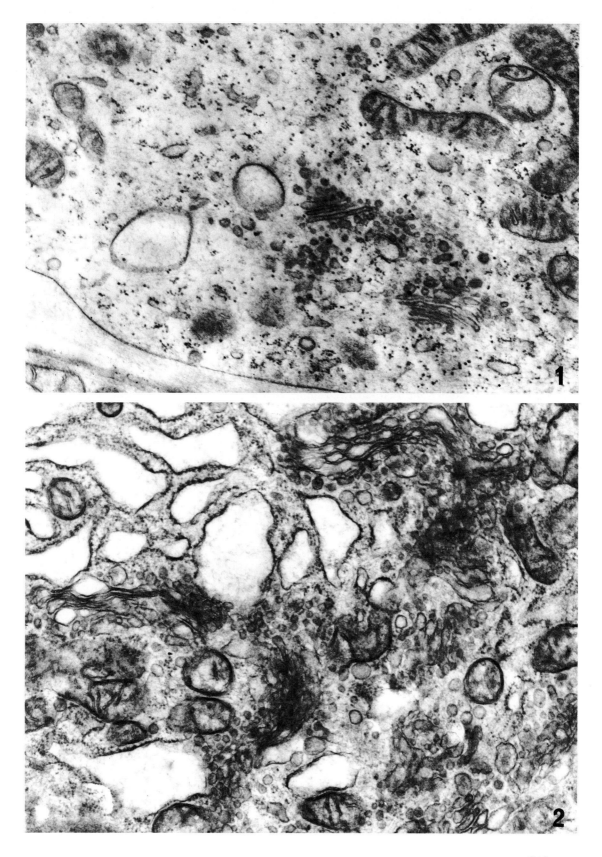

1

2

343

Lipid and lipoprotein in Golgi complex

In certain cell types the Golgi complex has frequently been implicated in the transport and secretion of lipid and/or lipoproteins. The best-known example of this is the Golgi complex of rat hepatocytes where electron microscopists have long noted the occurrence of occasional electron-dense 'granules' (80–100 nm diameter) (*Plate 150, Fig. 1*). In animals such as the rabbit, where the lipid is saturated, electron-lucent 'granules' occur instead of electron-dense ones. It is now clear that such granules (both electron-lucent and electron-dense varities) comprise very low-density lipoproteins. It would appear that such a difference in electron density between the very low-density lipoproteins reflects the saturated and unsaturated fatty acid content of the lipid in the diet and, hence, the lipoprotein.

Although the precise sites at which the steps in lipoprotein synthesis occur are debatable, the bulk of the evidence suggests that the synthesis occurs in the endoplasmic reticulum. The material is probably modified in the Golgi complex and then transported and secreted into the space of Disse and ultimately the blood stream.

A variety of hepatotoxic agents and experimental situations which ultimately produce a fatty liver also produce an increase in the size and number of lipid droplets in the endoplasmic reticulum. Such membrane-bound droplets are called liposomes, and the manner in which they are formed is dealt with later*. In such situations, however, alterations in the lipid or lipoprotein contents within the Golgi complex are also noted. For example, Reynolds (1963) has reported that 30 minutes after the administration of carbon tetrachloride to rats the Golgi complex is transformed into a cluster of dilated vacuoles devoid of coarse electron-dense particles. It is said that in rat livers perfused with free fatty acid for 90 minutes a few hepatocytes accumulate liposomes and that such cells appear to 'lack an organized system of membranes recognizable as the Golgi region' (Hamilton *et al.*, 1966, 1967). Similarly, in rat livers after administration of a choline-deficient diet (Amick and Stenger, 1964; Estes and Lombardi, 1969), puromycin (Jones *et al.*, 1967) and orotic acid (Jatlow *et al.*, 1965) disrupted or dilated particle-free Golgi complexes are found.

In the liver of cortisone-treated rabbits (*Plate 150, Fig. 2*), Mahley *et al.* (1968) found that by two days typical Golgi complexes were extremely rare or hard to find but by four to six days there was a dramatic increase in Golgi complexes containing electron-lucent particles. On the basis of their observation and a review of the literature they concluded that '(1) the appearance of liposomes in and near the hepatocyte Golgi apparatus is indicative of a degree of impaired very low density lipoprotein synthesis and/or secretion which, if not reversed, can lead to widespread accumulation of liposomes and development of fatty liver; and (2) that disappearance of typical Golgi apparatus, or Golgi apparatus devoid of any lipid particles, is indicative of a major or prolonged block in very low density lipoprotein synthesis and/or secretion'.

---

*The occurrence of lipid in endoplasmic reticulum is dealt with later (page 526). This topic is so closely linked with the subject dealt with here that it is recommended that both essays are read conjointly.

Plate 150

Fig. 1. Numerous electron-dense granules, representing very low-density lipoproteins, are seen in Golgi vacuoles (arrows). From a normal suckling rat hepatocyte. × 29 000

Fig. 2. Numerous electron-lucent particles, representing very low-density lipoproteins, are seen in Golgi vacuoles (arrows). From a cortisone-treated rabbit hepatocyte. × 52 000 (*From Mahley, Gray, Hamilton and Lequire, 1968*)

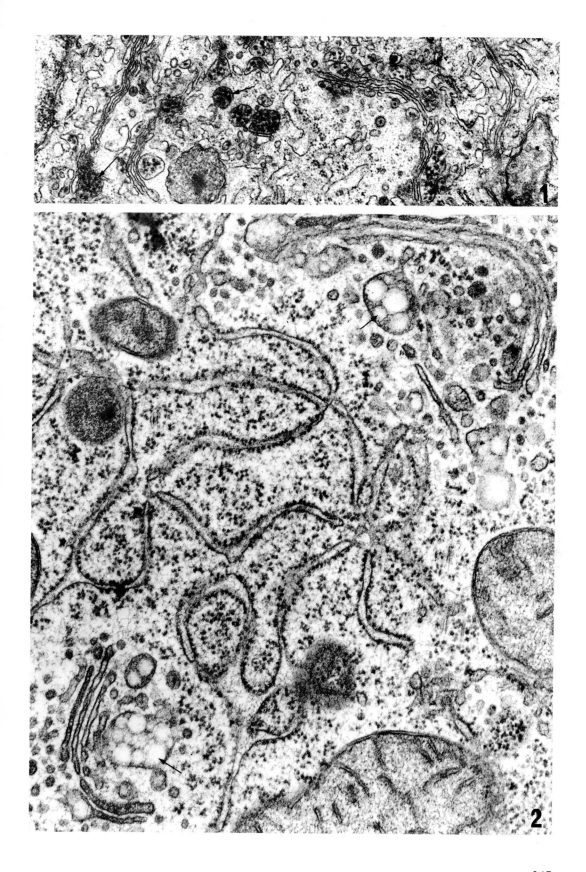

It is now well established that fatty acid esterification occurs in the endoplasmic reticulum of many cell types (Stein and Shapiro, 1959; Hultin, 1961; Tzur and Shapiro, 1964) and that during uptake of lipid, osmiophilic or non-osmiophilic lipid may be demonstrated in this system and also often in the Golgi complex. Perhaps the model studied most extensively here is the intestinal epithelial cell (see Plate 236 in Chapter 6) where, during lipid transport, lipid may be demonstrated both in the endoplasmic reticulum and in the Golgi complex (Palay and Karlin, 1959; Onoe and Ohno, 1963; Fawcett, 1966)★. The concept that emerges from these studies and studies on lipid uptake by various other tissues such as adipose, mammary, hepatic, cartilage, cardiac and skeletal muscle (Stein and Stein, 1967a, b; Ghadially et al., 1970; Scow, 1970; Mehta and Ghadially, 1973; Ghadially, 1983) is that, although some cells (Kajihara, et al., 1975) can pick up lipid droplets directly by a process of pinocytosis or micropinocytosis (e.g. Kupffer cells and polymorphonuclear neutrophils), generally and in the majority of instances the lipid is first hydrolysed and the fatty acids are then picked up by the cell (or diffuse through the cell membrane). The fatty acids are then re-esterified to triglycerides in the endoplasmic reticulum and at a later stage of the process lipid appears in the Golgi complex.

An example of this is seen in the chondrocytes of articular cartilage, where a few lipid droplets normally occur in the cytoplasm (Collins et al., 1965, Ghadially et al., 1965). In the rabbit, depot lipid is well saturated and hence usually presents in the chondrocytes and elsewhere as electron-lucent material. In this animal, if a lipid rich in unsaturated fatty acid (e.g. corn oil) is injected into the joint, electron-dense material (presumably lipidic in nature) soon appears in the Golgi complex and large osmiophilic lipid droplets accumulate in the cytoplasm (Mehta and Ghadially, 1973). On the other hand, if autologous fat (obtained from the omentum) rich in saturated fatty acids is injected into the joint, the Golgi complex becomes distended with lucent material and numerous electron-lucent lipid droplets are found in the cytoplasm (Ghadially et al., 1970) (Plate 151). Besides the lipid in the Golgi complex, elongated electron-lucent areas were sometimes found in the cisternae of the rough endoplasmic reticulum, in the perinuclear cisternae and apparently lying free in the cytoplasm. It would therefore appear that resynthesis of the lipid was probably occurring within the endoplasmic reticulum.

A question that arises is whether the chondrocytes pick up both the fatty acids and glycerol and reunite these to form lipid or whether only the fatty acid is taken into the cell and esterified by endogenously produced glycerol. The latter suggestion appears to be correct for light microscopic autoradiographic studies (Sprinz and Stockwell, 1976) show that numerous silver grains are located over fat-laden chondrocytes after intra-articular injection of trioleate which has been labelled in the fatty acid moiety of the molecule but not following injection of glyceryl-labelled trioleate. Thus, it would appear that after hydrolysis the labelled glycerol moiety is not picked up by the chondrocyte.

★It is interesting to recall that a long while ago light microscopic studies had led Cramer and Ludford (1925) to conclude that the Golgi complex was in some way concerned with resynthesis of fat during intestinal lipid absorption.

Plate 151

Fig. 1. Chondrocyte from articular cartilage of a rabbit after the injection of corn oil into the joint. Electron-dense lipidic droplets are seen within Golgi vacuoles (arrow). Similar but larger electron-dense lipid droplets found in the cytoplasm are illustrated in *Plate 412.* × 27 000 (*From Mehta and Ghadially, 1973*)

Fig. 2. Chondrocyte from articular cartilage of a rabbit after the injection of autologous lipid into the joint, showing a large round electron-lucent lipid droplet (L). The contents of the dilated Golgi complex (G) are remarkably electron lucent and resemble the lipid droplet in the cytoplasm. × 31 000 (*From Ghadially, Mehta and Kirkaldy-Willis, 1970*)

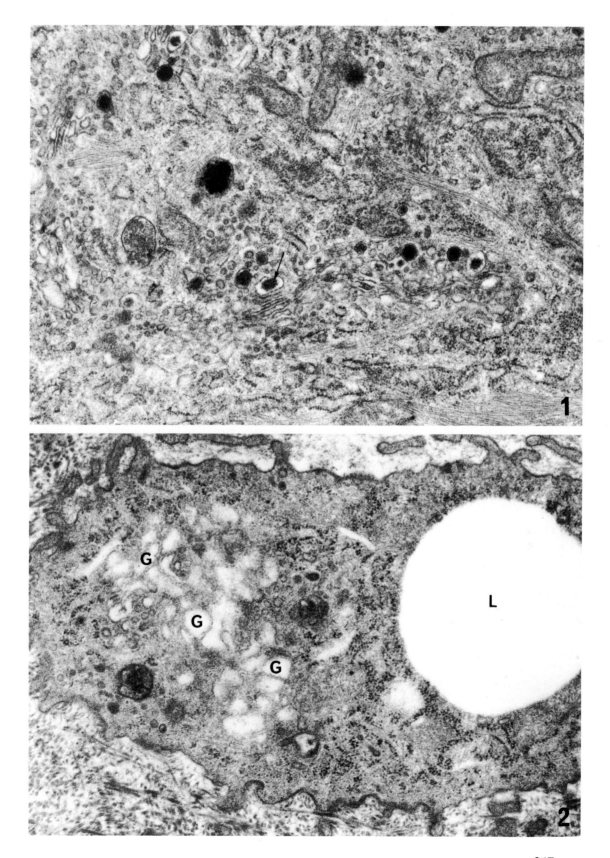

Mucous granules in normal and neoplastic cells

In this section of the text we deal with one of the two common types of secretory granules produced by exocrine glands, namely, the mucous granules produced by mucin-secreting or goblet cells. Serous granules produced by acinar cells are dealt with in the next section of the text (pages 352–357). These granules are, as a rule, easily distinguished from each other because the mucous granule is usually electron-lucent and its contents reticulated, while the serous granule is usually homogeneous and electron-dense, but naturally occurring and artefactually produced variations of morphology do occur, so that at times it is difficult to tell them apart. The manner in which secretory granules are produced has already been dealt with (*Plate 143* and pages 330–332), so this will not be repeated here.

There are variations in the chemical composition, staining reactions and ultrastructural morphology of mucous granules (sometimes referred to as 'mucous droplets' or 'mucigen droplets') but correlations between the morphology of a granule and its chemical composition have yet to be established. Most mucous granules present as single-membrane-bound structures containing an electron-lucent reticulated or flocculent material (*Plates 152* and *153*). Mucous granules are hydrophilic, so they tend to swell and coalesce during specimen preparation (Bloom and Fawcett, 1975) and the ensheathing membrane is at times ruptured. This is perhaps not entirely an *in vitro* phenomenon, for mucous granules near the free surface of the cell just prior to discharge may also imbibe water and swell and fuse.

It is important to recognize that not all mucous granules are electron-lucent. Indeed, the granules found in mucus-secreting cells are so pleomorphic that it would take innumerable illustrations to show all the forms and sizes that these granules can assume. Fortunately in a mucous cystadenoma of the ovary I studied, the cells contained an almost complete repertoire of granule types (*Plate 152*). It will be noted from the illustration that besides the 'typical' mucous granules there are also medium density granules, quite electron-dense granules and granules with a dark core (bull's-eye granules). This illustration is presented because it is a convenient way of showing the varieties and developmental stages of mucous granules, but it must be stressed that in normal tissues one finds only one or two versions of the granule in a cell, the commonest being the large lucent granule.

Plate 152
Mucous cystadenoma of the ovary showing mucous granules of varying morphology. Note large pale granules with a reticular (A) or particulate (B) content, dense granules (C) and an assortment of 'bull's-eye' granules with a central or eccentric core (arrows) set in a light or dense matrix. × 15 000 (*From Ghadially, 1985*)

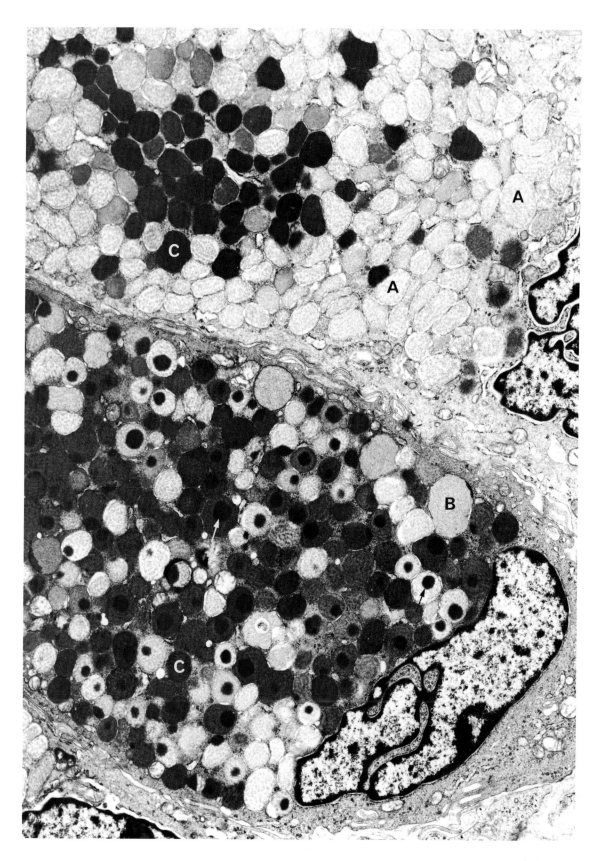

However, several varieties of lucent granules occur, in some the contents are flocculent, in others finely particulate, and in yet others reticular. The reticular pattern itself can vary markedly, from barely discernible to clearly recognizable to so exaggerated (*Plate 153, Fig. 3*) that at a casual glance one wonders whether one is looking at granules of basophil leucocytes or mast cells.

In adenocarcinoma also, one finds several varieties of granules, but in a given tumour only one or two varieties of granules are as a rule seen. In well differentiated adenocarcinomas, the granules are similar to those described above. In poorly differentiated tumours, the granules may be quite small (e.g. *Plate 153, Fig. 3* and *Plate 432* in Chapter 13) and rather dense (particulate content), or they may be reduced to lucent vacuoles containing small amounts of flocculent or particulate material which probably represents a much diluted or altered mucus produced by the tumour. Finally, even such vacuoles are lost and the diagnosis of adenocarcinoma is impossible to make or has to rest in other findings.

An interesting sequence of changes in the morphology of mucous granules has been demonstrated in the colonic mucosa during transformation from the normal to the adenomatous and finally to the cancerous state (Mughal and Filipe, 1978). In the normal mucosa, the mucous granules are large and lucent and the contents faintly reticulated, but as the neoplastic change progresses, the bull's-eye granules and dense granules begin to appear. However, such changes are not specific for the neoplastic state.

Plate 153

Mucous granules of varying morphology are depicted here. Note that mucous granules in malignant cells can be quite small as compared to those in mucous cells of benign tumours and normal mucous cells.

Fig. 1. Goblet cell from human colon showing typical lucent mucous granules (M) with easily discernible reticulation. The granule indicated by an asterisk (★) has an average diameter of 1.7 μm. × 19 000

Fig. 2. Cystadenoma of ovary. Same as *Plate 152*. Depicted here are dense mucous granules (D) with easily discernible reticulation. Also present are lucent mucous granules (L) with flocculent contents. The granule indicated by an asterisk (★) is approximately 0.8 μm in diameter. × 38 000

Fig. 3. Amphicrine tumour (mucinous carcinoid) of stomach. Same case as *Plate 174*. Seen here are mucous granules with an exaggerated reticular pattern (arrowheads). Also present are mucous granules with flocculent content (thick arrows) and intermediate forms (thin arrows) between these two varieties. The granule indicated by an asterisk (★) is approximately 0.3 μm in diameter. × 48 000

Fig. 4. Adenocarcinoma of appendix. The lucent mucous granules (M) seen here have a particulate content. The granule indicated by an asterisk (★) is approximately 0.5 μm in diameter. × 21 000

Fig. 5. Carcinoma of breast. The lucent mucous (M) granules seen here have a flocculent content. The granule indicated by an asterisk (★) is approximately 0.2 μm in diameter. × 83 000

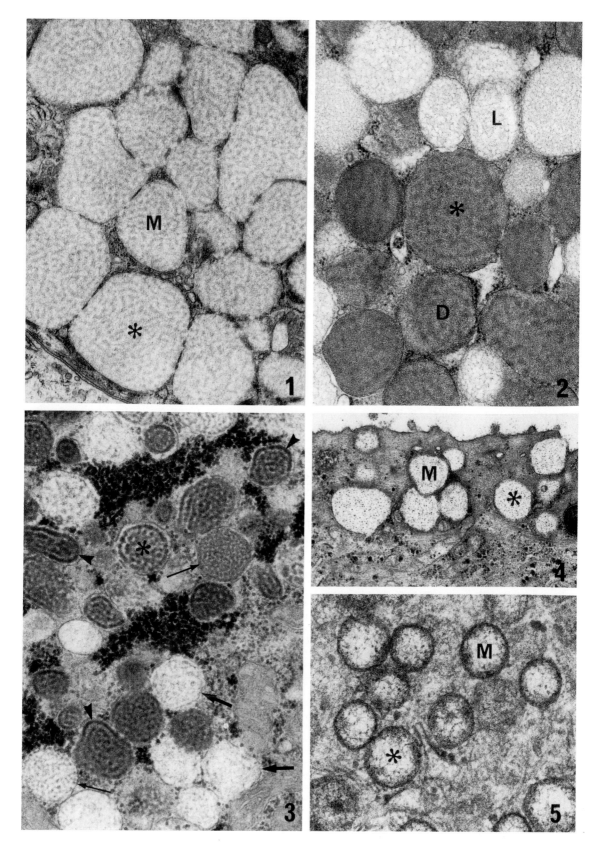

Serous and zymogen granules in normal and neoplastic cells

Secretory cells may be classified according to the physicochemical properties of their secretory product. Since secretory granules usually have a characteristic ultrastructural morphology, it is possible to identify these cells and their tumours. In the previous section of the text (pages 348–351), we dealt with mucin-secreting cells and mucous adenocarcinoma. Here we deal with acinar cells and their neoplasms, characterized by a serous or zymogenic secretion which is rich in protein*. As one would expect, such cells are well endowed with rough endoplasmic reticulum to produce the 'export protein' stored awhile in their secretory granules. The secretory granules produced by acinar cells (also called 'acinic cells' or 'serous cells') in serous salivary glands and mixed salivary glands are called 'acinar granules' or 'serous granules'. Those produced by the acinar cells of the exocrine pancreas are called 'zymogen granules' and at times also 'acinar granules'. Tumours of acinar cells from both these sites were called 'acinous cell carcinoma' or 'acinic cell carcinoma', but in the recent literature the term 'acinar cell carcinoma' is generally employed.

In glutaraldehyde-fixed material (post-fixed with osmium and sections double stained with uranium and lead), the serous granules of salivary glands have a homogeneous electron-dense appearance†; a few paler granules with a particulate substructure are also seen. These are probably immature granules. The size of serous granules varies, but in tumours the average diameter is somewhat smaller and there is also much greater variation in size (*Plate 154*). These granules are bounded by a single membrane but this is difficult to visualize because of the electron density of the contents. The membrane is easily visualized in immature granules (condensing vacuoles of the Golgi complex) which are of medium density.

Studies on normal serous cells of the parotid gland show that there is a rapid loss of enzymic protein (up to 70 per cent) from the serous granules during osmium fixation but not when glutaraldehyde is the primary fixative (Amsterdam and Schramm, 1966). The same phenomenon has been demonstrated by Erlandson and Tandler (1972) in cases of acinic cell carcinoma of the parotid gland. They found that with osmium fixation 'the secretory granules were irregular in outline and their contents extracted to various degrees' and they also state that 'the delimiting membrane of the granules was often disrupted and showed a tendency to curl into miniature scrolls at the broken ends'. The level of preservation of these granules appears to depend not only on the method of fixation but also upon various other factors such as: (1) delay in fixation; (2) tissue anoxia; and (3) biology and developmental history of the tumour (Erlandson and Tandler, 1972).

*Mucous secretion is viscid and relatively-speaking carbohydrate-rich compared with serous secretion which is watery and protein-rich. Zymogenic secretion is akin to serous secretion in that it too is protein-rich, the difference being that zymogen is a pro-enzyme which is activated into an enzyme after secretion. The term 'acinar granules' covers both serous and zymogen granules. (They look alike and both are protein-rich and carbohydrate poor.) In keeping with this, tumours of salivary glands containing serous granules and tumours of exocrine pancreas containing zymogen granules are called 'acinar cell tumours'. It will be evident that in the pathological literature the term 'acinar cell' is used in a restricted fashion, for it excludes mucous cells which too form acini and hence strictly speaking qualify as acinar cells.
†An exception to this are the acinar granules of the submaxillary gland where the granules have a dense core (central or eccentric) set in a less dense homogeneous fibrillogranular matrix (Tandler and Erlandson, 1972).

Plate 154

Fig. 1. Acinar cell carcinoma of parotid gland showing characteristic electron-dense secretory granules. × 5000 (*Electron micrograph supplied by Dr R. A. Erlandson*)

Fig. 2. Acinar cell carcinoma of parotid gland. Same case as *Fig. 1*. Besides the electron-dense serious granules (G) the cells also contain less dense granules with a particulate content (arrowheads) which may be looked upon as immature granules. Also present are some vacuoles (V) which may or may not be condensation vacuoles (i.e. an even earlier stage of granulogenesis) × 11 000 (*From Erlandson and Tandler, 1972*)

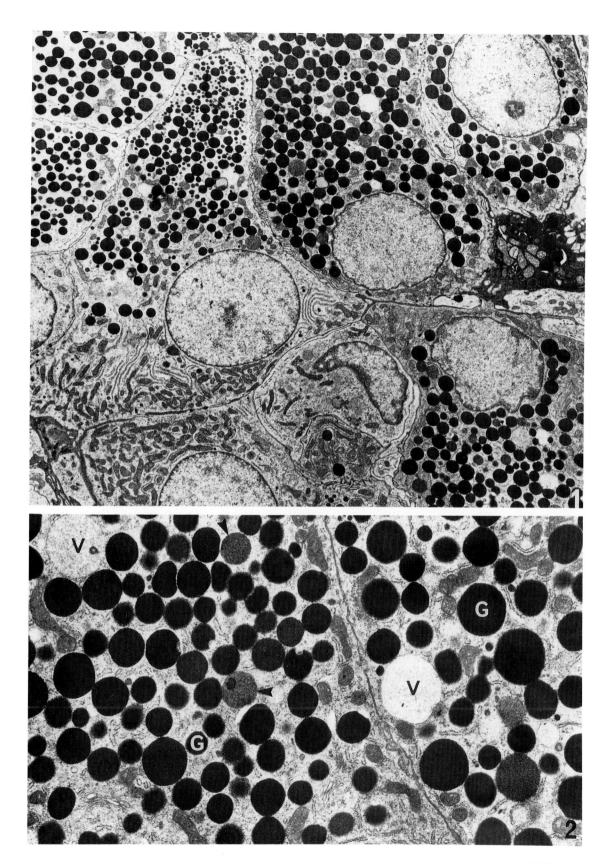

Whether the above considerations apply to all acinar granules and whether the choice of buffer affects the issue is not too clear. I have some old blocks of human pancreatic tissue which was fixed in osmium (cacodylate buffer) where zymogen granules are quite dense and well preserved (see Plate 430 in Chapter 13) and Fawcett (1966) illustrates (his Fig. 73) an acinar cell of the Brunner's gland (fixed in collidine buffered osmium) in the mouse with dense well preserved secretory granules.

It is important to be able to distinguish acinar granules from mucous granules in tumours so that one can arrive at a correct diagnosis. In this connection, it is worth noting that some of the dense mucous granules seen in mucin-secreting cells and their carcinomas bear some resemblance to the electron-dense acinar granules found in acinar cells and their tumours. Further, bull's eye granules are also at times seen in acinar cells. But when one is cognizant of such facts and bears in mind the changes engendered by preparative procedures and the neoplastic state there is usually little difficulty in arriving at a correct diagnosis.

The variations in morphology of acinar cell granules found in some tumours will now be described and illustrated, for these granules are the main feature on which the ultrastructural diagnosis of these neoplasms rest.

The main diagnostic feature of acinar cell carcinoma of the parotid gland is the occurrence of electron-dense serous granules and prominent rough endoplasmic reticulum, but one also finds some lucent and medium-density granules which are immature granules (Plate 154). There seems to be an inverse relationship between these two features, for rough endoplasmic reticulum is prominent in cells that do not contain many granules but when granules are plentiful the rough endoplasmic reticulum is sparse★. The illustrations in some of the published studies (for references see Ghadially, 1985) show well-preserved electron-dense granules acceptable as serous granules, but in others the granules appear extracted or quite pale and one is left wondering as to whether one is looking at poorly preserved serous granules or mucous granules.

Acinar cell carcinoma of the pancreas may occur in a pure form or it may contain a mixture of acinar and ductal elements. Ultrastructurally, the cells of this neoplasm (for references see Ghadially, 1985) are characterized by electron-dense zymogen granules (an occasional, not too dense, immature granule is also present) and also a fair amount of rough endoplasmic reticulum in cells that are not heavily loaded with granules (Plate 155). Thus, they bear a resemblance to normal pancreatic acinar cells. However, the zymogen granules in acinar cell carcinoma are generally smaller and more pleomorphic than the granules in normal pancreatic acinar cells (compare Plate 155 with Plate 430, Figs. 1 and 2).

These tumours have also been produced in various experimental animals (see Bockman et al., 1978; Iwanij et al., 1982). The origin of these tumours in animals, including man, is thought to be from either altered acinar cells or ductal cells. Clinically and/or histologically, this tumour is at times misdiagnosed as an islet cell tumour, carcinoid or other primary or secondary

★This appears paradoxical, but the same is evident also in the normal acinar cells of salivary glands and pancreas. One may speculate that this appearance may be due to the plane of sectioning, sometimes passing through granule-rich areas, and at other times through areas rich in rough endoplasmic reticulum or as an alternative one may suggest that as the granules accumulate the rough endoplasmic reticulum regresses.

Plate 155

Fig. 1. Metastatic acinar cell carcinoma of pancreas. Many of the tumour cells are loaded with electron-dense zymogen granules. Note the variations in the size and shape of these granules. × 4700 (From a block of tissue supplied by Dr K. O. Hewan-Lowe)

Fig. 2. Metastatic acinar cell carcinoma. Same case as Fig. 1 showing zymogen granules at a higher magnification. × 16 500 (From a block of tissue supplied by Dr K. O. Hewan-Lowe)

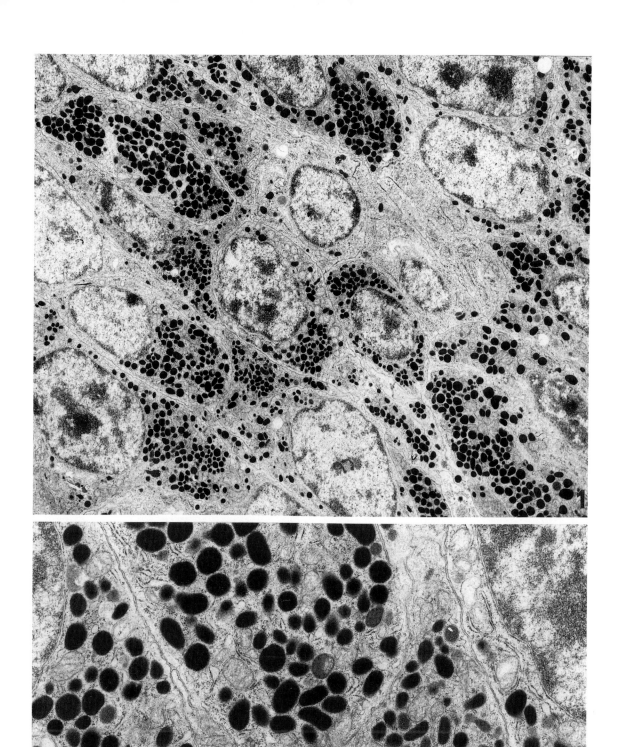

adenocarcinoma. An example of this is the tumour reported by Hewan-Lowe (1983) which was diagnosed as: (1) 'cholangiocarcinoma' on the basis of clinical and laboratory findings; (2) 'metastatic adenocarcinoma' on histological examination of tumour tissue found adjacent to the common bile duct and in a lymph node from the porta hepatis; and (3) 'acinar cell carcinoma of pancreas; metastasis from an occult primary' on the basis of ultrastructural study of the tumour tissue found adjacent to the common bile duct.

Similarly, Johannessen (1977) reported a case of acinar cell carcinoma of the pancreas, which was histologically diagnosed as such by one pathologist, but the diagnosis was changed to insulinoma by another pathologist, Electron microscopy of tumour tissue retrieved from a paraffin block showed characteristic electron-dense zymogen granules and abundant rough endoplasmic reticulum which unequivocally established the diagnosis of acinar cell carcinoma.

The ultrastructure of the lacrimal gland has been described by several workers (Kühnel, 1968; Egeberg and Jensen, 1969; Weingeist, 1973; Ruskell, 1975; Iwamoto and Jakobiec, 1982). The epithelial cells contain a basally located nucleus, abundant Golgi complex and serous granules which range in size from 0.7–3 μm but most are about 1–1.5 μm in size. These granules are generally electron-dense but some are paler and show a fine particulate substructure. One may surmise that the latter are immature granules. However, there is some difference of opinion here for some believe that the paler granules in some of the cells are mucous granules.

In the intraocular choristoma we studied (*Plate 156*), cells containing indubitable mucous granules were not found. The secretory granules were usually quite electron-dense. There were, however, variations in size (0.4–1 μm) and shape which ranged from round to oval or elongated. Less dense to quite pale granules (more likely to be immature granules or condensing vacuoles rather than mucous granules) were also at times seen, as also bull's eye or targetoid granules which had a dense centre and a paler periphery. At higher magnification, all granules which were not too dense showed a particulate substructure and a limiting membrane.

This tumour was at first mistakenly diagnosed (with the light microscope) as a medulloepithelioma (diktyoma). However, it did not show (with the electron microscope) cells with neuronal and glial differentiation as expected in a medulloepithelioma but it did contain acini, ducts and dilated ducts or cysts. The tumour, in fact, bore much resemblance to the lacrimal gland and as mentioned previously it contained electron-dense serous granules. These findings are quite incompatible with the diagnosis of medulloepithelioma but compatible with the diagnosis of intraocular lacrimal gland choristoma.

Plate 156

Intraocular lacrimal gland choristoma (*From Ghadially, Chisholm and Lalonde, 1986*)

Fig. 1. The cells contain small (S) and large (L) electron-dense secretory granules and larger less electron-dense to lucent granules (G) which may be interpreted as immature granules or condensing vacuoles, where the secretory product has not been sufficiently concentrated to form mature electron-dense secretory granules. × 11 000

Fig. 2. Same case as *Fig. 1.* Secretory granules of a somewhat different morphology than those shown in *Fig. 1* are depicted here. Some of these granules are oval or elongated (arrows) while two others (arrowheads) have a dense core which is difficult to discern because of the high overall density of the granules. × 45 000

Fig. 3. Same case as *Figs. 1 and 2.* Bull's eye or targetoid secretory granules are depicted in this electron micrograph. They have a dense core set in a medium density particulate matrix. × 40 000

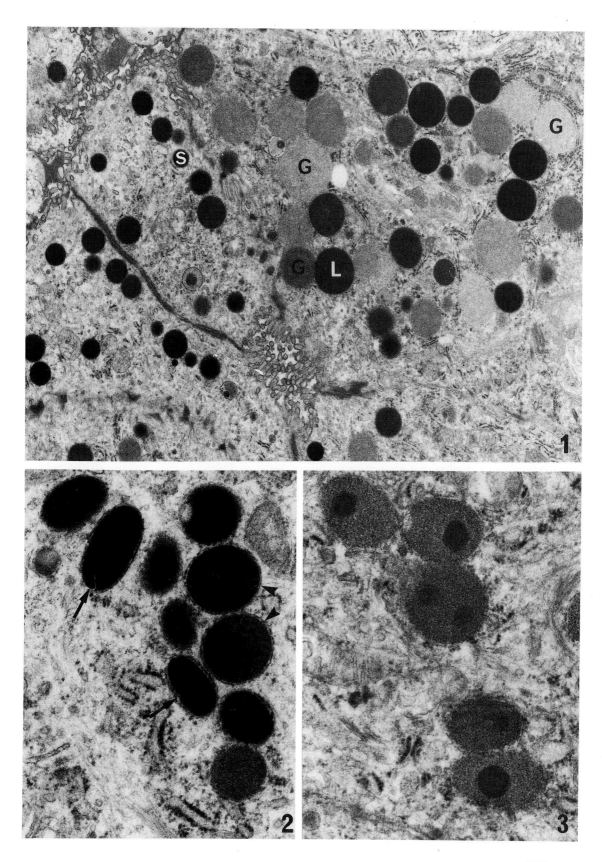

Secretory granules (myelinosomes) in normal and neoplastic type II alveolar cells

The type II alveolar cell (also called 'granular pneumocyte', 'great alveolar cell' and 'septal cell') is a secretory cell which contributes to the surfactant layer essential for lowering the surface tension and stabilizing the size of the alveolus. These cells (normal and neoplastic) are easily identified because they contain secretory granules (*Plate 157*) which present as single-membrane-bound bodies containing whorled (at times stacked) osmiophilic membranes. Hence, these secretory granules of characteristic morphology are best referred to as 'myelinoid bodies' or 'myelinosomes' (Ghadially, 1982), but they are frequently referred to by various other names also, such as 'cytosomes', 'multilamellar bodies', 'lamellar bodies' and 'osmiophilic lamellar bodies'.

Numerous studies on normal type II alveolar cells attest the fact that these myelinosomes contain acid phosphatase and that they evolve from multivesicular bodies with an electron-lucent or electron-dense matrix (for references *see* page 606). The probable sequence of events seems to be as follows (*see Plate 260* in Chapter 7). The light variety of multivesicular body is converted to the dense variety. Next, a few osmiophilic membranes (myelinoid membranes) appear in the matrix of the dense multivesicular body. As the amount of membranous material increases, the number of vesicles in the body diminishes until the fully mature myelinoid body packed with stacks or whorls of electron-dense membranes (myelin figures) is formed. This then moves to the surface of the cell and its contents (lipids, mainly phospholipids) are discharged like any other merocrine secretion.

The precise manner in which the multivesicular bodies form in the type II alveolar cell is not clear, but it is thought that vesicles containing the secretory material are pinched off from the rough endoplasmic reticulum and after their probable passage through the Golgi complex a cluster of vesicles is encompassed within a single limiting membrane, to form the multivesicular body.

Be that as it may, the characteristic morphology of the secretory granules of the type II alveolar cell is useful in diagnostic electron microscopy of tumours, because in the correct histopathological setting it acts as a marker for the neoplastic type II alveolar cell (*Plate 157*). This plus other related features (*Plates 158* and *159*) which assist in the diagnosis of bronchiolo-alveolar carcinoma★ and alveolar cell carcinoma are dealt with below.

Alveolar cell carcinoma is a subtype of bronchiolo-alveolar carcinoma characterized by the overwhelming abundance of neoplastic type II alveolar cells in a tumour showing a bronchiolo-alveolar pattern of growth (i.e. neoplastic cells growing along alveolar walls). Metastatic deposits composed of type II alveolar cells are also known to occur.

Alveolar cell carcinoma is an adenocarcinoma, hence, as expected one finds: (1) intercellular lumina bounded by cells united by tight junctions and desmosomes; (2) occasional intracellular lumina; and (3) a few or many microvilli. However, the distinction of alveolar cell carcinoma from other tumours rests on the demonstration of myelinosomes (*Plate 157*) which are the

---

★I am referring here to the mixed cell type which besides type II alveolar cells contains also Clara cells and/or mucous cells. For classification of bronchiolo-alveolar carcinoma and its subtypes *see* Chapter 32 in Ghadially (1985).

Plate 157

Fig. 1. Bronchiolo-alveolar carcinoma (mixed cell type). A type II alveolar cell containing characteristic secretory granules. Mature granules (arrows) contain little besides myelin figures; immature granules contain myelin figures (or a stack of myelinoid membranes) and vesicles (arrowheads). × 23 000

Fig. 2. Cerebellar metastasis from an alveolar cell carcinoma. Same case as *Plate 159*. This tumour cell contains myelinosomes (arrows) more or less similar to those seen in type II alveolar cells. × 42 000 (*From Ghadially, Harawi and Khan, 1985*)

Fig. 3. Lymph node metastasis from alveolar cell carcinoma (autopsy material). A neoplastic type II alveolar cell showing somewhat altered (postmortem changes) but still quite characteristic secretory granules containing myelin figures (arrows). × 12 000

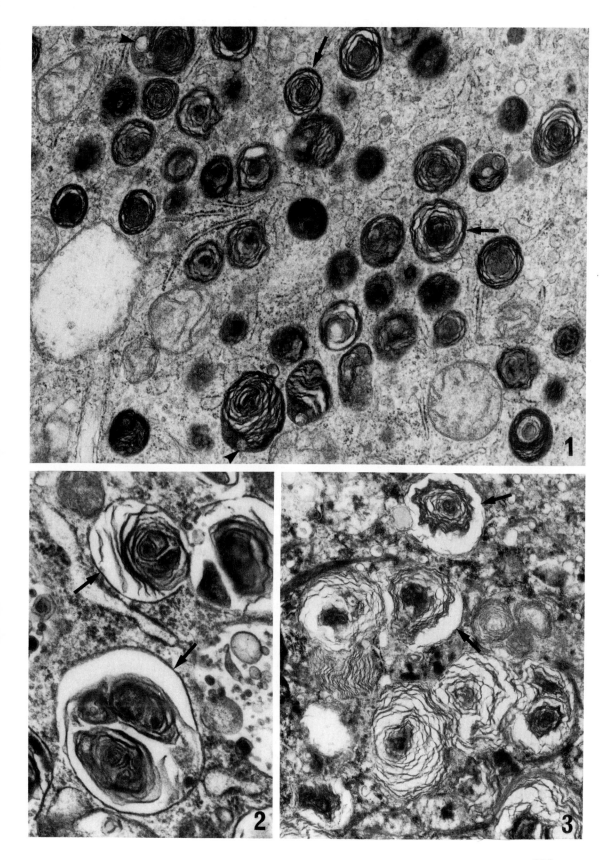

characteristic secretory granules of these cells. These granules have permitted the identification of the neoplastic type II alveolar cell not only in the primary lesion, but also in extrapulmonary metastatic deposits by electron microscopy of tissue or cytological preparations (Coalson *et al.*, 1970; Woyke *et al.*, 1972; Johnston and Frable, 1976; Hammar *et al.*, 1980; Ghadially, 1985).

However, some caution is required before myelinosomes found in a cell are accepted as secretory granules of the type II alveolar cell because myelinosomes are found in other sites and situations. It is now well known that lipidic residues in lysosomes usually present as low or medium density droplets and/or electron-dense granules, but when certain lipids (usually phospholipid) are hydrated they form stacks or whorls of myelinoid membranes which we call 'myelin figures'; and bodies containing such figures are called 'myelinosomes'.

Myelinosomes on their own (i.e. out of context with history and histological findings) are diagnostic of little or nothing because: (1) a common artefact of glutaraldehyde fixation (*Plate 264*) is the formation of myelinoid membranes and whorls composed of such figures (i.e. myelin figures). These, however, as a rule, occur in mitochondria and extracellular sites; (2) myelinosomes and myelinosiderosomes (*Plates 268 and 278*) are seen in phagocytic cells which have ingested erythrocytes after a haemorrhage; (3) myelinosomes containing whorled or stacked membranes are seen in a variety of lipidoses (*Plate 267*) and mucopolysaccharidoses; and (4) a large number of drugs produce myelinosomes (e.g. tripanol, chloroquine and amiodarone)⋆ (*Plate 270*).

We noted earlier that the myelinosomes in the type II alveolar cell evolve from multivesicular bodies and that at a stage in their evolution one can see myelin figures in company with vesicles. This type of structure (i.e. vesicles and myelin figures in the myelinosome) is a strong marker for the normal, hyperplastic or neoplastic type II alveolar cell (*Plate 157, Fig. 1*). Such structures are not illustrated in many published ultrastructural studies on alveolar cell carcinoma, perhaps because they have not been looked for. However, such bodies are at times seen in type II alveolar cells of alveolar cell carcinoma and bronchiolo-alveolar carcinoma.

In the correct histopathological setting, the finding of myelinosomes (with or without vesicles) tells us that we are looking at a type II alveolar cell, but it does not tell us whether it is a normal, hyperplastic or neoplastic cell. A study of other features such as the cell nucleus and nucleolus and close correlation with histological findings (including semithin sections from the block from which the ultrathin section was obtained) are essential before one decides that one is looking at a neoplastic type II alveolar cell and not a normal or hyperplastic version from adjacent pulmonary tissue. Of course, in an extrapulmonary metastasis one can more confidently identify the neoplastic type II alveolar cell.

We have discussed the importance of myelinosomes and the manner in which one evaluates them before arriving at a diagnosis of alveolar cell carcinoma. We will now look at two other markers found in type II alveolar cells which when sighted (particularly in a metastasis), should alert one to the possibility that the tumour may be an alveolar cell carcinoma. These two features are: (1) intranuclear tubular inclusions (*Plates 46–48* in Chapter 1) which in human material are seen almost exclusively in hyperplastic and neoplastic type II alveolar cells; and (2) pulmonary surfactant (*Plate 158*) which is found not only in the normal lung and primary

⋆For references and details about items 1–4 *see* pages 614–622 and 626.

Plate 158

Fig. 1. Bronchiolo-alveolar carcinoma. Within an alveolus bounded by tumour cells lie glycocalyceal bodies (arrowheads) and surfactant (arrows) which presents as a stack or whorl of highly ordered membranes (periodicity 39 nm). Note that these membranes (and also the ones shown in *Figs. 2 and 3*) have a trilaminar structure but this can be demonstrated only at higher magnifications. × 51 000

Fig. 2. Lung of a 1-day-old rat. Shown here is surfactant which in some areas presents a grid pattern. Surfactant of the type shown here is also at times referred to as 'tubular surfactant', the 'tubules' being square in cross section. × 31 000

Fig. 3. Lymph node metastasis from an alveolar cell carcinoma. Depicted here is a mass of surfactant (periodicity 32 nm) and necrotic debris found adjacent to several neoplastic type II alveolar cells. × 22 000 (*From Ghadially, Harawi and Khan, 1985*)

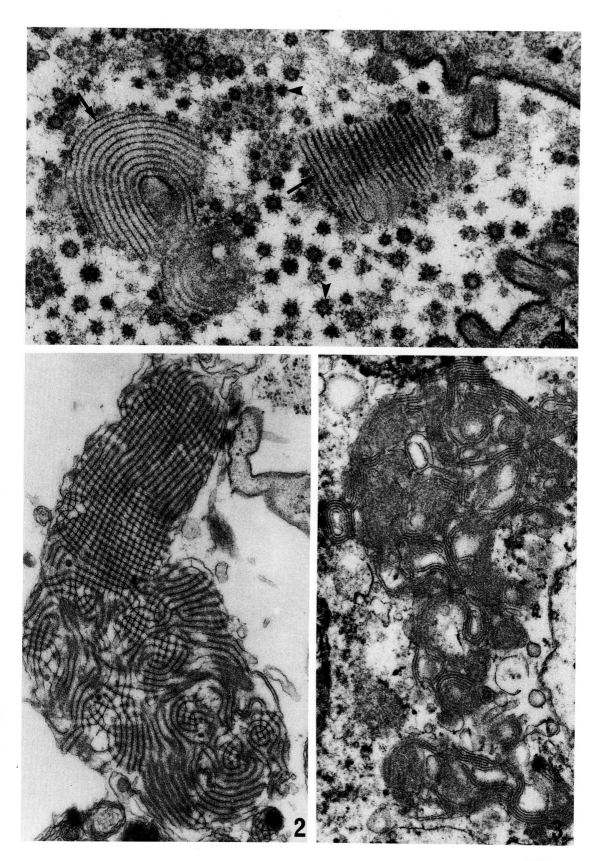

bronchiolo-alveolar carcinoma but also in metastatic deposits*.

I will illustrate these points by two cases (Ghadially *et al.*, 1985). The first case was a tumour mass involving the pleura and peripheral part of the lung found at autopsy. Grossly, the tumour was diagnosed as a mesothelioma. Histology of this tumour and metastatic deposits in hilar lymph nodes led to the diagnosis of 'adenocarcinoma (probably bronchiolar) or mesothelioma'. Ultrathin sections from the pleural mass (collected because it was thought to be the primary) showed many obviously malignant cells containing intranuclear tubular inclusions (*Plate 46* in Chapter 1), but no features supporting the diagnosis of mesothelioma. In the lymph node metastasis also, the prominent feature was the occurrence of numerous intranuclear tubular inclusions, and the occasional occurrence of material which reminded one of pulmonary surfactant (*Plate 158, Fig. 3*). Only after a diligent search in many blocks were cells containing several indubitable myelinosomes (*Plate 157, Fig. 3*) found, and thus the diagnosis of alveolar cell carcinoma was established. The possibility of a bronchiolo-alveolar carcinoma is largely but not completely excluded by the fact no other neoplastic cell type besides the type II alveolar cell was found in the material studied.

The second case was a biopsy from a cerebellar tumour. The patient had a persistent right lower lobe infiltrate which on clinical and radiological grounds was thought to be due to a neoplasm. No lung biopsy was performed. The cells in the cerebellar tumour contained many single-membrane-bound structures in which lay material resembling pulmonary surfactant (*Plate 159*). Myelinosomes similar to those seen in the secretory granules of type II alveolar cells were, at first, not detected but after much searching in several sections a rare cell (*Plate 157, Fig. 2*) containing such myelinosomes was found. On the basis of these findings a diagnosis of 'metastatic alveolar cell carcinoma' was made. The patient died in another hospital and no autopsy was performed. The diagnosis of 'alveolar cell carcinoma' rather than 'bronchiolo-alveolar carcinoma' is preferred, because no other neoplastic cell type besides the type II alveolar cell was found. However the possibility of a selective metastasis from a bronchiolo-alveolar carcinoma cannot be totally excluded.

These two cases show the value of intranuclear tubular inclusions, surfactant-like material and myelinosomes (i.e. secretory granules of the type II alveolar cell) in arriving at a diagnosis of alveolar cell carcinoma. In alveolar cell carcinoma, we have a truly remarkable tumour. It is so difficult to identify with the light microscope that some doubt its very existence. Yet it has such a characteristic set of ultrastructural markers that electron microscopists can detect it and its metastasis with a high level of confidence.

*Pulmonary surfactant has quite a characteristic morphology. In electron micrographs it presents as grids, stacks or whorls of membranes. It is the crystalline phase of a polar lipid–water system. The lipidic phase of the surfactant is derived from the myelinosomes secreted by the type II alveolar cells. At times continuity between the released myelinosome and surfactant is seen. This provides visual confirmation that the latter is derived from the former. Surfactant contains phospholipids including dipalmitoyl phosphatidylcholine. Hammar *et al.* (1980) have presented excellent illustrations showing metastatic type II alveolar cells and surfactant in cerebrospinal fluid.

Plate 159

Fig. 1. Cerebellar metastasis from an alveolar cell carcinoma. This tumour cell is packed with single-membrane-bound structures containing laminated membranes reminiscent of surfactant (periodicity approximately 27 nm) and electron-dense granules and vesicles. × 15 500 (*From Ghadially, Harawi and Khan, 1985*)

Figs. 2 and 3. Cerebellar metastasis from an alveolar cell carcinoma. Same specimen as *Fig. 1*. Higher-power views of the structures containing surfactant-like material (periodicity approximately 25 nm), granules and vesicles. × 65 000, × 65 000 (*From Ghadially, Harawi and Khan, 1985*)

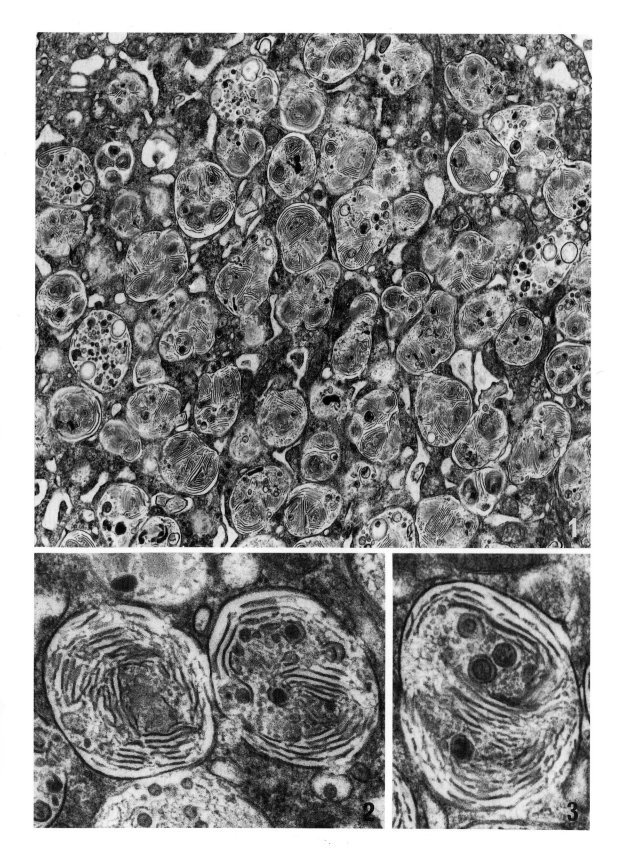

363

Neuroendocrine (APUD) granules and uranaffin reaction in normal and neoplastic cells

Neuroendocrine cells and their tumours contain secretory granules which are usually readily distinguishable from other varieties of secretory granules (e.g. mucous and serous granules) on the basis of size and ultrastructural morphology. There are also a few neurosecretory granules which have so characteristic a morphology that one can identify a specific cell type and its tumour, for example insulin granules in insulinoma (*Plate 166*) and noradrenaline granules, which occur almost exclusively in phaeochromocytoma (*Plate 171, Fig. 2*).

In this section of the text we shall deal not only with neuroendocrine granules, but we shall also review briefly the classification, nomenclature and embryological derivation of cells variously referred to as 'dispersed neuroendocrine cells', 'neuroendocrine cells' or 'APUD cells'. The acronym 'APUD' stands for 'amine precursor uptake and decarboxylation', but over the years it has become apparent that peptide hormone production is an even more important common feature of these cells than the secretion of biogenic amines. Ultrastructurally, these cells are characterized by the presence of granules called 'APUD granules' or 'neuroendocrine granules'. According to Pearse (1982), by 1969 about 40 types of APUD cells (including 18 gastroenteropancreatic APUD cells) had been identified. In the second edition of this book (Ghadially, 1982), I chose to adopt terms like 'APUD cells' and 'APUDomas', but over the years terms with the prefix 'APUD' have been dropped and terms such as 'neuroendocrine cells' and 'neuroendocrinoma' have been substituted. The text that follows adopts this changed nomenclature.

At one stage it was thought that all neuroendocrine cells were of neural crest origin, but the current view (for references *see* Gould, 1982) is that: (1) some neuroendocrine cells (e.g. melanocytes, Merkel cells, thyroid C cells and cells in the adrenal medulla and paraganglia) are of neural crest origin; (2) some neuroendocrine cells (e.g. in pineal body, adenohypophysis and hypothalamus) are derived from the neural tube or neural ridge; and (3) some other neuroendocrine cells (e.g. neuroendocrine cells in bronchi, gastrointestinal tract, pancreas and parathyroid) in common with epithelial cells of the gut and bronchi are either of endodermal derivation or derive from the 'neuroendocrine programmed ectoblast' as proposed by Pearse and Takor Takor (1979).

In the past neuroendocrine cells have been referred to (depending on site and staining reactions) by various terms, such as 'argentaffin cells', 'argyrophilic cells', 'chromaffin cells' and 'Kultschitzky cells'. The tumours from these cells* include: (1) carcinoids (pages 380–385); (2) islet cell tumours and other pancreatic neuroendocrine tumours (pages 372–379); (3) pituitary adenomas (pages 390–391); (4) parathyroid adenomas; (5) medullary thyroid carcinoma (*Plate 160*); (6) trabecular carcinoma of skin; (7) phaeochromocytoma (chromaffin paraganglioma)

---

*The melanocyte is also considered to be a member of the neuroendocrine system, but melanocytes and melanomas are best considered separately (Chapter 9).

Plate 160

Fig. 1. Medullary carcinoma of thyroid gland. The cells contain innumerable neuroendocrine granules (arrows). × 8200 (*From Ghadially, 1985*)

Fig. 2. A higher-power view of the same specimen as *Fig. 1*. These electron-dense neuroendocrine granules with a slender halo range in size from about 130–300 nm. Such granules have been shown to contain calcitonin and procalcitonin. × 54 000 (*From Ghadially, 1985*)

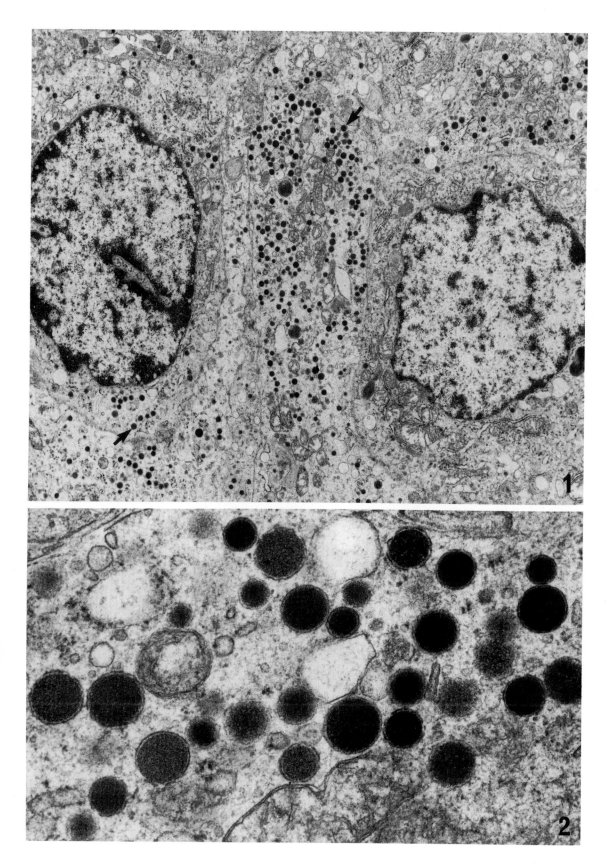

365

(*Plate 171*); and (8) chemodectoma (non-chromaffin paraganglioma) (*Plate 161*), but some of them have been classified under various terms with a functional connotation, such as 'gastrinoma', 'glucagonoma', 'insulinoma' and 'calcitoninoma'.

Although the term 'neuroendocrinoma' is useful, for it brings together a confusing collection of diverse neoplasms into a comprehensible group, it does not appear practical to pursue the classification of these tumours on the basis of hormone produced too far, for in many instances more than one hormone is produced or stored by a tumour.

In this book the terms 'neuroendocrine tumour' or 'neuroendocrinoma' cover all tumours (benign, malignant or of uncertain aggressiveness) of neuroendocrine cells, while the term 'neuroendocrine carcinoma' specifically designates the malignant variants. These are generic designations which are not intended to replace time-hallowed terms such as 'islet cell tumour', 'GI carcinoid', or 'phaeochromocytoma' which denote well-defined tumours regardless of hormonal activity.

A forte of the electron microscopist is his ability to diagnose confidently a neuroendocrinoma when histological and histochemical tests have failed to establish the diagnosis, probably because of the paucity of secretory granules in the tumour. Neuroendocrinomas have been discovered by electron microscopy when one was not even suspected on the basis of clinical and histopathological findings (more about this later). Further, our concepts regarding the histogenesis of some tumours have been altered by the neuroendocrine concept and electron microscopy. For example, we now know that: (1) the medullary carcinoma of the thyroid (*Plate 160*) is a calcitonin-producing neuroendocrine carcinoma of C-cells (for references *see* reviews by Ibanez, 1974; Johannessen, *et al.*, 1978); (2) the trabecular carcinoma of the skin is a neuroendocrine carcinoma of Merkel cells (for references *see* Zak *et al.*, 1982; Katenkamp and Wätzig 1984; Voigt *et al.*, 1985); and (3) the oat cell carcinoma of the lung is a neuroendocrine carcinoma, with a behaviour and prognosis probably different from that of other anaplastic carcinomas of the lung (*see* pages 380–383).

These feats are possible because neuroendocrine cells and their tumours contain granules which are as a rule readily identifiable on the basis of their size and ultrastructural morphology.

Plate 161

Fig. 1. Carotid body tumour. Numerous small dense cored neuroendocrine granules (arrowheads) and some much larger neuroendocrine granules (arrows). × 19 000

Fig. 2. Same case as *Fig. 1.* Higher-power view showing a large dense granule (arrow) and several dense core granules (arrowheads). Note the lucent space (i.e. 'halo') between the dense core and the 'loose-fitting' membrane. × 53 000

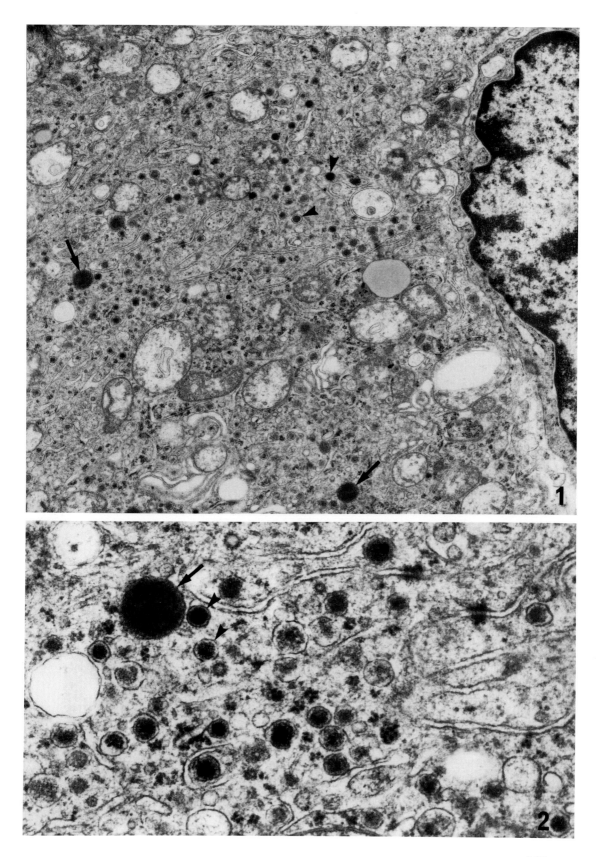

Such neuroendocrine granules include: (1) small, round, uniformly electron-dense granules 100–250 nm in diameter; (2) dense core granules 100–250 nm in diameter which, as their name implies, have a dense core, but the periphery is lucent or of medium density*; (3) larger uniformly electron-dense granules measuring 200–400 nm in diameter; (4) uniformly, electron-dense granules which are pleomorphic (round, oval, elongated, pear-shaped, dumb-bell-shaped or egg-shaped); (5) electron-lucent granules containing an electron-dense crystalline core (beta cell granules or insulin granules); and (6) large (200–450 nm) electron-lucent granules with an eccentrically placed dense core (noradrenaline granules).

Although one can often diagnose a neuroendocrinoma with the electron microscope at a glance, there are some pitfalls which one must guard against. As we have seen, neuroendocrine granules are, by and large, electron-dense structures bound by a single membrane and as such there is a real danger of mistaking lysosomes for neuroendocrine granules or vice versa. Here the saving grace is that neuroendocrine granules show only small variations in size and morphology, whereas lysosomes tend to be pleomorphic, in size and content. Small osmiophilic lipid droplets may at times cause problems, but these are not as a rule bound by a membrane and to the experienced eye at least, the texture is quite different. Further, lipid droplets vary quite a bit in size, which contrasts with the rather restricted size range of neuroendocrine granules.

If sufficient numbers of neuroendocrine granules are present in the specimen, there is usually no difficulty in deciding what one is looking at, but when very few 'dense granules' are present, the distinction between a neuroendocrine granule and say for example, a lysosome, a lipid droplet or a rather small serous secretory granule becomes difficult or impossible. In such instances, immunohistochemistry (light microscopy) or immunocytochemistry (electron microscopy) may help (by demonstrating specific peptides or neurotransmitter substances or neuron specific enolase) or one can try the uranaffin reaction† (Payne et al., 1983, 1984) (Plates 162 and 163).

*The dense core granule is sometimes looked upon as a dense granule lying in an ill-fitting membrane or a loose-fitting vesicle. The 'clear space' between the dense core and the limiting membrane is often referred to as the 'halo'. The dense core granule is often called a 'neurosecretory granule' or 'neurosecretory-like granule' because it closely resembles some of the neurosecretory granules seen in neurons, nerve fibres and nerve endings. As is to be expected, such granules are seen also in tumours like ganglioneuroma and neuroblastoma (see Plate 399 in Chapter 12).

†For this, tissue fixed in formaldehyde or glutaraldehyde can be used as also post-fixed tissues stored in buffer for a short or prolonged period of time. The tissue is not osmicated, but it is washed in several changes of 0.9 per cent NaCl at 4°C for 72 hours. It is then reacted with a 4 per cent aqueous solution of uranyl acetate (pH 3.9) at 4°C for 48 hours. After three rinses in 0.9 per cent NaCl (15 minutes each) it is dehydrated, infiltrated and embedded in plastic in the usual way for electron microscopy.

Plate 162
Uranaffin reaction on a dog pancreas. Granules in exocrine and endocrine pancreatic cells are compared here. Note how densely the neuroendocrine granules (arrows) in the islet cells have stained (i.e. +ve reaction) and how one can discern the crystalline core in the insulin granules. The electron-density of these granules is similar to the electron-density of heterochromatin (H) in the nuclei. The rough endoplasmic reticulum (R) is well visualized because of intense staining of ribosomes (not resolved at this low magnification) on its surface. In contrast to these uranaffin +ve structures are the zymogen granules (Z) which are much less electron-dense (i.e. −ve reaction). × 8000

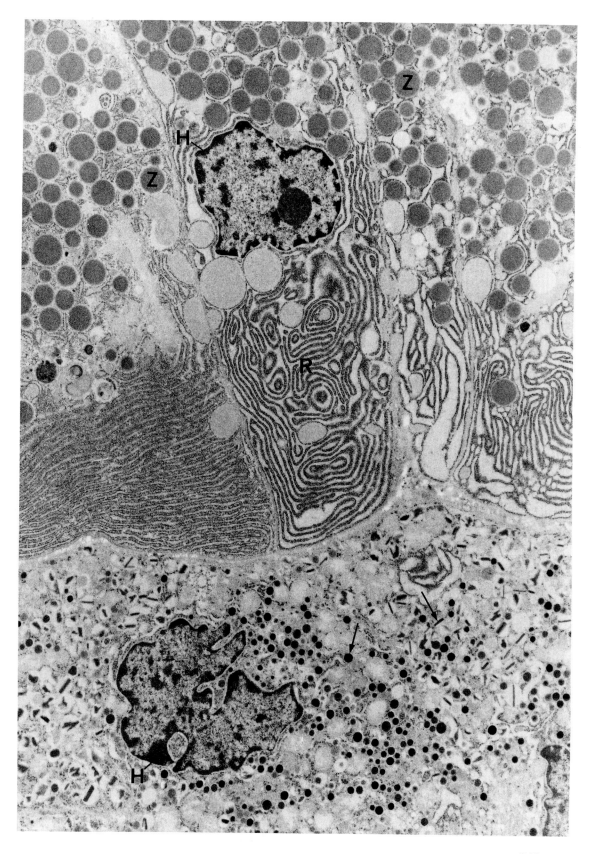

369

The uranaffin positive structures (which stain with uranium and hence appear electron-dense) include nuclei (chromatin DNA) and nucleolus (RNA), ribosomes (RNA) and neuroendocrine granules (staining thought to be due to high concentrations of adenosine triphosphate (ATP), diphosphate (ADP) or monophosphate (AMP) in these granules). Other structures such as exocrine secretory granules and lysosomes are uranaffin negative (*Plate 162*). It is fortunate that ribosomes stain with this reaction for one can use them as an inbuilt control (*Plate 163*). A positive granule is one which is as electron-dense as a ribosome, any granule showing less density is negative.

A comparative study (Nagle *et. al.*, 1986) on the relative values of immunohistochemical techniques and the uranaffin reaction showed that in poorly differentiated neuroendocrine tumours 7 out of 16 were negative for all anti-sera tested, but they all showed a few positive granules with the uranaffin reaction. This is only to be expected because if only a few scattered neuroendocrine granules are present the immunohistochemical reaction products associated with them would either not be resolved or even if resolved one would probably not be able to confidently assert (with the light microscope) that neuroendocrine granules were present. The uranaffin reaction appears to be a promising technique, but only time can determine its true practical value.

Apart from the secretory granules discussed above, there are no other ultrastructural features in neuroendocrinomas which are of specific diagnostic import. However, in passing one may note that these tumours usually contain: (1) a Golgi complex and a modest amount of rough endoplasmic reticulum, which has a tendency to form small stacks; (2) desmosomes with a modest number of converging tonofilaments, but only very rarely are a few tonofibrils seen lying free in the cytoplasm; and (3) on rare occasions intracellular and/or intercellular lumina with associated tight junctions and desmosomes.

Neuroendocrine cells are very widely distributed and one occasionally finds such cells 'accidentally included'* in a variety of neoplasms (e.g. in mucous adenocarcinoma) but this presents no diagnostic problems once it is recognized that the mere presence of a few neuroendocrine cells does not in itself automatically establish the diagnosis of neuroendocrinoma (Lillie and Glenner, 1960), nor must the presence of a rare granule resembling a neuroendocrine granule in one or two cells of a difficult to diagnose tumour make one jump to the diagnosis of neuroendocrinoma.

*For example, neuroendocrine cells form an integral element in 3.1 per cent of gastric and 2.5 per cent of intestinal carcinomas (Kubo and Watanabe, 1971). Some authors regard the occurrence of neuroendocrine cells in such situations as evidence of multidirectional differentiation (from a stem cell capable of producing mucous secreting cells and neuroendocrine cells) and not as 'accidentally included' cells. (For more details *see* pages 392–395.)

Plate 163
Uranaffin reaction on a carcinoid of ileum. (Same case as *Plates 170 and 172*). The neuroendocrine granules are intensely stained (thick arrows), so are the polyribosomes (arrowheads), heterochromatin (H) and perichromatin granules (thin arrows). A lipofuscin granule (L) is not stained. Note that membranes are not visualized because the specimen was not osmicated. × 28 000

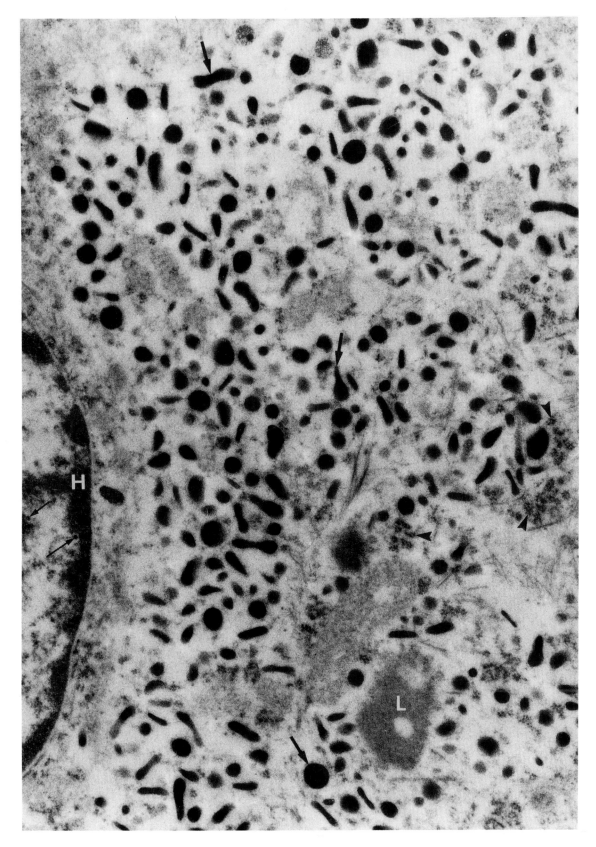

371

Neuroendocrine granules in normal and neoplastic pancreatic neuroendocrine cells

At one time it was thought that neuroendocrine cells in the pancreas occurred only in the islets, but we now know that quite a variety of neuroendocrine cells are also found dispersed in the pancreas (i.e. outside the islets).

There has been much confusion regarding the number of cell types present in the normal islets and the nomenclature of these cells, but it is now generally agreed that morphologically three or perhaps four cell types may be recognized in the islets. They are: (1) the alpha cell (A cell) containing dense core granules. The halo around the core is quite lucent in osmium fixed material but of a medium density after glutaraldehyde fixation; (2) the beta cell (B cell) with its highly characteristic granules containing a crystalline core; (3) the chromophobic cell (C cell) which lacks granules; and (4) the delta cell (D cell) which has granules of variable size and density where the appearance varies from light and punctate to flocculent to dense and compact.

In the past, most workers regarded chromophobic cells and delta cells as a stage of development or secretory cycle of the alpha cell*; therefore all non-beta granulated (i.e. without crystalline core) cells were designated alpha cells (Greider and Elliott, 1964; Like, 1967; Toker, 1967; Waisman, 1969). This situation began to change with the advent of immunofluorescence techniques and the term 'A$_1$ cells' (probably the same as D cells) was given to cells which presumably produced gastrin and 'A$_2$ cells' (probably the same as A cells) to cells which presumably produce glucagon (for references *see* Grieder *et al.*, 1970). Other authors however have contended that the converse is correct (for references and discussion *see* Zeitoun and Lehy, 1970). This controversy stems from the difficulty of establishing a correlation between cells which give a positive Hellman-Hellerström reaction and their corresponding ultrastructural appearance.

There seems little point in continuing with this classification (i.e. A$_1$ and A$_2$ cells) and arguing whether it is the A$_1$ or the A$_2$ cell which is the equivalent of the D cell. The situation has now become even more complex, for Capella *et al.* (1977) find that up to seven types of neuroendocrine cells occur in the pancreas. According to these authors these include: 'glucagon A cells, insulin B cells, somatostatin D cells, pancreatic peptide F cells and 5-hydroxytryptamine EC cells. In addition D$_1$ cells which have been proposed as the cell type producing VIP and possible P cells of unknown function'. Also now identified is a gastrin G cell, which was at first confused with D cells. It will be noted that we are now talking about the

---

*It has become difficult to retain the original terms 'alpha' and 'beta' cells, because we now have cells going up to G and more (e.g. P cells) and because it is incongruous to mix the Greek and English alphabet. The current tendency is to avoid these terms as far as possible and use the English equivalents. However, terms like 'beta cell tumour', 'beta granulated cells' and 'non-beta granulated cells' are often retained (presumably because they roll off the tongue better than the English equivalents) and the terms 'alpha' and 'beta' cells have at times to be used when dealing with the older literature.

Plate 164

Human pancreatic islet (fixed in osmium (cacodylate buffer) and stained with uranium and lead). Note A cell (A) containing dense core granules with a lucent halo and B cells (B) containing granules with a crystalline core. Compare with·glutaraldehyde fixed material shown in *Plate 165*. × 26 000 (*From Ghadially, 1985*)

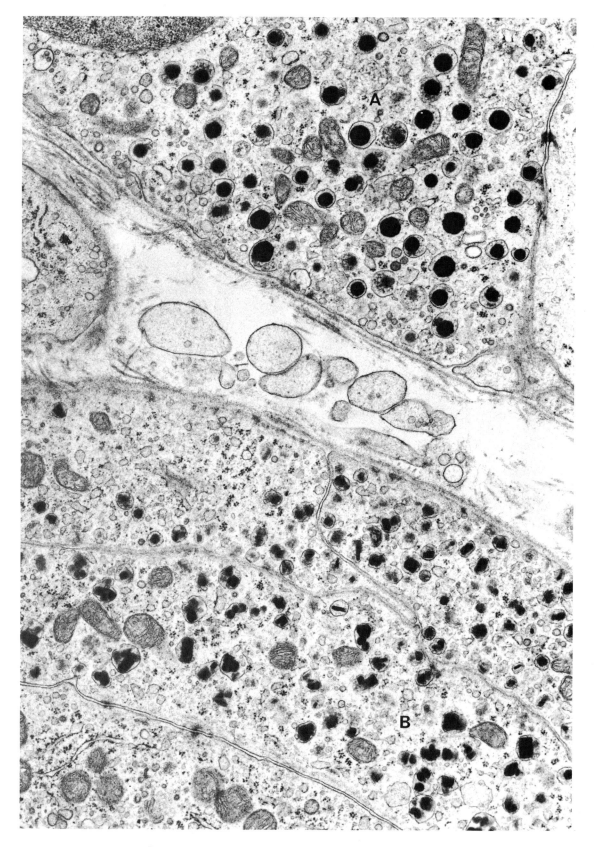

pancreas as a whole and not just the islets. In fact, all the cells mentioned in this paragraph except A, B, C and D cells (which occur in the islet) occur as cells dispersed in the pancreas and most are also found in the gastrointestinal tract. For example, EC cells are found principally in the intestines, while G cells are found in the stomach and duodenum.

As may be expected, in most instances the problem of identifying and classifying the neoplasms of these cells on the basis of granule morphology is difficult or impossible, because what slight differences there are in granule size and morphology are altered or obliterated in neoplastic cells. Nevertheless, it is interesting to know about the kind of granules seen in neuroendocrinomas of the pancreas, and this is what we will deal with now.

Innumerable studies on insulinomas (beta cell tumour) have been published but there are only a few in which correlations between radioimmunoassay, histology and ultrastructure have been attempted. The outstanding paper here is by Creutzfeldt et al. (1973), who studied 28 insulinomas in this fashion. They found that in 13 cases the tumour cells contained typical beta cell granules while in another seven cases both typical and atypical granules (i.e. granules of various morphology but lacking a crystalline core) were found. These 20 cases could be diagnosed as 'insulinomas' by electron microscopic appearances alone. In another four cases they found atypical granules only, while in the remaining four cases the tumours were virtually agranular; here the diagnosis rested on clinical and biochemical findings.

Plate 165

Fig. 1. Human pancreatic islet. Same case as *Plate 164* but fixed in glutaraldehyde, post-fixed in osmium and stained with uranium and lead. The halo of the A cell granules shown here is of medium density and not lucent as seen in *Plate 162*. This is because some proteinaceous material leaches out during osmium fixation. × 60 000 (*From Ghadially, 1985*)

Fig. 2. From same block of tissue as *Fig. 1.* A D cell showing granules of varying size and density. × 35 000

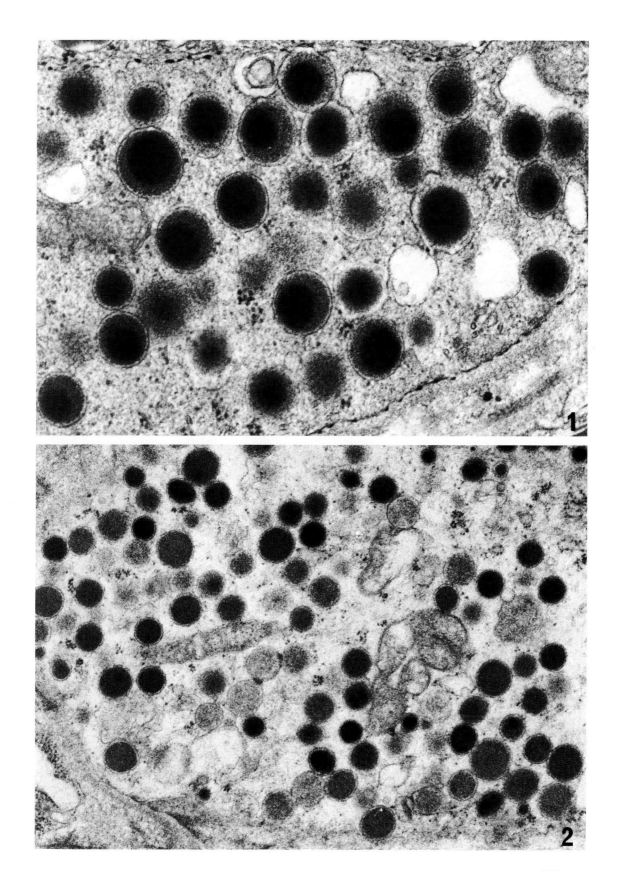

375

The insulinoma illustrated in *Plate 166* comes from a patient who had a severe hyperinsulinaemic hypoglycaemia. The tumour cells showed a variety of granules such as dense core granules, dense granules and granules whose contents were of a low density. Such granules are of no diagnostic value for one can find occasional examples of such granules not only in B cells but also in a variety of other neuroendocrine cells including A cells and D cells. Careful search however did reveal a few granules with a crystalline core and this establishes unequivocally the diagnosis of insulinoma.

The difficulty of finding crystal-containing granules in some insulinomas can be explained on the basis of what is known about the mechanics of insulin secretion and tumour biology. It is thought that when insulin is produced and secreted rapidly, it is not stored in granules, at least not long enough to crystallize. In such circumstances typical beta granules are not seen (Fawcett *et al.*, 1969). The concentration of insulin or proinsulin-like compounds is lower in insulinomas than in normal islet tissue (Creutzfeldt *et al.*, 1973), the raised level of insulin in the blood probably reflects a reduced capacity of tumour cells to store insulin which is rapidly released in an uncontrolled fashion either via the granular or pre-granular route.

An islet cell carcinoma which produced insulin and glucagon has been reported by Boden *et al.* (1977). Immunoreactive glucagon could be extracted from all parts of the tumour but immunoreactive insulin was present in only one area of the tumour. Thus it seems likely that there was a dual population of cells in this tumour.

Indeed the general consensus of most students of human islet cell tumours has been that when multiple hormones are produced each stems from a separate cell (e.g. Bordi and Bussolati, 1974). In contrast to this is the report by Amherdt *et al.* (1971) on the ultrastructure of a transplantable islet cell tumour of the hamster which contained insulin, glucagon and catecholamines. A heterogeneous population of granules (70–250 nm) was seen in the tumour cells so the authors suggest that either multihormone synthesis was occurring in individual cells or that 'one or several of the hormones found in the tumours may have been synthesized elsewhere and accumulated accidentally in this particular tissue'.

On the basis of radioimmunoassay and clinical data at least three well-defined categories of functionally distinct islet cell tumours are known to occur besides the insulin producing beta cell tumour. These are: (1) the so-called 'ulcerogenic tumour' of the Zollinger-Ellison syndrome; (2) the so-called 'diarrhoeogenic tumour' of the Verner-Morrison syndrome; and (3) the quite rare glucagonoma.

Several hormones such as gastrin, cholecystokinin, glucagon and secretin or combinations of these have been implicated in the production of these syndromes but the unequivocal association between a hormone and the neoplastic proliferation of a particular cell type has not been established in all instances.

Plate 166

Fig. 1. Insulinoma from a patient with marked hyperinsulinaemic hypoglycaemia. The tumour cells show pleomorphic granules of little diagnostic value, except one (arrow) which has a crystalline core. × 26 000 (*From Ghadially, 1985*)

Fig. 2. Same tumour as *Fig. 1*, showing granules with crystalline cores (arrows). × 64 000. (*From Ghadially, 1985*)

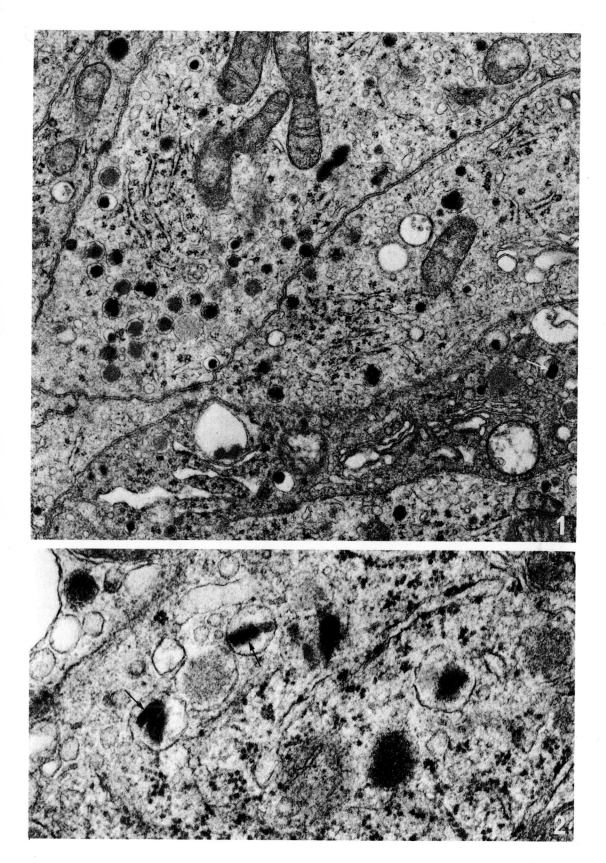

However, gastrin (produced by a gastrinoma) appears to be the principal hormone involved in the production of the Zollinger–Ellison sydrome (*Plate 167*). The cells in this tumour contain pleomorphic granules like D cells so at one time it was thought that a D cell tumour was the most likely candidate for the production of this syndrome (for references *see* Grieder *et al.*, 1974), but it is now clear that gastrinomas arise from G cells which are found in the stomach, duodenum and pancreas.

The situation regarding the diarrhoeogenic tumour seems more complex, for quite a few hormones have been implicated in the production of the Verner-Morrison syndrome such as secretin, gastrin and glucagon (Zollinger *et al.*, 1968; Sircus, 1969; Cleator *et al.*, 1970; Barbezat and Grossman, 1971). Grieder *et al.* (1974) studied 34 ulcerogenic tumours and five diarrhoeogenic tumours. They could find no constant morphological, histochemical or ultrastructural difference between these two types of neoplasm.

A glucagonoma producing hyperglucagonaemia (the patient had mild diabetes and dermatitis) is described by McGavran *et al.* (1966). They described this as an alpha cell carcinoma but the dense granules (average diameter 200 nm) did not have a halo around them. However, subsequent studies (reviewed by Kostianovsky, 1980 and Ruttman *et al.*, 1980) have confirmed that the principal cell in the glucagonoma is the alpha cell of the pancreatic islet. An islet cell tumour producing ACTH, glucagon and gastrin has been described by Belchetz *et al.* (1973). Two cell types were seen, one containing dense granules 120–200 nm in diameter and the other containing dense granules 330–500 nm in diameter. Neither type of granule had a halo around it. However, in a tumour thought to be a metastasizing ACTH secreting islet cell carcinoma Rawlinson (1973) found that the cells contained granules (180–200 nm in diameter) with a central electron-dense core and halo. Secretion of more than one hormone is a recognized feature of quite a few islet cell tumours (Law *et al.*, 1965; O'Neal *et al.*, 1968; Kostianovsky, 1980; Ruttman *et al.*, 1980).

It will be apparent from the above that the electron microscopist can confidently identify only certain cases of insulinomas when at least a few characteristic beta cell granules with a crystalline core are present. In the absence of this finding the tumour can still be an insulinoma or a tumour producing a variety of other hormones. For more precise distinction, immunohistochemical and radioimmunological methods are needed to characterize the hormones produced by pancreatic neuroendocrinomas (Polak *et al.*, 1976; Heitz *et al.*, 1979; Ruttman *et al.*, 1980). On the basis of the principal hormone produced, these tumours can then usually be classified as: gastrinomas, vipomas, glucagonomas, somatostatinomas and PP-omas, or as tumours producing two or more hormones.

Plate 167

From a bulldog with Zollinger–Ellison syndrome. The dog had peptic ulceration and a 1 cm diameter tumour in the caudal pole of the pancreas. Serum gastrin level was 770 pg/ml. Normal (human) is 0–100 pg/ml. (*Tissue for electron microscopy supplied by Drs S. Holt and R. Ghadially*)

Fig. 1. Low-power view showing neuroendocrine granules in neoplastic G cells. × 13 000

Fig. 2. Higher-power view of granules. Most of the granules are electron-dense. They vary in size and have a slender halo (arrows). In some granules (arrowheads) the contents are not so electron-dense × 37 000

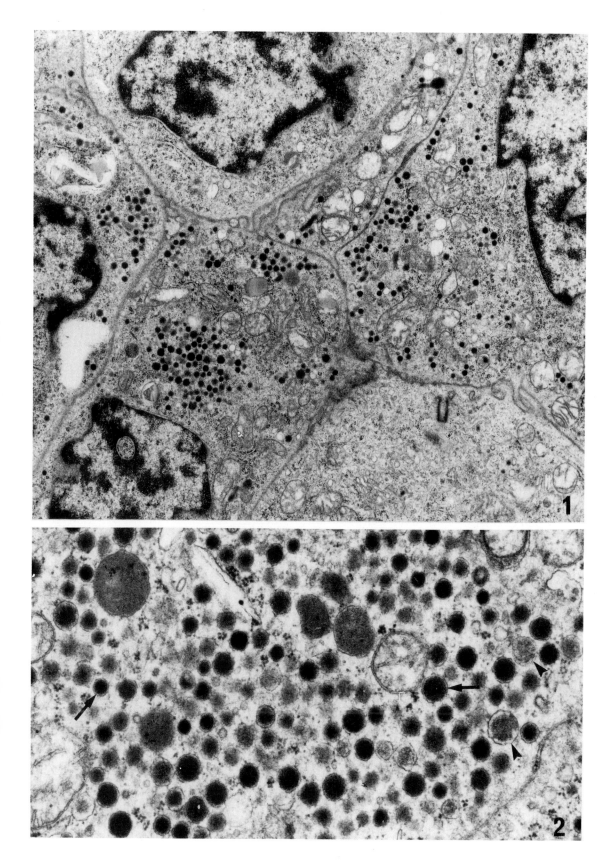

379

Neuroendocrine granules in carcinoids

At one time it was thought that the carcinoid was a distinctive tumour of the terminal ileum and vermiform appendix and that it originated from Kultschitzky cells (now called 'enterochromaffin cells' or 'EC cells'). These cells are characterized by quite dense secretory granules some of which are spherical while others are pear-shaped, dumb-bell-shaped, oval or elongated. A very slender halo or no halo is evident.

Carcinoids are now considered to be a variety of neuroendocrinoma; some, but perhaps not all arise from EC cells, but about such matters one cannot be too certain for eleven varieties of neuroendocrine cells are said to occur in the gut (Dobbins, 1978) and some three varieties are said to occur in the human fetal lung (Capella et al., 1978). Besides this there is the usual vexatious problem of morphological variations engendered by the neoplastic process which make it quite difficult to relate a given neuroendocrinoma to its presumed precursor cell.

However certain broad patterns of biological behaviour and granule morphology are worth noting (Williams and Sandler, 1963; Black, 1968; Orloff, 1971; Rosai et al., 1976). One can divide carcinoid tumours into three groups: (1) foregut carcinoids (stomach duodenum, thymus, and bronchus) (*Plates 168* and *169*). Main product 5-HTP, may secrete histamine. Associated with peptic ulcer, Cushing's syndrome or pluriglandular adenomatosis. Secretory granules said to be small and uniformly round (argyrophil +ve, argentaffin −ve); (2) midgut carcinoids (jejunum, ileum, appendix and right hemicolon) (*Plate 170*). Main product serotonin. Associated with the classic malignant carcinoid syndrome. Granules said to be large and pleomorphic (argyrophil +ve, argentaffin +ve); (3) hindgut carcinoids (left hemicolon and rectum). No known secretory product. Almost never associated with endocrine disturbances. Granules said to be large and round by electron microscopic examination (argentaffin −ve, argyrophil −ve).

It is now clear that while a majority (95 per cent) of the carcinoid tumours occur in the gastrointestinal tract (including pancreas, gall-bladder and very rarely in the liver), some (5 per cent) also occur in various other sites such as the: (1) bronchus* (Hosoda et al., 1970; Fu et al., 1974; Capella et al., 1979; Gillespie et al., 1979; Keane et al., 1980; Mills et al., 1982); (2) kidney (Stahl and Sidhu, 1979); (3) ovary (Qizilbash et al., 1974; Robboy et al., 1975; Ranchod et al., 1976; Livnat et al., 1977; Hart and Regezi, 1978; Ulbright et al., 1982; Talerman, 1984); (4) thymus (Levine and Rosai, 1976; Rosai et al., 1976; Kaneko et al., 1980; Fetissof et al., 1982; Huntrakoon et al., 1984); (5) testis (Talerman et al., 1978); and breast† (Cubilla and Woodruff, 1977; Kaneko et al., 1982). Most well differentiated carcinoids are easily diagnosed by electron microscopy, but from the morphology of the granules it is not possible to say in which organ the tumour arose. Let us now look at atypical or poorly differentiated carcinoids.

The small cell undifferentiated (oat cell) carcinoma of the bronchus is now regarded as a poorly differentiated neuroendocrinoma (carcinoid) and not a tumour derived from the basal cells of the bronchial mucosa as had been universally accepted in the past. Although the endocrine nature of this tumour was suspected as a result of the light microscopic studies of Azzopardi (1959) and the multifarious hormonal disturbances seen in patients bearing this

---

*We now know that some of the tumours designated as 'bronchial adenoma' are in fact carcinoid tumours and that the term adenoma is a misnomer because these tumours show low grade malignancy. Ultrastructural study can easily distinguish these from the truly benign adenoma arising from the mucous glands (Pritchett and Key, 1978).
†The carcinoid of the breast is a controversial tumour, the very existence of such an entity is doubted by some (*see* Ghadially, 1985). Two recent immunohistochemical studies, one supporting the idea that such an entity exists (Sariola et al., 1985) and another refuting (Santini et al., 1985) the idea have been published.

Plate 168
Bronchial carcinoid showing numerous neuroendocrine granules. × 9800 (*From Ghadially, 1985*)

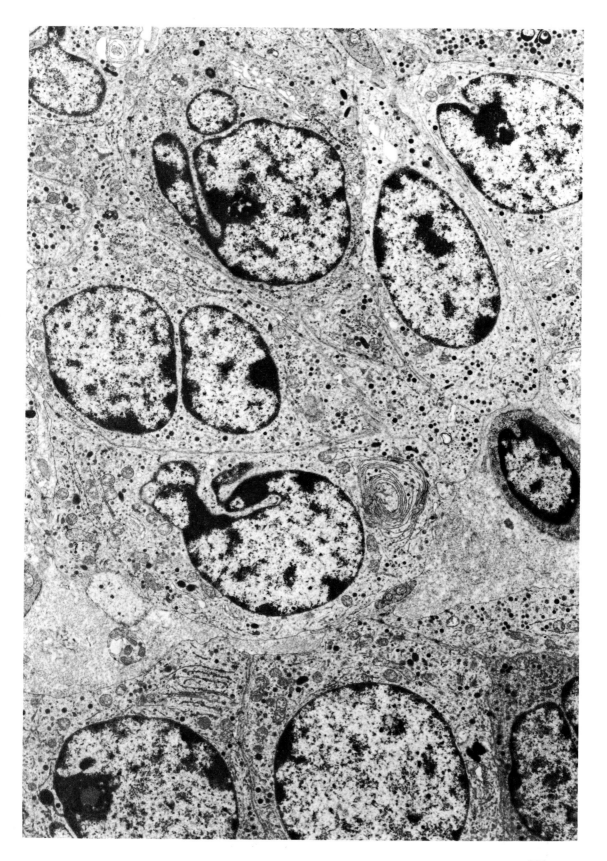

neoplasm, it was the demonstration (Bensch et al., 1968) of neuroendocrine granules (dense core granules called 'neurosecretory granules' or 'neurosecretory-like granules' by some workers) and the demonstration (Hattori et al., 1972) of substantial amounts of serotonin in extracts from the tumour, which established the idea that the well-known oat cell carcinoma of the bronchus is in fact a poorly differentiated carcinoid.

Intermediate forms where it has been difficult (by light microscopy) to decide whether a given tumour is an oat cell carcinoma or a carcinoid (so-called 'atypical carcinoid') have long been known to histopathologists. This conceptual dilemma is now resolved, for we can look upon these (carcinoids, atypical carcinoids and oat cell carcinomas) as one tumour differing only in degrees of differentiation and malignancy. The degree of differentiation can be assessed by the number of secretory granules present in a given tumour (Arrigoni et al., 1972). Rarity of secretory granules or their absence in a majority of tumour cells deserve the designation of 'oat cell carcinoma' or 'anaplastic carcinoid'. Somewhat more granules would be seen in the so-called 'atypical carcinoid', while plentiful granules in virtually all tumour cells would be designated as 'carcinoid of the lung' or 'carcinoid of the bronchus' (i.e. one variety of the so-called 'bronchial adenoma').

The diagnostic problem of distinguishing oat cell carcinoma (anaplastic carcinoid) from other anaplastic pulmonary neoplasms is of growing practical importance, for this affects prognosis and therapy. This problem can be solved by electron microscopy, but an adequate sample of the tumour tissue must be available for study. The finding of occasional dense core granules would establish the diagnosis of oat cell carcinoma (anaplastic carcinoid) while their total absence would favour the idea that it was an anaplastic carcinoma from some non-neuroendocrine cell line.

As a result of ultrastructural studies it has become apparent that several oat cell carcinomas or small cell carcinomas found in various non-pulmonary sites (e.g. larynx, salivary glands, oesophagus, colon, pancreas, uterine cervix and prostate) also contain neuroendocrine granules. Therefore, they too are now classified as 'anaplastic carcinoids' or 'neuroendocrine carcinomas' (for references see Rosai et al., 1976 and Davis et al., 1983). Plate 169, Fig. 2 shows neuroendocrine granules in a lymph node metastasis from an anaplastic carcinoid of the oesophagus. On the basis of light microscopy various diagnoses such as anaplastic carcinoma, lymphoma and amelanotic melanoma were offered. Ultrastructural study of the lesion in the lymph node revealed the presence of dense core granules. About one in three or four cells had one or two granules in the cytoplasm but in a few instances as many as five such granules were present and this is shown in Plate 169, Fig. 2. Quite a few desmosomes were seen but no tight junction or intercellular or intracellular lumen formation was detected.

Plate 169

Fig. 1. Bronchial carcinoid. Same case as *Plate 168.* Most of the granules are small and round; some have a barely discernible halo. There is however one granule which is tending towards a dumb-bell shape (arrow). × 58 000 (*From Ghadially, 1985*)

Fig. 2. Metastatic deposit in a lymph node from an anaplastic carcinoid of the oesophagus. Note the characteristic neuroendocrine granules. The granule indicated by an arrow is 135 nm in diameter. × 63 000 (*From Ghadially, 1985*)

382

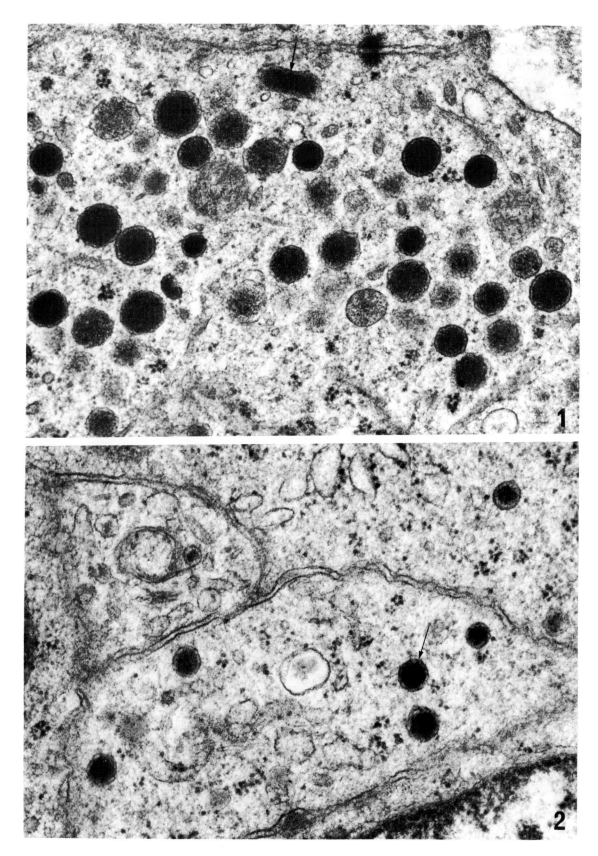

Finally, a note about the proposed changes in the nomenclature of carcinoid tumours is worth recording. All agree that the term 'carcinoid' is so well entrenched that it would be futile to try to replace it. Many people think of a carcinoid as a tumour with a very low level of aggressiveness and it is true that the well differentiated variety may take almost a decade to metastasize. At the other end of the spectrum, we have the highly malignant small cell carcinomas (and some intermediate size cell carcinomas) of the bronchus and other sites, which as we have seen are anaplastic or malignant carcinoids. The question then arises as to what one should call these malignant tumours? A current suggestion is that they should be called 'neuroendocrine carcinomas' and that the term 'carcinoid' should be retained for the almost but not quite benign tumours in this group. Criticisms against this suggestion would be that: (1) one does not as a rule use two quite different terms to describe the benign and malignant version of a given tumour, to do so would destroy the identity of the group; and (2) the term 'neuroendocrine carcinoma' is a broad term which covers all malignant neuroendocrine tumours like the medullary carcinoma of the thyroid and Merkel cell carcinoma of the skin, so this too would destroy the identity of the group of tumours we call 'carcinoids'.

The truth of the matter is that with advances in knowledge about neuroendocrine tumours the term 'carcinoid' has become somewhat redundant. One can now either redefine it (i.e. restrict it to only relatively non-aggressive tumours), qualify it (e.g. 'well-differentiated carcinoids', 'atypical carcinoids', 'anaplastic carcinoids', 'malignant carcinoids',* etc.) or drop it completely. The last suggestion though logical would probably be impossible to implement. Several suggestions for restricting or modifying the use of the term 'carcinoid' have been put forward (e.g. Williams et al., 1980; DeLellis et al., 1984), but none is entirely satisfactory.

*I find this an acceptable solution to the problem.

Plate 170

Lymph node (supraclavicular) metastasis from a carcinoid of ileum. Same case as Plates 163 and 172.

Fig. 1. Low-power view of tumour showing cells containing numerous neuroendocrine granules. × 5700

Fig. 2. Higher-power view showing pleomorphic granules. Some of the granules are rounded (thin arrows) while others are elongated (thick arrows) or pear-shaped (arrowheads). In a carcinoid, this kind of granule morphology is suggestive of a mid-gut carcinoid. × 19 500

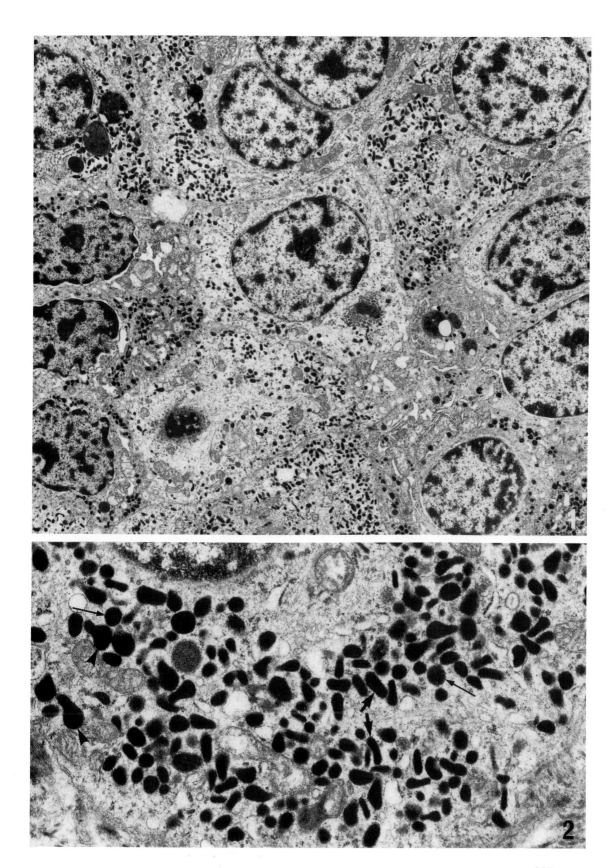

Adrenaline and noradrenaline granules in normal and neoplastic cells

Adrenaline and noradrenaline granules occur principally in the adrenal medulla and in chromaffin paragangliomas. On the basis of the chromaffin reaction, paragangliomas are classically divided into two groups; the chromaffin paragangliomas and non-chromaffin paragangliomas. The non-chromaffin paragangliomas arise from chemoreceptor tissue adjacent to parasympathetic nerves and are sometimes called 'chemodectomas'; the best known example being the carotid body tumour (*see below*). Non-chromaffin paragangliomas as a rule are non-functional and do not secrete pressor substances. The classic chromaffin paraganglioma is the phaeochromocytoma of the adrenal gland. It comprises about 90 per cent of all chromaffin paragangliomas or phaeochromocytomas (also called chromaffinoma), the remainder spring from extra-adrenal chromaffin tissue associated with sympathetic nerves (e.g. organs of Zuckerkandl). These tumours are often functional and generally contain more noradrenaline than adrenaline. We will now examine the phaeochromocytoma of the adrenal medulla (*Plate 171*).

There is quite a close morphological and histochemical resemblance between a phaeochromocytoma and the adrenal medulla. Two principal types of secretory granule-containing (catecholamine granules★ or chromaffin granules) cells are found in the normal adrenal medulla and phaeochromocytoma (Misugi *et al.*, 1968; Tannenbaum, 1970; DeLellis *et al.*, 1973). With the electron microscope, these granules present as: (1) quite large round or elongated medium-density granules with a particulate substructure (a very thin halo is usually discernible). These granules contain adrenaline; and (2) a small electron-dense granule lying in a large lucent vacuole. One might regard this as a variety of dense core granule with an unusually large halo, often the electron-dense granule is eccentrically placed or abuts the enveloping membrane. These granules (up to about 450 nm in overall diameter) contain noradrenaline.

The normal adrenal medulla contains more adrenaline than noradrenaline but phaeochromocytomas usually contain more noradrenaline than adrenaline (Wurtman, 1965; Tannenbaum *et al.*, 1966), and this correlates well with the population of the two cell types seen with the electron microscope. This is evidenced by the work of Tannenbaum (1970), who studied 14 phaeochromocytomas. In five cases of noradrenaline-containing phaeochromocytomas, cells containing granules with large haloes were found, but in two cases of 'biochemically pure' adrenaline-containing phaeochromocytomas oval or elongated granules about 270 nm long were seen. This is about 100 nm larger than the corresponding adrenaline granules in the normal adrenal medulla. Tannenbaum (1970) designated seven cases as 'mixed' type of phaeochromocytoma, for they contained both types of cells. Biochemical analysis of tumour homogenates correlated well with morphological findings. Thus, one might be able to guess what hormone is being produced by looking at ultrathin sections of a phaeochromocytoma, the main limiting factor being the smallness of the sample examined with the electron microscope.

★Catecholamine granules occur in: (1) sympathetic nerve endings (size 40–50 nm); (2) synaptosomes in brain (size about 130 nm); and (3) chromaffin cells in the adrenal medulla and elsewhere (size 50–450 nm).

Plate 171

Fig. 1. Phaeochromocytoma. A cell containing adrenaline granules. × 20 000 (*From Ghadially, 1985*)
Fig. 2. Phaeochromocytoma. Same case as *Fig. 1*. A cell containing noradrenaline granules. × 21 000 (*From Ghadially, 1985*)

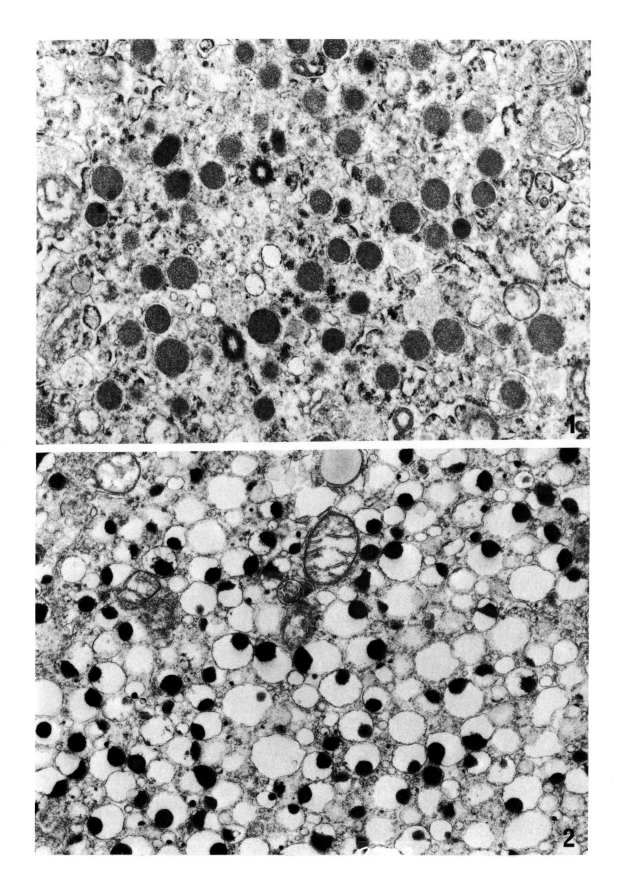

Some general comments about non-chromaffin paragangliomas have already been presented in the opening passages of this section. The best known tumour in this group is the carotid body tumour (*Plate 161*) which ordinarily presents no great diagnostic problem, although its biological behaviour is at times unpredictable. The neuroendocrine granules in the carotid body tumour are quite pleomorphic (Grimley and Glenner, 1967; Macadam, 1969; Alpert and Bochetto, 1974; Capella and Solcia, 1971) but most of them are of the small dense core variety. A few large dense granules and rare dumb-bell-shaped granules are also present. On the basis of granule morphology alone, it would be difficult to distinguish confidently this tumour from other neuroendocrinomas. Chemical analysis has shown adrenaline and noradrenaline in several examples of this tumour (for references *see* Hörtnagl *et al.*, 1973) and one can find at least a couple of reports (Crowell *et al.*, 1982; Gould *et al.*, 1983) where a few noradrenaline granules have been seen in carotid body tumours with the electron microscope. This is not what one expects from a tumour which gives a negative chromaffin reaction★ but one can explain this discrepancy by assuming that the number of catecholamine granules are too few to produce the characteristic brown colour of a positive reaction.

To the best of my knowledge noradrenaline granules have not been mentioned to occur in carcinoids, but granules vaguely resembling noradrenaline granules are seen in two reports on gastric carcinoids (*Fig. 6* in Soga *et al.*, 1972 and *Figs. 3* and *4* in Capella *et al.*, 1980) and granules bearing a strong resemblance to noradrenaline granules are seen in a reported carcinoid of the ileum (*Fig. 8* in Solcia *et al.*, 1980). I have seen these noradrenaline-like granules in two cases of malignant carcinoids of the ileum, one of which had involved the local lymph nodes while the other had spread further to para-aortic and right supraclavicular nodes. Histologically and ultrastructurally they were typical, indubitable carcinoids. The cells contained numerous large pleomorphic granules of the type usually found in midgut carcinoids, and also a few noradrenaline-like granules (*Plate 172*). I call these granules 'noradrenaline-like granules' because no biochemical studies were done to test for the presence of noradrenaline and hence we do not know whether these are genuine noradrenaline-containing granules or not. There is also a possibility that these noradrenaline-like granules derive by *in vivo* or *in vitro* (i.e. preparative artefact), modification (hydration?) of some of the normally occurring pleomorphic dense granules in the tumour. The occurrence of intermediate forms like rounded granules lying in not too large lucent vacuoles, and irregular-shaped granules with loose fitting membranes suggest that the noradrenaline-like granules may have been derived by modifications of the pleomorphic dense granules in the tumour. It remains for future work to decide whether these are genuine noradrenaline granules or not.

It will be apparent from the above that adrenaline granules cannot be confidently distinguished from other neuroendocrine granules, but noradrenaline granules have such a characteristic morphology that it would be difficult to confuse them with other structures. Thus, when a fair number of noradrenaline granules are sighted we know that we are almost certainly dealing with an adrenal or extra-adrenal phaeochromocytoma (i.e. chromaffin paragangliomas which can occur in diverse different sites), but when only a rare noradrenaline granule is present one should also consider the possibility of a non-chromaffin paraganglioma. Further one should remember that noradrenaline or noradrenaline-like granules may at times be found in some carcinoids.

★The classic chromaffin reaction demonstrates both adrenaline and noradrenaline (Pearse, 1972).

Plate 172

Figs 1. and 2. Carcinoid of ileum. Same case as *Plates 163* and *170*. Most of the neuroendocrine granules in these tumour cells present as round (R), elongated (E), and pear-shaped (P) electron-dense granules, but a few have the morphology of noradrenaline granules (arrows). Granules showing an intermediate morphology (arrowheads) are also present. × 38 000, × 64 000

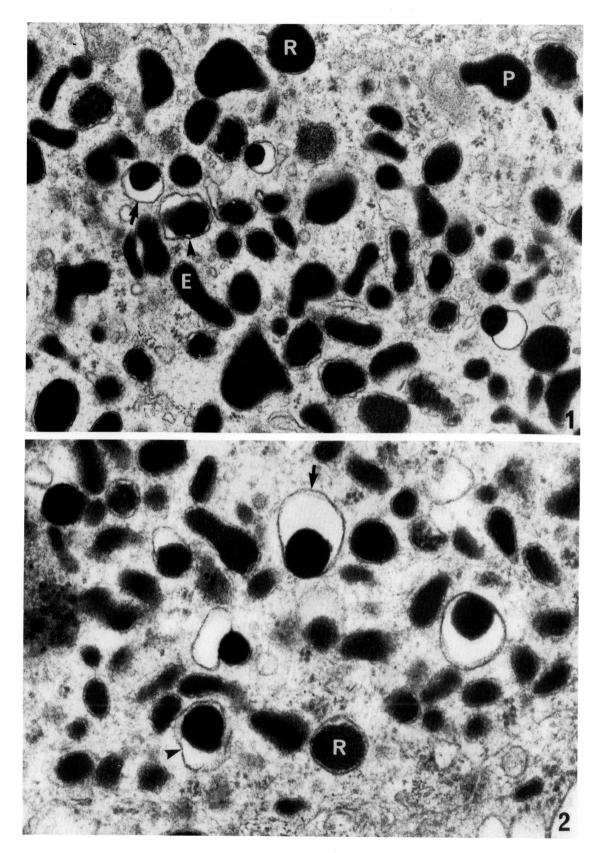

389

Misplaced exocytosis

Misplaced exocytosis is a phenomenon seen in the sparsely granulated prolactin cell adenoma of the pituitary gland, but not in any other pituitary adenoma (Horvath and Kovacs, 1976; Kovacs *et al.*, 1984). On the basis of hormone production★ and ultrastructural findings, Horvath and Kovacs (1976) have delineated five principal† classes of pituitary adenomas: (1) GH cell adenomas (subdivided into densely granulated and sparsely granulated varieties); (2) PRL cell adenomas (subdivided into densely granulated and sparsely granulated varieties); (3) mixed GH and PRL cell adenomas; (4) ACTH–MSH cell adenomas; and (5) undifferentiated cell adenomas (subdivided into oncocytic and non-oncocytic varieties).

In most varieties of pituitary adenomas, the cell type constituting these tumours cannot be confidently identified from morphology alone, because the secretory granules (neuroendocrine granules) they contain do not have a specific enough morphology to begin with, and variations in number and size of these granules engendered by the neoplastic state and the rate of secretion of the hormone by a given example of a tumour, complicates interpretation of the appearances seen. However, there are certain quite characteristic ultrastructural features in the sparsely granulated PRL cell adenomas and the sparsely granulated GH cell adenomas‡ which permit the electron microscopist to diagnose them with some confidence.

This diagnostic feature in the case of the sparsely granulated prolactin cell adenoma is the occurrence of what Kovacs and Horvath (1974) call 'misplaced exocytosis'. Exocytosis (i.e. secretion) of secretory product no doubt occurs in all or virtually all neuroendocrinomas, but this is a difficult phenomenon to detect, probably because the granule contents disperse instantly or shortly after release from the cell. In any case one expects neuroendocrine granule contents (formed or otherwise) to be released at the base of neuroendocrine cells close to the capillaries in the stroma on which the cells rest§. The term 'misplaced exocytosis' is used because the formed spherical granule content in the sparsely granulated PRL cell adenoma is released between the lateral borders of the cells. This phenomenon is so common that in a single small field (*Plate 173*) several examples of misplaced exocytoses may be found.

Other features of the sparsely granulated PRL cell adenoma include: (1) secretory granules which are spherical, oval or elongated and which range in size from 100–350 nm (majority between 200–250 nm); (2) a well developed rough endoplasmic reticulum; and (3) a prominent Golgi complex. As noted earlier, there also occurs (very rare) a densely granulated PRL cell adenoma where the granules range in size from 300–600 nm (majority between 350–450 nm) and where exocytosis of granules is not a prominent feature but a few exocytosed granules may be found. One may surmise that here the granules are stored and not released at a rapid rate and hence they grow to a larger size than the granules in the sparsely granulated PRL cell adenoma.

★The abbreviations commonly employed, and used here, are as follows: GH, growth hormone; PRL, prolactin; ACTH, adrenocorticotrophic hormone; and MSH, melanocyte stimulating hormone.
†For a more detailed classification covering very rare tumours like the thyrotroph cell adenomas and the mammosomatotroph cell adenomas *see* Kovacs *et al.* (1974).
‡The GH cell adenoma is identified by the presence of filamentous globular bodies (*see Plate 388*).
§The manner in which secretory products leave the pituicytes and enter the blood stream has been studied by several workers. The widely accepted view (Farquhar and Rhinehart, 1954a, b; Green and Van Breeman, 1955; Farquhar and Wellings, 1957; Ichikawa, 1959, Lever and Peterson, 1960; Lölich and Knezevic, 1960; Farquhar, 1961a,b; Sano, 1962; Schelin, 1962; Salazar and Peterson, 1964) is that the membrane of the granule fuses with the basal cell membrane and the contents are discharged (i.e. merocrine secretion) from the base of the cell so that a naked granule or material derived from it is seen between the basal cell membrane and the basal lamina.

Plate 173
From a sparsely-granulated prolactin-cell adenoma (Grade IV) obtained from a 49-year old woman who had a 16-year history of amenorrhoea and galactorrhoea (prolactin level, 7000 ng/ml; normal, less than 20 ng/ml). (*From a block of tissue supplied by Drs E. Horvath and K. Kovacs*)
Fig. 1. Note the misplaced exocytoses (arrows) and the well developed Golgi elements (G) in these cells. × 21 000
Figs. 2. and 3. Higher-power views showing exocytosed prolactin granules lying between the cell membranes of adjacent cells. × 52 000, × 60 000

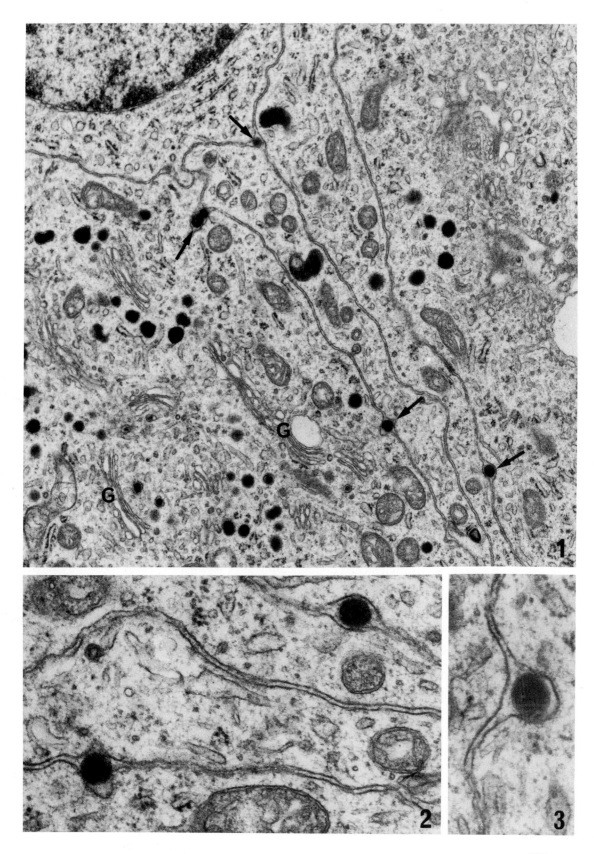

391

Amphicrine cells and amphicrine tumours

The term 'amphicrine cell' (Gk *amphi* – means both or double) denotes a cell that contains, produces, or co-expresses, two quite different types of secretory products or granules (e.g. mucous granules and neuroendocrine granules). There has been much debate as to whether such cells really exist (see below). The term 'amphicrine tumour'* usually implies that the tumour contains two different and distinct secretory-cell populations (e.g. mucous cells and neuroendocrine cells). This term is also used to cover tumours apparently composed of, or containing, amphicrine cells. Amphicrine tumours are found mainly but not exclusively in the GI tract.

It is said that about 2.5–20 per cent of gastric adenocarcinomas (Kubo and Watanabe, 1971; Smith and Haggitt, 1984) and 3–13 per cent of intestinal adenocarcinomas (Kubo and Watanabe, 1971; Azzopardi and Pollock, 1963) contain neuroendocrine cells. Conversely, the presence of stainable mucin in some cases of otherwise typical carcinoids has been known to histopathologists for over 60 years (Cordier, 1924; Siburg, 1929).

The questions that arise are: (1) should one classify a histologically typical carcinoid which contains very few mucous cells as an amphicrine tumour? and (2) conversely, should an obvious mucinous adenocarcinoma where a rare neuroendocrine cell is detected be called an amphicrine tumour? I do not think so, because the former (item 1) look like (histologically) and behave like carcinoids, while the latter (item 2) look like and behave like mucinous adenocarcinomas. Further one can explain away such a phenomenon by evoking the popular hypothesis of 'accidental inclusion' of a prevalent normal cell type in a neoplasm growing in that part.

However, there occur tumours where substantial proportions of both cell types are present and one is then at a loss to know whether to call the tumour a 'carcinoid' or an 'adenocarcinoma'. It is to describe such tumours that the term 'amphicrine tumours' is useful (*Plate 174*). Here, the 'accidental inclusion' theory is found lacking, for clearly in such tumours there is a proliferation of both cell types (i.e. both cell types are neoplastic and could presumably be derived from a common stem cell). Depending upon the predominant type of differentiation (mucinous or neuroendocrine) and whims of the authors various terms have been coined to describe these tumours. These include: 'mucous carcinoid', 'mucinous carcinoid', 'composite carcinoid', 'goblet cell carcinoid', 'carcinoma-carcinoid', 'adenocarcinoid', 'mixed carcinoid tumour', 'argentaffin cell adenocarcinoma' and 'argyrophil mucus-secreting adenocarcinoma'. It seems essential to distinguish these amphicrine tumours for many of them appear to be less aggressive than 'pure' adenocarcinomas but somewhat more aggressive than the well differentiated carcinoid. One may speculate that the greater the content of neuroendocrine cells the more benign the tumour is likely to be.

*If the term 'amphicrine tumour' is to be of any use it has to be restricted. Multiple hormone production is common enough in neuroendocrine tumours but there would be little point in calling them all 'amphicrine tumours'. One would not want to call a phaeochromocytoma an 'amphicrine tumour' even though it has cells containing adrenaline granules and noradrenaline granules because they are closely related products (catecholamines) and multiple secretory products *per se* will not do otherwise even a fibrosarcoma would qualify as an amphicrine tumour for its cells secrete precursors of collagen (procollagen) and proteoglycans.

Plate 174

Amphicrine tumour (mucous carcinoid of stomach). Cells containing pleomorphic mucous granules (arrows) (shown at higher magnification in *Plate 153, Fig. 3*) and cells containing neuroendocrine granules (arrowheads) are seen here. × 20 000 (*From a block of tissue supplied by Dr P. Marcus*)

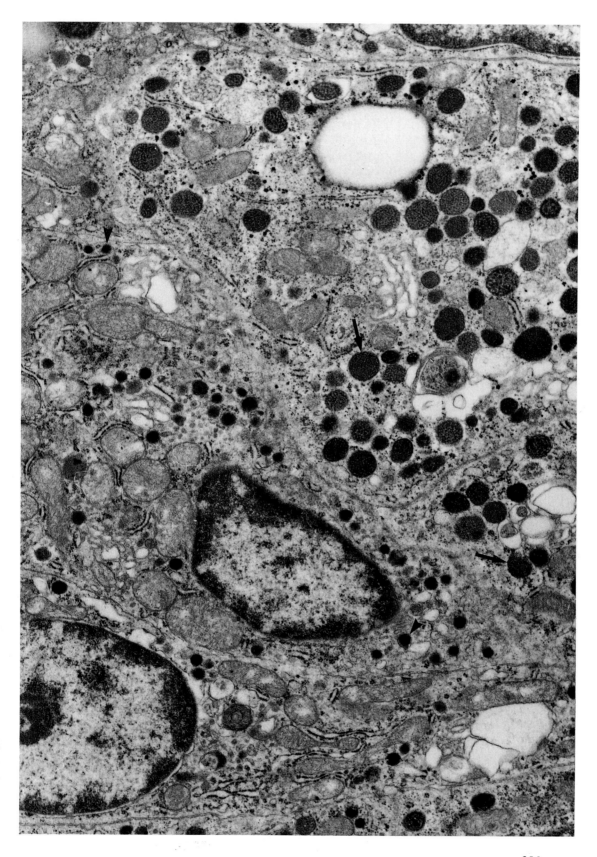

Amphicrine tumours have been reported to occur in the: (1) oesophagus (Chong *et al.*, 1979; Gould *et al.*, 1984); (2) stomach (Azzopardi and Pollock, 1963; Soga *et al.*, 1971; Chejfec and Gould, 1977; Rogers and Murphy, 1979; Morgan *et al.*, 1983; Gould *et al.*, 1984); (3) gall bladder (Wisniewski and Toker, 1972); (4) intestines (mainly colon) (Gibbs, 1963; Bates and Belter, 1967; Hernandez and Reid, 1969; Toker, 1969; Hernandez and Fernandez, 1974; Lyss *et al.*, 1981; Peonim *et al.*, 1983; Gould *et al.*, 1984; Smith and Haggitt, 1984); (5) appendix (Klein, 1974; Subbuswamy *et al.*, 1974; Cooper and Warkel, 1978; Warkel *et al.*, 1978; Warner and Seo, 1979; Isaacson, 1981; Merino *et al.*, 1983); (6) nasal mucosa (enteric type) (Schmid *et al.*, 1979); (7) lung (Wilson *et al.*, 1985); and (8) prostate (Capella *et al.*, 1981).

In the above-mentioned instances the tumours expressed mucin and neuropeptides. Other tumours acceptable as amphicrine tumours include: (9) thyroid tumours containing mucin and calcitonin (Zaatari *et al.*, 1983; Golouh *et al.*, 1985); (10) thyroid tumours containing thyroglobulin and calcitonin (largely by immunostaining) (for references *see* LiVolsi, 1987); and (11) strumal ovarian carcinoids containing thyroglobulin and calcitonin (Snyder and Tavassoli, 1986).

An example of an amphicrine tumour of stomach whose light microscopic morphology was that of a carcinoid, but where electron microscopy showed large numbers of both neuroendocrine cells and mucus cells, is shown in *Plate 174*. Whether both mucous granules and neuroendocrine granules are present in any single cell (i.e. amphicrine cell) of such tumours is difficult to determine. Much caution is required in arriving at such a conclusion for oblique sectioning of cell membranes (and hence failure to visualize them) of adjacent cells may create the impression that one rather than two cells are present, and this would lead one to imagine, erroneously, that neuroendocrine granules and mucous granules were present in the same cell (*Plate 175*). Yet another problem is that some mucous granules can be quite small and fairly dense and hence resemble neuroendocrine granules. Therefore when some dense granules are seen in company with typical mucous granules one cannot be absolutely certain that one is looking at two different types of granules (i.e. exocrine and endocrine) in a cell.

Most authors avoid the issue and speak only about exocrine and endocrine cells in amphicrine tumours. However, there are at least three reports (Hernandez and Fernandez, 1974; Abt and Carter, 1976; Schmid *et al.*, 1979) where the authors attempt to prove with the aid of photomicrographs and/or electron micrographs that true amphicrine cells are present, while there are three other reports (Black and Haffner, 1968; Warkel *et al.*, 1978; Cooper and Warkel, 1978) where the authors criticize such work and feel that unequivocal proof that amphicrine cells exist is still lacking. Despite much searching I have not been able to find any indubitable amphicrine cells in the material I have studied. According to some authors, however, (Ratzenhofer and Leb, 1965; Ratzenhofer *et al.*, 1969; Ratzenhofer, 1977; Ratzenhofer and Aubock, 1980) amphicrine cells are a separate species of cells found in both normal and pathological gastroenteric epithelium and Chejfec and Gould (1984) state that 'In our own laboratory we have studied a group of gastrointestinal and bronchopulmonary neoplasms with a significant number of amphicrine cells which by light and electron microscopy examination had apical mucosubstance vacuoles and basal neurosecretory granules'.

Plate 175

Figs. 1 and 2. Same case as *Plate 174*. Depicted here are cells which could be mistaken for amphicrine cells, because mucous granules (arrows) and neuroendocrine granules (small arrowheads) apparently occur in the same cell. However, the two types of granules are set apart (i.e. not intimately mixed together) and there is a vague cytoplasmic density in *Fig. 1* (between large arrowheads) which suggests, if not proves, that obliquely sectioned cell membranes are present. Similarly in *Fig. 2* the differences in texture of the area containing neuroendocrine granules and the area containing mucous granules makes one suspect that two separate cells (rather than one amphicrine cell) are present. × 38 000, × 62 000 (*From a block of tissue supplied by Dr P. Marcus*)

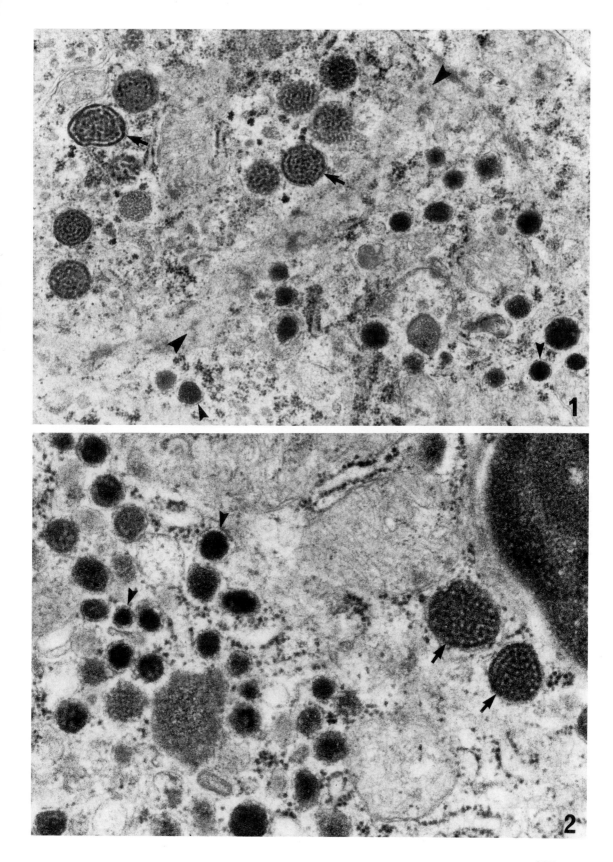

Granules of mast cells and basophilic leucocytes

The mast cell was recognized as a discrete connective tissue cell different from the basophilic leucocyte by Paul Ehrlich as early as 1877. He coined the term 'Mastzellen' (well-fed cell) because the abundance of metachromatic granules suggest a 'well-fed' or 'overnourished' state. However, several investigators (e.g. Selye, 1965) consider the basophil as a circulating form of mast cell and a collective non-committal term 'metachromatic cell' is at times used to cover both mast cells and basophils.

There are several morphological differences (*see below*) between human mast cells and basophils; the principal one being that the granules in basophils have a particulate content while those in mast cells are pleomorphic and often contain membranous formations with a scroll-like pattern.

There are, however, considerable variations of granule morphology and composition in various species. It would appear that the granules of basophilic leucocytes of some species resemble tissue mast cells of the same and other species in their: (1) ultrastructural morphology (Fedorko and Hirsch, 1965); (2) content of sulphated glycosaminoglycans (mucopolysaccharides) (Jorpes, 1947; Olsson *et al.*, 1970); and (3) enzyme content as demonstrated by histochemical methods (Ackerman, 1963).

Mast cells have been found in fishes, amphibians, amphisbaena, tuatara, lizards, crocodiles, snakes, turtles, birds and a large variety of mammals (for references *see* Sottovia-Filho, 1974). The numerous morphological variations and the interpretations placed on them defy epitomizing in this brief essay. We will therefore concentrate on the ultrastructural morphology of human basophils and mast cells with occasional reference to such cells in other species.

First let us look at similarities between these cells (for references supporting the statements in this paragraph *see* Dvorak and Dvorak, 1979; Zucker-Franklin, 1980). Both basophils and mast cells of humans contain metachromatic granules. The granules of both contain histamine and heparin, the latter being responsible for the metachromasia of the granules. A variety of agents★ and stimuli are known to produce degranulation of both basophils and mast cells. Both basophils and mast cells bind IgE by means of specific receptors which when cross-linked by anti-IgE or a variety of ligands cause the cells to degranulate and participate in immediate hypersensitivity reactions. And it is said that in most animals there is a reciprocal relationship between the number of mast cells and circulating basophils.

It has long been accepted that the basophil leucocyte is of bone marrow origin, but the mast cell derives from some connective tissue element. However, there is now compelling evidence which refutes this idea and shows that both these cells derive from the bone marrow (Breton-Gorius and Reyes, 1976; Hatanaka *et al.*, 1979; Kitamura *et al.*, 1979) and Zucker-Franklin (1980) has shown that an intermediate cell type which contains the characteristic scroll-containing granule of the mast cell and typical particle-containing granule of the basophil occurs in patients with myeloproliferative diseases. Nevertheless on the basis of morphological differences it is possible in a majority of instances to distinguish the basophil leucocyte from the mast cell. These differences may be summarized as follows: (1) the basophil is smaller and the shape and heterochromatin distribution of its lobated nucleus resembles that of other polymorphonuclear leucocytes. The nucleus of the mast cell is usually small and rounded or oval. Heterochromatin aggregation is usually not so prominent; (2) the mast cell is

★Most studies, however, have been carried out on mast cells. The list of agents that can cause degranulation of mast cells is quite large (*see* Selye, 1965). It includes: low pH, hypertonic solutions, emulsifying agents, dextran, compound 48/80, protamine sulphate, some venoms, vitamin A and ACTH.

Plate 176

Fig. 1. Mast cell from human bronchial mucosa. × 19 000

Fig. 2. Higher-power view showing scroll-like membranous formations in mast cell granules. × 54 000

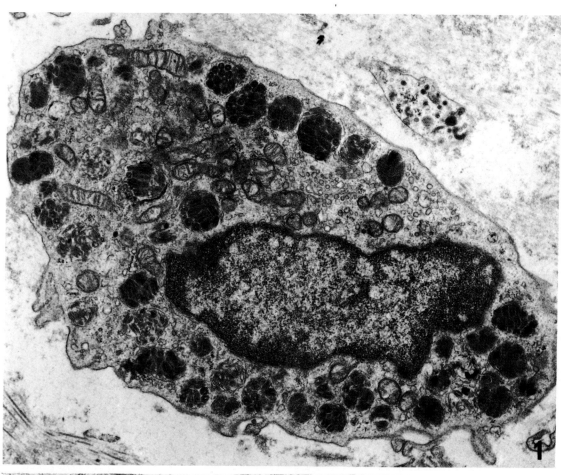

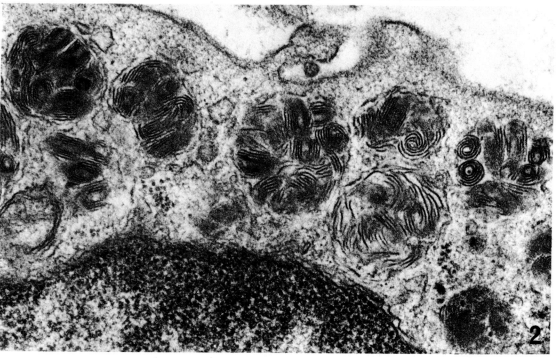

usually better endowed with cell processes; and (3) there are differences in the ultrastructural morphology of their granules.

The characteristic granule of the human mast cell (*Plates 176* and *177*) contains lamellar membranous structures which are often but not invariably rolled up in a manner reminiscent of a cylindrical papyrus scroll★. Such granules have been seen in mast cells but not in basophilic leucocytes (Stoeckenius, 1956; Hibbs *et al.*, 1960; Weinstock and Albright, 1967; Brinkman, 1968; Kobayasi *et al.*, 1968; Dobbins *et al.*, 1969; Orr, 1977; Ts'ao *et al.*, 1977). Thus if such granules are seen, the cell should be called a mast cell and not a basophil. It should, however, be noted that scrolls and other varieties of lamellar formations are at times difficult to discern (except at the periphery of the granule) because they are sometimes set in an electron-dense matrix (*Plate 177, Fig. 2*).

Besides the scroll-containing granules mentioned above the mast cell also contains granules whose contents are particulate or crystalline. These types of granules have been seen in the mast cells of humans, guinea pigs and some other species. In contrast to the mast cell the granules in the human basophil leucocyte (*Plate 178*) are fewer and not so pleomorphic. They are rounded single membrane-bound structures containing electron-dense particles (11–26 nm diameter) embedded in a less-dense matrix (Watanabe *et al.*, 1967; Zucker-Franklin, 1967; Miura *et al.*, 1968; Dvorak *et al.*, 1970; Keyhani and Breton-Gorius, 1972; Anzil *et al.*, 1974; Hastie, 1974). Granules containing finer particles are more abundant in immature basophils. In the mature basophil granules the peripheral row or rows of particles are concentrically arranged. Therefore in certain planes of sectioning they present a 'membranous' appearance which might tempt one to think that the cell is a mast cell.

Granules acceptable as mast cell granules or basophil leucocyte granules are at times seen lying free in the intercellular matrix, particularly in pathological states where accumulations of mast cells occur (e.g. urticaria). It is difficult to be certain in any given instance whether this is a biologically significant *in vivo* phenomenon or an artefact of handling and processing the tissue. However, it seems likely that such an event does occur *in vivo* for phagocytosed mast cell granules have been seen in other cells particularly macrophages (Hill, 1957; Smith and Lewis, 1958). The manner in which mast cells discharge their granules or granule contents has been the subject of many studies. Two types of degranulation are thought to occur; a slow release of contents in physiological conditions and some chronic inflammatory states and a fast massive release of granule contents as seen in anaphylactic states.

The type of mast cell degranulation which occurs in anaphylaxis (Lawson *et al.*, 1977; Taichman, 1971) can also be induced by compound 48/80 (Röhlich *et al.*, 1971) and by polymyxin B (Lagunoff, 1973). Here a fusion of the limiting membrane of a group of granules and the fusion of the membrane of a more superficially placed granule with the cell membrane creates a labyrinth, channel or tunnel through which partially or more or less completely disintegrated granule contents are discharged from the cell†. This mechanism of degranulation of mast cells is similar in humans and in some other species (Röhlich *et al.*, 1971; Taichman, 1971; Lagunoff, 1972, 1973; Trotter and Orr, 1973; Lawson *et al.*, 1977), and it is also similar to

---

★Scrolls are not found in all species. For example, they are not seen in the mast cell of the rat. Immature mast cell granules in the rat have a particulate content whereas in the mature state the granule is homogeneously electron-dense.
†The appearance created is similar to the degranulating eosinophil depicted in *Plate 286*.

Plate 177

Fig. 1. Mast cell from normal human abdominal skin. Membranous formations with scroll-like (arrow) and crystalloid (arrowhead) patterns are present in the granules. × 52 000

Fig. 2. Mast cell from a carcinoma of breast. Some of the granules of this mast cell are highly electron-dense, others have a particulate content. Membranous formations can be seen at the periphery of some of the granules. × 59 000

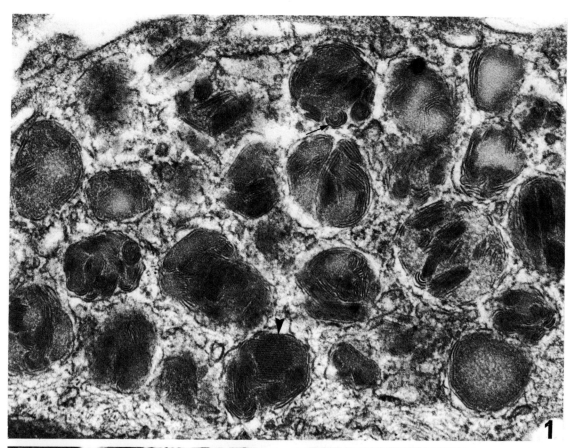

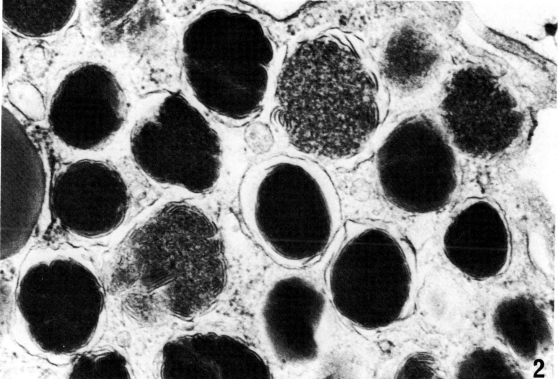

that seen in basophilic leucocytes undergoing anaphylactic degranulation (Dvorak and Dvorak, 1975; Dvorak et al., 1976; Hastie et al., 1977).

It has however, been shown that basophilic leucocytes can degranulate slowly and not in an explosive fashion (Dvorak and Dvorak, 1975, 1979; Dvorak et al., 1976). Here, no fusion between granule membrane and cell membrane occurs; instead, a chain of transport vesicles containing granular material is seen between the granule and the cell membrane, and it is thought that these carry granule contents to the exterior. It would appear that this is a more physiological method of degranulation, but it may also be operational in delayed-type hypersensitivity reactions. It is thought that this slow release type of mechanism also operates in mast cells in the lung of patients with fibrotic lung disorders (Kawanami et al., 1979).

Mast cells are primarily connective tissue cells usually located near the walls of blood vessels. However, it would appear that after partial or more or less complete degranulation they migrate to and eventually through various epithelia. Such migratory mast cells have been seen between epithelial cells in: (1) kidney, bladder and ureter of rats with magnesium deficiency (Cantin and Veilleux, 1972); (2) kidney tubules in cases of chronic glomerulonephritis, pyelonephritis, malignant nephrosclerosis, chronic renal allograft rejection and analgesic nephropathy (Colvin et al., 1974); (3) oropharynx, larynx, trachea, bronchi and bronchioles in rats (Kent, 1966); (4) human pulmonary alveoli (also seen in alveolar lumina) in cases of fibrotic lung disease (Kawanami et al., 1979); (5) human mouth and oesophagus (Colvin et al., 1974); (6) human ovarian tumours (Colvin et al., 1974), human nasal polyps and tonsils (Feltkamp-Vroom et al, 1975; Feltkamp-Vroom, 1977); (7) normal human and rat stomach (also found in gastric juice) (Cambel et al., 1952; Brinkman, 1968); (8) small intestine of rats infested with Nippostrongylus (Miller, 1971; Miller and Jarrett, 1971); (9) normal human jejunum and jejunum of humans with Zollinger-Ellison syndrome (Dobbins et al., 1969; Toner and Ferguson, 1971); and (10) abomasum of cattle and sheep with various parasitic infestations (Murray et al., 1968).

As is to be expected the histological and ultrastructural characteristics of these partially or totally degranulated mast cells differ markedly from those of mast cells in connective tissues. The remaining granules show altered tinctorial properties and may present as acidophilic globules at light microscopy. Cells containing such granules are referred to as 'Schollen-leukocyten' or 'globule leucocytes' (Colvin et al., 1974). Yet others show little besides large vacuoles in their cytoplasm. The formation of a globule leucocyte is not a pathological phenomenon but increased numbers of these cells are seen in some pathological states.

It will be apparent to the reader that the mast cell is essentially a secretory cell and its granules can be looked upon as secretory granules*. There is, however, evidence that the mast cell (and also basophils) is also a phagocytic cell that can phagocytose ferritin, viruses, nuclei and plastic spheres (Padawer, 1971). Many lysosomal enzymes have also been demonstrated in the granules of mast cells and basophils, in addition of course to heparin and histamine (Lagunoff and Benditt, 1963). Serotonin is found in the mast cell of rats but not in humans and most other species.

---

*It has been suggested that regeneration of granules can occur after discharge of granules (Fawcett, 1955; Hill, 1957; Fasske and Themann, 1969).

Plate 178

Fig. 1. Human basophil leucocyte from peripheral blood showing characteristic granules and a nucleus with abundant marginally placed heterochromatin. × 23 000

Fig. 2. High-power view of basophil granules showing particulate contents. × 100 000

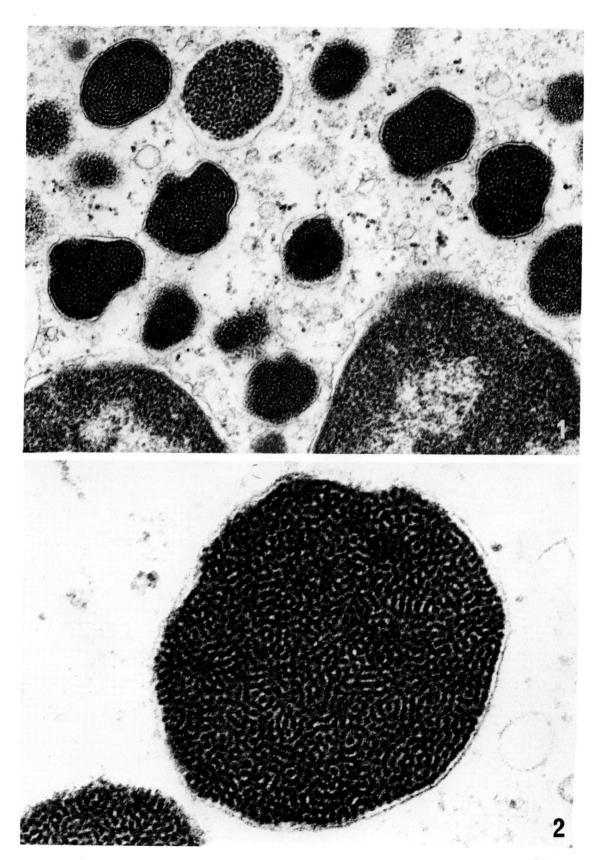

401

References

Abt, A. B. and Carter, S. L. (1976). Goblet cell carcinoid of the appendix. *Arch. Path. Lab. Med.* **100,** 301

Ackerman, G. A. (1963). Cytochemical properties of the blood basophilic granulocyte. *Ann. N.Y. Acad. Sci.* **103,** 376

Adams, J. B. and Rienits, K. G. (1961). The biosynthesis of chondroitin sulphates. Influence of nucleotides and hexosamines on sulphate incorporation. *Biochem. biophys. Acta* **51,** 567

Alpert, L. I. and Bochetto, J. F. (1974). Carotid body tumor: Ultrastructural observations. *Cancer* **34,** 564

Amherdt, M., Orci, L., Track, N. S., Lambert, A. E., Kanazawa, Y. and Stauffacher, W. (1971). An ultrastructural study of the islet cell tumor of the golden hamster. *Horm. metab. res.* **3,** 252

Amick, C. J. and Stenger, R. (1964). Ultrastructural alterations in experimental acute hepatic fatty metamorphosis. *Lab. Invest.* **13,** 128

Amsterdam, A. and Schramm, M. (1966). Rapid release of the zymogen granule protein by osmium tetroxide and its retention during fixation by glutaraldehyde. *J. Cell Biol.* **29,** 199

Anzil, A. P., Blinzinger, K. and Herrlinger, H. (1974). Hexagonal arrangement of intragranular particles in human basophilic leucocytes. *Acta Haemat.* **52,** 189

Arrigoni, M. G., Woolner, I. B. and Bernatz, P. E. (1972). Atypical carcinoid tumors of the lung. *J. Thorac. Cardiovasc. Surg.* **64,** 413

Azzopardi, J. G. (1959). Oat cell carcinoma of the bronchus. *J. Path. Bact.* **78,** 513

Azzopardi, J. G. and Pollock, D. J. (1963). Argentaffin and argyrophil cells in gastric carcinoma. *J. Path. Bact.* **86,** 443

Barbezat, G. O. and Grossman, M. I. (1971). Cholera-like diarrhoea induced by glucagon plus gastrin. *Lancet* **1,** 1025

Bates, H. R. and Belter, L. F. (1967). Composite carcinoid tumor (argentaffinoma-adenocarcinoma) of the colon: report of two cases. *Dis. Colon Rect.* **10,** 467

Beams, H. W. and King, R. L. (1933). The Golgi apparatus in the developing tooth, with special reference to polarity. *Anat. Rec.* **57,** 29

Belchetz, P. E., Brown, C. L., Makin, H. L. J., Trafford, D. J. H., Stuart Mason, A., Bloom, S. R. and Ratcliffe, J. G. (1973). ACTH, glucagon and gastrin production by a pancreatic islet cell carcinoma and its treatment. *Clin. endocr.* **2,** 307

Bensch, K. G., Corrin, B., Pariente, R. and Spencer, H. (1968). Oat-cell carcinoma of the lung; its origin and relationship to bronchial carcinoid. *Cancer* **22,** 1163

Bensley, R. R. (1951). Facts versus artefacts in cytology: the Golgi apparatus. *Exp. Cell Res.* **2,** 1

Bernhard, W. (1969). Ultrastructure of the cancer cell. In *Handbook of Molecular Cytology.* Ed. by A. Lima-de-Faria. Amsterdam and London: North Holland Publ.

Black, W. C. (1968). Enterochromaffin cell types and corresponding carcinoid tumours. *Lab. Invest.* **19,** 473

Black, W. C. and Haffner, H. E. (1968). Diffuse hyperplasia of gastric argyrophil cell and multiple carcinoid tumors. *Cancer* **21,** 1080

Bloom, W. and Fawcett, D. W. (1975). *A Textbook of Histology.* Philadelphia, London, Toronto: W. B. Saunders Co.

Bockman, D. E., Black, O., Mills, L. R. and Webster, P. D. (1978). Origin of tubular complexes developing during induction of pancreatic adenocarcinoma by 7, 12-dimethybenz(a)anthracene. *Am. J. Path.* **90,** 645

Boden, G., Owen, O. E., Rezvani, I., Elfenbein, B. I. and Quickel, K.E. (1977). An islet cell carcinoma containing glucagon and insulin. Chronic glucagon excess and glucose homeostasis. *Diabetes* **26,** 120

Bordi, C. and Bussolati, G. (1974). Immunofluorescence, histochemical and ultrastructural studies for the detection of multiple endocrine polypeptide tumours of the pancreas. *Virchows Arch. B. cell Path.* **17,** 13

Bostrom, H. and Aquist, F. (1952). Utilization of S^{35}-labelled sodium sulphate in the synthesis of chondroitin sulphuric acid, taurine, methionine and cystine. *Acta chem. Scand.* **6,** 1557

Bothe, A. E., Dalton, A. J., Hastings, W. S. and Zillessen, F. O. (1950). A study of Golgi material and mitochondria in malignant and benign prostatic tissue. *J. natn. Cancer Inst.* **11,** 239

Bowen, R. H. (1929). The cytology of glandular secretion. *Q. Rev. Biol.* **4,** 299

Breton-Gorius, J. and Reyes, F. (1976). Ultrastructure of human bone marrow cell maturation. *Int. Rev. Cytol.* **46,** 251

Brinkman, G. L. (1968). The mast cell in normal human bronchus and lung. *J. Ultrastruct. Res.* **23,** 115

Cajal, R. Y. (1914). Algunas variaciones fisiologicas y pathologicas del aparato reticular de Golgi. *Trab. Lab. Inv. Madrid* **12,** 127

Cambel, P., Conroy, C. E. and Sgouris, J. T. (1952). Gastric mast cell diapedesis in the albino rat. *Science* **115,** 373

Cantin, M. and Veilleux, R. (1972). Globule leukocytes and mast cells of the urinary tract in magnesium-deficient rats. *Lab. Invest.* **27,** 495

Capella, C. and Solcia, E. (1971). Optical and electon microscopical study of cytoplasmic granules in human carotid body, carotid body tumours and jugular tumours. *Virchows Arch. B Cell Path.* **7,** 37

Capella, C., Gabrielli, M., Polak, J. M., Buffa, R., Solcia, E. and Bordi, C. (1979). Ultrastructural and histological study of 11 bronchial carcinoids. *Virchows Arch. A Path. Anat. Histol.* **381,** 313

Capella, C., Hage, E. Solcia, E. and Usellini, L. (1978). Ultrastructural similarity of endocrine-like cells of the human lung and some related cells of the gut. *Cell tiss. Res.* **186,** 25

Capella, C., Usellini, L., Buffa, R., Frigerio, B. and Solcia, E. (1981). The endocrine component of prostatic carcinomas, mixed adenocarcinoma-carcinoid tumours and non-tumour prostate. Histochemical and ultrastructural identification of the endocrine cells. *Histopathology,* **5,** 175

Capella, C., Solcia, E., Frigerio, B., Buffa, R., Usellini, L. and Fontana, P. (1977). The endocrine cells of the pancreas and related tumours. *Virchows Arch. A Path. Anat. Histol.* **373,** 327

Capella, C., Polak, J. M., Timson, C. M., Frigerio, B. and Solcia, E. (1980). Gastric carcinoids of argyrophil ECL cells. *Ultrastruct. Path.* **1,** 411

Castor, C. W., Prince, R. K. and Hazelton, M. J. (1966). Hyaluronic acid in human synovial effusion. *Arthritis Rheum.* **9,** 783

Chejfec, G. and Gould, V. E. (1977). Malignant gastric neuroendocrinomas. Ultrastructural and biochemical characterization of their secretory activity. *Human Path.* **8,** 433

Chejfec, G. and Gould, V.E. (1984) (Editorial). Amphicrine cells. *Ultrastruct. Path.,* **7,** iii

Chong, F. K., Graham, J. H. and Madoff, I. M. (1979). Mucin-producing carcinoid ("Composite Tumor") of upper third esophagus. *Cancer* **44,** 1853

Cleator, I. G. M., Thomson, C. G., Sircus, W. and Coombes, M. (1970). Bio-assay evidence of abnormal secretin-like and gastrin-like activity in tumour and blood in cases of 'choleraic diarrhoea'. *Gut* **11,** 206

Coalson, J. J., Mohr, J. A., Pirtle, J. K., Dee, A. L. and Rhoads, E. R. (1970). Electron microscopy of neoplasms of the lung with special emphasis on the alveolar cell carcinoma. *Am. Resp. Dis.* **101,** 181

Collins, D. H., Ghadially, F. N. and Meachim, G. (1965). Intracellular lipids of cartilage. *Ann. rheum. Dis.* **24,** 123

Colvin, R. B., Dvorak, A. M. and Dvorak, H. F. (1974). Mast cells in the cortical tubular epithelium and interstitium in human renal disease. *Human Path.* **5,** 315

Cooper, P. H. and Warkel, R. L. (1978). Ultrastructure of the goblet cell type of adenocarcinoid of the appendix. *Cancer* **42,** 2687

Cordier, R. (1924). Les cellules argentaffines dans les tumeurs intestinales. *Arch.Int. Med. Exp.* **1,** 59

Cramer, W. and Ludford, R. J. (1925). On cellular changes in intestinal fat absorption. *J. Physiol.* **60,** 342

Creutzfeldt, W., Arnold, R., Creutzfeldt, C., Deuticke, U., Frerichs, H. and Track, N. S. (1973). Biochemical and morphological investigations of 30 human insulinomas. *Diabetologia* **9,** 217

Crowell, W. T., Grizzle, W. E. and Siegel, A. L. (1982). Functional carotid paragangliomas. *Arch. Path. Lab. Med.* **106,** 599

Cubilla, A. L. and Woodruff, J. M. (1977). Primary carcinoid tumor of the breast. A report of eight patients. *Am. J. Surg. Path.* **1,** 283

Dalton, A. J. (1959). Organization in benign and malignant cells. *Lab. Invest.* **8,** 510

Dalton, A. J. (1961). Golgi apparatus and secretion granules. In *The Cell,* Vol. 2, p. 603. Ed. by J. Brachet and A. E. Mirsky, New York: Academic Press

Dalton, A. J. (1964). An electron microscopical study of a series of chemically induced hepatomas. In *Cellular Control, Mechanisms and Cancer,* p. 211. Ed. by P. Emmelot and O. Muhlbock. New York: American Elsevier

Dalton, A. J. and Edwards, J. E. (1942). Mitochondria and Golgi apparatus of induced and spontaneous hepatomas in the mouse. *J. Natn. Cancer Inst.* **2,** 565

Dalton, A. J. and Felix, M. D. (1954a). Cytologic and cytochemical characteristics of the Golgi substance of epithelial cells of the epididymis *in situ,* in homogenates and after isolation. *Am. J. Anat.* **94,** 171

Dalton, A. J. and Felix, M. D. (1954b). In *The Fine Structure of Cells,* Proc. 8th Int. Congr. Cell Biol., Leiden, 1954, p. 274. New York: Interscience

Dalton, A. J. and Felix, M. D. (1956). A comparative study of the Golgi complex. *J. biophys. biochem. Cytol.* **2,** 79

Davis, B. H., Ludwig, M. E., Cole, S. R. and Pastuszak, W. T. (1983). Small cell neuroendocrine carcinoma of the urinary bladder: Report of three cases with ultrastructural analysis. *Ultrastruct. Path.* **4,** 197

Decker, B., McGuckin, W. F., McKenzie, B. F. and Slocumb, C. H. (1959). Concentration of hyaluronic acid in synovial fluid. *Clin. Chem.* **5,** 465

DeLellis, R. A., Dayal, Y. and Wolfe, H. J. (1984). Editorial: Carcinoid tumors. Changing concepts and new perspectives. *Am. J. Surg. Path.* **8,** 295

DeLellis, R. A., Merk, F. B., Deckers, P., Warren, S. and Balogh, K. (1973). Ultrastructure and *in vitro* growth characteristics of a transplantable rat pheochromocytoma. *Cancer* **32**, 227

Dobbins, W. O. (1978). Diagnostic Pathology of the Intestine and Colon. In *Diagnostic Electron Microscopy* Vol. 1, pp. 253–339. Ed. by B. F. Trump and R. T. Jones, New York: John Wiley & Sons

Dobbins, W. O., Tomasini, J. T. and Rollins, E. L. (1969). Electron and light microscopic identification of the mast cell of the gastrointestinal tract. *Gastroenterology* **56**, 268

Dvorak, H. F. and Dvorak, A. M. (1975). Basophilic leucocytes: structure, function and role in disease. *Clin. Haematol.* **4**, 651

Dvorak, A. M. and Dvorak, H. F. (1979). The Basophil. *Arch. Pathol. Lab. Med.* **103**, 551

Dvorak, A. M., Dickersin, G. R., Connell, A., Carey, R. W. and Dvorak, H. F. (1976). Degranulation mechanisms in human leukemic basophils. *Clin. Immunol. Immunopath.* **5**, 235

Dvorak, H. F., Dvorak, A. M., Simpson, B. A., Richerson, H. B., Leskowitz, S. and Karnosky, M. J. (1970). Cutaneous basophil hypersensitivity. II A light and electron microscopic description. *J. Exp. Med.* **132**, 558

Dziewiatkowski, D. (1951). Isolation of chondriotin sulfate-S^{35} from articular cartilage of rats. *J. biol. Chem.* **189**, 187

Egeberg, J. and Jensen, O. A. (1969). The ultrastructure of the acini of the human lacrimal gland. *Acta Ophthalmol.* **47**, 400

Ehrlich, P. (1877). Beiträge zur Kenntniss der Anilinfärbungen und ihrer Verwendung in der mikroskopischen Technik. *Arch. Mikros. Anat.* **13**, 263

Epstein, M.A. (1957a). The fine structure of the cells in mouse sarcoma 37 ascitic fluids. *J. biophys. biochem. Cytol.* **3**, 567

Epstein, M. A. (1957b). The fine structural organization of Rous tumor cells. *J. biophys. biochem. Cytol.* **3**, 851

Erlandson, R. A. and Tandler, B. (1972). Ultrastructure of acinic cell carcinoma of the parotid gland. *Arch. Path.* **93**, 130

Estes, L. and Lombardi, B. (1969). Effect of choline deficiency on the Golgi apparatus of rat hepatocytes. *Lab. Invest.* **21**, 374

Farquhar, M. G. (1961a). Origin and fate of secretory granules in cells of the anterior pituitary gland. *N.Y. Acad. Sci. Trans.* **23**, 346

Farquhar, M. G. (1961b). Fine structure and function in capillaries of the anterior pituitary gland. *Angiology* **12**, 270

Farquhar, M. G. and Rinehart, J. F. (1954a). Electron microscopic studies of the anterior pituitary gland of castrate rats. *Endocrinology* **55**, 516

Farquhar, M. G. and Rinehart, J. F. (1954b). Cytologic alterations in the anterior pituitary gland following thyroidectomy: An electron microscopic study. *Endocrinology* **55**, 857

Farquhar, M. G. and Wellings, S. R. (1957). Electron microscopic evidence suggesting secretory granule formation within the Golgi apparatus. *J. Biophys. Biochem. Cytol.* **3**, 319

Fasske, E. and Themann, H. (1969). Elektronenmikroskopische experimentelle Untersuchungen zur Entladung der Gewebsmastzellen. *Virchows Arch. Abt. B. Zellpath* **4**, 126

Fawcett, D. W. (1955). An experimental study of mast cell degranulation and regeneration. *Anat. Rec.* **121**, 29

Fawcett, D. W. (1966). *An Atlas of Fine Structure. The Cell, its Organelles and Inclusions.* Philadelphia. London: Saunders

Fawcett, D. W., Long, J.A. and Jones, A. L. (1969). The ultrastructure of endocrine glands. *Rec. Prog. Horm Res.* **25**, 318

Fedorko, M. E. and Hirsch, J. G. (1965). Crystalloid structure in granules of guinea pig basophils and human mast cells. *J. Cell Biol.* **26**, 973

Feltkamp-Vroom, T. M. (1977). Mast cells in atopic and non-atopic subjects. *Scand. J. resp. Dis. Supp.* **98**, 8

Feltkamp-Vroom, T. M., Stallman, P. J., Aalberse, R. C. and Reerink-Brongers, E. E. (1975). Immunofluorescence studies on renal tissue, tonsils, adenoids, nasal polyps and skin of atopic and nonatopic patients with special reference to IgE. *Clin. Immunol. Immunopath.* **4**, 392

Fetissof, F., Boivin, F. and Jobard, P. (1982). Microfilamentous carcinoid of the thymus: correlation of ultrastructural study with Grimelius stain. *Ultrastruct. Path.* **3**, 9

Fewer, D., Threadgold, J. and Sheldon, H. (1964). Studies on cartilage. V. Electron microscopic observations on the autoradiographic localization of S^{35} in cells and matrix. *J. Ultrastruct. Res.* **11**, 166

Flickinger, C. J. (1970). The fine structure of the nuclear envelope in amebae: alterations following nuclear transplantation. *Exp. Cell Res.* **60**, 225

Fu, Y-S., McWilliams, N. B., Stratford, T. P. and Kay, S. (1974). Bronchial carcinoid with choroidal metastasis in an adolescent. *Cancer* **33**, 707

Ghadially, F. N. (1978). Fine Structure of Joints. In *The Joints and Synovial Fluid*. Ed. by Leon Sokoloff. New York: Academic Press

Ghadially, F. N. (1980). The articular territory of the reticuloendothelial system. *Ultrastruct. Path.* **1**, 249

Ghadially, F. N. (1982). *Ultrastructural Pathology of the Cell and Matrix*. London: Butterworths

Ghadially, F. N. (1983). *Fine Structure of Synovial Joints*. London: Butterworths

Ghadially, F. N. (1985). *Diagnostic Electron Microscopy of Tumours*, 2nd Edn. London: Butterworths

Ghadially, F. N. and Parry, E. W. (1966). Ultrastructure of a human hepatocellular carcinoma and surrounding non-neoplastic liver. *Cancer* **19**, 1989

Ghadially, F. N. and Roy, S. (1967). Ultrastructure of synovial membrane in rheumatoid arthritis. *Am. rheum. Dis.*, **26**, 426

Ghadially, F. N. and Roy, S. (1969). *Ultrastructure of Synovial Joints in Health and Disease*. London: Butterworths

Ghadially, F. N., Chisholm, I. A. and Lalonde, J-M. A. (1986). Ultrastructure of an intraocular lacrimal gland choristoma. *J. Submicrosc. Cytol.* **18**, 189

Ghadially, F. N., Harawi, S. and Khan, W. (1985). Diagnostic ultrastructural markers in alveolar cell carcinoma. *J. Submicrosc. Cytol.* **17**, 269

Ghadially, F. N., Meachim, G. and Collins, D. H. (1965). Extracellular lipid in the matrix of human articular cartilage. *Ann rheum. Dis.* **24**, 136

Ghadially, F. N., Mehta, P. H. and Kirkaldy-Willis, W. H. (1970). Ultrastructure of articular cartilage in experimentally produced lipoarthrosis. *J. Bone Jt Surg.* **52A**, 1147

Gibbs, N. M. (1963). The histogenesis of carcinoid tumours of the rectum. *J. clin. Path.* **16**, 206

Gillespie, J. J., Luger, A. M. and Callaway, L. A. (1979). Peripheral spindled carcinoid tumor: A review of its ultrastructure, differential diagnosis, and biologic behavior. *Human Path.* **10**, 601

Godman, G. C. and Lane, N. (1964). On the site of sulfation in the chondrocyte. *J. Cell Biol.* **21**, 353

Golgi, C. (1898). Sur la structure des cellules nerveuses des ganglions spinaux. *Archo ital. biol.* **30**, 278

Golouh, R., Us-Krasovec, M., Auersperg, M., Jancar, J., Bondi, A. and Eusebi, V. (1985). Amphicrine — composite calcitonin and mucin-producing — carcinoma of the thyroid. *Ultrastructur. Path.*, **8**, 197

Gould, V. E. (1982). Neuroendocrine tumors in 'miscellaneous' primary sites: Clinical, pathologic and histogenic implications. In *Progress in Surgical Pathology*, Vol. 4, Chapter 10, Ed. by C. Fenoglio and M. Wolff. New York: Masson Publishing Co.

Gould, V. E., Memoli, V. A. and Warren, W. H. (1983). Case 5: Metastatic paraganglioma in lung (primary in left carotid body). *Ultrastruct. Path.* **5**, 299

Gould, V. E., Jao, W., Chejfec, G., Banner, B. F., and Bonomi, P. (1984). Neuroendocrine carcinomas of the gastrointestinal tract. *Seminars in Diagnostic Pathol.* **1**, 13

Grabner, G., Boltz, B. and Förster, O. (1980). Macrophage-like properties of human hyalocytes. *Invest. Ophthal.* **19**, 333

Green, J. D. and Van Breemen, V. L. (1955). Electron microscopy of the pituitary and observations on neurosecretion. *Am. J. Anat.* **97**, 177

Greider, M. H. and Elliott, D. W. (1964). Electron microscopy of human pancreatic tumors of islet cell origin. *Am. J. Path.* **44**, 663

Greider, M. H., Bencosme, S. A. and Lechago, J. (1970). The human pancreatic islet-cells and their tumors. I. The normal pancreatic islets. *Lab. Invest.* **22**, 344

Greider, M. H., Rosai, J. and McGuigan, J. E. (1974). The human pancreatic islet cells and their tumors. II. Ulcerogenic and diarrheagenic tumors. *Cancer* **33**, 1423

Grimley, P. M. and Glenner, G. G. (1967). Histology and ultrastructure of carotid body paragangliomas. *Cancer* **20**, 1473

Haguenau, F. and Bernhard, W. (1955). L'appareil de Golgi dans les cellules normales et cancereuses de vertèbres. *Arch Anat. microsc. Morph. exp.* **44**, 27

Haguenau, F. and Lacour, F. (1955). Cytologie electronique de tumeurs hypophysaires experimentals; leur appareil de Golgi. In *The Fine Structure of Cells*, Proc. 8th Int. Congr. Cell Biol., Leiden, 1954, p. 316. New York: Interscience.

Hamerman, D. and Sandson, J. (1963). Unusual properties of hyaluronate-protein isolated from pathological synovial fluids. *J. clin. Invest.* **42**, 1882

Hamilton, R. L., Regen, D. M. and LeQuire, V. S. (1966). Electron microscopic studies of lipoprotein transport in the perfused rat liver. *Fedn Proc.* **25**, 361

Hamilton, R. L., Regen, D. M., Gray, M. E. and Lequire, V. S. (1967). Lipid transport in liver. I. Electron microscopic identification of very low density lipoproteins in perfused rat liver. *Lab. Invest.* **16**, 305

Hammar, S. P., Bockus, D., Remington, F., Hallman, K. O., Winterbauer, R. H., Hill, L. D., Bauermeister, D. E., Jones, H. W., Mennemeyer, R. P. and Wheelis, R. F. (1980). Langerhans cells and serum precipitating antibodies against fungal antigens in bronchioloalveolar cell carcinoma: Possible association with pulmonary eosinophilic granuloma. *Ultrastruct. Path.* **1**, 19

Hart, W. R. and Regezi, J. A. (1978). Strumal carcinoid of the ovary. *Am. J. Clin. Path.* **69**, 356

Hastie, R. (1974). A study of the ultrastructure of human basophil leukocytes. *Lab. Invest.* **31**, 223

Hastie, R., Levy, D. A. and Weiss, L. (1977). The antigen-induced degranulation of basophil leukocytes from atopic subjects studied by electron microscopy. *Lab. Invest.* **36**, 173

Hatanaka, K., Kitamura, Y. and Nishimune, Y. (1979). Local development of mast cells from bone marrow-derived precursors in the skin of mice. *Blood* **53**, 142

Hattori, S., Matsuda, M., Tateishi, R., Nishihara, H. and Horai, T. (1972). Oat cell carcinoma of the lung: clinical and morphological studies in relation to its histogenesis. *Cancer* **30**, 1014

Heitz, Ph. U., Kasper, M., Polak, J. M. and Klöppel, G. (1979). Pathology of the endocrine pancreas. *J. Histochem. Cytochem.* **27**, 1401

Hernandez, F. J. and Fernandez, B. B. (1974). Mucus-secreting colonic carcinoid tumors: Light- and electron microscopic study of three cases. *Dis. Colon Rect.* **17**, 387

Hernandez, F. J. and Reid, J. D. (1969). Mixed carcinoid and mucus-secreting intestinal tumors. *Arch. Path.* **88**, 489

Hewan-Lowe, K. O. (1983). Acinar cell carcinoma of the pancreas: metastases from an occult primary tumor. *Arch. Path. Lab. Med.* **107**, 552

Hibbs, R. G., Burch, G. E. and Phillips, J. H. (1960). Electron-microscopic observations on the human mast cell. *Am. Heart J.* **60**, 121

Hill, M. (1957). Secretion of heparin by mast cells. *Nature* **180**, 654

Hogan, M. J., Alvarado, J. A. and Weddell, J. E. (1971). *Histology of the Human Eye. An Atlas and Textbook*. Philadelphia, London: W. B. Saunders

Hörtnagl, H., Hörtnagl, H., Propst, A., Schwingshackl, H., Weiser, G. and Winkler, H. (1973). Catecholamine storage in liver metastases of a malignant carotid body tumour. *Virchows Arch. B Cell Path.* **12**, 330

Horvath, E. and Kovacs, K. (1976). Ultrastructural classification of pituitary adenomas. *Can. J. Neurol. Sci.* **3**, 9

Horwitz, A. L. and Dorfman, A. (1968). Subcellular sites for synthesis of chondromucoprotein of cartilage, *J. Cell Biol.* **38**, 358

Hosoda, S., Nakamura, W., Suzuki, H., Hoshino, M. and Karasawa, K. (1970). A bronchial carcinoid having low serotonin concentration. *Arch. Path.* **90**, 320

Howatson, A. F. and Ham, A. W. (1955). Electron microscope study of sections of two rat liver tumors. *Cancer Res.* **15**, 62

Howatson, A. F. and Ham, A. W. (1957). The fine structure of cells. *Can. J. Biochem. Physiol.* **35**, 549

Hultin, T. (1961). On the functions of the endoplasmic reticulum. *Biochem. Pharmac.* **5**, 359

Huntrakoon, M., Lin, F., Heitz, P. U. and Tomita, T. (1984). Thymic carcinoid tumor with Cushing's syndrome. *Arch. Path. Lab. Med.* **108**, 551

Ibanez, M. L. (1974). Medullary carcinoma of the thyroid gland. *Path. Ann.* **9**, 263

Ichikawa, A. (1959). Electron microscope study on secretion of the rat adenohypophysis. *Acta Anat. Nipp.* **34**, 460

Isaacson, P. (1981). Crypt cell carcinoma of the appendix (so-called adenocarcinoid tumor). *Am. J. Surg. Path.* **5**, 213

Ito, S. (1969). Structure and function of the glycocalyx. *Fedn. Proc.* **28**, 12

Iwamoto, T. and Jakobiec, F. A. (1982). A comparative ultrastructural study of the normal lacrimal gland and its epithelial tumors. *Human Path.* **13**, 236

Iwanij, V., Hull, B. E. and Jamieson, J. D. (1982). Structural characterization of a rat acinar cell tumor. *J. Cell Biol.* **95**, 727

Jasswoin, G. (1924). On the structure and development of the enamel in mammals. *Q. Jl microsc. Sci.* **69**, 97

Jatlow, P., Adams, W. R. and Handschumacher, R. E. (1965). Pathogenesis of orotic acid-induced fatty change in the rat liver. Light and electron microscopic studies. *Am. J. Path.* **47**, 125

Johannessen, J. V. (1977). Use of paraffin material for electron microscopy. *Path. Ann.* **12**, 189

Johannessen, J. V., Gould, V. E. and Jao, W. (1978). The fine structure of human thyroid cancer. *Human Path.* **9**, 385

Johnston, W. W. and Frable, W. J. (1976). The cytopathology of the respiratory tract. *Am. J. Path.* **84**, 372

Jones, A. L., Rudermann, N. B. and Herrera, M. G. (1967). Electron microscopic and biochemical study of lipoprotein synthesis in the isolated perfused rat liver. *J. Lipid. Res.* **8**, 429

Jorpes, J. E. (1947). The origin and the physiology of heparin: The specific therapy in thrombosis. *Ann. Int. Med.* **27**, 361

Kajihara, H., Totović, V. and Gedigk, P. (1975). Zur Ultrastruktur und Morphogenese des Ceroidpigmentes. 1. Fettphagocytose und Bildung von lipidhaltigen Lysosomen in den Kupfferschen Sternzellen der Rattenleber nach intravenöser Injektion hochungesättigter Lipide. *Virchows Arch. B. Cell Path.* **19,** 221

Kaneko, H., Ishikawa, S., Sumida, T., Sekiya, M., Toshima, M., Kobayashi, H. and Naka, Y. (1980). Ultrastructural studies of a thymic carcinoid tumor. *Acta Pathol., Jpn* **30,** 651

Kaneko, H., Sumida, T., Sekiya, M., Toshima, M., Kobayashi, H. and Naito, K. (1982). A breast carcinoid tumor with special reference to ultrastructural study. *Acta Path., Jpn* **32,** 327

Katenkamp, D. and Wätzig, V. (1984). Multiple neuroendocrine carcinomas (so-called Merkel cell tumours) of the skin. *Virchows Arch. A Pathol. Anat.* **404,** 403

Kawanami, O., Ferrans, V. J., Fulmer, J. D. and Crystal, R. G. (1979). Ultrastructure of pulmonary mast cells in patients with fibrotic lung disorders. *Lab. Invest.* **40,** 717

Keane, J., Fretzin, D. F., Jao, W. and Shapiro, C. M. (1980). Bronchial carcinoid metastatic to skin. Light and electron microscopic findings. *J. Cut. Pathol.* **7,** 43

Kent, J. F. (1966). Distribution and fine structure of globule leucocytes in respiratory and digestive tracts of the laboratory rat. *Anat. Rec.* **156,** 439

Keyhani, E. and Breton-Gorius, J. (1972). Etude au microscope électronique de la formation et de la maturation des granulations des leucocytes basophiles de la moelle osseuse de l'homme et du cobaye. *Acta anat.* **82,** 337

Kirkman, H. and Severinghaus, A. E. (1938). A review of the Golgi apparatus. *Anat. Rec.* **70,** 557

Kitamura, Y., Shimada, M., Go, S., Matsuda, H., Hatanaka, K. and Seki, M. (1979). Distribution of mast cell precursors in hematopoietic and lymphopoietic tissues of mice. *J. exp. Med.* **150,** 482

Klein, H. Z. (1974). Mucinous carcinoid tumor of the vermiform appendix. *Cancer* **33,** 770

Kobayasi, T., Midtgard, K. and Asboe-Hansen, G. (1968). Ultrastructure of human mast-cell granules. *J. Ultrastruct. Res.* **23,** 153

Kostianovsky, M. (1980). Endocrine pancreatic tumors: Ultrastructure. *Ann. Clin. Lab. Sci.* **10,** 65

Kovacs, K. and Horvath, E. (1974). Amphophil adenoma of the human pituitary gland with masses of cytoplasmic microfilaments. *Endokrinologie* **63,** 402

Kovacs, K., Horvath, E. and McComb, D. J. (1984). Fine structure of pituitary tumors. In *Ultrastructure of Endocrine Cells and Tissues.* Ed. by P. M. Motta. Boston: Martinus Nijhoff

Kubo, T. and Watanabe, H. (1971). Neoplastic agentaffin cells in gastric and intestinal carcinomas. *Cancer* **27,** 447

Kühnel, W. (1968). Vergleichende histologische, histochemische und elektronenmikroskopische Untersuchungen an Tränendrüsen. *Z. Zellforsch.* **89,** 550

Lagunoff, D. (1972). The mechanism of histamine release from mast cells. *Biochem. Pharmacol.* **21,** 1889

Lagunoff, D. (1973). Membrane fusion during mast cell secretion. *J. Cell Biol.* **57,** 252

Lagunoff, D. and Benditt, E. P. (1963). Proteolytic enzymes of mast cells. *Ann. N. Y. Acad. Sci.* **103,** 185

Law, D. H., Liddle, G. W., Scott, H. W. Jr. and Tauber, S. D. (1965). Ectopic production of multiple hormones (ACTH, MSH and gastrin) by a single malignant tumor. *New Engl. J. Med.* **273,** 292

Lawson, D., Raff, M. C., Gomperts, B., Fewtrell, C. and Gilula, N. B. (1977). Molecular events during membrane fusion. A study of exocytosis in rat peritoneal mast cells. *J. Cell Biol.* **72,** 242

Lever, J. D. and Peterson, R. (1960). Cellular identities in the pars distalis of the rat pituitary. *N. Y. Acad. Sci. Trans.* **22,** 504

Levine, G. D. and Rosai, J. (1976). A spindle cell variant of thymic carcinoid tumor. *Arch. path. Lab. Med.* **100,** 293

Like, A. A. (1967). The ultrastructure of the secretory cells of the islets of Langerhans in man. *Lab. Invest.* **16,** 937

Lillie, R. D. and Glenner, G. G. (1960). Histological reaction in carcinoid tumors of the human gastrointestinal tract. *Am. J. Path.* **36,** 623

Livnat, E. J., Scommegna, A., Recant, W. and Jao, W. (1977). Ultrastructural observations of the so-called strumal carcinoid of the ovary. *Arch. Pathol. Lab. Med.* **101,** 585

LiVolsi, V. A. (1987) (Editorial). Mixed thyroid carcinoma: A real entity. *Lab. Invest.,* **57,** 237

Löblich, H. J. and Knezevic, M. (1960). Elektronenoptische Untersuchungen nach akuter Schädigung des Hypophysen-Zwischenhirnsystems. *Beitr. zur Path. Anat.* **122,** 1

Ludford, R. J. (1929). Vital staining of normal and malignant cells; staining of malignant tumours with trypan blue *Proc. R. Soc., B* **104,** 493

Ludford, R. J. (1952). Pathological aspects of cytology. In *Cytology and Cell Physiology,* 2nd ed., p. 373. Ed. by G. Bourne. London and New York: Oxford University Press

Lyss, A. P., Thompson, J. J. and Glick, J. H. (1981). Adenocarcinoid tumor of the colon arising in preexisting ulcerative colitis. *Cancer* **48,** 833

Macadam, R. F. (1969). The fine structure of a human carotid body tumour. *J. Path.* **99,** 101

McGavran, M. H., Unger, R. H., Recant, L., Polk, H. C., Kilo, C. and Levin, M. E. (1966). A glucagon secreting alpha cell carcinoma of the pancreas. *New Engl. J. Med.* **274,** 1408

Mahley, R. W., Gray, M. E., Hamilton, R. L. and Lequire, V. S. (1968). Lipid transport in liver. II. Electron microscopic and biochemical studies of alterations in lipoprotein transport induced by cortisone in the rabbit. *Lab. Invest.* **19,** 358

Martinez, A., Argüelles, F., Cervera, J. and Gomar, F. Jr. (1977). Sites of sulfatation in the chondrocytes of the articular cartilage of the rabbit. A study by quantative radioautography of high resolution. *Virchows Arch. B Cell Path.* **23,** 53

Mehta, P. N. and Ghadially, F. N. (1973). Articular cartilage in corn oil induced lipoarthrosis. *Ann. rheum. Dis.* **32,** 75

Merino, M. J., LiVolsi, V. A., Edmonds, P. R. and Duray, P. (1983). Carcinoid tumors of the appendix. *Lab. Invest.* **48,** 57A

Miller, H. R. P. (1971). Immune reactions in mucous membranes. II. The differentiation of intestinal mast cell during helminth expulsion in the rat. *Lab. Invest.* **24,** 339

Miller, H. R. P. and Jarrett, W. F. H. (1971). Immune reactions in mucous membranes. 1. Intestinal mast cells response during helminth expulsion in the rat. *Immunology* **20,** 277

Mills, S. E., Walker, A. N., Cooper, P. H. and Kron, I. L. (1982). Atypical carcinoid tumor of the lung. *Am. J. Surg. Path.* **6,** 643

Misugi, K., Misugi, N. and Newton, W. A. (1968). Fine structural study of neuroblastoma, ganglioneuroblastoma and pheochromocytoma *Arch. Path* **86,** 160

Miura, A. B., Shibata, A., Onodera, S., Suzuki,, A., Sakamoto, S. and Suzuki, C. (1968). The ultrastructure of basophile leukocytes in human chronic myelogenous leukemia. *Tohoku J. Exp. Med.* **96,** 87

Morgan, J. E., Kaiser, C. W., Johnson, W., Doos, W. G., Dayal, Y., Berman, L., and Nabseth, D. (1983). Gastric carcinoid (gastrinoma). *Cancer* **51,** 2332

Mughal, S. and Filipe, M. I. (1978). Ultrastructural study of the normal mucosa-adenoma-cancer sequence in the development of familial polyposis coli. *J. Natn. Cancer Inst.* **60,** 753

Murray, M., Miller, H. P. R. and Jarrett, W. F. H. (1968). The globule leukocyte and its derivation from the subepithelial mast cell. *Lab. Invest.* **19,** 222

Nagle, R. B., Payne, C. M. and Clark, V. A. (1986). Comparison of the usefulness of histochemistry and ultrastructural cytochemistry in the identification of neuroendocrine neoplasms. *Am. J. Clin. Path.* **85,** 289

Nakayama, I., Nickerson, P. A. and Skelton, F. R. (1969). An ultrastructural study of the adrenocorticotrophic hormone-secreting cell in the rat adenohypophysis during adrenal cortical regeneration. *Lab. Invest.* **21,** 169

Neutra, M. and Leblond, C. P. (1966a). Synthesis of the carbohydrate of mucus in the Golgi complex as shown by electron microscope radioautography of goblet cells from rats injected with glucose-H^3. *J. Cell Biol.* **30,** 119

Neutra, M. and Leblond, C. P. (1966b). Radioautographic comparison of the uptake of galactose-H^3 and glucose-H^3 in the Golgi region of various cells secreting glycoproteins or mucopolysaccharides. *J. Cell Biol.* **30,** 137

Oberling, Ch. and Bernhard, W. (1961). The morphology of the cancer cells. In *The Cell,* Vol. 5, p. 405. Ed. by J. Brachet and A. E. Mirsky. New York: Academic Press

Olsson, I., Berg, B., Fransson, L. A. and Nordén, A. (1970). The identity of the metachromatic substance of basophilic leucocytes. *Scand. J. Haemat.* **7,** 440

O'Neal, L. W., Kipnis, D. M., Luse, S. A., Lacey, P. E. and Jarett, L. (1968). Secretion of various endocrine substances by ACTH-secreting tumors-gastrin, melanotropin, norepinephrine, serotonin, parahormone, vasopressin, glucagon. *Cancer* **21,** 1219

Onoe, T. and Ohno, K. (1963). Role of endoplasmic reticulum in fat absorption. In *Intracellular Membranous Structure,* Vol. 14. Ed. by S. Seno and E. V. Cowdry. Okayama: The Japan Society for Cell Biology

Orloff, M. J. (1971). Carcinoid tumors of the rectum. *Cancer* **28,** 175

Orr, T. S. C. (1977). Fine structure of the mast cell with special reference to human cells. *Scand. J. resp. Dis. Suppl.* **98,** 1

Padawer, J. (1971). Phagocytosis of particulate sustances by mast cells. *Lab. Invest.* **25,** 320

Palay, S. L. and Karlin, L. J. (1959). An electron microscopic study of the intestinal villus. II. The pathway of fat absorption. *J. biophys. biochem. Cytol.* **5,** 373

Payne, C. M., Nagle, R. B. and Borduin, V. (1984). Methods in laboratory investigation. An ultrastructural cytochemical stain specific for neuroendocrine neoplasms. *Lab. Invest.* **51,** 350

Payne, C. M., Nagle, R. B., Borduin, V. F. and Kim, A. (1983). An ultrastructural evaluation of the cell organelle specificity of the uranaffin reaction in two human endocrine neoplasms. *J. Submicrosc. Cytol.* **15,** 833

408

Pearse, A. G. E. (1972). *Histochemistry*, Vol. 2. 3rd Ed. London: Churchill-Livingstone

Pearse, A. G. E. (1974). The APUD cell concept and its implications in pathology. *Path. Ann.* **9**, 27

Pearse, A. G. E. (1982). This week's citation classic. *Current Contents* **19**, (May 10) 24

Pearse, A. G. E. and Takor Takor, T. (1979). Embryology of the diffuse neuroendocrine system and its relationship to the common peptides. *Fed. Proc.* **38**, 2288

Peonim, V., Thakerngpol, K., Pacharee, P. and Stitnimankarn, T. (1983). Adenosquamous carcinoma and carcinoidal differentiation of the colon. *Cancer* **52**, 1122

Peterson, M. R. and Leblond, C. P. (1964). Uptake by the Golgi region of glucose labelled with tritium in the 1 or 6 position, as an indicator of synthesis of complex carbohydrates. *Exp. Cell Res.* **34**, 420

Polak, J. M., Bloom, S. R., Adrian, T. E., Heitz, Ph. U., Bryant, M. G. and Pearse, A. G. E. (1976). Pancreatic polypeptide in insulinomas, gastrinomas, vipomas and glycagonomas. *Lancet* **1**, 328

Pritchett, P. S. and Key, B. M. (1978). Mucous gland adenoma of the bronchus: ultrastructural and histochemical studies. *Ala. J. Med. Science.* **15**, 43

Qizilbash, A. H., Trebilcock, R. G., Patterson, M. C. and Lamont, K. G. (1974). Functioning primary carcinoid tumor of the ovary. *Am. J. Clin. Path.* **62**, 629

Rambourg, A. (1971). Morphological and histochemical aspects of glycoproteins at the surface of animal cells. *Int. Rev. Cytol.* **31**, 57

Rambourg, A., Marraud, A. and Chretien, M. (1973). Tri-dimensional structure of the forming face of the Golgi apparatus as seen in the high voltage electron microscope after osmium impregnation of the small nerve cells in the semilunar ganglion of the trigeminal nerve. *J. Microscopy* **97**, 49

Ranchod, M., Kempson, R. L. and Dorgeloh, J. R. (1976). Strumal carcinoid of the ovary. *Cancer* **37**, 1913

Ratzenhofer, M. (1977). Uber enterale Hyperplasien und Geschwulste der disseminierten endokrinen (parakrinen) Hellen Zellen Feyrters unter besonderer Berucksichtigung amphikriner Zellwucherungen. *Verh. Dtsch. Ges. Pathol.* **61**, 7

Ratzenhofer, M. and Aübock, L. (1980). The amphicrine (endo-exocrine) cells in the human gut, with a short reference to amphicrine neoplasia. *Acta Morphol. Acad. Sci. Hung.* **28**, 37

Ratzenhofer, M. and Leb, D. (1965). Uber die Feinstrukter der argentaffinen und der anderen Erscheinungsformen der 'Hellen Zellen' Feyrter's im Kaninchen-Magen. *Z. Zellforsch.* **67**, 113

Ratzenhofer, M., Aübock, L. and Becker, H. (1969). Elektronen- und fluoreszenzmikroskopische Untersuchungen der Appendicite neurogene. *Verh. Dtsch. Ges. Path.* **53**, 218

Rawlinson, D. G. (1973). Electron microscopy of an ACTH secreting islet cell carcinoma. *Cancer* **31**, 1015

Reynolds, E. S. (1963). Liver parenchymal cell injury. I. Initial alterations of the cell following poisoning with carbon tetrachloride. *J. Cell Biol.* **19**, 139

Robboy, S. J., Norris, H. J. and Scully, R. E. (1975). Insular carcinoid primary in the ovary. *Cancer* **36**, 404

Rogers, L. W. and Murphy, R. C. (1979). Gastric carcinoid and gastric carcinoma. *Am. J. Surg. Path.* **3**, 195

Röhlich, P., Anderson, P. and Uvnäs, B. (1971). Electron microscope observations on compound 48/80-induced degranulation in rat mast cells. Evidence for sequential exocytosis of storage granules. *J. Cell Biol.* **51**, 465

Rosai, J., Levine, G., Weber, W. R. and Higa, E. (1976). Carcinoid tumors and oat cell carcinomas of the thymus. *Pathology Annual* **11**, 201

Roy, S. (1967). Ultrastructure of synovial membrane in osteoarthritis. *Ann. rheum. Dis.* **26**, 517

Roy, S. and Ghadially, F. N. (1967a). Ultrastructure of normal rat synovial membrane. *Ann. rheum. Dis.* **26**, 26

Roy, S. and Ghadially, F. N. (1967b). Synthesis of hyaluronic acid by synovial cells. *J. Path. Bact.* **93**, 555

Ruskell, G. L. (1975). Nerve terminals and epithelial cell variety in the human lacrimal gland. *Cell Tiss. Res.* **158**, 121

Ruttman, E., Klöppel, G., Bommer, G., Kiehn, M. and Heitz, Ph. U. (1980). Pancreatic glycagonoma with and without syndrome. *Virchows Arch. A Pathol. Anat. Histol.* **388**, 51

Salazar, H. and Peterson, R. R. (1964). Morphologic observations concerning the release and transport of secretory products in the adenohypophysis. *Am. J. Anat.* **115**, 199

Sano, M. (1962). Further studies on the theta cell of the mouse anterior pituitary as revealed by electron microscopy, with special reference to the mode of secretion. *J. Cell Biol.* **15**, 85

Santini, D., Bazzocchi, F., Pileri, S., Govoni, E., Taffurelli, M., Grassigli, A., Marrano, D. and Martinelli, G. (1985). Mammary carcinoma with argyrophilic cells: An immunohistochemical and ultrastructural study. *Tumori* **71**, 331

Sariola, H., Lehtonen, E. and Saxén, E. (1985). Breast tumors with a solid and uniform carcinoid pattern. Ultrastructural and immunohistochemical study of two cases. *Path. Res. Pract.* **178**, 405

Schelin, U. (1962). Chromophobe and acidophile adenomas of the human pituitary gland. *Acta Path. Microbiol. Scand.* Supp. 158

409

Schmid, K. O., Aübock, L. and Albegger, K. (1979). Endocrine-amphicrine enteric carcinoma of the nasal mucosa. *Virchows Arch. A. Path. Anat. Histol.* **383,** 329

Scow, R. O. (1970). Transport of triglyceride. Its removal from blood circulation and uptake by tissues. In *Parenteral Nutrition,* p. 294. Ed. by H. C. Meng and D. L. Law. Springfield, Illinois: Charles C. Thomas

Selby, C. C., Biesele, J. J. and Grey, C. E. (1956). Electron microscope studies of ascites tumor cells. *Ann. N.Y. Acad. Sci.* **63,** 748

Selye, H. (1965). The blood basophil. In *The Mast Cells.* Washington: Butterworths

Severinghaus, A. E. (1937). Cellular changes in the anterior hypophysis with special reference to its secretory activities. *Physiol. Rev.* **17,** 556

Sheldon, H. and Kimball, F. B. (1962). Studies on cartilage. III. The occurrence of collagen within vacuoles of the Golgi apparatus. *J. Cell Biol.* **12,** 599

Sheldon, H. and Robinson, R. A. (1960). Studies on cartilage. II. Electron microscope observations on rabbit ear cartilage following the administration of papain. *J. Biophys. biochem. Cytol.* **8,** 151

Siburg, F. (1929). Uber einin Fall von Sogenanntem Karzinoid des Rektums mit ausgedehnter Metastasenbildung. *Frankfurt Ztschr. Pathol.* **37,** 254

Sircus, W. (1969). Peptide secreting tumours with special reference to the pancreas. *Gut* **10,** 506

Smith, D. E. and Lewis, Y. S. (1958). Phagocytosis of granules from disrupted mast cells. *Anat. Rec.* **132,** 93

Smith, D. M. and Haggitt, R. C. (1984). The prevalence and prognostic significance of argyrophil cells in colorectal carcinomas. *Am. J. Surg. Path.* **8,** 123

Snyder, R. R. and Tavassoli, F. A. (1986). Ovarian strumal carcinoid: Immunohistochemical, ultrastructural, and clinicopathologic observations. *Int. J. Gynecol. Pathol.,* **5,** 187

Soga, J. and Tazawa, K. (1971). Pathologic analysis of carcinoids. *Cancer* **28,** 990

Soga, J., Tazawa, K., Aizawa, O., Wada, K. and Tuto, T. (1971). Argentaffin cell adenocarcinoma of the stomach: An atypical carcinoid? *Cancer* **28,** 999

Soga, J., Tazawa, K., Wada, K., Fujimaki, M., Saito, K. and Ikarashi, K. (1972). Argyrophil cell carcinoid of the stomach – A light- and electron microscopic observation. *Acta Path. Jap.* **22,** 541

Solcia, E., Capella, C., Buffa, R., Fiocca, R., Frigerio, B. and Usellini, L. (1980). Identification, ultrastructure and classification of gut endocrine cells and related growths. *Invest. Cell Path.* **3,** 37

Sottovia-Filho, D. (1974). Morphology and histochemistry of mast cells of snakes. *J. Morph.* **142,** 109

Sprinz, R. and Stockwell, R. A. (1976). Changes in articular cartilage following intraarticular injection of tritiated glyceryl trioleate. *J. Anat.* **122,** 91

Stahl, R. E. and Sidhu, G. S. (1979). Primary carcinoid of the kidney. *Cancer* **44,** 1345

Stein, Y. and Shapiro, B. (1959). Assimilation and dissimilation of fatty acids by the rat liver. *Am. J. Physiol.* **196,** 1238

Stein, Y. and Stein, Y. (1967a). Lipid synthesis, intracellular transport, storage and secretion. I. Electron microscopic radioautographic study of the liver after injection of tritiated palmitate or glycerol in fasted and ethanol-treated rats. *J. Cell Biol.* **33,** 319

Stein, Y. and Stein, Y. (1967b). The role of the liver in the metabolism of chylomicrons, studied by electron microscopic autoradiography. *Lab. Invest.* **17,** 436

Stoeckenius, W. (1956). Zur Feinstruktur der Granula Menschlicher Gewebsmastzellen. *Exp. Cell Res.* **11,** 656

Subbuswamy, S. G., Gibbs, N. M., Ross, C. F. and Morson, B. C. (1974). Goblet cell carcinoid of the appendix. *Cancer* **34,** 338

Suzuki, T. (1957). Electron microscopic cytohistopathology. III. Electron microscopic studies on spontaneous mammary carcinoma of mice. *Gann* **48,** 39

Taichman, N. S. (1971). Ultrastructural alterations in guinea pig mast cells during anaphylaxis. *Int. Arch. Allergy and Appl. Immunol.* **40,** 934

Talerman, A. (1984). Carcinoid tumors of the ovary. *J. Cancer Res. Clin. Oncol.* **107,** 125

Talerman, A., Gratama, S., Miranda, S. and Okagaki, T. (1978). Primary carcinoid tumor of the testis. *Cancer* **42,** 2696

Tandler, B. and Erlandson, R. A. (1972). Ultrastructure of the human submaxillary gland. IV. Serous granules. *Am. J. Anat.* **135,** 419

Tannenbaum, M. (1970). Ultrastructural Pathology of Adrenal Medullary Tumors. *Path. Ann.* **5,** 145

Tannenbaum, M., Spiro, D. and Lattimer, J. K. (1966). Norephinephrine and epinephrine secreting tumors of the adrenal medulla. An electron microscopic and biochemical study. *Am. J. Path.* **48,** 48A (abstract)

Toker, C. (1967). Some observations on the ultrastructure of a malignant islet cell tumor associated with duodenal ulceration and severe diarrhea. *J. Ultrastruct. Res.* **19,** 522

Toker, C. (1969). Observations on the composition of certain colonic tumors. *Cancer* **24,** 256

410

Toner, P. G. and Ferguson, A. (1971). Intraepithelial cells in the human intestinal mucosa. *J. Ultrastruct. Res.* **34**, 329

Trelstad, R. L. (1970). The Golgi apparatus in chick corneal epithelium: changes in intracellular position during development. *J. Cell Biol.* **45**, 34

Trotter, C. M. and Orr, T. S. C. (1973). A fine structure study of some cellular components in allergic reactions. I. Degranulation of human mast cells in allergic asthma and perennial rhinitis. *Clin. Allergy* **3**, 411

Ts'ao, C., Patterson, R., McKenna, J. M. and Suszko, I. M. (1977). Ultrastructural identification of mast cells obtained from human bronchial lumens. *J. Allerg. Clin. Immunol.* **59**, 320

Tzur, R. and Shapiro, B. (1964). Dependence of microsomal lipid synthesis on added protein. *J. Lipid Res.* **5**, 542

Ulbright, T. M., Roth, L. M. and Ehrlich, C. E. (1982). Ovarian strumal carcinoid. *Am. J. Clin. Path.* **77**, 622

Voigt, J. J., Alsaati, T., Gorguet, B., Caveriviere, P., Scarna, H., Bugat, R. and Delsol, G. (1985). Carcinome à cellules de Merkel de la peau. *Ann. Path.* **5**, 195

Waisman, J. (1969). Alpha cell granules in a pancreatic neoplasm. *Arch. Path.* **88**, 672

Warkel, R. L., Cooper, P. H. and Helwig, E. B. (1978). Adenocarcinoid, a mucin-producing carcinoid tumor of the appendix. *Cancer* **42**, 2781

Warner, T. F. C. S. and Seo, I. S. (1979). Goblet cell carcinoid of appendix. *Cancer* **44**, 1700

Watanabe, I., Donahue, S. and Hoggatt, N. (1967). Method for electron microscopic studies of circulating human leucocytes and observations on their fine structure. *J. Ultrastruct. Res.* **20**, 366

Weingeist, T. A. (1973). The glands of the ocular adnexa. In *Ocular Fine Structure for the Clinician*. Ed. by K. M. Zinn, *Int. Ophthalmol. Clin.* **13**, 243

Weinstock, A. and Albright, J. T. (1967). The fine structure of mast cells in normal human gingiva. *J. Ultrastruct. Res.* **17**, 245

Whur, P., Herscovics, A. and Leblond, C. P. (1969). Radioautographic visualization of the incorporation of galactose 3H and mannose 3H by rat thyroids *in vitro* in relation to the stages of thyrogolobulin synthesis. *J. Cell Biol.* **43**, 289

Williams, E. D. and Sandler, M. (1963). The classification of carcinoid tumours. *Lancet* **1**, 238

Williams, E. D., Siebenmann, R. E. and Sobin, L. H. (1980). *Histological Typing of Endocrine Tumors*. International Classification of Tumors No. 23. Geneva: World Health Organization

Wilson, T. S., McDowell, E. M., Marangos, P. J. and Trump, B. F. (1985). Histochemical studies of dense-core granulated tumors of the lung. *Arch Path. Lab. Med.* **109**, 613

Wisniewski, M. and Toker, C. (1972). Composite tumor of the gallbladder exhibiting both carcinomatous and carcinoidal patterns. *Am. J. Gastroenterol.* **58**, 633

Woyke, S., Domagala, W. and Olszewski, W. (1972). Alveolar cell carcinoma of the lung: An ultrastructural study of the cancer cells detected in the pleural fluid. *Acta Cytol.* **16**, 63

Wurtman, R. J. (1965). Catecholamines. *New Engl. J. Med.* **273**, 637

Zaatari, G. S., Saigo, P. E. and Huvos, A. G. (1983). Mucin production in medullary carcinoma of the thyroid. *Arch. Pathol. Lab. Med.,* **107**, 70

Zagury, D., Uhr, J. W., Jamieson, J. D. and Palade, G. E. (1970). Immunoglobulin synthesis and secretion. II. Radioautographic studies of sites of addition of carbohydrate moieties and intracellular transport. *J. Cell Biol.* **46**, 52

Zak, F. G., Lawson, W., Statsinger, A. L., Marquet, E. and Sobel, H. J. (1982). Intracellular amyloid in trabecular (Merkel cell) carcinoma of skin: ultrastructural study. *Mt. Sinai J. Med.* **49**, 46

Zeitoun, P. and Lehy, T. (1970). Utilization of paraffin-embedded material for electron microscopy. *Lab. Invest.* **23**, 52

Zollinger, R. M., Tompkins, R. K., Amerson, J. R., Endahl, G. L., Kraft, A. R. and Moore, F. T. (1968). Identification of the diarrheoagenic hormone associated with non-beta islet cell tumors of the pancreas. *Ann. Surg.* **168**, 502

Zucker-Franklin, D. (1967). Electron microscopic study of human basophils. *Blood* **29**, 878

Zucker-Franklin, D. (1980). Ultrastructural evidence for the common origin of human mast cells and basophils. *Blood* **56**, 534

5

Endoplasmic reticulum

Introduction

The organelle now known as the 'endoplasmic reticulum' was first noted by Porter *et al.* (1945) in whole mounts of cultured cells examined with the electron microscope, where it presented as a network of tubular strands and vesicles of varying size and form. It was later named the endoplasmic reticulum (Porter and Thompson, 1948; Porter and Kallman, 1952) because it appeared confined to the main mass of the cell cytoplasm (endoplasm) and did not extend to the cell periphery (ectoplasm). However, such a distribution is not seen in sectioned material, nor is the reticular form easily appreciated. Nevertheless, it is now quite clear that the organelle does in fact often extend close to the cell membrane, and although one has at times to stretch the meaning of the word 'reticulum', this organelle, in its well developed form at least, consists of a system of interconnected cavities and passages and not a series of isolated sacs or vesicles.

Numerous electron microscopic studies now attest to the fact that virtually all the cells of higher plants and vertebrates contain elements of the endoplasmic reticulum (*see* reviews by Palade, 1955 and Porter, 1961). In some cells the organelle is quite simple and is represented by a few vesicles, tubules or cisternae. In others it is quite large and complex and occupies a major volume of the cell cytoplasm (*Plate 179*).

Two main morphological types of endoplasmic reticulum are recognized: the granular or rough endoplasmic reticulum, and the agranular or smooth endoplasmic reticulum. The rough or granular endoplasmic reticulum is so named because its cytoplasmic surface is studded with loops, rows or spirals of ribosomes (called polyribosomes). The smooth endoplasmic reticulum or agranular endoplasmic reticulum, as its name implies, is not associated with ribosomes. This, however, is the main but not the only morphological difference because, while the rough endoplasmic reticulum has a marked tendency to form lamellar cisternae, the smooth endoplasmic reticulum tends to present as fine branching tubules and vesicles. Cell types which have abundant rough endoplasmic reticulum usually have little smooth endoplasmic reticulum and *vice versa*. An exception to this is the hepatocyte where both forms of endoplasmic reticulum are fairly well represented and continuities between the two can frequently be demonstrated.

It is generally accepted that the main function of the rough endoplasmic reticulum (*Plate 179*) is the production of secretory or 'export' protein, and that most of the protein required for endogenous cellular needs is produced by polyribosomes lying free in the cytoplasm. No such common function can be ascribed to the smooth endoplasmic reticulum. It is believed to be involved in a variety of tasks such as: (1) the synthesis of steroid hormones in certain endocrine cells; (2) the detoxification of drugs and metabolism of cholesterol, lipoproteins and perhaps also glycogen in liver cells; (3) the release and recapture of calcium ions in muscle during contraction and relaxation; (4) the transport of ions in the chloride cells of fishes; (5) the secretion of chloride ions by oxyntic cells of the stomach; and (6) lipid transport in intestinal epithelium (Porter, 1961; Fawcett, 1966). It is worth noting, however, that some doubts exist regarding the nature of the smooth membrane systems seen in certain cells such as the chloride cells and intestinal epithelial cells, because at least some of the tubules and vesicles seen here are invaginations of the plasma membrane (*see* page 426).

(*see* page 426)

Plate 179

Fig. 1. Pancreatic acinar cells from a child with islet cell adenoma, showing the graceful arrays of rough endoplasmic reticulum (R) characteristic of this cell type. Note also the poorly formed myelin figure (arrow). This is an artefact of glutaraldehyde fixation which has at times been mistaken for a pathological lesion. ×20 000

Fig. 2. A group of transversely cut cisternae (C) of the rough endoplasmic reticulum, showing ribosomes at irregular intervals along the cytoplasmic surface of the membranes. A group of polyribosomes (P) is seen in an area where the section has passed tangential to the membrane. From same case as *Fig. 1.* ×58 000

Fig. 3. Tangentially cut cisternae showing polyribosomes. From a plasma cell found in human bronchial mucosa. ×58 000

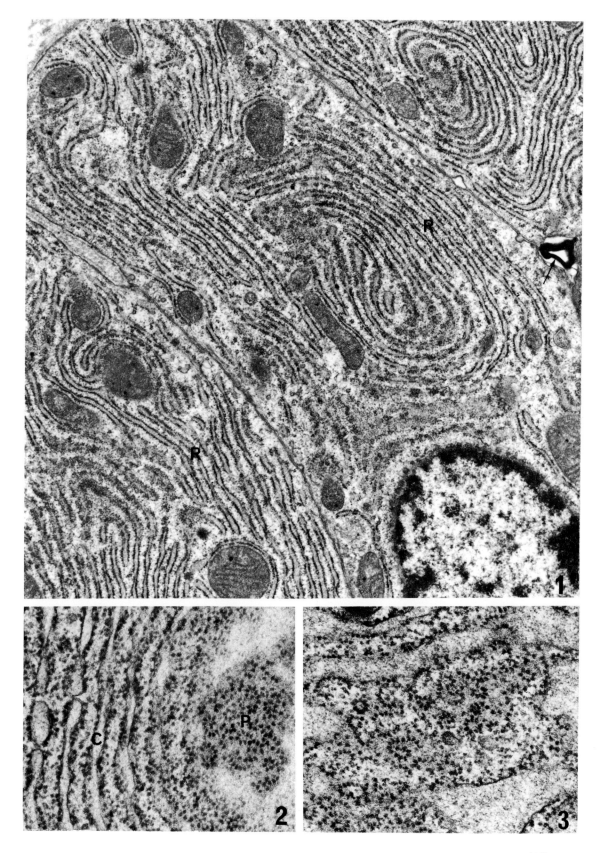

415

Rough endoplasmic reticulum

The term 'granular' or 'rough endoplasmic reticulum' is used to describe a system of ribosome-studded membranes found in the cytoplasm of many cells (*Plates 179–182*). The morphology of this organelle varies markedly in different cell types. In its well developed form, the rough endoplasmic reticulum may be looked upon as a system of vesicular and tubular elements which frequently expand to form flat saccular structures called 'cisternae'. Such cisternae may be solitary, occur in loosely arranged groups, as closely packed parallel stacks, or as gracefully curved or concentric arrays of evenly spaced lamellae. The rough endoplasmic reticulum creates a complex two-phase system in the cell separated by a membrane. Outside the system lies the cytoplasmic matrix, and within it the proteinaceous products elaborated by the polyribosomes of the rough endoplasmic reticulum.

Since the membrane-bound passages of the rough endoplasmic reticulum have often been found to be continuous with the perinuclear cistern, and the outer membrane of the nuclear envelope (*Plate 18*) is frequently studded with some polyribosomes, Porter (1961) has looked upon the nuclear envelope as a stable subdivision of the endoplasmic reticulum. He states, 'the nuclear envelope appears in section as a large lamellar or cisternal unit of the endoplasmic reticulum enclosing the nucleus'. Further support for such a concept comes from the observation that after mitosis the nuclear envelope seems to be re-formed from the endoplasmic reticulum. Annulate lamellae (Chapter 6), which bear much resemblance to the nuclear envelope, have also been looked upon as a variety of endoplasmic reticulum.

The amount of rough endoplasmic reticulum and its morphology in various cell types are quite variable. The greatest development of this organelle is seen in cells which produce an abundant, protein-rich secretion. Some others contain a more modest amount of rough endoplasmic reticulum, while almost all cells contain at least a few elements of this organelle. In pancreatic acinar cells and plasma cells singularly well endowed with rough endoplasmic reticulum the cytoplasm is packed with arrays of closely stacked cisternae (*Plates 179* and *180*) but in synovial cells and chrondrocytes (*Plate 181*) the not-so-abundant complement of rough endoplasmic reticulum is represented by a system of irregular sacs and vesicles. Fibroblasts also usually contain a fair amount of rough endoplasmic reticulum but this depends (as in other cells) on the state of secretory activity of the cells. The rough endoplasmic reticulum is quite well developed in fibroblasts actively engaged in procollagen synthesis and secretion but in resting fibroblasts (called 'fibrocytes' by some) there is a relative paucity of this organelle (*Plate 182*).

Plate 180

Plasma cells from the subsynovial tissue of a rheumatoid joint (*From Ghadially and Roy, 1969*)

Fig. 1. Plasma cells showing abundant arrays of rough endoplasmic reticulum (R), which produces the cytoplasmic basophilia characteristic of this cell, and a well developed juxtanuclear Golgi complex (G) which presents at light microscopy as a clear crescentic area called the 'Hof'. A lymphocyte (L) with scant cytoplasm and a small portion of a macrophage (M) containing lysosomes are also seen in this electron micrograph. ×11 000

Fig. 2. Plasma cell showing cisternae (C) of the rough endoplasmic reticulum which are moderately distended with proteinaceous secretory product. On the surface of the tangentially cut cisternae can be seen numerous polyribosomes (arrows). ×28 000

Fig. 3. A plasma cell showing vesiculation of the rough endoplasmic reticulum. Note that the vesicles (V) contain secretory product which is fairly electron-dense. There is no evidence here that vesiculation has been produced by an ingress of water, for the contents appear neither diluted nor lucent. ×28 000

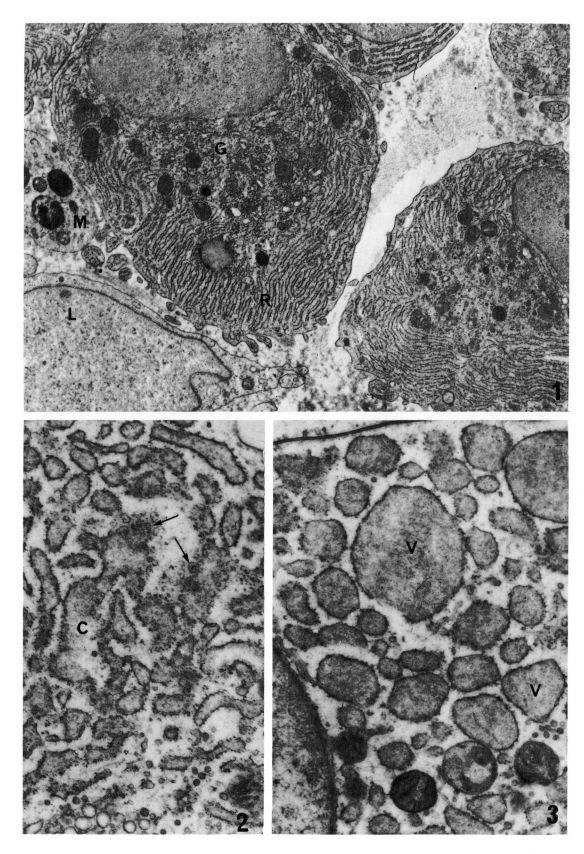

417

Although the main function of the rough endoplasmic reticulum is the production of secretory or export proteins, it also produces some which are used endogenously. Thus there is evidence that, when hypertrophy of the rough or smooth endoplasmic reticulum occurs, the proteins constituting the new membranes are produced by the rough endoplasmic reticulum. The hydrolytic enzymes of primary lysomes are also produced in the rough endoplasmic reticulum.

In normal sections through the cisternae the ribosomes do not appear uniformly spaced along the membranes*. The reason for this becomes apparent when tangential cuts revealing the surface of the cisternae are examined, for now most of the ribosomes are seen to occur in groups forming rosettes, linear arrays, loops or spirals (*Plate 179*). Such collections of ribosomes are spoken of as polysomes or polyribosomes. Ribosomes and polyribosomes occur not only on the membranes of the rough endoplasmic reticulum but also free in the cytoplasm. Polyribosomes consist of ribosomes (12–20 nm diameter) held together by a fine strand of messenger RNA (about 1–1.5 nm thick). (*See* page 438 for more details.)

It is now generally accepted that polyribosomes lying free in the cytoplasm are engaged in the synthesis of proteins for endogenous cellular needs, in contrast to those attached to the rough endoplasmic reticulum which are concerned mainly with the production of export protein.

Cells which produce a protein-rich secretion (e.g. pancreatic acinar cells and plasma cells) are well endowed with rough endoplasmic reticulum while fast-growing populations of cells, such as cells in culture, embryonic cells and tumour cells, are often characterized by numerous polyribosomes lying free in the cytoplasmic matrix. Similarly, in erythroblasts (normoblasts), where the haemoglobin produced is stored and not exported, numerous polyribosomes occur in the cytoplasm but rough endoplasmic reticulum is either absent or represented by an occasional small vesicle covered by sparse ribosomes.

Light microscopists have long known that the cytoplasm of all cells is not uniformly eosinophilic and that certain cell types contain basophilic material or discrete basophilic bodies in their cytoplasm. This has been referred to by various terms such as the 'chromidial substance', 'chromophilic substance' or 'ergastoplasm'. It is now clear that the electron microscopic equivalent of this is the rough endoplasmic reticulum and cytoplasmic ribosomes. Thus, the cytoplasmic basophilia and pyroninophilia of plasma cells reflect the abundant rough endoplasmic reticulum in these cells, while the Nissl bodies or Nissl substance of neurons, are revealed to be areas within the cytoplasm containing parallel arrays of rough endoplasmic reticulum and clusters of polyribosomes in the intervening cytoplasmic matrix.

*Erroneous statements contrary to this easily observed fact are common enough. For example, in the well known pathology text for students, Robbins (1974) states, 'As is well known, the rough ER is studded with an evenly spaced array of ribosomal granules'.

Plate 181

Fig. 1. Section through a human type B synovial cell, showing numerous profiles of rough endoplasmic reticulum, with moderately dilated cisternae (C) and a small Golgi complex (G). Although this cell is well endowed with rough endoplasmic reticulum as compared with the type A synovial cell (*Plate 145*) which contains only rare small vesicles studded with ribosomes, the endoplasmic reticulum here (type B cell) does not attain the level of development and organization found in plasma cells (*Plate 180*) or pancreatic acinar cells (*Plate 179*). ×30 000

Fig. 2. A zone 2 chondrocyte from the articular cartilage of a rabbit. These cells are also fairly well endowed with rough endoplasmic reticulum. The cisternae (C) are moderately distended with medium-density material. ×37 000 (*From Ghadially and Roy, 1969*)

418

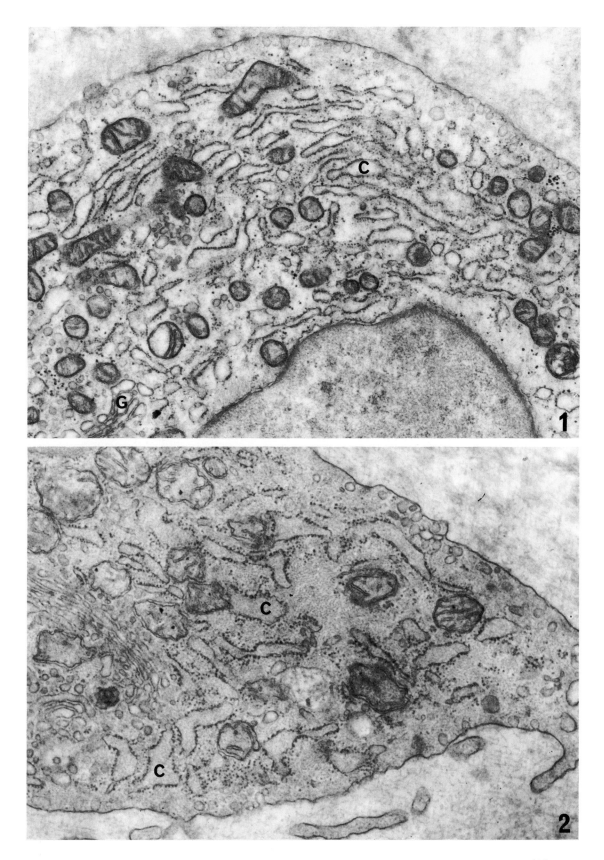

419

This basophilic reaction depends on the RNA in the ribosomes and is not related to the membranes themselves. Cells in which there is a paucity of rough endoplasmic reticulum and ribosomes show an eosinophilic cytoplasm at light microscopy. Since both the membranes of the smooth endoplasmic reticulum and the cytoplasm are eosinophilic the presence of modest amounts of smooth endoplasmic reticulum cannot be discerned by light microscopy. However, when the smooth membranes are abundant the cytoplasmic eosinophilia is quite intense. In instances where the smooth endoplasmic reticulum has a focal rather than a diffuse distribution within the cell, it may present as eosinophilic bodies in the cytoplasm*.

In certain cells, such as hepatocytes and pancreatic acinar cells, the cisternae are quite narrow and often appear almost empty or contain but a sparse amount of medium-density material. In others, such as fibroblasts, chondrocytes and synovial cells, the sacs of the endoplasmic reticulum are invariably more distended (*Plates 181–182*). In plasma cells every conceivable variation may be found, but more often than not the cisternae are moderately distended. Occasionally, the rough endoplasmic reticulum in these cells is reduced to a collection of vesicles loaded with secretory products (*Plate 180*).

The manner in which secretory products leave the rough endoplasmic reticulum and the cell have been subject of much debate. The best-known and most widely held thesis is that material formed in the rough endoplasmic reticulum is transported to the Golgi complex where it is condensed and/or modified in various ways, and packaged into single-membrane-bound vacuoles which then travel to the cell membrane and the contents are discharged from the cell in a variety of ways.

At one time it was thought that connections existed between the rough endoplasmic reticulum and the cell membrane (Epstein, 1957a) and that secretory products were perhaps discharged via openings of the cisternae on the cell surface. This view has lost favour, for such openings are rarely if ever seen. However, line drawings of 'typical cells' showing such connections are commonly encountered in many elementary treatises on the cell†.

Conflicting opinions have been expressed by workers who have studied the manner in which procollagen is secreted by fibroblasts and chondrocytes to form the matrical collagen fibrils‡. The commonly held idea is that procollagen produced by the rough endoplasmic reticulum passes via the Golgi complex to the cell exterior as a merocrine secretion. However, Ross and Benditt (1965) have suggested that the rough endoplasmic reticulum approaches close to the cell membrane and discharges its contents into the matrix via vesicles budding from the cisternae. Other workers have proposed that a shedding of cell processes or segments of the cell containing rough endoplasmic reticulum and secretory material may occur to release procollagen into the matrix (Porter and Pappas, 1959; Godman and Porter, 1960; Chapman, 1962; Porter, 1964).

*Eosinophilic granularity of the cytoplasm can also be due to the presence of numerous mitochondria (page 260) or numerous lysosomes (page 684)
†This myth is perpetuated in a drawing on Plate XI in *Dorland's Illustrated Medical Dictionary*, 25th Edition.
‡For details about collagen synthesis *see* page 1222.

Plate 182

Fig. 1. Fibroadenoma of breast. A fibroblast showing a few profiles of rough endoplasmic reticulum. ×23 000 (*From Ghadially 1980a*)

Fig. 2. Non-ossifying fibroma of bone. A fibroblast showing abundant rough endoplasmic reticulum. ×30 000 (*From Ghadially 1980a*)

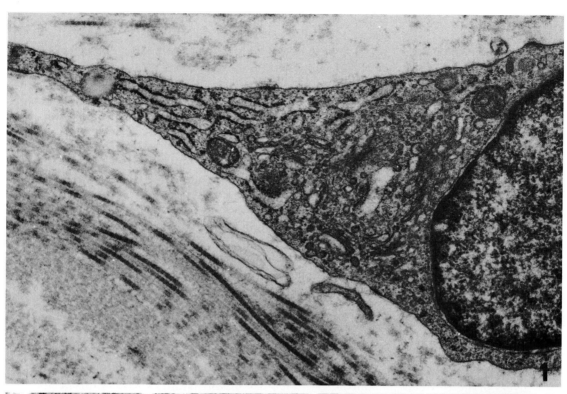

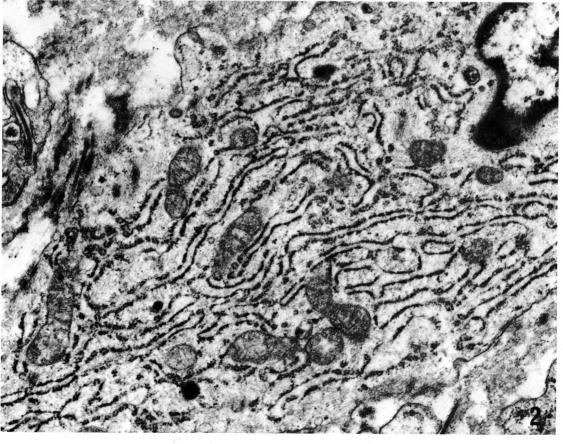

Smooth endoplasmic reticulum

As its name implies, the agranular or smooth-surfaced endoplasmic reticulum is distinguished from the rough endoplasmic reticulum by the absence of attached ribosomes. Although continuities between the rough and smooth endoplasmic reticulum are frequently demonstrable in many cell types (*Plate 183 Fig. 1; Plate 202*), they are morphologically and functionally distinct (*see* reviews by Porter, 1961, and Fawcett, 1981). The smooth endoplasmic reticulum usually presents as a meshwork of branching tubules and/or vesicles. Relatively thick sections are needed to demonstrate the tubular pattern. Unlike the rough endoplasmic reticulum, the smooth endoplasmic reticulum rarely forms cisternae. It is worth noting that this is a delicate system which, at least in some cell types (e.g. steroid-producing cells), is easily affected by preparative procedures. Glutaraldehyde fixation is, as a rule, more likely to preserve the tubular formations while in osmium-fixed material the tubules tend to break up into vesicles. The smooth endoplasmic reticulum in hepatocytes, however, is not so sensitive to preparative procedures. In the tubular epithelial cells of rat kidney fixed by glutaraldehyde perfusion many focal aggregates of branching smooth-membrane-bound tubules are found (*Plate 183, Fig. 2*), but kidney tissue preserved by immersion in fixatives usually shows scant smooth endoplasmic reticulum (Newstead, personal communication).

Although the structure of the smooth endoplasmic reticulum is somewhat similar in most cell types, its enzyme content and functions differ. In the liver the smooth endoplasmic reticulum occupies focal areas of cytoplasm, usually in company with glycogen rosettes (*Plate 183, Fig. 1*). If the glycogen is abundant then the smooth endoplasmic reticulum is difficult to visualize. The smooth endoplasmic reticulum becomes somewhat more prominent and its association with glycogen more evident in animals fasted for a day or two. This close association of glycogen and smooth endoplasmic reticulum led Porter and Bruni (1959) and others to suggest that the smooth endoplasmic reticulum was perhaps involved in glycogenesis or glycogenolysis. Biochemical studies on microsomal fractions have, however, failed to support this idea. It would appear that the main enzymes of glycogen metabolism lie in the cytoplasmic matrix or elsewhere, but not in the endoplasmic reticulum. (An exception to this is glucose-6-phosphatase, which is associated with the endoplasmic reticulum (Ernster *et al.*, 1962).) However, Rothschild (1963) has pointed out that enzymes may be detached from the endoplasmic reticulum and released into the 'soluble fraction' during isolation procedures. In any case, the significance of so distinct and constant an association between smooth endoplasmic reticulum and glycogen, which has been observed repeatedly in many species, still awaits clarification. That such an association is not a prerequisite of glycogen synthesis or breakdown is attested by the fact that in other situations such as brown adipose tissue and the glycogen body of birds (Revel *et al.*, 1960) the smooth endoplasmic reticulum is quite rudimentary. Similarly, as noted elsewhere (pages 100 and 288), glycogen deposits are at times found in nuclei or mitochondria, and it has been suggested that glycogen may be synthesized in such sites without any obvious assistance from the smooth endoplasmic reticulum.

Plate 183

Fig. 1. Cow hepatocyte, showing cytoplasmic zones occupied by rough (R) and smooth (S) endoplasmic reticulum. Glycogen rosettes (G) occur almost exclusively in association with the smooth endoplasmic reticulum. Continuity between the rough and smooth endoplasmic reticulum can just be discerned (arrow) at this low magnification. ×36 000

Fig. 2. Numerous smooth-membrane-bound ramifying tubules are seen in this tubular epithelial cell of a rat kidney perfused with glutaraldehyde. ×54 000 (*Dr J.D. Newstead, unpublished electron micrograph*)

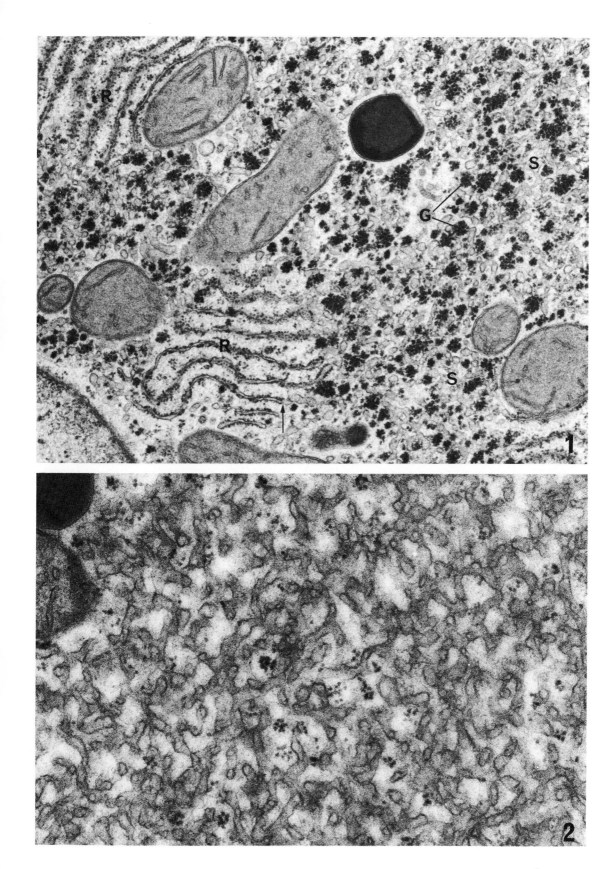

The smooth endoplasmic reticulum in the hepatocyte appears to be involved in cholesterol metabolism (Fawcett, 1964; Jones and Armstrong, 1965) and detoxification of drugs (page 458).

An extensively developed smooth endoplasmic reticulum occurs in cells engaged in the production and secretion of steroid hormones★. Examples include: (1) the interstitial (Leydig) cells of the testis (Christensen and Fawcett, 1961; Christensen, 1965); (2) cells of the adrenal cortex (Brenner, 1966; Long and Jones, 1967a, b; McNutt and Jones, 1970); and (3) corpus luteum (Yamada and Ishikawa, 1960; Enders, 1962; Enders and Lyons, 1964). Biochemical studies have long indicated that the cells of the above-mentioned organs synthesize steroid from acetate via cholesterol (Morris and Chaikoff, 1959; Werbin and Chaikoff, 1961; Armstrong *et al.*, 1964; Srere *et al.*, 1968). Christensen and Fawcett (1961) suggested that it was the smooth endoplasmic reticulum in such cells which was involved in the biosynthesis of cholesterol, and cell fractionation studies have since confirmed that the needed enzymes do reside in this organelle (Goldblatt, 1969).

Many interesting correlations exist between the amount of smooth endoplasmic reticulum and the biosynthesis of cholesterol by the adrenal cortex of different species. For example, the hamster adrenal cortex, which is poorly endowed with smooth endoplasmic reticulum, does not appear to use cholesterol as a precursor for steroid hormone production (Marks *et al.*, 1958; Schindler and Knigge, 1959). The guinea-pig adrenal cortex, which is richly endowed with smooth endoplasmic reticulum, is said to produce 40 per cent of the cholesterol used for steroid production but the rat adrenal cortex, with a relatively poorly developed smooth endoplasmic reticulum, depends almost entirely upon plasma cholesterol for steroid synthesis (Christensen, 1965; Jones and Fawcett, 1966).

In striated muscle the morphology and distribution of smooth endoplasmic reticulum (often called sarcoplasmic reticulum), shows many variations, depending upon species and type of muscle. Generally speaking, fast-acting muscle tends to have a well-developed sarcoplasmic reticulum (*Plate 184*). Examples include: (1) the muscle of the swim bladder of the toad-fish (Fawcett and Revel, 1961; Fawcett, 1966); (2) the cricothyroid muscle of the bat (Revel, 1961); (3) the flight muscle of the dragon-fly (Smith, 1961); (4) the extrinsic eye muscle of *Fundulus heteroclitus* (Reger, 1961); and (5) the remotor muscle of the lobster (Rosenbluth, 1969).

In most skeletal muscles of mammals, the sarcoplasmic reticulum is not as abundant as in the examples stated above. Here it occurs as a sparse laciform network of fine tubules around each myofibril†. In the region of the A-bands the tubules of the system are longitudinally orientated (i.e. parallel to the myofibrils) but they are somewhat dilated and anastomose freely in the region of the H-bands (H-band sacs). At regular intervals along the myofibrils the longitudinally orientated tubules of the smooth endoplasmic reticulum join transversely orientated channels of the smooth endoplasmic reticulum called the 'terminal cisternae'. In longitudinal sections of skeletal muscle fibres (*Plate 185*), three vesicular profiles (collectively referred to as a triad) are seen at regularly repeating intervals. The outer two represent sections through the transversely orientated cisternae of the smooth endoplasmic reticulum, while the inner, more slender, tubular or vesicular profile represents a section through a T-tubule.

★Tumours of steroid secreting cells are also usually well endowed with smooth endoplasmic reticulum. This plus the presence of mitochondria with tubulovesicular cristae are of value in distinguishing tumours of steroid secreting cells. (For details *see* Ghadially, 1985.)
†It is difficult to explain the relationships of the sarcoplasmic reticulum without the aid of diagrams. Excellent drawings and a singularly lucid account of the subject may be found in Bloom and Fawcett (1975).

Plate 184
Flight muscle of dragon-fly, showing abundant smooth endoplasmic reticulum (S). (Compare with *Plate 84*.) Note also the close association of mitochondria with smooth endoplasmic reticulum and lipid droplets (L). ×20 000

424

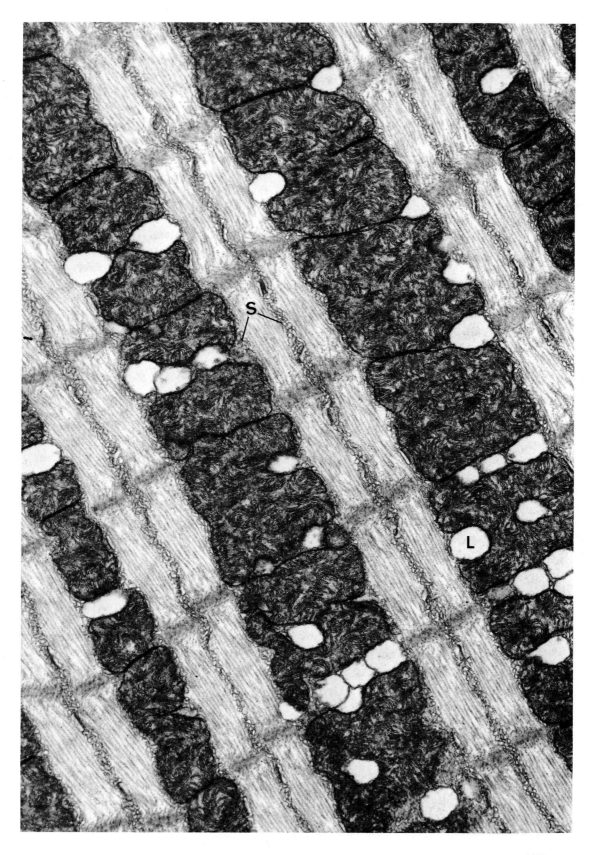

425

These T-tubules have now been demonstrated to be tubular invaginations of the plasma membrane into the muscle fibre of many species. The location of the triads with respect to the cross-banded pattern of the myofibrils varies from species to species. In mammals the triads occur at the junction of I- and A-bands. In the frog, the triads are found at the Z-line.

Cardiac muscle is poorly endowed with smooth endoplasmic reticulum as compared with skeletal muscle (turtle heart is singularly deficient in this respect (Fawcett and Selby, 1958)), but the T-system tubules are much greater in diameter and run at the level of the Z-line. There are no terminal cisternae and hence no triads, but small expansions of the sarcoplasmic reticulum form a close association with the sarcolemma and T-tubules. The latter association presents as diads at the Z-line.

It is now clear that the coupling of excitation and contraction is mediated by the T-system tubules and the sarcoplasmic reticulum (Smith, 1966), but details of the sequence of events that occur during contraction and relaxation of muscle fibres has received various interpretations. It would appear that on arrival of an impulse a wave of depolarization is set up which spreads over the sarcolemma and into the T-system tubules. This explains why, on the arrival of an impulse, the myofibrils throughout the muscle fibre contract simultaneously. It is thought that in the resting state most of the calcium ions reside in the smooth endoplasmic reticulum, a point supported by the fact that electron-dense granular material is often seen there (*Plate 185*). When the depolarization wave reaches the triads, calcium ions diffuse out of the smooth endoplasmic reticulum and activate the dephosphorylation of ATP, with resultant muscle contraction (which is looked upon as a repetitive making and breaking of successive cross-links between myosin and actin filaments, *see* pages 842–845 for more details).

In the apical cytoplasm of intestinal mucosa a fair amount of smooth endoplasmic reticulum is present. (There is argument as to whether the vesicles and tubules seen in this region truly represent smooth endoplasmic reticulum or whether they are pinocytotic vesicles and invaginations of the plasma membrane (Sjostrand, 1974).) During fat absorption, lipid droplets appear in this system of tubules and vesicles and are transported to the Golgi complex and thence to the lateral surface of the cell.

Teleosts living in the sea excrete via the gills large amounts of sodium chloride taken in with the sea water. These cells contain a much branched system of agranular cytoplasmic tubules (Newstead, 1971) which at one time were considered to be elements of the smooth endoplasmic reticulum. This interpretation is not acceptable because these tubules are continuous with the cell membrane but not the rough endoplasmic reticulum in these cells (Newstead, personal communication). The mechanisms in sodium chloride excretion are poorly understood but both sodium (Mizuhira *et al.*, 1970) and chloride (Petrik, 1968) ions have been demonstrated in the smooth endoplasmic reticulum of the chloride cells of eel gills and it is thought that this organelle plays an important part in the transport of these ions.

Other cells in which a conspicuous amount of smooth endoplasmic reticulum is found include the retinal pigment cells (Porter and Yamada, 1960), gastric cells (Ito, 1961), cells of sebaceous glands (Palay, 1958), and Clara cells of mice and rats (but not humans) (Ghadially, 1985).

Plate 185
Human skeletal muscle showing sparse, smooth endoplasmic reticulum (arrow). At the junction of the I- and A-bands lie the triads, consisting of a T-tubule (T) bounded on either side by the terminal cisternae or lateral sacs (S) of the smooth endoplasmic reticulum, containing moderately electron-dense material. ×65 000

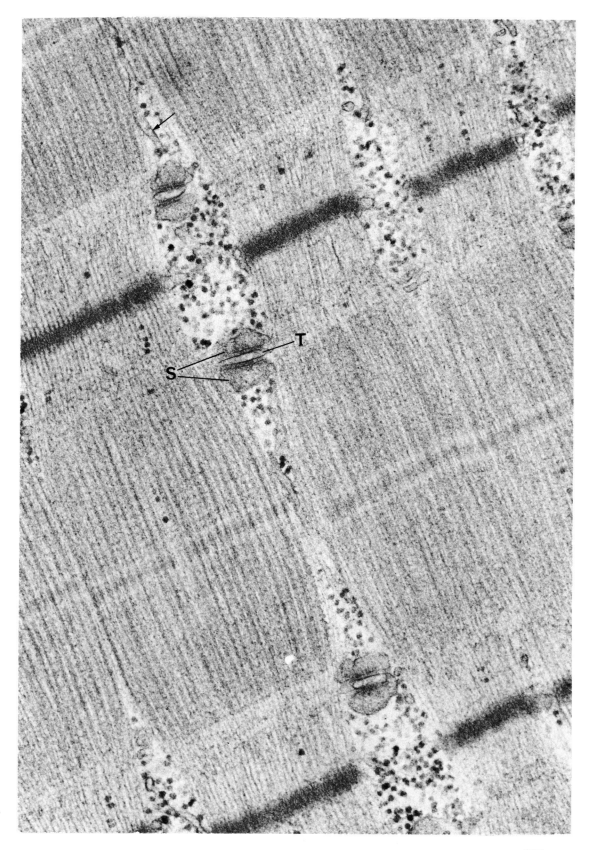

427

Dilatation and vesiculation of endoplasmic reticulum due to ingress of water

Dilatation and vesiculation of the rough endoplasmic reticulum can be due to an ingress of water (dealt with in this section) or storage of secretory products (dealt with on page 434). The two are usually distinguishable by the fact that in the former instance the contents are diluted and hence appear more electron-lucent than normal; while in the latter instance, they may have a normal density or appear somewhat more electron-dense if the secretory product becomes more concentrated. However, there are times when it is difficult to decide which of the two phenomena one is witnessing and there is also the possibility that a rough endoplasmic reticulum distended with secretory product may suffer further dilatation by ingress of water. Ingress of water and solutes into the cell may lead to dilatation and vesiculation of various membrane-bound compartments, such as the rough and smooth endoplasmic reticulum, Golgi complex and mitochondria. It should be noted that when the rough endoplasmic reticulum suffers dilatation and vesiculation it tends to become degranulated and hence comes to resemble smooth endoplasmic reticulum; under similar circumstances the Golgi complex also loses its characteristic morphology and becomes indistinguishable from other membranous components.

Dilatation of the rough endoplasmic reticulum is often described as 'dilatation of the cisternae of the rough endoplasmic reticulum'. Since not all the elements of the rough endoplasmic reticulum occur as cisternae, the shorter term 'dilatation of rough endoplasmic reticulum' seems more desirable. The term 'enlargement of the rough endoplasmic reticulum' is sometimes used (e.g. Pfeiffer *et al.*, 1971) but this seems undesirable as it might be confused with an increase in the amount of rough endoplasmic reticulum in the cell. Singularly confusing is the term 'cytoplasmic lakes' used by Ward *et al.* (1971) to describe dilated rough endoplasmic reticulum, for it could create the erroneous impression that cytoplasmic material is contained within dilated rough endoplasmic reticulum.

Dilatation of the rough endoplasmic reticulum may be quite modest in degree so that there is only a slight increase in width of the cisternae, or it may be quite marked so that the cell assumes a cribriform appearance (*Plate 186*). When the term 'dilated rough endoplasmic reticulum' is used, one assumes that the reticular nature of the organelle is not totally lost and that the enlarged cavities are still more or less continuous with each other. The term 'vesiculation' implies that the rough endoplasmic reticulum has broken up into numerous discrete vesicles (*Plate 187*) or somewhat larger vacuoles, pools or lakes. However, a clear distinction between dilatation and vesiculation is often not possible for, in another plane of sectioning, continuity might be demonstrable between such pools and lakes.

Plate 186

Human synovial intima. Two weeks history of traumatic lipohaemarthrosis of the knee joint (fracture and separation of upper tibial epiphysis with liberation of fat and blood into the joint). This low-power view shows an area of synovial membrane where there is a marked dilatation (D) of the endoplasmic reticulum, which gives the cells a cribriform appearance. Joint space (J). Note that the mitochondria are not swollen, if anything, they are somewhat pyknotic. ×12 000 (*From Ghadially and Roy, 1969*)

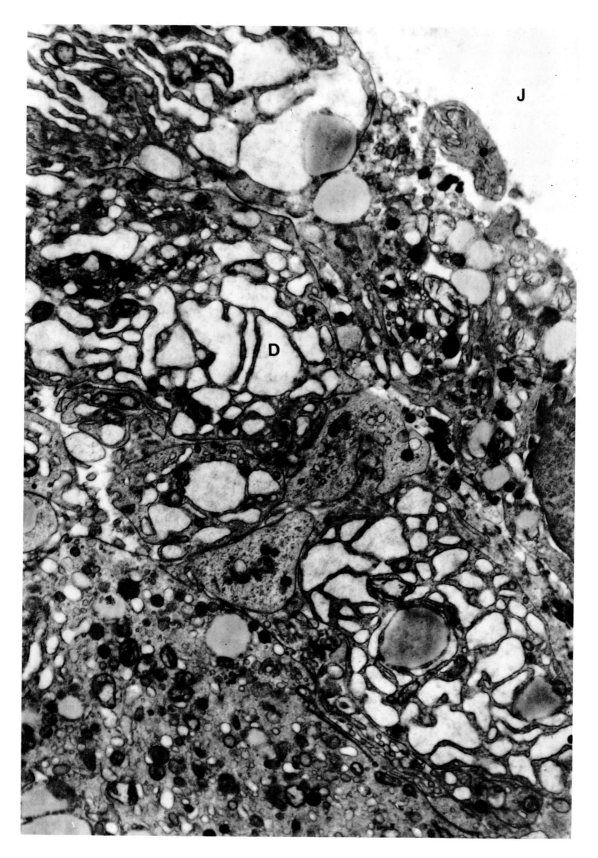

429

Dilatation and vesiculation of the endoplasmic reticulum due to ingress of water into the cell is part and parcel of cloudy swelling, a ubiquitous change that occurs in cells subjected to various noxious influences. It therefore follows that dilatation of rough endoplasmic reticulum, like swollen mitochondria, will frequently be encountered. Vesiculation of rough endoplasmic reticulum which represents a more advanced lesion is encountered somewhat less frequently, but even so it is common enough. One of the finest examples of this lesion is seen in the liver, where the endoplasmic reticulum breaks up into numerous small vesicles (*Plate 187*)*.

David (1964) lists various conditions where vesiculation of hepatocyte endoplasmic reticulum has been reported to occur. These include: starvation, kwashiorkor, choline deficiency, hormone administration, oxygen lack, scurvy, hepatitis, yellow fever, enteromelia, biliary obstruction, irradiation and administration of various drugs such as carbon tetrachloride, phosphorus, ethionine, dinitrophenol and dimethylnitrosamine.

Like mitochondrial swelling (pages 240–249), dilatation of the rough endoplasmic reticulum can also be produced artefactually by poor techniques of tissue collection and processing, such as the use of hypotonic fixative solutions. Distinction between the two may at times be difficult or impossible. However, when cells showing dilated or vesiculated rough endoplasmic reticulum are found in company with others not so affected, one can be reasonably certain that it is not an artefact of tissue collection or preparation.

The vesicles produced by fragmentation of the rough endoplasmic reticulum in hepatocytes (*Plate 187*) are usually sparsely populated by ribosomes and vesicles without ribosomes are also seen. Such appearances are probably the result of degranulation of the rough endoplasmic reticulum (page 436) and also involvement of the smooth endoplasmic reticulum and Golgi complex in vesicle formation.

It has already been noted (page 422) that the smooth endoplasmic reticulum is a delicate structure easily affected by fixative procedure, and that in certain cells such as the steroid-secreting cells it usually presents as a collection of small smooth-walled vesicles rather than a system of ramifying tubules. Ingress of fluid in such cells results in the production of larger irregular-bordered vacuoles (*Plate 188*). Dilatation and vesiculation of the smooth endoplasmic reticulum has also been noted in a variety of pathologically altered muscle tissue (Mair and Tomé, 1972).

It was noted earlier that dilatation and vesiculation of the endoplasmic reticulum and mitochondrial swelling constitute the main changes in 'cloudy swelling'. This condition has been the subject of long-standing interest and controversy. Virchow (1858), in his classic studies on parenchymatous inflammation, concluded that cells could absorb exudate from blood vessels and become swollen, cloudy and granular.

*It is interesting to note that the endoplasmic reticulum breaks up into small vesicles when cells are homogenized. The microsomal fraction prepared from normal hepatocytes contains ribosome-studded vesicles similar to those shown in *Plate 187*.

Plate 187
Marked mitochondrial swelling and vesiculation (V) of the rough endoplasmic reticulum is seen in one of the hepatocytes in this electron micrograph. An adjacent hepatocyte shows a more modest mitochondrial swelling and dilatation (D) of the rough endoplasmic reticulum. From the liver of a rat bearing a subcutaneous carcinogen-induced sarcoma. *See also Plate 107.* ×45 000 (*Ghadially and Parry, unpublished electron micrograph*)

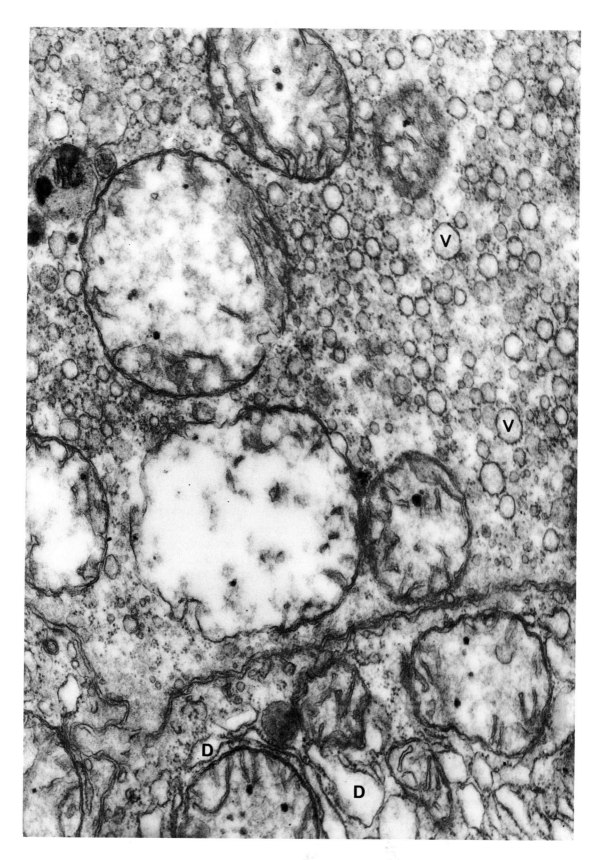

431

As early as 1914 at least three workers (Anitschkow, 1914; Ernst, 1914; Fahr, 1914) brought forward evidence in support of the idea that mitochondrial swelling was a factor responsible for the granularity of the cytoplasm, and this has since been reiterated by many light and electron microscopists. Remarkable were the careful observations of Anitschkow (1914) who noted that in cloudy swelling at first the mitochondria stained deeply with mitochondrial stain but, as swelling progressed, the mitochondria became sharp contoured spheres, where only the periphery appeared stained but the central portion took up no dye. The idea that other cytoplasmic constituents also participated in the formation of vesicles and granules was not denied; in fact, most workers subscribed to the idea that the 'granules' were also derived from various other cytoplasmic structures, particularly the Golgi complex.

With the advent of the electron microscope and the discovery of the endoplasmic reticulum, it is now known that the 'other cytoplasmic structure' which gives rise to multiple vesicles is mainly the endoplasmic reticulum, but no doubt the Golgi complex also participates in this change. Indeed, one of the earliest studies on the endoplasmic reticulum (Fawcett and Ito, 1958) performed on spermatids *in vitro* showed that with the passage of time the cisternae of the endoplasmic reticulum break up into vesicles. This behaviour has since been observed in many cultured cells★.

However, the time-hallowed controversies regarding the nature of the granules in cloudy swelling, and the mechanisms by which such changes are produced, have by no means ended. Some observers stress the importance of the mitochondria in the production of this phenomenon† while others consider dilatation and vesiculation of the endoplasmic reticulum more significant.

No simple generalization can be made, but certain points are worth considering. In hepatocytes vesiculation of the endoplasmic reticulum produces structures too small to be resolved by the light microscope. This probably contributes to the general cloudiness of the cytoplasm, but the marked granularity is probably due to the abundant swollen mitochondria. However, in cells not so richly endowed with mitochondria, and where the endoplasmic reticulum breaks up into quite sizeable vacuoles (*Plate 188*), the swollen endoplasmic reticulum may well contribute to the granularity of the cytoplasm seen with the light microscope.

Regarding the sequence of events in cloudy swelling, it would perhaps be reasonable to generalize that in most examples studied, some degree of dilatation of the endoplasmic reticulum precedes detectable mitochondrial swelling. Indeed, it is possible to have quite marked swelling of endoplasmic reticulum with mitochondria appearing almost normal in size or even pyknotic (*Plate 186*). However, the earliest change heralding cloudy swelling does seem to lie in the mitochondrion for there is a rapid loss of matrical dense granules (page 238).

★The mere act of detaching a monolayer of cultured fibroblasts with a rubber policeman can produce dilatation and vesiculation of the rough endoplasmic reticulum (Lucky *et al.*, 1975).
†This section of the text should be read in conjunction with the section on swollen mitochondria (page 240) where cloudy swelling is also discussed.

Plate 188
Adrenal cortical cells from a case of Cushing's disease, showing many irregular-shaped vacuoles (V) derived from the smooth endoplasmic reticulum. Only occasional mitochondria (★) show some swelling. The smooth-endoplasmic-reticulum-derived vacuoles are distinguished from lipid droplets (not present in this electron micrograph) which usually have a round smooth contour and are not bounded by a membrane. ×9000 (*Ghadially and Larsen, unpublished electron micrograph*)

432

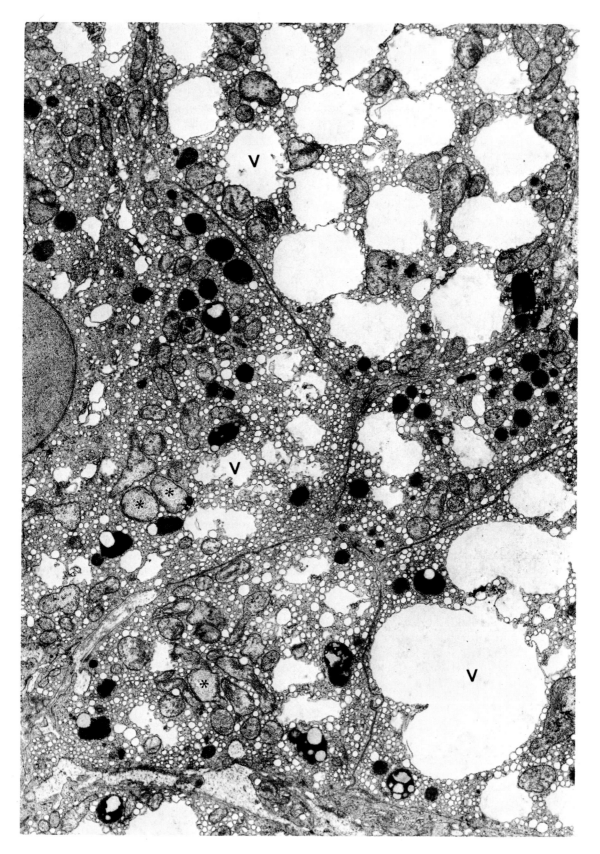

433

Dilatation and vesiculation of rough endoplasmic reticulum due to storage of secretory products

As noted previously dilatation and vesiculation of the rough endoplasmic reticulum can be due to an ingress of water (dealt with on page 428) or storage of secretory products. In the former instance the contents are diluted and hence tend to be more electron-lucent than normal; in the latter instance the contents may appear normal or concentrated (i.e. more electron-dense). Such concentration of secretory products may lead to the formation of proteinaceous granules or crystals in the rough endoplasmic reticulum (page 530). Many cells, such as fibroblasts, chondrocytes, synovial cells and plasma cells seem to have a tendency to store the secretory products awhile within the elements of the rough endoplasmic reticulum, so as a rule these tend to appear somewhat more dilated than say the rough endoplasmic reticulum in hepatocytes or pancreatic acinar cells. However, in quite a few situations cells with gross dilatation and vesiculation of the rough endoplasmic reticulum have been found and since they contain normal looking or condensed contents it has been argued that this cannot be due to an ingress of water.

The various theories proposed to explain this phenomenon include: (1) a rate of synthesis of secretory products in excess of that which can be handled by the transport mechanism; (2) a defect in the transport system, such as a mechanical or enzymic abnormality in the rough endoplasmic reticulum which hinders the egress of normal amounts of secretory material; and (3) the production of an abnormal secretory product with which the normal transport mechanism is unable to cope.

There are no studies which support or refute the above mentioned hypotheses but it is generally assumed that the dilatation and vesiculation of the rough endoplasmic reticulum found in reactive plasma cells (*Plate 180*) (e.g. those seen in the rheumatoid synovial membrane) probably reflect heightened immunoglobulin production and that here we have an example where the secretory products are being produced at a rate faster than the export mechanism can cope with.

On the other hand, the view frequently expressed in the case of tumours is that dilatation or vesiculation of the rough endoplasmic reticulum probably reflects an enzymic or mechanical defect in the rough endoplasmic reticulum of the neoplastic cell.

In certain skeletal dysplasias (Maynard *et al.*, 1972; Cooper *et al.*, 1973a, b) such as metaphyseal dysostosis and pseudochondroplasia (a variety of spondyloepiphyseal dysplasia) there is a marked dilatation and vesiculation of the rough endoplasmic reticulum in chondrocytes. Biopsies from epiphyseal plate and iliac crest show that a large number, if not virtually all chondrocytes are so affected. In pseudoachondroplasia the stored product presents as laminated inclusions in the rough endoplasmic reticulum (page 542) but in metaphyseal dysostosis the product is flocculent and only moderately electron-dense (*Plate 189*).

In these conditions it is thought that there is a genetic defect in the rough endoplasmic reticulum (probably an enzyme defect) and that the dilatation and vesiculation results from a relative decrease in the egress of normal protein or that an abnormal protein is synthesized by these chondrocytes with which the normal transport mechanism is unable to cope.

Plate 189

Figs. 1 and 2. Chondrocytes from the epiphyseal cartilage of a case of metaphyseal dysostosis. Note the dilated and vesiculated (V) rough endoplasmic reticulum containing a medium density material. ×23 000; ×40 000

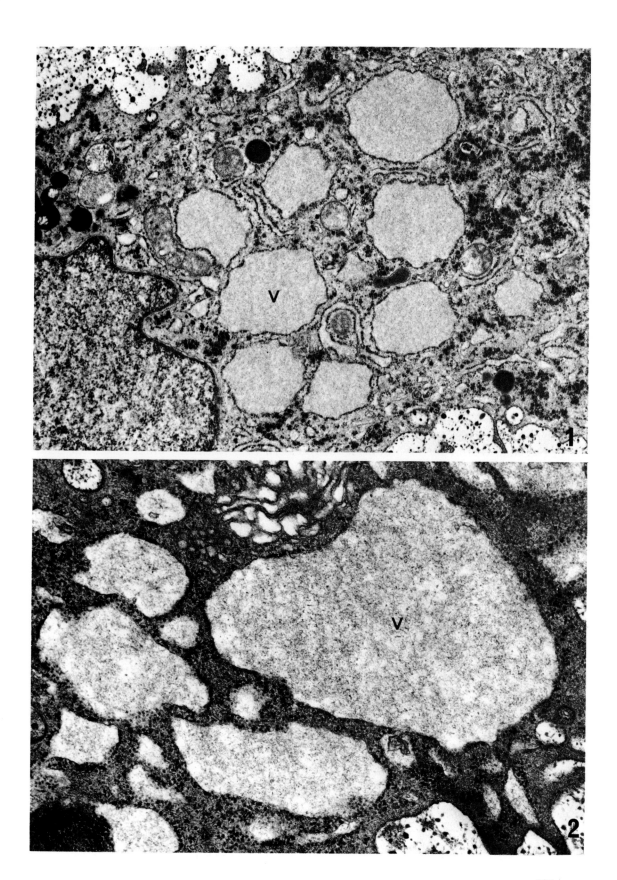

Degranulation of rough endoplasmic reticulum

Degranulation of the rough endoplasmic reticulum is a distinct morphological change but it is usually accompanied by other morphological alterations, such as dilatation and vesiculation of the rough endoplasmic reticulum and disaggregation of polyribosomes (page 438). Collectively· these changes are referred to as disorganization of rough endoplasmic reticulum. Such changes have been studied extensively in the hepatocytes of experimental animals subjected to various noxious influences.

In the phenomenon called 'degranulation of rough endoplasmic reticulum' the membranes of the rough endoplasmic reticulum appear sparsely populated by ribosomes. Since numerous ribosomes are often found lying free in the cytoplasm, it looks as though the ribosomes have dropped off the rough endoplasmic reticulum into the cytoplasmic matrix. Such an idea is supported by biochemical studies, for in the liver of carbon-tetrachloride-poisoned rats, where degranulation of rough endoplasmic reticulum is a prominent early change (*Plate 190*), there is a shift of RNA from the microsomal fraction (containing endoplasmic reticulum) into the supernatant fluid (containing cytoplasmic matrix) (Reynolds and Yee, 1967; Slater and Sawyer, 1969). Degranulation of the rough endoplasmic reticulum is associated with a loss of polyribosome configuration so that solitary ribosomes are seen in the cytoplasmic matrix (*Plate 190*).

Examples of degranulation of hepatocyte rough endoplasmic reticulum suggesting a dropping off of ribosomes are seen in rats after the administration of: (1) ethionine (Villa-Trevino *et al.*, 1964; Baglio and Farber, 1965a; Wood, 1965); (2) carbon tetrachloride (Smuckler *et al.*, 1962; Reynolds, 1963; Krishan and Stenger, 1966); (3) monobromotrichloromethane (Bini *et al.*, 1978); (4) α-naphthylisothiocyanate (Steiner and Baglio, 1963); and (5) puromycin and various other drugs (Reid *et al.*, 1970).

Degranulation of the type described above is an early, relatively mild lesion. The same noxious agent (e.g. carbon tetrachloride) can produce more drastic alterations of membrane structure such as vesiculation, fragmentation or dissolution of the membranes of the rough endoplasmic reticulum, accompanied by a general decrease in ribosomes, both attached to and lying free in the cytoplasm.

One would expect that changes of the type mentioned above would disturb protein synthesis, and there is ample biochemical evidence that protein synthesis is in fact impaired by drugs which produce this change. For example, it has been shown that after carbon tetrachloride poisoning the synthesis of several export proteins is depressed (Smuckler *et al.*, 1962), and cell fractionation studies show that the defect is related to polyribosome disaggregation and a decreased capacity to incorporate amino acids (Smuckler and Benditt, 1963).

Plate 190

Fig. 1. Rat hepatocyte 1 hour after the administration of carbon tetrachloride, showing vesiculation (V) of rough endoplasmic reticulum and numerous solitary ribosomes, no doubt derived from disaggregated polyribosomes. Most of these ribosomes can be interpreted as lying free in the cytoplasm but some, seen on a dense background, could still be attached to tangentially cut membranes. ×34 000

Fig. 2. Normal rat hepatocyte, showing numerous polyribosomes (arrows) on tangentially cut cisternae of the rough endoplasmic reticulum. Note the paucity of free ribosomes in the cytoplasmic matrix compared with *Fig. 1*. ×29 000

436

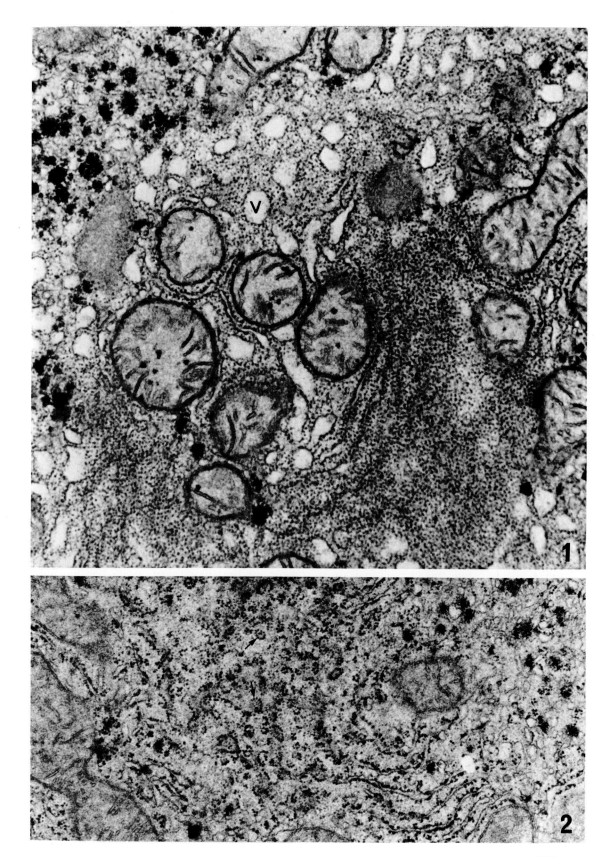

437

Disaggregation of polyribosomes

As already noted (page 418), ribosomes lying free in the cytoplasm or attached to the membrane of the rough endoplasmic reticulum may occur either as solitary particles or in groups showing various configurations. Such aggregates of ribosomes, which usually present as rosettes, loops or spirals, are referred to as polyribosomes. It is now well established that such polyribosomes comprise ribosomes attached to a fine strand (single molecule) of messenger RNA. The number of ribosomes in a polyribosome is approximately proportional to the number of amino acid residues in the polypeptide chain that is to be synthesized. Thus the peptide chains of haemoglobin which contain only about 150 amino acid residues are synthesized by polyribosomes possessing five or six ribosomes; but much larger polyribosomes composed of 60–100 ribosomes synthesize the major chains of myosin which contain about 1800 amino acid residues.

Current concepts envisage that protein synthesis is accomplished by polyribosomes. The ribosomes are believed to be attached to specific sites on a strand of messenger RNA that has the encoded information which determines the amino acid sequence for the specific protein being synthesized. The ribosomes are thought to move along the length of the messenger RNA and to be released when the specific polypeptide chain has been completed. Many studies on various mammalian and other cells now support the concepts stated above (Jacob and Monod, 1961; Goodman and Rich, 1963; Hardesty *et al.*, 1963; Marks *et al.*, 1963; Rich *et al.*, 1963; Staehelin and Noll, 1963; Warner *et al.*, 1963).

In the phenomenon variously referred to as loss of 'polyribosomal configuration', 'disaggregation of polyribosomes' and 'disaggregation of ribosomes', it is believed that polyribosomes break up and/or are not re-formed, so that one finds many solitary ribosomes in the cell but few or no characteristic polyribosomal forms (*Plates 190–192*). Two well known models where disaggregation of polyribosomes bound to the rough endoplasmic reticulum occur are the carbon-tetrachloride-poisoned rat hepatocyte and the fibroblast of vitamin-C-deficient guinea-pigs. In both instances there is a disaggregation of membrane-bound polyribosomes, but while in the former instance the ribosomes drop off the membranes (degranulation) in the latter instance they do not.

It will be recalled (page 436) that a prominent, widespread, early alteration of hepatocyte morphology after carbon tetrachloride administration is a degranulation of rough endoplasmic reticulum and a disaggregation of polyribosomes (*Plate 190*). It has now been shown that after carbon tetrachloride poisoning the synthesis of several 'export' proteins is depressed (Smuckler *et al.*, 1962) and this is believed to be related to the disaggregation of hepatocellular polyribosomes (Smuckler and Benditt, 1963).

Plate 191

Disaggregation of polyribosomes produced in synovial cells by immobilizing a rabbit knee joint is illustrated here. *Fig. 1* is from the control joint, and *Fig. 2* from the contralateral immobilized (in a plaster cast) joint of the same animal

Fig. 1. Numerous polyribosomes (P) showing various configurations are seen on the surface of tangentially cut membranes of the rough endoplasmic reticulum. ×70 000

Fig. 2. The polyribosomes have disaggregated (as evidenced by the lack of characteristic configurations as seen in *Fig. 1*) to form solitary ribosomes (R), but they are still attached to the vesiculated (V) rough endoplasmic reticulum. ×65 000

438

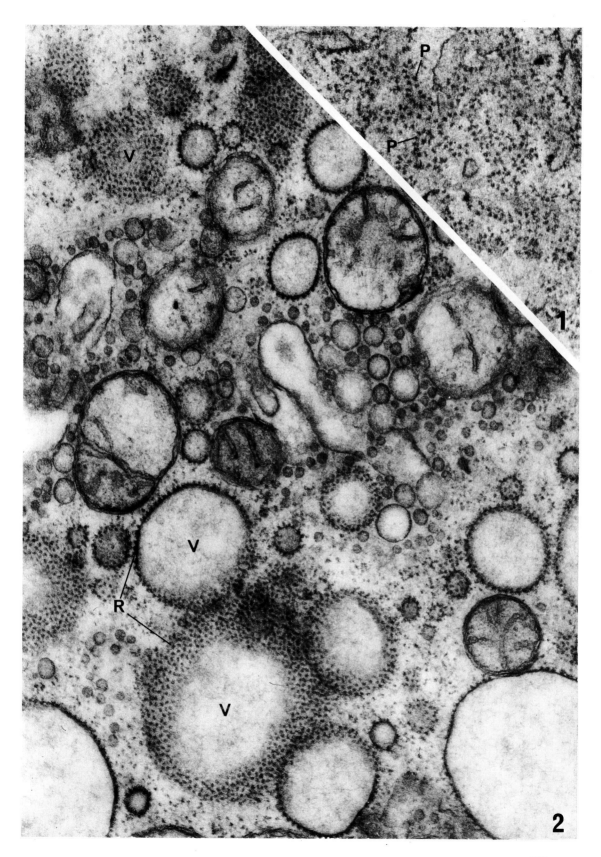

Singularly interesting also is the situation seen in the scorbutic guinea-pig where there is a pathological alteration of connective tissue associated with an impaired procollagen synthesis in fibroblasts and a paucity of collagen fibrils in the matrix. (Details of biochemical changes that occur in the scorbutic fibroblast are beyond the scope of this text; the reader should refer to Schubert and Hamerman, 1968.) Ultrastructural studies on the fibroblasts from the healing wounds of such animals have shown that the characteristic lesion seen is a disaggregation of polyribosomes (Ross and Benditt, 1964). In healthy guinea-pigs numerous polyribosomes showing spiral and parallel linear configurations abound on the surface of the rough endoplasmic reticulum, but in the scorbutic animal this characteristic configuration is lost and numerous solitary ribosomes, still attached to the membranes, are seen. Vesiculation of the rough endoplasmic reticulum also occurs, but such vesicles are well populated by solitary ribosomes. Thus in the scorbutic fibroblast, disaggregation of polyribosomes is not accompanied by degranulation of the rough endoplasmic reticulum, as is the case in the carbon-tetrachloride-injured hepatocyte.

A similar disaggregation of polyribosomes without degranulation of the vesiculated rough endoplasmic reticulum is found (*Plate 191*) in the synovial membrane of the immobilized rabbit knee joint (Ghadially, unpublished). This correlates well with the marked synovial atrophy and regressive changes that occur in the immobilized joint.

It can be shown that, just as disaggregation of polyribosomes attached to the rough endoplasmic reticulum indicates an impaired 'export' protein production, disaggregation of polyribosomes lying free in the cytoplasm is associated with depressed endogenous protein production.

For example, in normoblasts and young reticulocytes where active haemoglobin synthesis is in progress, numerous polyribosomes occur in the cytoplasm, but as the cell matures such ribosomal clusters are replaced by solitary ribosomes (*Plate 192, Figs. 1 and 2*), and by the time the mature well haemoglobinized erythrocyte has evolved even these disappear from the cytoplasm (Hardesty *et al.*, 1963; Marks *et al.*, 1963; Warner *et al.*, 1963; Rifkind *et al.*, 1964). Similarly, cells in culture show numerous polyribosomes in their cytoplasm which presumably produce cytoplasmic proteins to keep pace with cell division. In virus-infected cells where cell division is halted a disaggregation of polyribosomes occurs and the cytoplasm is at times filled with innumerable solitary ribosomes (Rich *et al.*, 1963).

Numerous studies, including autoradiographic ones on cultured cells, have shown that there is a marked depression of protein synthesis during mitosis, and under such circumstances there is also a disaggregation of polyribosomes (Scharff and Robbins, 1966) (*Plate 192, Fig. 3*). These authors have also noted a disaggregation of polyribosomes in cells arrested in metaphase by colchicine.

Thus it is now well established that disaggregation of polyribosomes is a useful morphological indicator of depressed or arrested protein synthesis.

Plate 192

Fig. 1. A late normoblast from human bone marrow, showing numerous polyribosomes (arrow) in its cytoplasm. ×50 000

Fig. 2. Cytoplasm of a late reticulocyte from peripheral blood, showing numerous solitary ribosomes (arrow). ×50 000

Fig. 3. Ehrlich ascites tumour cell in mitosis, showing chromosomes (C) and numerous solitary ribosomes (arrow) in the cytoplasm. Compare with *Plate 197*, which shows an Ehrlich ascites tumour cell with abundant polyribosomes in the cytoplasm. ×50 000

440

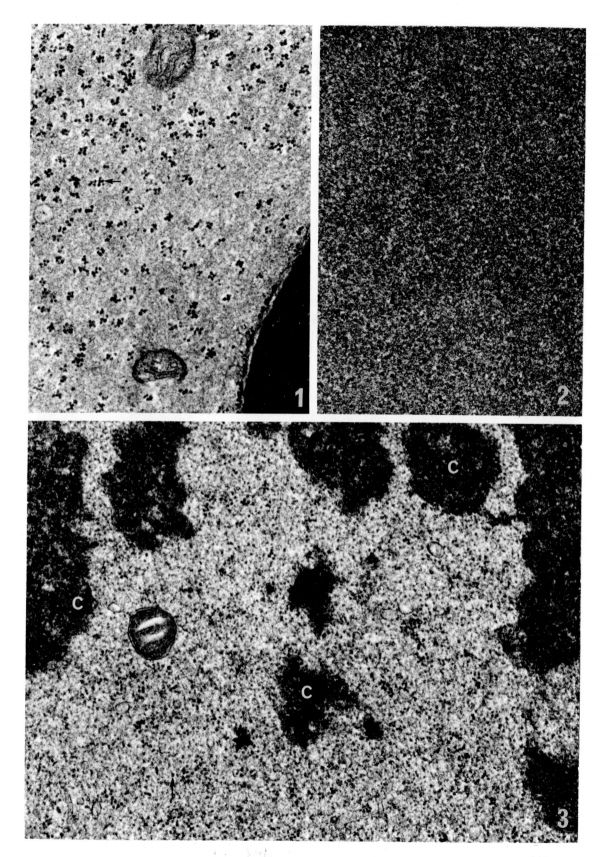

441

Helical polyribosomes and ribosome crystals

As pointed out earlier (pages 418 and 438), polyribosomes usually present as linear, spiral or rosette-like structures. In some instances, however, polyribosomes showing a helical configuration have been found, and in rarer instances ribosomes arranged in crystalline arrays have also been noted. Ribosome crystals have at times been seen in company with helical polyribosomes, so it is convenient to consider these together.

Helical polyribosomes have been seen in: (1) developing mother pollen cells of *Ipomoea purpurea* (L) Roth (Echlin, 1965); (2) cotton embryo (Jensen, 1968); (3) *Entamoeba invadens* (Siddiqui and Rudzinska, 1963, 1965); (4) *E. histolytica* (Rosenbaum and Wittner, 1970); (5) intestinal cells of rat fetus (Behnke, 1963); (6) muscle cells of *Rana pipiens* embryo (Waddington and Perry, 1963); (7) follicular cells and oocytes of rat ovary (Ghiara and Taddei, 1966); (8) chick embryo cells subjected to hypothermia (Byers, 1967; Maraldi and Barbieri, 1969); (9) cultures of chick embryo liver cells treated with vinblastine and subjected to hypothermia (Maraldi *et al.*, 1970); (10) several types of cells in culture (HeLa, kidney, conjunctiva) (Scharff and Robbins, 1966; Weiss and Grover, 1968; Suzuki *et al.*, 1969); (11) virus infected cells (Djaczenko *et al.*, 1970) (*Plate 193*); (12) fibroblast cultures treated with vincristine (Krishan and Hsu, 1969); (13) a mutant of *Escherichia coli* treated with vinblastine (Kingsbury and Voelz, 1969); (14) *in vitro* single beating rat myocardial cell (Cedergren and Harary, 1964); (15) ribosome pellets isolated from normal rat liver (Benedetti *et al.*, 1966); (16) intact or regenerating rat liver after administration of lasiocarpine or aflatoxin (Monneron, 1969); (17) Taper hepatoma ascites cells (Fritzler *et al.*, 1973); and (18) the companion cells of the phloem of *Acer pseudoplatanus* (Wooding, 1968).

In intact normal rat liver helical polyribosomes have not been seen, and in ribosomal pellets obtained after fractionation only an occasional example of such polyribosomes has been recorded. Therefore it is particularly interesting to note the observation made by Monneron (1969) that within 10 minutes of administration of lasiocarpine or aflatoxin numerous helical polyribosomes develop and that they disappear within a few hours. Since the time required by the normal liver to make a ribosome is much longer than 10 minutes and since administration of actinomycin D at a dose level sufficient to block synthesis of 45 S RNA does not prevent the formation of helical polyribosomes by lasiocarpine, it would appear that a change in the nature of messenger RNA linking the ribosomes together is probably responsible for the helical form of the polyribosomes rather than an alteration in the ribosomes. Monneron (1969) therefore suggests that under these experimental conditions a transient (perhaps abnormal) messenger RNA is produced. Similarly, Jensen (1968) also suggests that helical polyribosomes produced during cotton embryogenesis are related to the production of a special transient messenger RNA (informosome).

Plate 193
Green monkey kidney cell in culture, infected with herpesvirus (V) showing helical polyribosomes (arrows). ×67 000

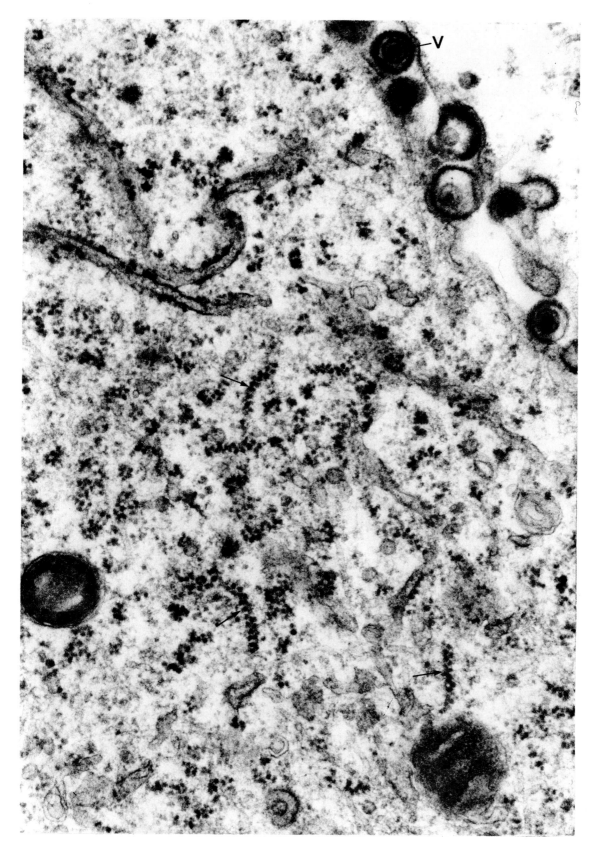

443

In various species of *Entamoeba* studied so far, classically formed mitochondria, Golgi complex and rough endoplasmic reticulum have not been found but helical polyribosomes and crystalline arrays of helical polyribosomes occur (these large ribonucleoprotein-containing bodies are the equivalent of the chromatid bodies seen in *Entamoeba* with the light microscope). Regarding this situation, Rosenbaum and Wittner (1970) state that 'the absence in *E. histolytica* of most of the usual cytoplasmic organelles and the presence of highly organized and apparently dynamic RNP material in helical form suggests the possibility that these structures may have a multifaceted and extremely labile role in the economy of amoeba'. Furthermore, since many helical polyribosomes were seen in close association with autophagic and phagocytic vacuoles which demonstrated acid phosphatase activity, they suggest that 'enzymic protein synthesis may be occurring in association with the larger bodies themselves and that the newly synthesized protein may be carried via the short helices to digestive vacuoles'. Thus, the helical polyribosome of *E. histolytica* becomes analogous to a primary lysosome of man and other animals, which transports hydrolytic enzymes made in the rough endoplasmic reticulum, to the autophagic vacuole.

In *Entamoeba*, ribosomal crystals appear to be derived by parallel alignment of helical polyribosomes but other forms of ribosomal crystals not derived in this manner also seem to occur. Thus in chick embryos subjected to hypothermia (Byers, 1967; Maraldi and Barbieri, 1969) and in cultures of embryonic chick hepatocytes subjected to hypothermia (Barbieri *et al.*, 1970), square tetramer ribosome crystals are readily produced but helical polyribosomes rarely occur (*Plate 194*). However, in chick hepatocyte cultures treated with vinblastine and then subjected to hypothermia, numerous helical polyribosomes and square tetramer crystals were found, although it was noted that while the number of helical polyribosomes increased with increasing doses of vincristine the population of ribosome crystals remained constant. Maraldi *et al.* (1970) therefore concluded that 'these data which demonstrate a different ribosome behaviour owing to the same treatments (neoformation of polyribosome helices and ribosome crystallization) may suggest the existence at least of two distinct ribosome classes, the one functionally active in protein synthesis, the other inactive'.

The idea that there are two classes of ribosomes; i.e. newly formed inactive ones which can form crystals and older ones which cannot is supported by studies on chicken bone marrow subjected to hypothermia (Brunelli *et al.*, 1977). These authors found that crystals formed in immature cells and sometimes in differentiated cells as long as they were capable of mitosis, but they were absent in fully differentiated cells.

Byers (1971) has isolated intracellular ribosome crystals from hypothermic chick embryos and also succeeded in producing such crystals and tetramers of ribosomes from solitary ribosomes *in vitro*. He states that 'the polypeptide synthesizing activity of these ribosomes was found to be unimpaired by their constraint in the tetrameric configuration'.

Plate 194

From a liver of a nine-day-old chick embryo subjected to 12 hours of hypothermia.

Fig. 1. Hepatocyte showing a short helical polyribosome (H) and ribosome crystals (C). The square tetramer arrangement of ribosomes can just be discerned. ×58 000

Fig. 2. Ribosomes showing square tetramer arrangement. ×84 000

Fig. 3. The square tetramer configuration of ribosomes (arrow) in the crystal is evident only in a certain plane of sectioning. ×84 000

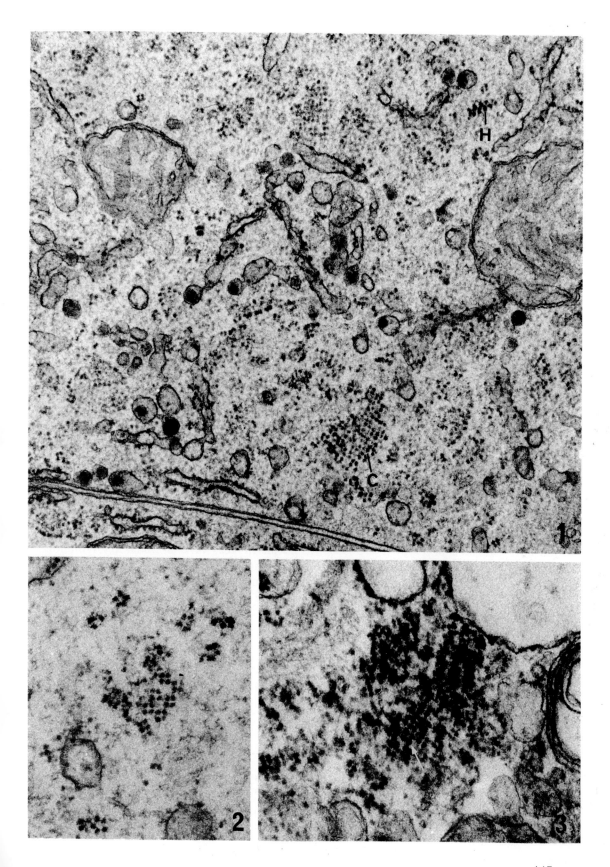

445

Ribosome–lamella complex

Various terms such as 'ribosome-lamella complex', 'polysome-lamella complex', 'granulo-lamellar structures', 'granulo-filamentous body' and 'granulo-lamella complex' have been employed to describe hollow cylindrical or tubular structures composed of spiral or concentric lamellae studded with ribosomes. In sections they present as circular, oval or linear arrays of lamellae and ribosomes. These structures are usually about 2–5 µm long (diameter 0.5–1 µm) but some measuring 10–13 µm have also been described.

Terms such as 'granule-lamella complex' and 'granulo-lamellar structures' are needlessly non-committal because cytochemical reactions (pyroninophilic and susceptible to ribonuclease) and ultrastructural morphology leave little doubt that the 'granules' are in fact ribosomes. Except in rare instances (e.g. Hoshino, 1969) solitary ribosomes rather than polyribosomes are evident in this structure. Hence, the term 'ribosome-lamella complex' seems more apt than most others. The occurrence of concentric or spiral lamellae, rather than membranes with the characteristic trilaminar structure, distinguishes ribosome-lamella complexes from the 'ergastoplasmic Nebenkern' composed of whorled membranes studded with ribosomes and the glycogen body where membranous whorls interspersed with glycogen particles occur (*see* page 516). It has been suggested that the lamellae comprise an array of filaments deployed parallel to the long axis of the cylinder (Daniel and Flandrin, 1974), or that pairs of filaments (2.5 nm wide and spaced about 10.5 nm apart) are attached to a lamina about 2 nm in thickness (Chandra and Stefani, 1978).

Ribosome–lamella complexes have been seen in: (1) leukaemic cells of chronic lymphocytic leukaemia (Zucker-Franklin, 1963; Brunning and Parkin, 1975a; Cawley *et al.*, 1975; Woessner and Rozman, 1976; Catovsky, 1977; Katayama and Schneidner, 1977; Stefani *et al.*, 1977; Mirra *et al.*, 1981); (2) hairy cells of hairy cell leukaemia (Katayama *et al.*, 1972, 1973; Daniel and Flandrin, 1974; Katayama and Finkel, 1974; Schnitzer and Kass, 1974; Möbius *et al.*, 1975; Pilotti *et al.*, 1978; Rozman and Woessner, 1978; Turner and Kjeldsberg, 1978; Kamiyama *et al.*, 1979; Quan *et al.*, 1980; Rosner and Golomb, 1980); (3) blast cells in acute leukaemia (Komiyama *et al.*, 1976); (4) lymphoma cells of the pike (*Esox lucius*) (the laminae show 9.5 nm periodic striations) (Banfield *et al.*, 1976; Dawe *et al.*, 1976); (5) leukaemic cells of acute monoblastic leukaemia (Brunning and Parkin, 1975a; Feremans *et al.*, 1980); (6) neoplastic cells of lymphosarcoma and lymphosarcoma cell leukaemia (Anday *et al.*, 1973; Djaldetti *et al.*, 1974; Chandra and Stefani, 1978) (*Plate 195*); (7) neoplastic cells of non-Hodgkin's lymphomas (Henry, 1975; Perez-Atayde *et al.*, 1982a); (8) lymphocytes from a case of plasmacytic lymphadenopathy with polyclonal hypergammaglobulinaemia (Mikata *et al.*, 1984); (9) plasma cells of multiple myeloma and Waldenstrom's macroglobulinaemia (Brunning and Parkin, 1975a; Oikawa, 1975; Chandra and Stefani, 1978); (10) pericytes within the villous cores of 2 out of 10 human placentas (Sutherland *et al.*, 1980); (11) owl monkey cells infected with *Herpesvirus saimiri*[*] (Banfield *et al.*, 1977); (12) neoplastic cells of an adrenal cortical adenoma from a case of Cushing's syndrome (Hoshino, 1969); (13) neoplastic cells of parathyroid

[*]These structures which present as ribbons or cylinders of lamellae and ribosomes are somewhat different in appearance from the human ribosome–lamella complex. The lamellae are quite prominent and striated and many of the cylindrical ribosome–lamella complexes seem to be composed of but a single lamella studded with ribosomes.

Plate 195

Fig. 1. Lymphosarcoma cell leukaemia. Leukaemic cell displaying two ribosome-lamella complexes. ×22 000 (*From Djaldetti, Landau, Mandel, Har-Zaav and Lewinski, 1974*)

Fig. 2. Hairy cell leukaemia. Leukaemic cell showing obliquely and transversely cut ribosome-lamella complexes. ×39 000 (*From Djaldetti, 1976*)

Fig. 3. Lymphosarcoma cell leukaemia. Leukaemic cell displaying a transversely cut ribosome-lamella complex. ×37 000 (*From Djaldetti, Landau, Mandel, Har-Zaav and Lewinski, 1974*)

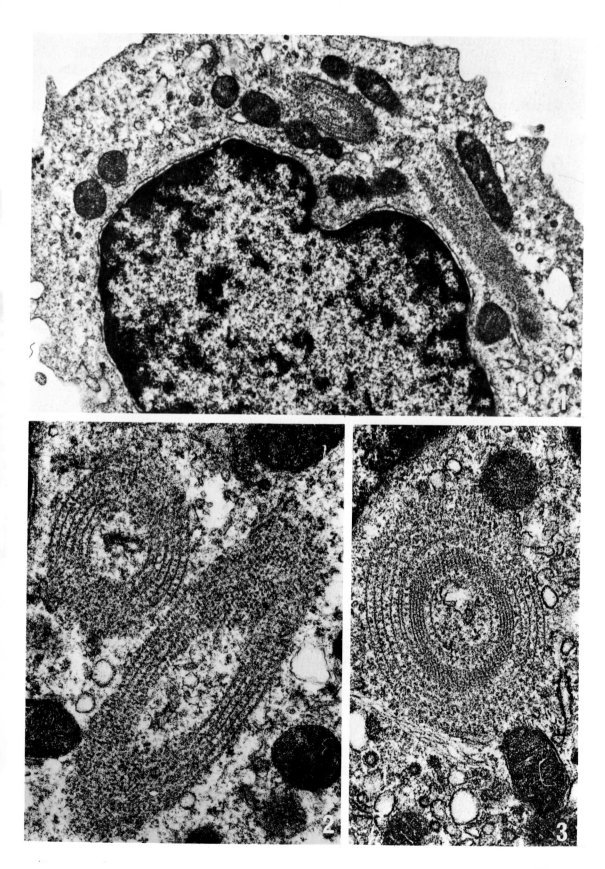

adenoma (Cinti and Osculati, 1982); (14) cells of benign hyperplasia of prostate (Ohtsuki et al., 1978); (15) plasma cells in the skin from a case of mycosis fungoides and plasmacytic infiltrate in a fibrosarcoma of the foot (Zimmerman et al., 1984); (16) mast cells in an iris biopsy from a case of Usher's syndrome (retinitis pigmentosa associated with deafness) and in the neoplastic cells from an alveolar soft part sarcoma (Bull and McCartney, 1986); (17) circulating Sézary's cells (Sebahoun et al., 1979); (18) neoplastic cells of abdominal paraganglioma (Nabarra et al., 1977); (19) neoplastic cells of cerebellar haemangioblastoma (Wassef et al., 1979); (20) neoplastic cells of astrocytoma and glioblastoma multiforme (Stinson, 1981; Gessaga, 1982; Perez-Atayde, 1982; Min, 1982); (21) neoplastic cells of insulinoma (Perez-Atayde et al., 1982b); and (22) neoplastic cells of hibernoma (Plate 196).

There also occur structures which bear some superficial resemblance to ribosome–lamella complexes in that an association between collections of filaments or lamellae and ribosomes or polyribosomes is seen but they lack the complex organization and hollow cylindrical form of the ribosome–lamella complex. Such structures have been seen in: (1) cells exposed to vinblastine sulphate (Krishan and Hsu, 1969; Krishan, 1970); (2) human glomerular epithelial cells (podocytes) from a transplanted kidney and a kidney from a case of nephrotic syndrome (Schuurmans Stekhoven and van Haelst, 1975); (3) cells of human meningioma (Tani and Higashi, 1972); (4) renal tubular epithelial cells of the spider monkey (Ateles geoffroyi), the Colombian squirrel monkey (Saimiri sciurea) and the olive baboon (Papio anubis) (Bulger, 1968); and (5) protoplasts of Triticum vulgare L. seedlings (Bartels and Weier, 1967).

The genesis of ribosome–lamella complexes is obscure but it would appear that they derive from the rough endoplasmic reticulum because a close association with the rough endoplasmic reticulum has been noted by quite a few authors. The most convincing illustrations of this are presented by Daniel and Flandrin (1974) who found that 'the majority of tubular inclusions were surrounded by rough endoplasmic reticulum' and 'occasionally ER was applied to the inner surface of the cylinder'. Various other cytoplasmic organelles (e.g. mitochondria and lysosomes) and inclusions (e.g. lipid droplet) are at times seen in the centre of this cylindrical structure.

It will be noted from the list presented above that the large majority of sightings of ribosome-lamella complex have been in leukaemic cells notably the hairy cells of hairy cell leukaemia. As a result of the report by Katayama et al. (1972) for a while it appeared that the ribosome-lamella complex might be a specific cytoplasmic marker of the hairy cell which would be diagnostic of hairy cell leukaemia. It is now abundantly clear that this is incorrect for ribosome-lamella complexes have been seen in other leukaemic disorders. Even so one should first think of hairy cell leukaemia if these structures are sighted for it is estimated (Daniel and Flandrin, 1974) that about half the cases of hairy cell leukaemia show ribosome-lamella complexes and that a few to almost 100 per cent of the cells may contain ribosome-lamella complexes. However, personal experience and a review of the cases published since the report by Daniel and Flandrin (1974) leads me to believe that much less than half the cases of hairy cell leukaemia show ribosome-lamella complexes.

Plate 196

Hibernoma (From a block of tissue supplied by Dr T.A. Seemayer)

Fig. 1. Longitudinal section through a ribosome–lamella complex, about 3.4 μm long. The appearance seen here is in keeping with the idea that this is a tubular or hollow cylindrical organelle. The wall of the cylinder presents as numerous ribosome-studded lamellar profiles. In the hollow of the cylinder lies cytoplasmic material (C) and a lipid droplet (L). ×40 000

Fig. 2. Obliquely and tangentially sectioned ribosome–lamella complexes are seen here. Note the lipid droplets (L) and mitochondria (M) lying within these structures. ×16 500

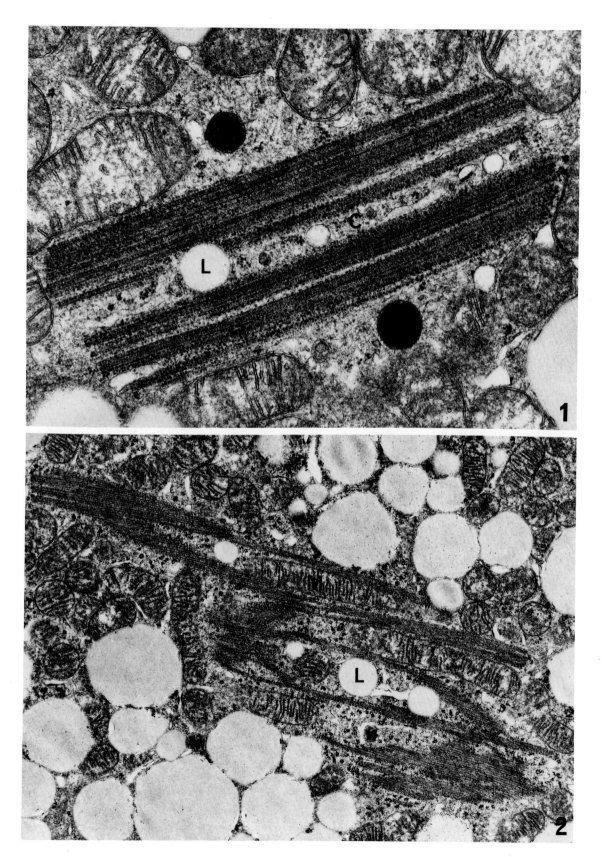

Endoplasmic reticulum and ribosomes in cell differentiation and neoplasia

The endoplasmic reticulum is a highly specialized structure which performs many distinct functions. Hence a well developed endoplasmic reticulum may be looked upon as an expression of cell differentiation and functional activity. Innumerable examples support this concept (*see* review by Porter, 1961). It is also now abundantly clear that immature or undifferentiated cells such as stem cells, blast cells, embryonic cells, and cells in culture have, as a rule, a poor complement of rough endoplasmic reticulum as compared with their normal, mature functioning counterparts. Such immature cells, particularly fast-growing populations of cells, generally also have an abundance of free polyribosomes in the cytoplasm. This presumably reflects the active synthesis of endogenous proteins needed for cell growth and division. The above-mentioned concepts also apply to tumours (*Plates 197–199*), where an inverse relationship has often been noted between the amount of rough endoplasmic reticulum present and the growth rate and malignancy of the tumour (Oberling and Bernhard, 1961; Bernhard, 1969; Ghadially, 1985).

One of the fastest-growing transplantable tumours is the Ehrlich ascites tumour⋆. This highly anaplastic tumour probably derived from a mouse breast carcinoma is now grown as a free cell suspension in the peritoneal cavity of mice. The cells of this tumour contain scant rough endoplasmic reticulum but abundant polyribosomes in the cytoplasm (*Plate 197*).

Perhaps the most frequently studied model illustrating the above-mentioned concept is the rat hepatoma (Dalton, 1964; Hruban *et al.*, 1965a; Ma and Webber, 1966; Flaks, 1968). Here, the cells of very well differentiated slow-growing examples of this tumour have been found to contain a well developed rough endoplasmic reticulum resembling that found in normal hepatocytes, but in highly anaplastic fast-growing variants only an occasional vesicle of rough endoplasmic reticulum is seen and the cytoplasm contains little besides some mitochondria and innumerable polyribosomes. In extreme examples of this kind there is little difficulty in drawing meaningful positive correlations between ultrastructural signs of anaplasia and growth rate or malignancy, but when intermediate examples of tumours with moderate degrees of anaplasia and differences in growth rates are compared exceptions or apparent exceptions to our concepts are soon found. Such differences may be real or may be due to the small sample examined with the electron microscope not being truly representative of the whole tumour mass.

⋆The history and origin of the Ehrlich tumour (solid and ascites forms) is shrouded in mystery. By about 1907 Ehrlich had at least nine murine transplantable tumours (carcinomas and sarcomas) in his laboratory. The Ehrlich ascites tumour (or tumours) is now so anaplastic that it is impossible to say whether it is a carcinoma or sarcoma but it is generally believed that the one used in most laboratories started off as an adenocarcinoma – probably an adenocarcinoma of the breast.

Plate 197

Ehrlich ascites tumour cell, showing scant cisternae of rough endoplasmic reticulum and numerous polyribosomes in the cytoplasm. ×32 000

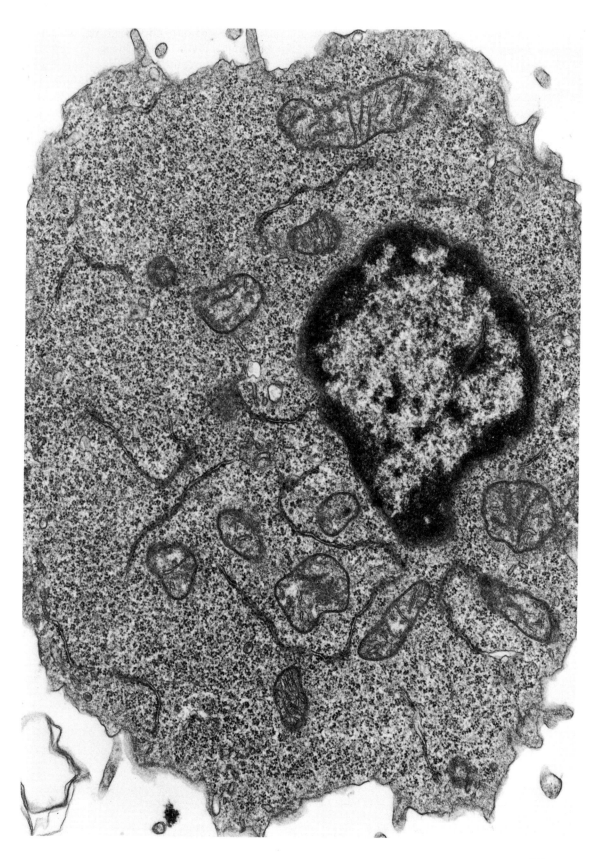

The thesis, presented above, namely that in malignant tumours the rough endoplasmic reticulum is, relatively speaking, not too abundant but polyribosomes lying free in the cytoplasm are, is found to be valid also in the case of fibrosarcomas and osteosarcomas. In rapidly growing malignant fibrosarcoma (*Plate 198*) the rough endoplasmic reticulum of the malignant fibroblast is not so abundant or well ordered as, for example, in the fibroblast from a benign lesion such as a non-ossifying fibroma of bone (*Plate 182*), but numerous polyribosomes lying free in the cytoplasm can be detected in many tumour cells (*Plate 198, Fig. 2*). Further, it will be noted that in the malignant fibroblast the rough endoplasmic reticulum is dilated and vesiculated and the contents are quite electron-dense suggesting perhaps that an impaired transport and condensation of secretory product had occurred or that an abnormal secretory material was being produced (pages 434 and 530).

In osteosarcoma a similar situation prevails, for here too the rough endoplasmic reticulum is often less abundant than in the normal osteoblast but it is dilated or vesiculated and the stored secretory product is likely to condense into structures known as 'intracisternal dense granules' (*Plate 237*).

It is said that the rough endoplasmic reticulum is developed to a greater degree in the keratinocytes of the keratoacanthoma as compared with the cells of the normal hair follicle from which such tumours arise (Prutkin, 1967). Similarly, Lipetz (1970) reports that 'crown gall cells of several plant species contain considerably more endoplasmic reticulum than their normal or hyperplastic counterparts' and that 'this characteristic appears to be stable in crown gall tissues grown *in vitro* for many years'. The significance of this situation in tumour tissue of plants is not clear but some crown gall cells, such as those of *Parthenocissus tricuspidata*, produce impressive amounts of peroxidase, presumably from the rough endoplasmic reticulum of the tumour cells (Lipetz and Galston, 1959).

Plate 198

(*From Ghadially, 1985, From a block of tissue supplied by Dr A.H. Cameron*)

Fig: 1. Neoplastic fibroblast from a fibrosarcoma. Note dilated and vesiculated rough endoplasmic reticulum with electron-dense contents (D). ×38 000

Fig. 2. Same case as *Fig. 1.* A neoplastic fibroblast showing numerous polyribosomes lying free in the cytoplasm (arrows). Note also the dilated rough endoplasmic reticulum with electron-dense contents (D) and polyribosomes lying on the surface of tangentially cut cisternae (arrowheads). ×18 000

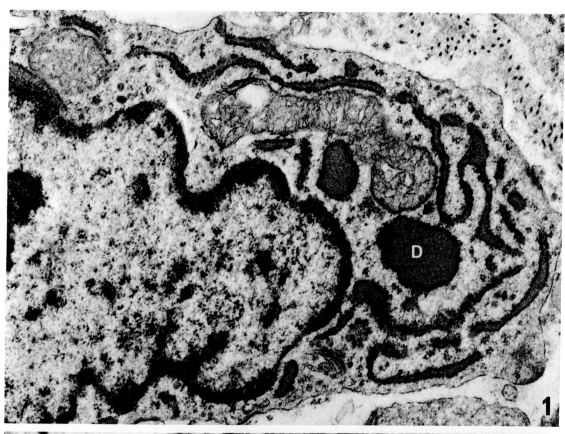

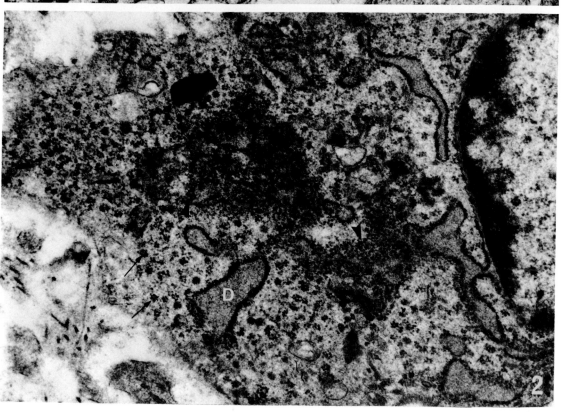

The rough endoplasmic reticulum in animal tumours (particularly adenomas and well differentiated examples of malignant tumours) can also be functionally active and form products characteristic of the cell of origin. There are numerous examples of this; for instance, the milk-producing mouse mammary tumours and thyroid tumours which contain abundant rough endoplasmic reticulum and actively produce secretory proteins (for references, *see* Bernhard, 1969). One of the best-known examples of this in man is the multiple myeloma (Skinnider and Ghadially, 1975) where the neoplastic cells (*Plate 199*) are usually well endowed with rough endoplastic reticulum★ and produce immunoglobulins or fragments thereof (e.g. Bence-Jones protein) in abundance. However, here also there is much variation in the morphology and amount of rough endoplasmic reticulum present, and one cannot correlate this too closely with the type or amount of immunoglobulin produced. (For discussion and references, *see* Zucker-Franklin, 1964.) Yet this may again reflect no more than the inescapable limitation imposed by the small samples that can be examined with the electron microscope.

It is also worth pointing out that, despite some claims to the contrary, none of the alterations seen in the endoplasmic reticulum of neoplastic cells can be regarded as characteristic of the neoplastic state. As a rule, such changes are similar to those found in embryonic tissues and reflect merely the well known increased growth rate, and poor functional capacity of tumour cells as a class.

The comments made regarding the rough endoplasmic reticulum relate mainly to tumours arising from cells fairly well endowed with rough endoplasmic reticulum to begin with. However, the remarks about the polyribosomes lying free in the cytoplasm are generally applicable to all tumours. If numerous polyribosomes are seen, it is an indication of rapid growth. This change goes hand in hand with hypertrophy and margination of the nucleolus and correlates well with the number of mitoses seen by light microscopy. It is worth noting that solitary ribosomes lying free in the cytoplasm have a converse connotation—namely a suppressed or deranged messenger RNA production and protein synthesis (page 440).

The smooth endoplasmic reticulum is not well represented in most cells and their tumours, except steroid secreting cells and their tumours. This and other features such as the occurrence of mitochondria with tubulovesicular cristae and lipid droplets helps distinguish tumours of steroid secreting cells from other tumours (Ghadially, 1985).

★Even so the rough endoplasmic reticulum is usually not quite as abundant as in normal or reactive plasma cells and in plasma cell leukaemia which may be considered a more malignant lesion of plasma cells, there is a further more evident reduction in the amount of rough endoplasmic reticulum (for illustrations supporting this, *see* Ghadially, 1985).

Plate 199
Plasma cells from a case of multiple myeloma. These neoplastic cells are well endowed with rough endoplasmic reticulum. ×10 500 (*Ghadially and Skinnider, unpublished electron micrograph*)

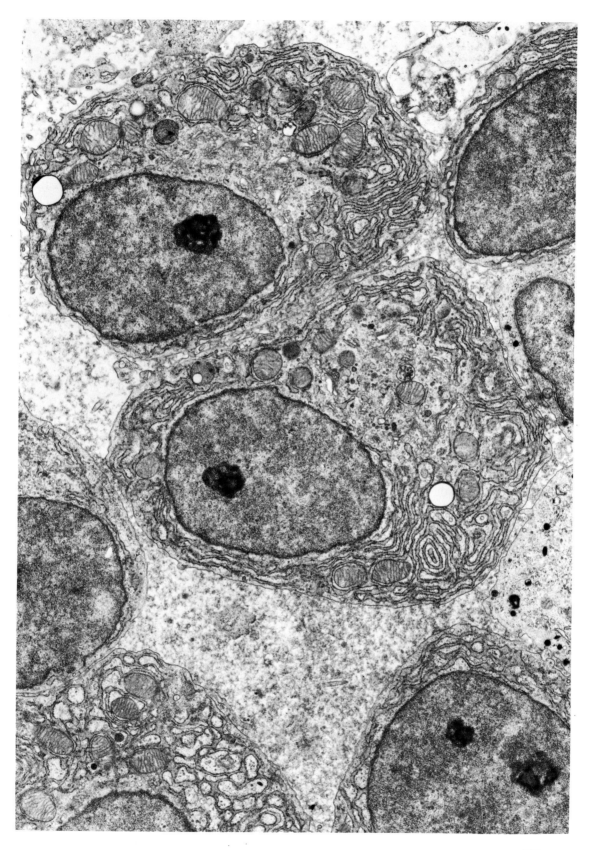

455

Hypertrophy of rough endoplasmic reticulum

Many studies indicate that the endoplasmic reticulum is a dynamic labile organelle which can readily undergo hypertrophy or atrophy, and this usually reflects a state of altered functional activity. Atrophy or involution of the rough endoplasmic reticulum and hypertrophy of smooth endoplasmic reticulum are dealt with later (pages 458 and 544). Here are examined only a few of the many instances where an increase in the amount of rough endoplasmic reticulum has been noted to occur. Such an increase always raises the question as to whether the increased rough endoplasmic reticulum is produced in existing cells or whether the existing cells are replaced by a new population of rough-endoplasmic-reticulum-rich cells. Of course, each example has to be evaluated on its own merits, but at times the speed at which the change occurs and the absence of signs of any undue cellular proliferative activity leads one to conclude that the former mechanism may be operative.

Ultrastructural morphometric studies on the pregnant rat liver (Hope, 1970) have shown that an increase in the volume proportion of rough endoplasmic reticulum occurs in hepatocytes, and this is also evident as an increase in RNA biochemically and as an increase in basophilia histologically. An important function of the rough endoplasmic reticulum in the liver is the synthesis of plasma proteins. Therefore, it would appear that the increased rough endoplasmic reticulum reflects the increased demand for plasma proteins known to occur during pregnancy as a result of the increased blood volume (hydraemia of pregnancy).

Atrophy of the rough endoplasmic reticulum occurs in the submaxillary gland of the rat when the duct is ligated. Removal of the ligature and resumption of secretory activity is accompanied by a reappearance of the rough endoplasmic reticulum. It has been noted (Tamarin, 1971a, b) that there is no evidence of overt cell proliferation and that the rough endoplasmic reticulum undergoes these changes within the existing population of cells.

Macrophages are poorly endowed with rough endoplasmic reticulum but when they engage in phagocytic activity a modest hypertrophy of the rough endoplasmic reticulum occurs, presumably needed for the synthesis of acid hydrolases and primary lysosomes★.

As noted earlier (page 338), two main types of synovial cells have been found in the synovial membrane of all species studied to date: a type A cell where the rough endoplasmic reticulum is scanty or virtually absent, and a type B cell which is well endowed with rough endoplasmic reticulum. In various pathological states such as traumatic arthritis, haemarthrosis and rheumatoid arthritis there is a marked increase of type B and intermediate cells well endowed with rough endoplasmic reticulum (*Plate 200*). This alteration can be appreciated also with the light microscope which shows that not only is there an increase in the number of pyroninophilic cells but there is also a marked increase in the intensity of staining. However, the true significance of this increase eludes us for it is not too clear what export protein the type B synovial cell normally produces; the various opinions expressed being that it produces: (1) some of the proteins found in the synovial fluid; (2) precursors of collagen; or (3) α_2-macroglobin (Ghadially, 1980b, 1983).

★*See* footnote on page 718.

Plate 200

Synovial cells showing marked hypertrophy of the rough endoplasmic reticulum. Long parallel arrays of cisternae (C) are seen. Such an arrangement is rarely, if ever, found in normal synovial intimal cells (compare with *Plates 145* and *181*). ×8500 (*From Ghadially and Roy, 1969*)

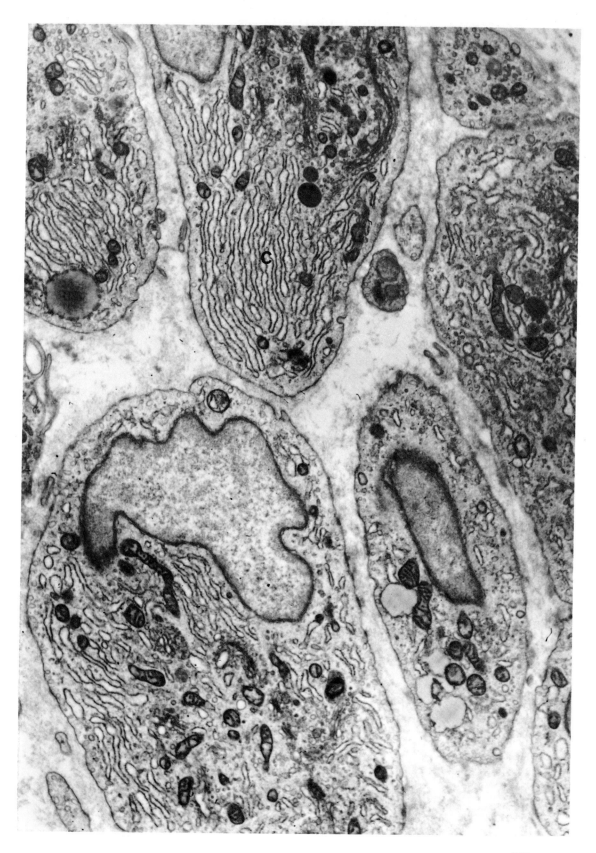

457

Hypertrophy of smooth endoplasmic reticulum in hepatocytes

Perhaps the most extensively studied example of smooth endoplasmic reticulum hypertrophy is that seen in the hepatocytes of phenobarbitone-treated rats and hamsters, where after a few doses of the drug almost every nook and cranny of the cell may be filled with a ramifying network of smooth-membraned branching tubules and vesicles. This change is associated with an increase in liver weight, an increase in the size of the microsomal fraction (in this case composed mainly of smooth endoplasmic reticulum membranes) and a concomitant rise in drug-metabolizing enzymes. Smooth endoplasmic reticulum hypertrophy (*Plates 201* and *202*) has now come to be regarded as an adaptive response (drug tolerance) by which an animal develops an enhanced ability to handle doses of drugs which would be fatal to normal animals.

Smooth endoplasmic reticulum hypertrophy shows many interesting morphological variations, depending on the drug used and the amount, frequency and duration of its administration. It may also at times be related to the species, age and sex of the animal. One can find a spectrum of changes varying from obvious degranulation of rough endoplasmic reticulum followed by a barely discernible or modest new smooth endoplasmic reticulum formation (e.g. after administration of some hepatocarcinogens) to overt hypertrophy of smooth endoplasmic reticulum without a marked reduction in the amount of rough endoplasmic reticulum (e.g. after administration of phenobarbitone; *Plate 202*). Phosphorus poisoning provides a further interesting variation, for here marked hypertrophy of the rough endoplasmic reticulum with concentric ribosome-studded membrane formations (*Plate 230*) is seen prior to smooth endoplasmic reticulum hypertrophy (*Plate 201*). Furthermore, one may observe that smooth endoplasmic reticulum hypertrophy may be diffuse and occur as large areas of branching tubules almost filling the cytoplasm (*Plate 201*), or it can be focal and present as small rounded aggregates of vesicular smooth endoplasmic reticulum in the cell.

With light microscopy focal zones of smooth endoplasmic reticulum hypertrophy may present as hyaline eosinophilic inclusions in the cytoplasm. Many of the drugs that produce this change also yield concentric membranous whorls of smooth membranes in the cytoplasm (*Plate 232, Fig. 1*). Smooth endoplasmic reticulum hypertrophy has occasionally been noted in a few pathological states such as viral hepatitis (Schaffner, 1966) and extrahepatic cholestasis (Steiner et al., 1962), but it has mainly been observed after the administration of a large variety of drugs, including many hepatocarcinogens. There is ample evidence that such changes occur not only in a variety of laboratory animals but also in man.

Drugs which have produced smooth endoplasmic reticulum hypertrophy in the liver include: (1) aflatoxin (Svoboda et al., 1966; Novi, 1977); (2) allylisopropylacetamide (Posalaki and Barka, 1968; Moses et al., 1970; Biempica et al., 1971); (3) β-3-furylalanine (Hruban et al., 1965b); (4) β-3-thienylalanine (Hruban et al., 1963); (5) butylated hydroxytoluene (Lane and Lieber, 1967); (6) carbon tetrachloride (Bassi, 1960; Ganote and Otis, 1969); (7) dichlorodiphenyltrichloroethane (DDT) (Ortega, 1966); (8) dieldrin (Hutterer et al., 1968); (9) dimethylnitrosamine (Emmelot and Benedetti, 1960, 1961; Svoboda and Higginson, 1963; Hadjiolov and Markov, 1973); (10) ethanol (Rubin et al., 1968); (11) ethionine (Wood, 1964, 1965; Meldolesi et al., 1967); (12) N-2-fluorenyldiacetamide (Mikata and Luse, 1964);

Plate 201
Two hepatocytes are seen in this electron micrograph. The cytoplasm of one of these (A) is packed with smooth endoplasmic reticulum, but the other (B) is not so affected. From the liver of a rat given yellow phosphorus. ×20 000 (*Ghadially and Bhatnagar, unpublished electron micrograph*)

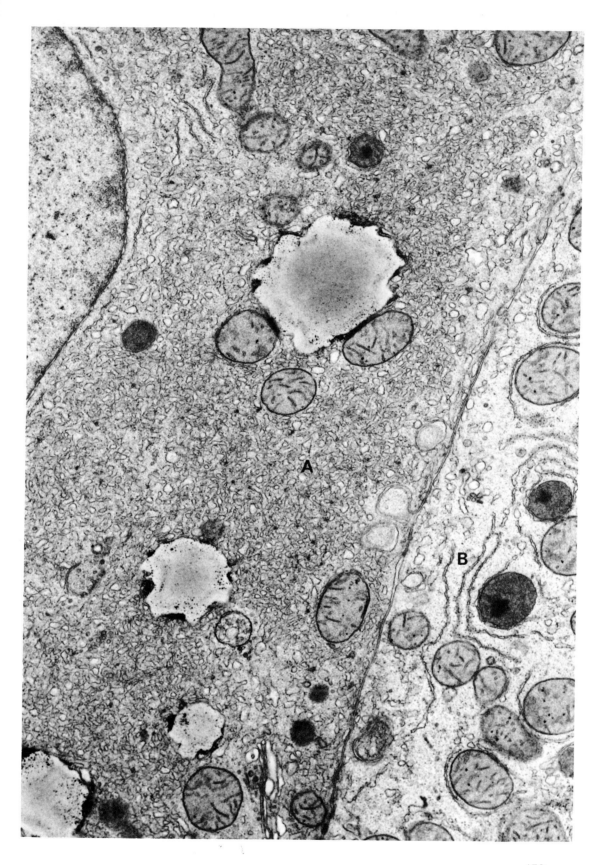

459

(13) 2-methyl-4-dimethylaminoazobenzene (Lafontaine and Allard, 1964); (14) 3-methyl-4-dimethylaminoazobenzene (butter yellow) (Porter and Bruni, 1959; Arcasoy et al., 1968, Hutterer et al., 1969); (15) naphthylisothiocyanate (Steiner and Baglio, 1963); (16) phenobarbitone (Remmer and Merker, 1963; Orrenius et al., 1965; Orrenius and Ericsson, 1966a, b; Burger and Herdson, 1966; Jones and Fawcett, 1966; Chiesara et al., 1967); (17) lasiocarpine (Svoboda and Higginson, 1963); (18) reserpine (Winborn and Seelig, 1970); (19) tannic acid (Arhelger et al., 1965); (20) thioacetamide (Ashworth et al., 1965; Kendry, 1968); (21) yellow phosphorus (Ganote and Otis, 1969); (22) 2-acetylaminofluorene (Flaks, 1971); (23) halothane (Ross and Cardell, 1972); (24) certain anthelmintic drugs and prednisolone (Cockrell et al., 1972); and (25) polychlorinated biphenyls (Nishizumi, 1970; Kimbrough et al., 1972; Amagase, 1975; Hinton et al., 1978).

An examination of the above-mentioned list of compounds shows that drugs with diverse pharmacological properties and chemical structure can produce smooth endoplasmic reticulum hypertrophy. However, most of these compounds are lipid soluble and since large doses of progesterone can also produce this change it has been suggested (Jones and Fawcett, 1966) that enzymes of the smooth endoplasmic reticulum are responsible for the degradation of both endogenous and exogenous lipid-soluble compounds. Such a concept is further supported (see review by Conney, 1965) by the observation that the livers of phenobarbitone-treated rats have a several-fold increased ability to hydroxylate testosterone, androsterone, oestradiol, progesterone and cortisone and that the hydroxylases involved are located in the microsomal fraction (Kuntzman and Jacobson, 1965; Orrenius et al., 1965). Smooth endoplasmic reticulum hypertrophy has been noted in viral hepatitis (Schaffner, 1966) and in extrahepatic cholestasis (Steiner et al., 1962). This may indicate an adaptive response to deal with endogenously produced toxic material (Barka and Popper, 1967).

Proliferation of smooth endoplasmic reticulum is now regarded as the morphological expression of drug-induced enzyme production in the liver. The newly formed smooth endoplasmic reticulum has frequently been seen to arise from the rough endoplasmic reticulum (Plate 202). This is in keeping with the idea that the proteins needed for new membrane synthesis are produced by the rough endoplasmic reticulum, as are the associated drug-metabolizing enzymes. The expanded smooth endoplasmic reticulum may then be looked upon as providing the surface for interaction of drugs and enzymes.

Various studies (Barka and Popper, 1967; Arcasoy et al., 1968; Hutterer et al., 1969) show that three stages may be identified in the response of the liver to drugs which produce smooth endoplasmic reticulum hypertrophy. The first stage (induction) is associated with liver enlargement, smooth endoplasmic reticulum hypertrophy, increase in microsomal protein fraction and formation of drug-handling enzymes. This is followed by a steady state of increased drug tolerance, the length of which may be fairly long as in the case of phenobarbitone and dieldrin, or quite short as in the case of 3-methyl-4-dimethylaminoazobenzene. Finally, a third stage (decompensation) may be reached where the activity of the drug-handling enzymes diminishes and the smooth endoplasmic reticulum is seen as focal clusters of tightly packed vesicles in the cell cytoplasm.

Plate 202
An area of smooth endoplasmic reticulum hypertrophy from the liver of a hamster that had received phenobarbitone. Note the continuity between the rough and the smooth endoplasmic reticulum (arrows). ×48 000 (*Ghadially and Bhatnagar, unpublished electron micrograph*)

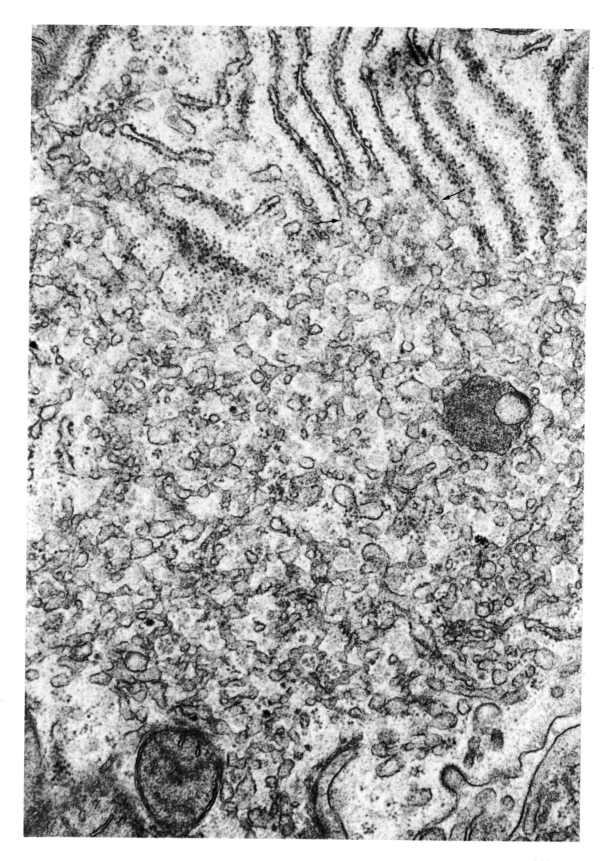

461

Confronting cisternae

Multilayered membranous formations derived from the nuclear envelope or the rough endoplasmic reticulum have been seen in mitotic and interphase cells. On closer examination they are found to comprise a pair or more of closely apposed cisternae (perinuclear cistern or cisternae of the rough endoplasmic reticulum) with electron-dense material (called 'the dense lamina') between them (*Plates 203–204*). The outermost membranes usually, but not invariably, bear a few or several ribosomes on their surface but the ribosomes trapped between the confronting membranes suffer disintegration and this probably produces the dense lamina. Sometimes confronting cisternae have been found in continuity with the nuclear envelope (*Plate 203, Fig. 1*) at other times with the rough endoplasmic reticulum, but there are times when no such connections are seen. On rare occasions they have been seen in continuity with annulate lamellae.

Generally only two 'fused' cisternae are seen but at times three (*Plate 204, Fig. 2*) or more cisternae are involved. Various terms such as 'paired cisternae', 'triple cisternae', 'pentalaminar membranous structures', 'confronting cisternae', 'spindle lamellae', 'lamellar bodies', 'peculiar membranes' and quite a few other terms have been used to describe these structures.

Of the various terms proffered 'confronting cisternae' appears to be the best for it clearly describes the situation that prevails and is applicable in all instances (i.e. it does not matter whether two or more cisternae are involved). However, the term 'confronting cisternae' poses a grammatical dilemma, because it is a single structure derived by the apposition of two or more cisternae. Hence, in the former sense it is singular, in the latter plural. It would, however, be grammatically incongruous to speak about a single example of this structure as 'a confronting cisternae'. Therefore a judicious choice of words is usually needed to describe this structure. Confronting cisternae are on rare occasions seen in the nucleus (*see Plate 22, Fig. 2*). Therefore one may speak about 'intracytoplasmic confronting cisternae' and 'intranuclear confronting cisternae'. In instances where one finds intranuclear confronting cisternae one also almost invariably finds intracytoplasmic confronting cisternae, but not *vice versa*.

Confronting cisternae have been seen in: (1) HeLa cells in culture (Epstein, 1961); (2) various rat hepatomas (Hruban *et al.*, 1965a; Chang and Gilbey, 1968); (3) colcemid-treated Chinese hamster cells (Brinkley *et al.*, 1967); (4) fibromyxosarcoma (Leak *et al.*, 1967); (5) phytohaemagglutinin stimulated lymphocytes (Procicchiani *et al.*, 1968); (6) KB cells in culture (derived from human epidermoid carcinoma) (Kumagawa *et al.*, 1968); (7) Wolffian duct cells during differentiation of the epididymis (Flickinger, 1969); (8) cells of human giant-cell tumour of bone, rhabdomyosarcoma, reticulum cell sarcoma and osteosarcoma (Hanaoka *et al.*, 1970; Hanaoka and Friedman, 1970; Nakanishi *et al.*, 1986); (9) leukaemic cells (chloroleukaemia of rat) and mesenchymal cells from forelimb of human embryos (Kelley, 1971); (10) nasopharyngeal carcinoma cells in culture (Vuillaume and de-Thé, 1973); (11) pulmonary adenomatosis of the Awassi sheep (Perk *et al.*, 1971); (12) a variety of cultured cells infected with herpesvirus (Nii *et al.*, 1968; King *et al.*, 1972; Hamdy *et al.*, 1974) (*Plate 22*); (13) cultured

---

Plate 203

Fig. 1. Confronting cisternae (arrows) are seen in a cell found in a malignant ascites produced by secondary deposits of melanoma. These cisternae are placed well away from the nucleus and are not connected to the nuclear envelope. ×16 000

Fig. 2. High-power view of confronting cisternae. Note the electron-dense material between the confronting faces (arrows). ×65 000

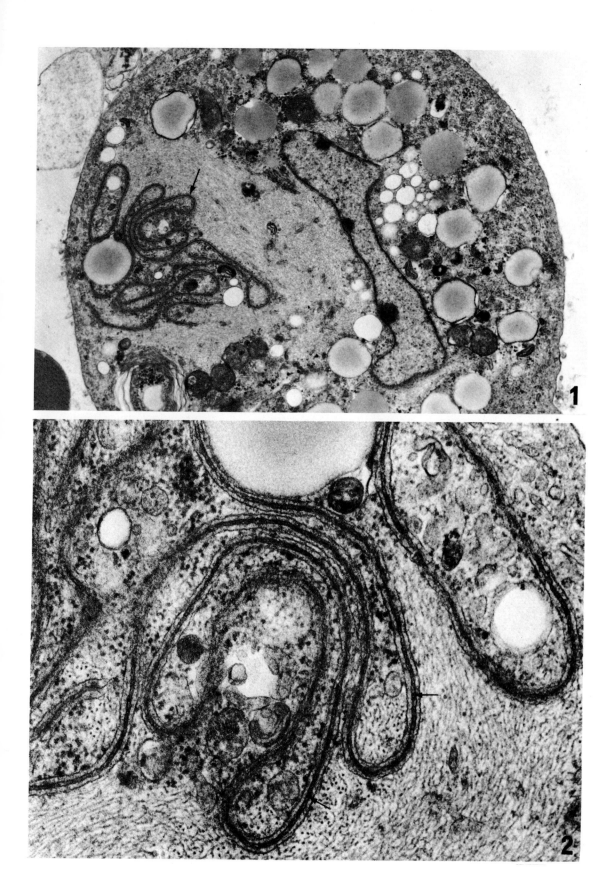

Burkitt lymphoma cells (Chandra and Stefani, 1976) (*Plate 227, Fig. 1*); (14) regenerating aortic cells after experimental injury (Taura, 1978); (15) rat adipocytes depleted of fat by prolonged low food intake (Napolitano and Gagne, 1963); (16) Walker carcinoma (Buck, 1961); (17) mitotic endothelial cells (Warren *et al.*, 1972); (18) normal human lymphocytes incubated with *Staphylococcus aureus* (Kuyama *et al.* 1985); (19) rat sarcoma (Porter, 1955); (20) cells in malignant ascites produced by metastasis from a cutaneous melanoma (*Plate 203*); (21) cells from malignant pleural effusions (Cappelli-Gotzos *et al.*, 1983); (22) rectal carcinoma (*Plate 204, Fig. 1*); and (23) malignant fibrous histiocytoma (*Plate 204, Fig. 2*).

It will be noted from the list presented above that confronting cisternae occur in rapidly dividing cells, both *in vitro* and *in vivo* but they have been seen more often in neoplastic and virus infected cells than in normal cells. Their association with mitosis has been stressed by some authors because they have been seen quite frequently in mitotic cells. However, they have now been seen often enough in interphase cells.

As is well known, during mitosis the nuclear envelope disintegrates*. Two mechanisms seem to have been identified. In some instances the envelope breaks up into vesicles, and in other cases it flakes off or scales off in layers (Barer *et al.*, 1961). One may therefore suggest that confronting cisternae may at times be formed from the nuclear envelope by: (1) folding upon itself; (2) reduplication; (3) fusion of broken segments; or (4) fusion with an adjacent cistern of the rough endoplasmic reticulum. One may argue that this is at least an atypical if not an overtly pathological event because not all cells in mitosis develop confronting cisternae.

Confronting cisternae seen in interphase cells may represent 'leftover' nuclear envelope segments from a previous mitosis, but it is equally likely that at times confronting cisternae develop by a falling together of cisternae of the rough endoplasmic reticulum in an interphase cell. Such distinctions are often difficult to make, for both the rough endoplasmic reticulum and the nuclear envelope are part of the same membrane system. Therefore, attempts to classify confronting cisternae on the basis of alleged origin from nuclear envelope or the rough endoplasmic reticulum are hardly a practical proposition.

Confronting cisternae generally occur either as short solitary segments, or as long meandering structures lying in the cytoplasm. Sometimes they form concentric whorls. A much rarer form (i.e. seen in only a few sites and situations) where the confronting cisternae form tubular structures (i.e. tubular confronting cisternae) is dealt with later (pages 466–477).

The so-called 'spine apparatus' in the spines on the dendrites of neurons and the so-called 'lamellar bodies' in bodies of neurons are, in fact, examples of confronting cisternae. These structures and confronting cisternae complexes found in Purkinji cells are described later (page 476).

---

*True for all human cells but not for all lower forms and plants.

Plate 204

Fig. 1. Carcinoma of rectum. The perinuclear cisterna is one of the two cisternae involved in the formation of this confronting cisternae. ×40 000

Fig. 2. Malignant fibrous histiocytoma. Confronting cisternae with one dense lamina (arrowhead) and two dense laminae (arrows) are seen here. The former derives from close apposition of two cisternae of the rough endoplasmic reticulum, while the latter derive from close apposition of three such cisternae. ×48 000

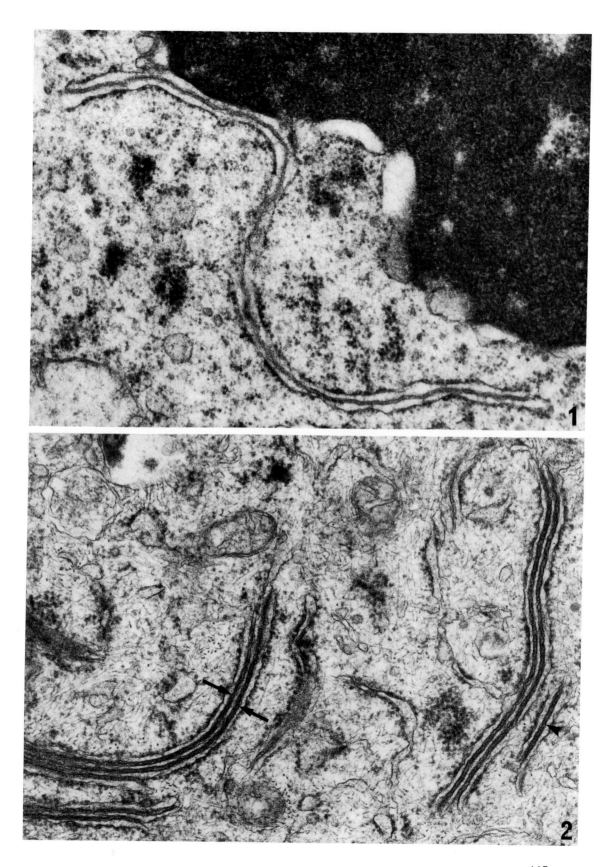

465

Tubular confronting cisternae

The common confronting cisternae (pages 462–465) generally occur as short segments or as long meandering sheets (lamellar formations) lying in the cell cytoplasm. In tubular confronting cisternae (*Plates 205–209*), we have a situation whereby the confronting cisternae form a tubular structure. Cytoplasmic matrix containing some small organelles like ribosomes lies within this tube-shaped structure. Sometimes these structures are referred to as 'cylindrical confronting cisternae'. This is an acceptable but a not too accurate term, for while in common parlance one speaks about 'solid cylinders' and 'hollow cylinders', in geometry the cylinder, like the sphere, designates a 'solid' form. A hollow cylinder is in fact a tube, so it is best to call these structures 'tubular confronting cisternae'.

Unfortunately, tubular confronting cisternae are commonly referred to in the literature on AIDS (acquired immune deficiency syndrome) as 'test-tube and ring-shaped structures' or 'test-tube and ring-shaped forms' or 'TRF'*. The penalty of naming a structure by the profiles it produces in sectioned material is that false ideas about its true morphology are soon created. For example, an excellent, informative review (Rácz et al., 1986) on the morphology of lymph nodes in AIDS is somewhat marred by the statement that: 'TRF are in longitudinal sections, cylindrical in shape with one end closed'; thus implying that these structures are indeed truly test-tube shaped. The same misconception is propagated by Orenstein (1983) who imagines that confronting cisternae are 'straight cylinders, often closed at one end like a test-tube whose 'lumen' communicates with the ground substance'. (By ground substance one presumes he means cytoplasmic matrix.) The fact of the matter is that these structures are 'tubes' (both ends open) and not 'test-tubes' (one end closed) as even a casual glance at a single electron micrograph proves (e.g. *Plate 205, Fig. 3* or *Plate 206, Fig. 1*). Further, our serial section study (Ghadially et al., 1987) (where more than 100 tubular confronting cisternae were followed in serial sections) did not reveal a single instance where one end was closed; all were tubules with both ends open.

Like any tubular structure (e.g. ribosome–lamella complex and manchette of spermatid) tubular confronting cisternae present: (1) a circular profile when cut transversely; (2) a profile composed of a pair of parallel 'lines' when cut longitudinally; (3) an oval profile when cut

---

*The 'credit' for this undesirable term is claimed by Sidhu (1983) who states: 'more intriguing was the presence of another structure which I have descriptively designated test-tube and ring-shaped forms'. Their (Sidhu et al., 1985) claim that tubular confronting cisternae are at times 'formed by the apposition of endoplasmic reticulum and the outer membrane of the mitochondrion' is quite untenable and is certainly not supported by their Fig. 11 as they claim.

Plate 205

Hepatocytes of a chimpanzee inoculated with serum from a patient with Non-A, Non-B hepatitis. (*From a block of tissue supplied by Dr H.P. Dienes*)

Fig. 1. Confronting cisternae showing a C-shaped profile. ×125 000

Figs. 2 and 3. Confronting cisternae showing various profiles. The ones seen at T and L represent transverse and longitudinal sections respectively through tubular structures. ×85 000; ×54 000

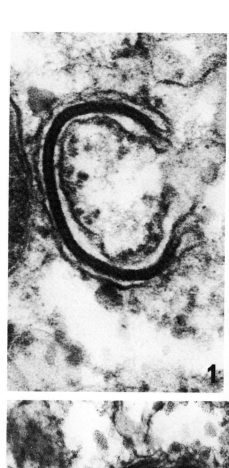

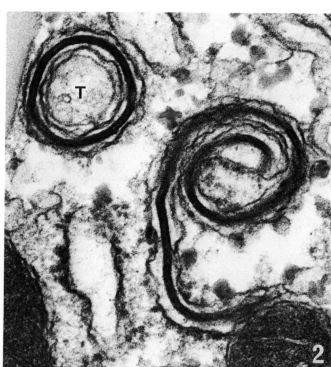

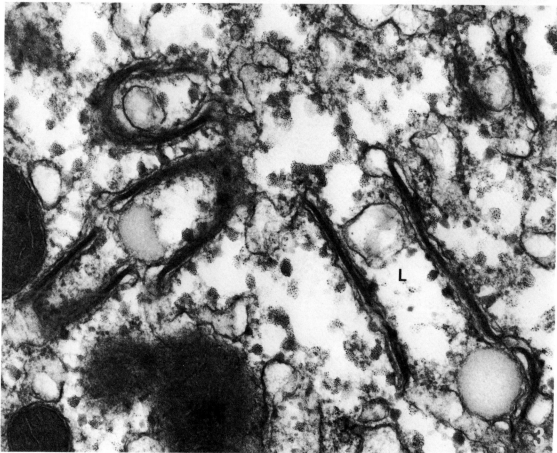

obliquely through the body of the tube; and (4) a test-tube-shaped or V-shaped profile when an oblique section passes through an open end of the tube.

Tubular confronting cisternae have been seen in: (1) the hepatocytes of chimpanzees inoculated with plasma or serum from cases of non-A, non-B hepatitis (but apparently not in human cases with this disease) (*Plate 205*) (O'Connell, 1977; Jackson *et al.*, 1979; Shimizu *et al.*, 1979; Pfeifer *et al.*, 1980); (2) hepatocytes of HBsAg carrier chimpanzees infected with the delta agent (Kamimura *et al.*, 1983); (3) lymphocytes from a Japanese case of adult T cell leukaemia (Shamoto *et al.*, 1981); (4) a case of multiple sclerosis (Prineas and Wright, 1978); (5) endothelial cells in cases of idiopathic fibrosing alveolitis, and collagen vascular diseases (Hammar *et al.*, 1984, 1985); (6) lymphocytes in lymph nodes and peripheral blood of cases of AIDS and to a lesser extent in persistent generalized lymphadenopathy which is thought to be a prodrome of AIDS (Ewing *et al.*, 1983a, b; Schaff *et al.*, 1983; Sidhu, 1983; Allegra *et al.*, 1984; Anderson *et al.*, 1984; Onerheim *et al.*, 1984; Orenstein *et al.*, 1984, 1985; Kostianovsky and Grimley, 1985; Lewis *et al.*, 1985; Sidhu *et al.*, 1985; Rácz *et al.*, 1986).

My measurements on tubular confronting cisternae in chimpanzee hepatocytes and in lymphoid cells in AIDS indicate that they have a fairly constant overall diameter* of about 225–300 nm and that they are usually about 1.2–1.5 μm long, but a few longer ones up to about 2.2 μm in length also occur. The thickness of the dense lamina between the confronting cisternae is about 20 nm, and at times this dense lamina shows a crystalline appearance (periodicity about 10 nm).

*These represent measurements taken on cross cut or longitudinally cut confronting tubular cisternae where the peripheral or outer cisterna of the confronting cisternae is not dilated. At times this cisterna is so dilated that it looks as if a dense lamina (and the cytoplasmic material 'within' it) has fallen into a markedly dilated or vesiculated cisterna of the rough endoplasmic reticulum.

Plate 206

Lymphoid cells from a lymph node of a patient with AIDS (*From Ghadially, Senoo, Fuse and Chan, 1987*)

Fig. 1. Profiles of eight tubular confronting cisternae cut in various planes are seen here. These include circular profiles produced by transverse sections (T) through tubular confronting cisternae, a V-shaped or test-tube-shaped profile produced by an oblique section (O) passing through an open end of confronting tubular cisternae and a parallel line profile representing a longitudinal section (L) through tubular confronting cisternae. ×38 000

Fig. 2. Several profiles more complex than those seen in *Fig. 1* are present here. One of them (arrow) is a T-shaped profile where two test-tube-shaped profiles of dense laminae and associated cytoplasmic material lie in a dilated sac of endoplasmic reticulum. Such an image could be due to a fusion of the outer membranes of two neighbouring confronting cisternae. Another profile (large arrowhead) shows two V-shaped dense laminae and some microtubules lying in a dilated cisterna. Yet another profile depicts an outer cisterna which is dilated and contains some microtubules (small arrowheads). The inset shows a profile produced by an oblique section through cylindrical confronting cisternae where the wall is the product of the apposition of three confronting cisternae (instead of the usual two) hence two dense laminae are seen in its wall. Because two dense laminae (instead of the usual one) are present these structures are referred to as 'double-walled tubular confronting cisternae'. ×36 000 Inset ×82 000

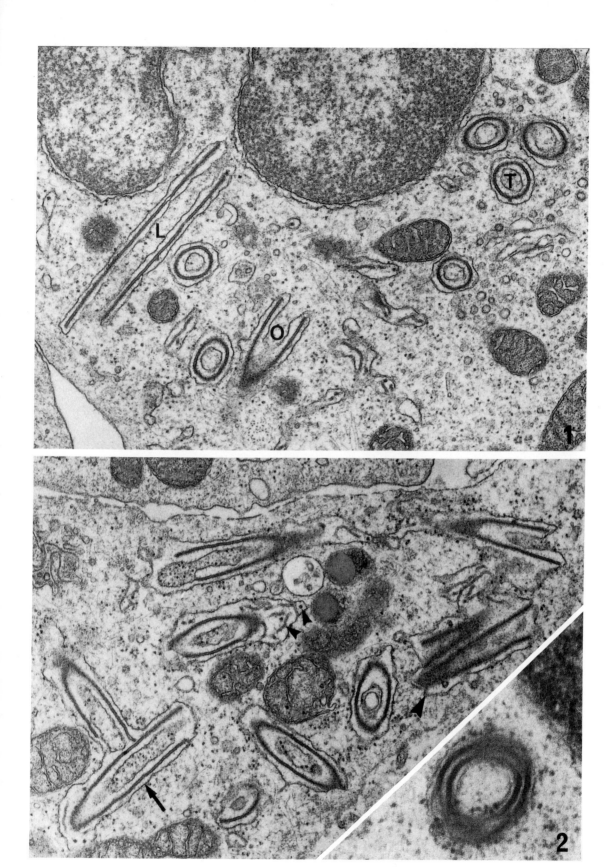

Most tubular confronting cisternae present the simple profiles described above, but there also occur variations worthy of note (*Plates 206, 208* and *209*). For example, one may find: (1) double walled profiles composed of three confronting cisternae with two dense laminae between them instead of the usual two cisternae with a single dense lamina; (2) branched (Y-shaped, T-shaped and cruciate) profiles of tubular confronting cisternae; (3) microtubules or microtubuloreticular structures lying outside the dense lamina or apparently within the hollow of the tubular confronting cisternae; and (4) broken profiles (C-shaped, S-shaped and others) which as we shall see represent sections through immature or developing tubular confronting cisternae.

Regarding the mode of formation of tubular confronting cisternae, I speculated (Ghadially, 1982) that, since short straight profiles and C-shaped profiles of confronting cisternae are seen (besides the various profiles expected from a tubular structure), the first step in the process must be the formation of ribbon-shaped confronting cisternae and that curling and fusion of the edges produces these tubular structures (*Plate 207, Figs. 1–3*). Regarding the mode of formation of these ribbons of confronting cisternae one may surmise that they develop (as do the common confronting cisternae) by close apposition of the cisternae of the rough endoplasmic reticulum and that the electron–dense lamina between them is derived from trapped ribosomes (page 462). The crystalline appearance at times seen here probably results from a crystallization of ribonucleoprotein (derived from disintegrated ribosomes) and perhaps other proteins in this region. However, this hypothesis (curling of a ribbon-shaped structure) based on the study of random sections of tubular confronting cisternae from the hepatocytes of chimpanzees inoculated with plasma or serum from patients with non-A, non-B hepatitis finds little support in our subsequent serial section studies (Ghadially *et al.*, 1987) on these structures in the AIDS lymph node.

Plate 207

Set of schematic diagrams (not to scale) depicting the probable mode of formation of tubular confronting cisternae. (*From Ghadially, Senoo, Fuse and Chan, 1987*)

Fig. 1. Ribbon-shaped confronting cisternae formed by the apposition of two cisternae of the rough endoplasmic reticulum. Note the ribosomes and polyribosomes (arrowheads) on the surface of the cisternae and the dense lamina (arrows) which probably derives from ribosomes trapped between the two cisternae.

Fig. 2. Depicted here is the idea that tubular confronting cisternae may form by simple curling of ribbon-shaped confronting cisternae. A shows a transverse section through ribbon-shaped confronting cisternae (similar to that shown in *Fig. 1*). B and C show how curling and fusion of the edges would produce tubular confronting cisternae as shown in D. A quite separate point is also illustrated in C. Sometimes one sees the profile of a dense lamina lying in a dilated cisterna. This could be due to a rearrangement and fusion of the membranes at the edge or margin of confronting cisternae. In the diagram only one edge (arrow) is 'closed', and other edge (arrowhead) is left 'open' to show that such an event does not always happen. Obviously for the dense lamina to fall into a dilated cisterna both edges would have to suffer membrane rearrangement and fusion.

Fig. 3. A is a three-dimensional model of the event shown in *Fig. 2*. Here we see a ribbon-shaped structure in the process of curling to produce a tubular structure. There is, however, no evidence that this actually happens. What does happen, however, is that the ribbon-shaped structure twists and spirals (B, C, D) to produce a tubular structure (E). Thus, at one stage of its development the immature tubular confronting cisternae has a spiralling slit in its wall. F shows how from an S-shaped ribbon, two tubular confronting cisternae develop.

Figs. 4 and 5. Two immature tubular confronting cisternae with slits in their walls. Sections through such immature tubular confronting cisternae will produce broken profiles as shown in these diagrams.

470

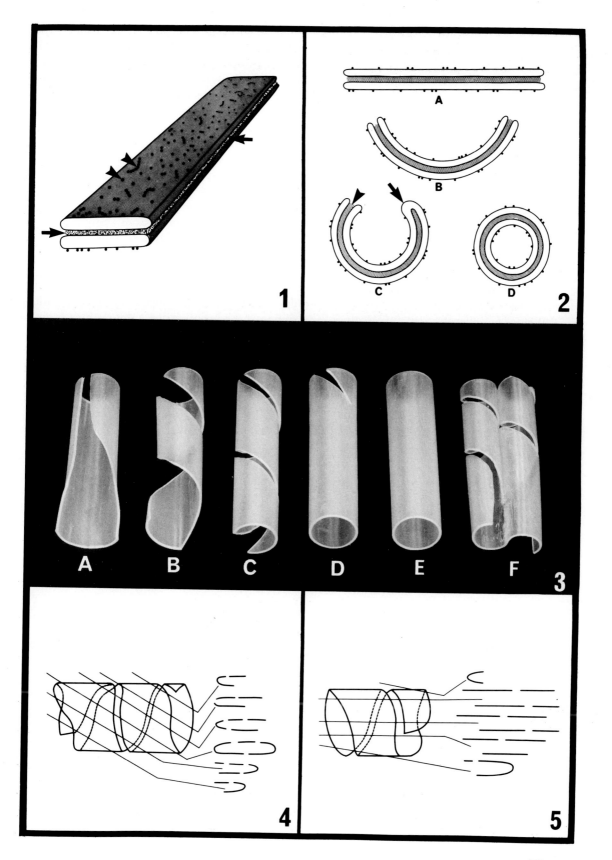

471

Although such a mechanism (i.e. simple curling) may at times be operative, more often than not it is a twisting and spiralling of the ribbon which produces the tubular form (*Plate 207, Fig. 3*). This spiralling was deduced by us from sets of serial sections through some tubular confronting cisternae (which we surmise are immature or developing forms) which show breaks or discontinuities in the various profiles (circular, oval, elliptical, etc.). These breaks or discontinuities when followed in serial sections show that at one stage of development tubular confronting cisternae have a spiralling slit or channel in their wall (*Plates 207 and 208*).

The fact that most tubular confronting cisternae give perfect profiles with no breaks, in serial sections along the entire dimension (length or width) of the structure indicates that fusion of the edges of the spiralling slit occurs and that the fully mature structure is indeed a tube composed of confronting cisternae.

A distinct and different profile (from all the ones described above) we found in our studies (*Plate 208*) was the S-shaped profile of confronting cisternae. Serial sections show that from such S-shaped ribbons ultimately arise two separate tubular confronting cisternae (*Plates 207 and 208*) presumably by a process of splitting of the S-shaped ribbon followed by a spiralling of the two ribbons derived in this fashion.

One may conclude by saying that our serial section study clearly demonstrates that the so-called 'test-tube and ring forms' are profiles derived from sectioned tubular confronting cisternae and that this structure evolves from ribbon-shaped confronting cisternae by a process of twisting and spiralling.

As mentioned earlier, in most instances tubular confronting cisternae present as discrete or solitary structures but sometimes the outer membrane of two adjacent structures is continuous (*Plate 206, Fig. 2*) suggesting that a fusion or budding process may be involved in the production of such profiles. At times the outer cisterna of the confronting cisternae is dilated and contains microtubules (*Plate 206, Fig. 2*) similar to those seen in microtubuloreticular structures (*see* pages 496–509) found in the endoplasmic reticulum.

Plate 208

From a lymph node of a patient with AIDS. Same case as *Plates 206* and *209* (*From Ghadially, Senoo, Fuse and Chan, 1987*)

Figs. 1–8. Serial sections through a lymphoid cell. In the bottom half of the illustrations one can see several immature confronting cisternae which present C-shaped or broken O-shaped profiles. If we follow the break (arrows) in one of these structures, from *Fig. 1* to *Fig. 8*, we find that the break varies in width and rotates through an angle of more than 180 degrees. This indicates that there is a spiralling slit or channel on this as yet not fully formed tubular structure. Note also the breaks (small arrowheads) in the obliquely cut immature confronting cisternae. In the top part of *Figs. 1–3* we see (large arrowheads) S-shaped profiles which turn into two C-shaped and broken O-shaped profiles as we follow this structure in serial sections (*Figs. 4–8*). This shows that two as yet incompletely formed tubular confronting cisternae are developing from an S-shaped ribbon of confronting cisternae. All at ×28 000

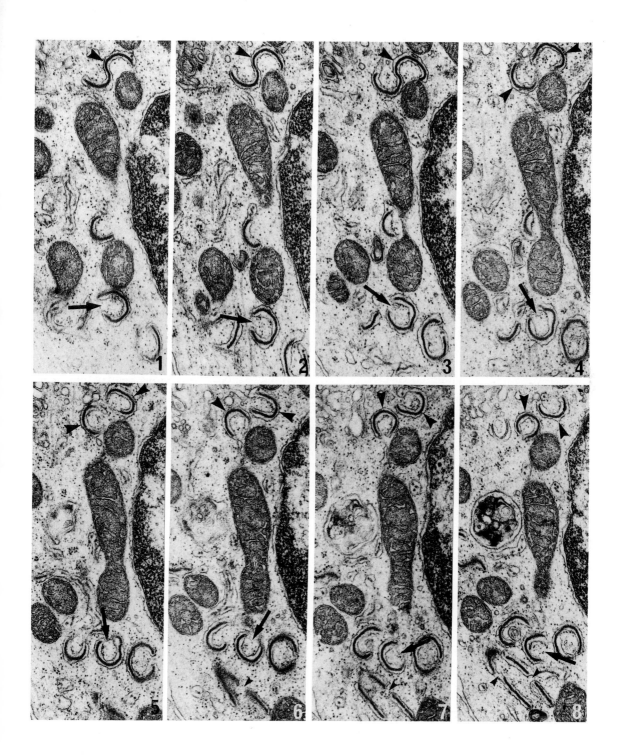

473

Microtubuloreticular structures (unfortunately, often referred to in the literature as 'tubuloreticular structures' or 'TRS') are also at times seen 'within' the tubular confronting cisternae (*Plate 209*). In such instances, no cytoplasmic material is seen within the tubular confronting cisternae and also the innermost ribosome-studded membrane in its interior is absent. One may interpret this as an expansion or dilatation of a microtubuloreticular structure-containing inner cisterna which has displaced cytoplasmic material or one may look upon this as a dilated cisterna produced by a process of membrane fusion (*Plate 207, Fig. 2c*) wherein lie the dense lamina of the confronting cisternae and a microtubuloreticular complex.

Let us now look at the significance and diagnostic value of cylindrical confronting cisternae in AIDS. Sidhu *et al.* (1985) consider them to be a specific ultrastructural marker for AIDS. In the correct clinicopathological setting this might be so, but this structure is not specific or diagnostic of AIDS because it has been seen in other conditions besides AIDS (see above). Further, its value as a diagnostic marker is limited because it is seen only in a minority of cases with AIDS and even fewer cases of persistent generalized lymphadenopathy. If we add up the data provided in papers by Ewing *et al.* (1983a), Anderson *et al.* (1984), Rozman and Feliu (1983), Onerheim *et al.* (1984) and Rácz *et al.* (1986) we find that only about 27 per cent of cases of AIDS and 14 per cent of cases with persistent generalized lymphadenopathy show tubular confronting cisternae in lymph nodes and/or peripheral blood. Orenstein *et al.* (1985) screened lymphocytes in the buffy coat of subjects at risk for AIDS. They found that 44 per cent of the cases were positive for microtubuloreticular structures and 20 per cent were positive for tubular confronting cisternae. They state that tubular confronting cisternae were never found in the absence of microtubuloreticular structures. According to these authors, follow-up of these cases suggests that the presence of these structures in 'peripheral blood lymphocytes may identify those pre–AIDS patients who will subsequently develop AIDS'. Similar views on the prognostic value of tubular confronting cisternae have been expressed by Anderson *et al.* (1984) and Sidhu (1983).

Plate 209

Fig. 1. Seen here are profiles of several tubular confronting cisternae. Microtubules (arrowheads) similar to those found in microtubuloreticular structures are seen within and outside the profiles of dense lamina. Also seen is a dilated cisterna containing microtubules (thin arrows) and linear profiles (thick arrows) of a longitudinally sectioned tubular dense lamina. ×42 000 (*From Ghadially, Senoo, Fuse and Chan, 1987*)

Fig. 2. This cell contains two microtubuloreticular structures lying in dilated endoplasmic reticulum (arrows) and longitudinally and transversely sectioned tubular confronting cisternae with broken profiles (breaks indicated by arrowheads). ×42 000 (*From Ghadially, Senoo, Fuse and Chan, 1987*)

474

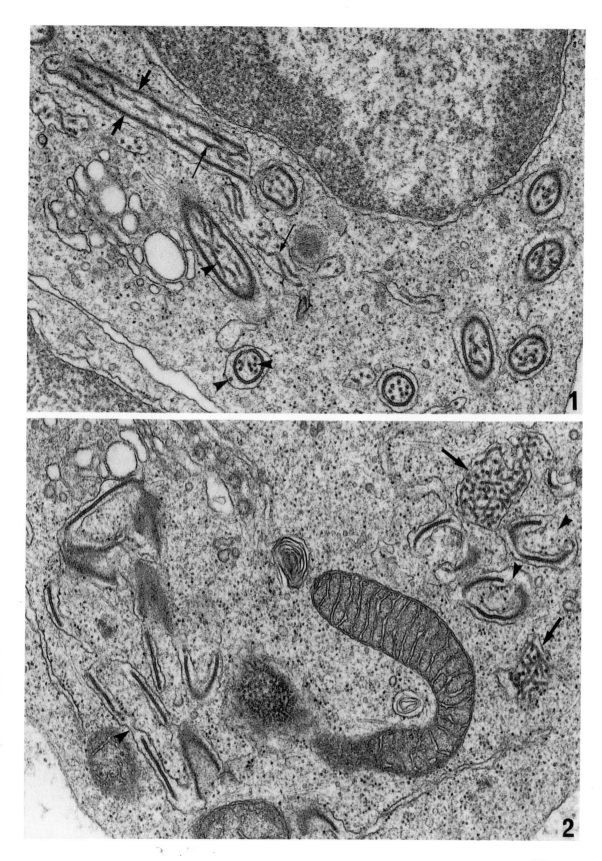

475

Confronting cisternae complex

The term 'confronting cisternae complex' was coined by us (Nimmo Wilkie and Ghadially, 1987) to describe structures or bodies composed of aggregates of confronting cisternae deployed in various ways (i.e. in parallel, random or rosette-like arrangements). These confronting cisternae complexes (*Plate 210*) were found by us in the Purkinje cells of the cerebellum of a dog that was clinically diagnosed as suffering from an 'inflammatory reticulosis' and who had been treated with prednisone, dexamethasone and chloramphenicol. At autopsy, the brain and spinal cord appeared normal. Histologically, the only abnormality was the presence of large (about 5–9 µm) eosinophilic inclusions in the Purkinje cells of the cerebellum. Ultrastructural studies were executed on cerebellar tissue retrieved from buffered formalin.

Confronting cisternae have on several occasions been seen in neurons. Thus, for example, the so-called 'spine apparatus' (Gray, 1959) in the spines on the dendrites of neurons are composed of three or four short cisternae with some dense material between them. In current terms, the spine apparatus would be classified as a stack of small confronting cisternae. Somewhat larger, more numerous stacks of confronting cisternae are at times seen in the cytoplasm of large neurons, like the Purkinje cells of the cerebellum. Herndon (1964) called them 'lamellar bodies' and he and others (e.g. Morales and Duncan, 1966) have argued that to some extent they are fixation artefacts.

Terms such as 'lamellar bodies' and 'spindle lamellae' have in the past been used to describe structures we now call 'confronting cisternae'. The non-specific term 'lamellar bodies' has also been used to describe several other structures such as: (1) myelin figures which are often an artefact of glutaraldehyde fixation (page 616); (2) lysosomes containing stacked or whorled myelinoid membranes (these are best referred to as myelinosomes. *See* pages 614–626); (3) secretory granules of type II pneumocytes (page 618); and (4) concentric whorls of rough and smooth endoplasmic reticulum such as those shown in *Plates 230* and *231*. Hence the term 'lamellar body' is best avoided and the structures in the Purkinje neurons should be referred to as stacks of confronting cisternae, while large inclusions (like the ones shown in *Plate 210*) composed of aggregates of stacks of confronting cisternae are best referred to as confronting cisternae complexes.

Cameron and Conroy (1974) found eosinophilic inclusion bodies (3–9 µm in diameter) in the Purkinje cells of the dog with neoplastic reticulosis of the central nervous system. The electron micrographs presented in this paper are derived from very poorly preserved formalin fixed tissue but even so one can see that these inclusions contain some stacks of confronting cisternae. It is possible that the inclusions we describe here are similar to those described by Cameron and Conroy (1974), but about this one cannot be certain..

It is difficult to believe that so refined and complex a structure like the confronting cisternae complex (*Plate 210*) is a fixation or postmortem artefact, although such factors may have modified its appearance. The aetiogenic agent or agents responsible for the production of confronting cisternae complexes and their mode of formation are obscure.

Plate 210

From formaldehyde-fixed cerebellar tissue obtained at autopsy on a dog. Illustrations show inclusion bodies found in Purkinji cells (*From Nimmo Wilkie and Ghadially, 1987*).

Fig. 1. Seen here are stacks of small confronting cisternae (between arrowheads) called 'lamellar bodies' by some workers and two profiles of confronting cisternae complexes which extend diagonally across the electron micrograph. These complexes contain almond-shaped cisternal profiles (arrows) set in a granular electron-dense matrix. ×60 000

Fig. 2. A confronting cisternae complex composed of aggregates of confronting cisternae (arrows) and multiple focal deposits of electron-dense material (arrowheads). ×24 000

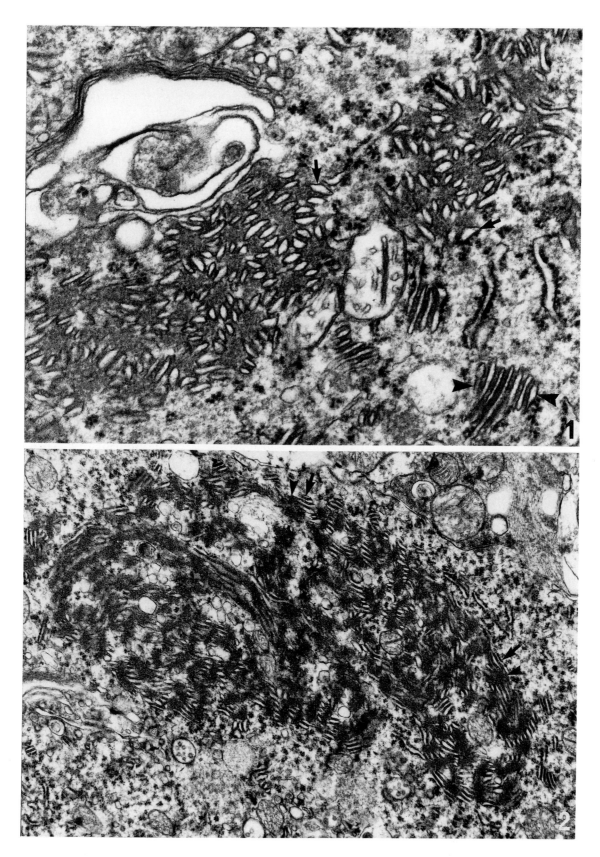

Tubule group: rough and smooth tubular aggregates and intracisternal tubules
(with a note on tubule group, microtubule group and membrane group)

For some time now a complex group or groups of structures derived from the endoplasmic reticulum, lying in the endoplasmic reticulum, in association with or in continuity with the endoplasmic reticulum, or lying free or apparently free in the cytoplasmic matrix have been the subject of much study, debate and nomenclatural chaos.

Since the publication of the second edition of this book (Ghadially, 1985), many more of these structures have been described and it seems to me that three groups of structures can now be identified: (1) the tubule group comprising structures composed principally of rough or smooth tubules; (2) the microtubule group comprising structures composed of various types of microtubules deployed in various different ways; and (3) the membrane group comprising structures composed of membranes (usually sheets or lamellae composed of paired membranes) deployed in various ways.

A major source of nomenclatural error and chaos stems from the haphazard use of the terms 'tubules' and 'microtubules'*. The classic tubulin microtubules have a diameter of about 22–27 nm so in the second edition of this book I proposed that hollow cylindrical structures of about this size or smaller should be called 'microtubules'; while structures of greater diameter should be called 'tubules'. A look at various such structures suggests that a convenient dividing point would be about 30 nm. Hence, hollow cylindrical structures under 30 nm are referred to in this book as 'microtubules', while structures above this size are called 'tubules'.

Let us now look at the tubule group which as its name implies contains members characterized by the presence of tubules (i.e. diameter greater than 30 nm). The members of this group include: (1) rough tubular aggregates; (2) smooth tubular aggregates; and (3) intracisternal tubules.

Various terms have been employed to describe members of the tubule group. These include, 'unusual aggregation of tubules', 'unusual lamellar bodies', 'tubuloampullary structures', 'glomiform inclusion', 'aggregates of cylindrical tubules', 'hexagonally packed tubules', 'tubule complex', 'intracytoplasmic lamellar bodies', 'crystalloid endoplasmic reticulum', 'aggregates of tubules', 'honeycomb structures' and 'parallel tubular arrays'†.

Most of these terms are good enough to describe a given structure but not good enough for general application because often the same term has been used to describe quite different structures. Therefore, I have coined the terms 'rough tubular aggregates' and 'smooth tubular

---

*I too was guilty of this in the first edition of this book. It is strongly recommended that at this stage the reader should consult page 938 where the differences between tubules and various microtubules (including the microtubules composed of tubulin) are fully explained.
†Structures such as those shown in *Plates 211* and *212* could quite correctly be called 'parallel tubular arrays' but this term must be strictly avoided because it has been widely used (to be accurate, misused!) to describe the parallel microtubular arrays found in natural killer lymphocytes (pages 492–495).

Plate 211

From an undiagnosed tumour.
Fig. 1. A rough tubular aggregate composed of parallel striated tubules. Ribosomes (arrowheads) may be just discerned between the tubules. ×59 000
Fig. 2. Some of the rough tubules follow a parallel course, others a curved course. Circular profiles (long arrows) derived from transverse sections through the tubules are also present. Note the ampullary dilatations (short arrows) and the rows of ribosomes (between arrowheads) between the tubules. ×64 000

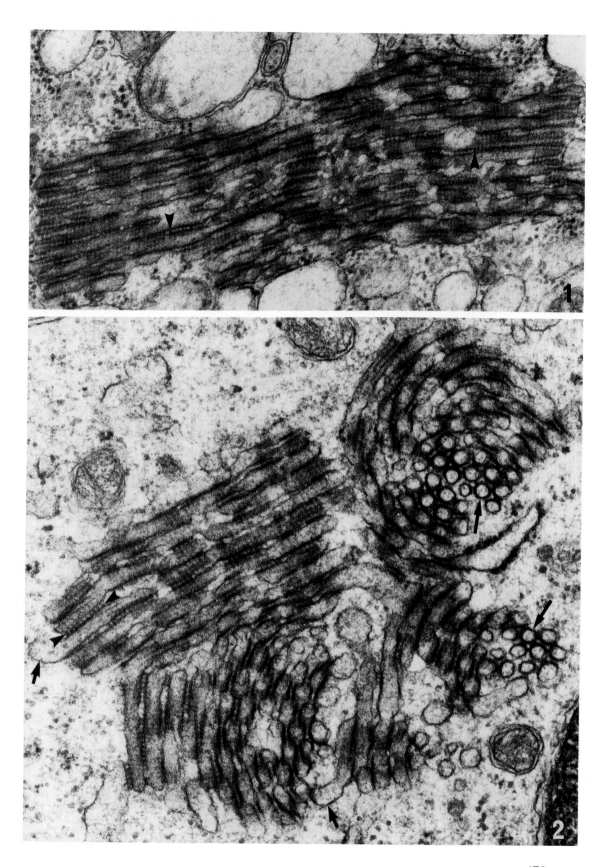

aggregates' which are adequate for describing most of these structures. In only a small minority of the reports, neither the description nor the illustrations permit one to make this distinction confidently.

A rough tubular aggregate may be defined as a structure composed of a group of ribosome-studded tubules lying in the cytoplasmic matrix. The tubules are called 'rough' because like the rough endoplasmic reticulum the surface of the tubules is studded with ribosomes. Indeed, continuity between the two can at times be demonstrated. The tubules of most of these aggregates found in human cells (neoplastic) show a striated appearance but those in the cells of other animals do not. Hence, the former are best (or more fully) referred to as 'striated rough tubular aggregates'. The striated appearance of the tubules may be explained by assuming that rings of ribosomes (like pearl bracelets) encircle the tubules. This is supported by the observation that in sectioned material the ribosomes lying on or between the tubules are in register with the dense bands creating the striated appearance. Ampullary dilatations of the tubules are also often seen. Most rough tubular aggregates are composed of bundles of parallel tubules. The bundles may all run in one direction or they may run at various angles up to about 90 degrees to each other. Some of the bundles may follow a curvilinear course (*Plate 211*).

Rough tubular aggregates (non-striated) have been seen in: (1) chief cells of the gastric mucosa of hibernating bats (*Myotis lucifugus lucifugus*) (Ito and Winchester, 1963); (2) cells of the digestive gland of a herbivore sacoglossan gastropod (*Alderia modesta*) (McLean, 1978); and (3) neurons of the hibernating dormouse (*Eliomys quercinus L.*) (Machín-Santamaría, 1978).

Striated rough tubular aggregates have been seen in neoplastic cells of: (1) a malignant stromal tumour (diameter of tubules, 85 nm) (Tokue *et al.*, 1985); (2) an acinar cell carcinoma (Bockus *et al.*, 1985); (3) solid and cystic acinar cell tumours of the pancreas★ (Arai *et al.*, 1986); (4) a neuroendocrine carcinoma of pancreas (producing gastrin and serotonin) and a neuroendocrine carcinoma of colon (producing VIP) (Payne, personal communication†); (5) an undiagnosed tumour thought to be either a malignant haemangiopericytoma or a neuroendocrine carcinoma (no neuroendocrine granules were detected by electron microscopy) (*Plate 211*); and (6) a phaeochromocytoma (Ghadially, unpublished observation).

In all the above-mentioned instances the rough tubular aggregates were composed largely of parallel tubules, but there is a report (Hruban *et al.*, 1976) where lupus-type microtubuloreticular structures are considered together with a structure which they call 'glomiform inclusion' (their Fig. 9) which seems to be composed of a bundle of rough tubules forming a knot or glomiform structure. It would appear that these inclusions are but a variation of the rough tubule aggregate which one may call a 'glomiform rough tubular aggregate'.

The significance of rough tubular aggregates is not known but since they have been seen in hibernating bats and dormice (but not in active animals) it has been suggested that they may represent a response of the rough endoplasmic reticulum to low environmental temperature

---

★The illustrations in the paper by Arai *et al.* (1986) show an indubitable rough tubule aggregate and another which could be a transected rough tubule aggregate or a smooth tubule aggregate. However, the authors think they are annulate lamellae. The solid and cystic acinar cell tumour of the pancreas occurs in young women as an abdominal mass causing little discomfort. The prognosis is excellent despite histological appearances suggesting malignancy. In some of these tumours neuroendocrine granules have been detected.
†Dr Payne has also sent me an electron micrograph which shows that the 'granules' seen on the rough tubules are uranaffin positive. This supports the idea that these structures are indeed ribosomes (*see page 368*).

Plate 212
From a giant cell carcinoma of the thyroid (*From Carstens, 1984*)
Fig. 1. A neoplastic cell showing a smooth tubular aggregate where most of the tubules are cut longitudinally. The continuity between the lumina (arrowhead) of some tubules and dilated rough endoplasmic reticulum (arrow) is clearly seen. ×53 000
Fig. 2. In this smooth tubular aggregate profiles of longitudinally cut (L) and transversely (T) cut tubules are evident. The latter show a honeycomb pattern. ×60 000

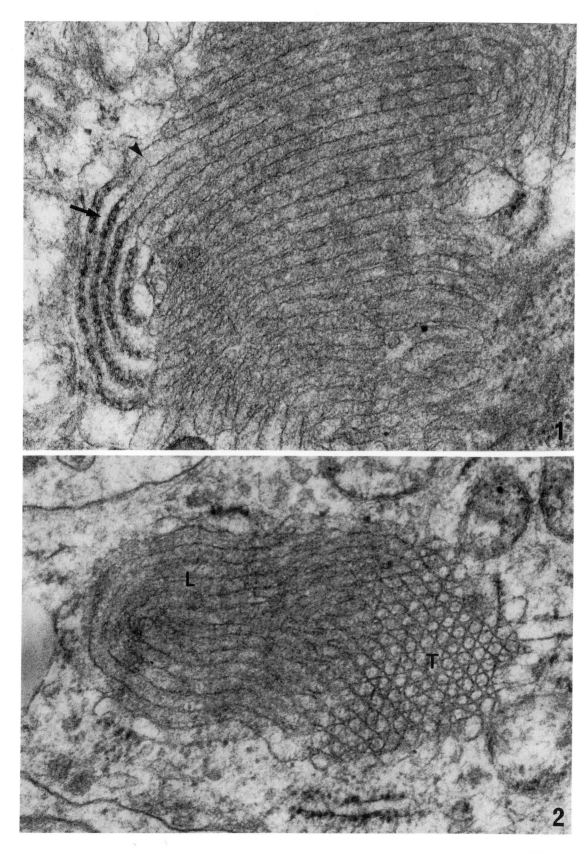

associated with hibernation. In humans, one may speculate that the rough tubular aggregate represents an abnormal proliferation of the rough endoplasmic reticulum engendered by the neoplastic state.

The second member of the group, namely the smooth tubular aggregate is composed of bundles of parallel tubules lying in the cytoplasmic matrix. The bundles may run in one direction or they may run at various angles (up to 90 degrees) to each other. Some bundles follow a curvilinear course. The tubules of the aggregate are at times seen to be continuous with the rough endoplasmic reticulum. Transverse sections through the parallel tubules present a honeycomb-like appearance.

Smooth tubular aggregates have been found in: (1) neurons in cerebellum of cats (Morales and Duncan, 1966); (2) compactin-resistent UT-1 cells (a cell line derived from Chinese hamster ovary) grown in a medium containing compactin (this includes the formation of smooth tubular aggregates (diameter of tubules, 83 nm) and undulating membranous formations) (Pathak *et al.*, 1986); (3) diseased cardiac and skeletal muscle cells (some aggregates presumably derive from cell membrane or its extension, the T-tubules, others perhaps from smooth endoplasmic reticulum), (for references *see* Maron and Ferrans, 1974 and Papadimitriou and Mastaglia, 1982); (4) cells of human corpus luteum (Crisp *et al.*, 1970); (5) neoplastic cells of colonic carcinoma (difficult to say whether they are rough or smooth tubules) (Toner, 1984); (6) pancreatic beta cells of rats and in a human malignant insulinoma (some ribosomes present on peripheral tubules of the aggregates) (Graf and Heitz, 1980); (7) neoplastic cells of granular cell tumour and giant cell tumour of thyroid(Carstens, 1984) (*Plate 212*); (8) neoplastic cells of osteosarcoma and other sarcomas (Alexander, 1984); (9) neoplastic cells of endometrial carcinoma (Gompel, 1971); (10) cloned Friend erythroleukaemia cells (Tandler, 1984); and (11) hepatocytes of a hamster after intrapleural injection of asbestos fibres (the tubules have an inner coat and a central filamentous core) (Sobel *et al.*, 1983).

The list is by no means complete for small aggregates of smooth tubules (half a dozen or so) are occasionally seen in a variety of tumours and other tissues (personal experience). The function of smooth tubular aggregates is not known, but one may speculate that they could be an indicator of hypertrophy or an aberrant reaction of the endoplasmic reticulum to neoplasia and other pathological states.

The third member of the tubule group (i.e. the intracisternal tubules) presents as solitary tubules or aggregates of tubules lying in dilated cisternae of the rough endoplasmic reticulum and its continuation, the perinuclear cistern.

Plate 213

Circulating leukaemic cells from a case of chronic lymphocytic leukaemia (*From Kostianovsky and Ghadially, 1987*)

Fig. 1. Groups of longitudinally cut and obliquely cut, single-walled tubules (diameters range from about 76–87 nm) are seen lying in dilated rough endoplasmic reticulum and dilated perinuclear cisterna. The contents of the tubules are largely lucent and flocculent, but there are also focal deposits of electron-dense material (arrows). Glycogen particles are rarely seen in leukaemic cells but this cell (and others in this and the next plate) contains quite prominent glycogen particles (arrowheads). ×65 000

Fig. 2. Groups of transversely cut single-walled tubules (arrowheads) measuring about 70–76 nm in diameter are seen lying in the dilated cisternae of rough endoplasmic reticulum. Also present are a couple of double-walled tubules (short arrows). Electron-dense material is present in some of the tubules (long arrows). ×72 000

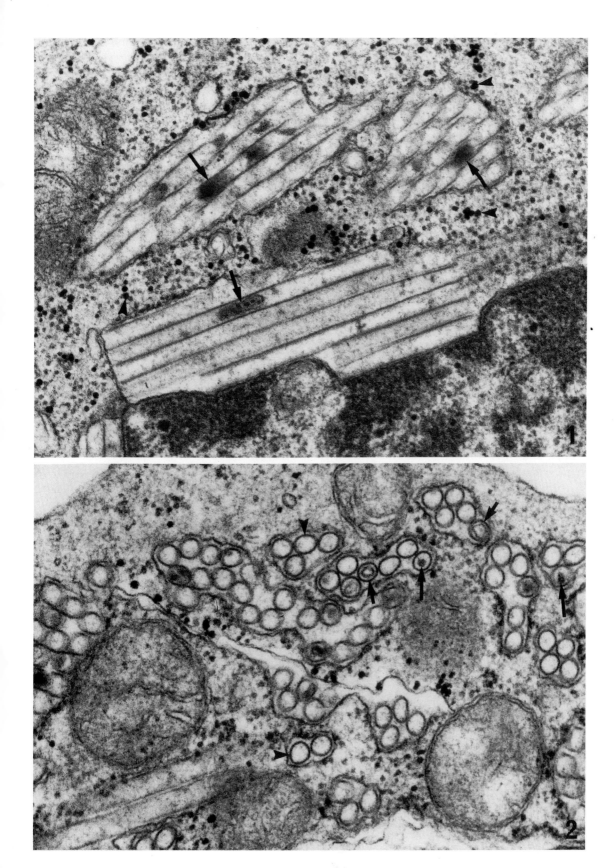

483

Intracisternal tubules have been seen in: (1) leukaemic cells from a case of 'pure' monocytic leukaemia ('true' histiocytic lymphoma) (Begin et al., 1981); (2) a canine ectopic thyroid adenoma (Cheville, 1972); and (3) leukaemic cells from a case of chronic lymphocytic leukaemia (Kostianovsky and Ghadially, 1987) (*Plates 213* and *214*).

In the monocytic leukaemic cells (item 1), solitary double-walled rough tubules (i.e. ribosome-studded walls) were found in dilated rough endoplastic reticulum. The evidence presented by Begin *et al.* (1981) indicates that these intracisternal tubules arise from the membranes of the rough endoplasmic reticulum.

In the canine ectopic thyroid adenoma (item 2) intracisternal smooth-walled tubules were found. The tubules were neither so numerous nor so 'rigid-looking' as the ones found by us (Kostianovsky and Ghadially, 1987) in the cells of chronic lymphocytic leukaemia (*Plates 213* and *214*). Only one illustration is presented by Cheville (1972) which shows groups of two or three tubules lying in dilated rough endoplasmic reticulum. No comment is made about the significance or mode of formation of these inclusions.

In the case we studied (item 3) only a few (<5 per cent) of the leukaemic lymphocytes contained inclusions. These inclusions presented as solitary tubules or aggregates of parallel tubules cut in various planes (*Plates 213* and *214*). They lay within dilated cisternae of the rough endoplasmic reticulum and perinuclear cistern. Some of the tubules were bounded by a single wall, while others were bounded by two walls. We also found a tubule bounded by three walls and another where a segment of the tubular profile was triple-walled and the remainder double-walled. The overall or external diameters of all tubules ranged from about 70–90 nm, except one, which measured about 100 nm in diameter.

Like cytomembranes, the single wall of the single-walled tubules and each wall of the multiple-walled tubules were osmiophilic in unstained sections. Further, their thickness (about 5.5–6.2 nm) was also similar to that of cytomembranes. Therefore, we are inclined to think that the walls of these tubules are composed of membranes. However, the expected trilaminar structure of cytomembranes was demonstrable neither in the walls of the tubules, nor in various cytomembranes such as the membranes of mitochondria and rough endoplasmic reticulum. As is well known the trilaminar structure of cytomembranes is not always demonstrable in routine preparations (*see* page 1046). Therefore, this does not rule out the idea that the walls of the tubules are composed of membranes. The contents of most tubules were largely lucent and flocculent. However, at times focal deposits of electron-dense material were also present in the tubules.

The mode of genesis and significance of intracisternal tubules is obscure. The idea that they represent some secretory product is not too attractive, particularly for item 2 where the tubules are studded with ribosomes, and at times appear to be continuous with and hence no doubt derived from the rough endoplasmic reticulum. One may therefore speculate that the smooth intracisternal tubules also probably arise by elongation of invaginations of the endoplasmic reticulum.

Plate 214

Circulating leukaemic cells from a case of chronic lymphocytic leukaemia. Same case as *Plate 213* (*From Kostianovsky and Ghadially, 1987*)

Fig. 1. Longitudinally cut and obliquely cut, solitary tubules and groups of tubules are seen lying in dilated cisternae of rough endoplasmic reticulum. These are double-walled tubules. Arrowheads indicate places where the double-wall is well demonstrated. ×78 000

Fig. 2. In the dilated perinuclear cisterna lie transversely cut single-walled tubules (S), double-walled tubules (D), and a tubule (T) where a part of the tubular profile is triple-walled and the remainder double-walled. This tubule has an external diameter of about 100 nm. ×100 000

Fig. 3. Nineteen double-walled tubules are seen in a dilated perinuclear cisterna (internal diameter about 57 nm, external diameter about 85 nm, thickness of double wall about 14 nm). The poorly defined structure indicated by an arrow is interpreted as a solitary triple-walled tubule lying in dilated rough endoplasmic reticulum. ×141 000

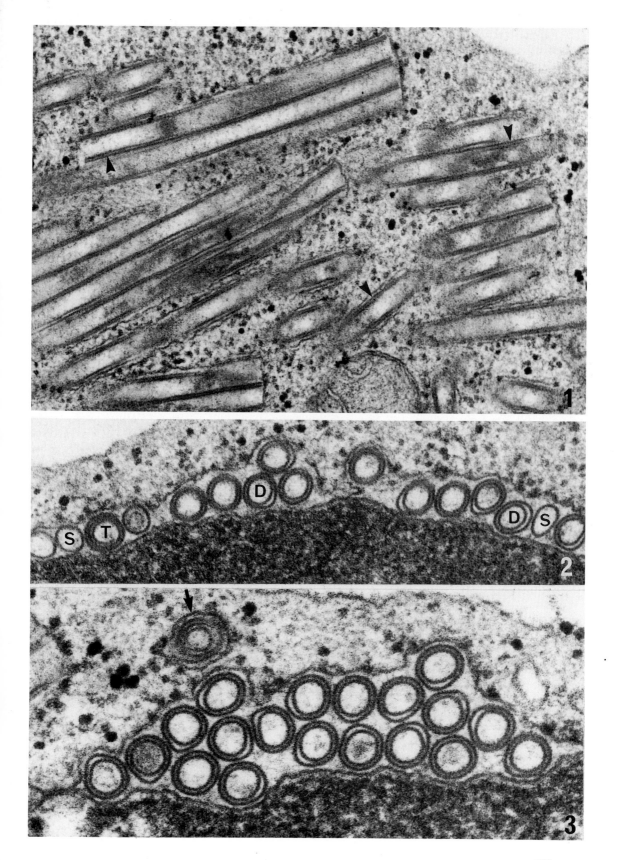

485

Microtubule group: ordered arrays of straight microtubules and randomly oriented microtubules in rough endoplasmic reticulum
(with a note on classification and nomenclature of members of microtubule group)

The term 'microtubule group' embraces a variety of structures composed mainly or entirely of a collection of microtubules* (12–30 nm in diameter). Members of this group may lie within the rough endoplasmic reticulum, in association with the rough endoplasmic reticulum or in the cell cytoplasm and rarely even in the nucleus. One member of this group (parallel microtubular arrays) lies in a vacuole, but it is not clear as to whether the membrane of the vacuole is derived from the endoplasmic reticulum or not. The members of this group display different microtubular patterns which permit us to distinguish between them. Each member of the group may be further characterized by noting where it has been most frequently or characteristically seen, so as to provide in each instance a standard or model against which others can be compared.

The members of the microtubule group are: (1) parallel arrays of straight or rod-like microtubules in the rough endoplasmic reticulum forming a crystalloid or crystalline structure (melanoma-type inclusion); (2) randomly oriented not so straight or curved microtubules in the rough endoplasmic reticulum (myxoid chondrosarcoma-type inclusion); (3) parallel microtubular arrays (natural killer lymphocyte-type inclusion). This inclusion is commonly referred to as 'parallel tubular arrays' (pages 492–495); (4) microtubuloreticular structures (lupus-type inclusion, chimpanzee hepatitis-type inclusion and others). These inclusions are commonly called 'tubuloreticular structures' (pages 496–509); (5) fuzzy or coated microtubular structures (viral infection-type inclusion) (pages 946–949).

In this section of the text we deal with items 1 and 2. In both types of inclusions, the microtubules are seen in the rough endoplasmic reticulum. In one instance (item 1) the microtubules are straight and rod-like and in transverse section a well-ordered crystalline structure is evident (*Plate 215*). The microtubules in the second group (item 2) do not show such a highly ordered arrangement (*Plates 216* and *217*). Bundles of short straight microtubules or a few or many slightly curved or irregularly wavy microtubules appear scattered in dilated rough endoplasmic reticulum. When the microtubules are relatively straight a pattern of striation can at times be discerned in both types of inclusions.

The microtubules (in items 1 and 2) are at times set in a medium density material filling the dilated rough endoplasmic reticulum. In other instances they are set in a light matrix and the microtubules appear to be covered by a fuzzy medium density coat. Such differences probably

---

*For reasons given on page 478, all hollow, cylindrical structures under 30 nm in diameter are referred to in this book as 'microtubules'; while structures above this size are called 'tubules'. It is important to realize that not all microtubules are composed of tubulin, and that a variety of microtubules exist (page 938). The distinction between the tubule group, microtubule group and membrane group is also explained on page 478.

Plate 215

Tumour cells from a metastatic melanoma (*From a block of tissue supplied by Dr B. Mackay*)

Fig. 1. Longitudinally cut straight, parallel microtubules are seen in some cisternae (arrows), while highly ordered (crystalline) circular profiles of transversely cut microtubules are seen in others (arrowheads). ×24 000

Fig. 2. Higher-power view of longitudinally (arrowhead) and transversely (arrow) cut microtubules in the rough endoplasmic reticulum. The former bear faint striations which may or may not be visible in the reproduction. ×60 000

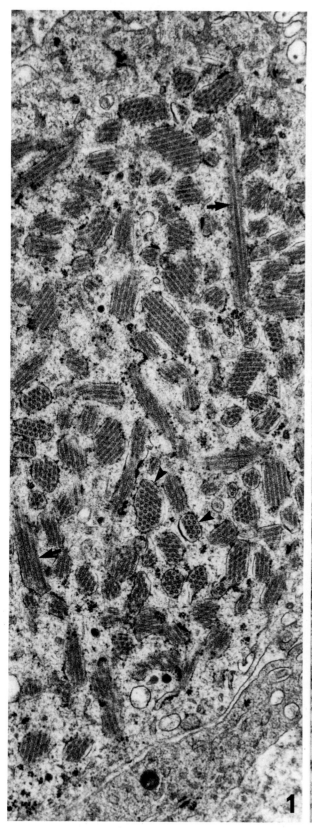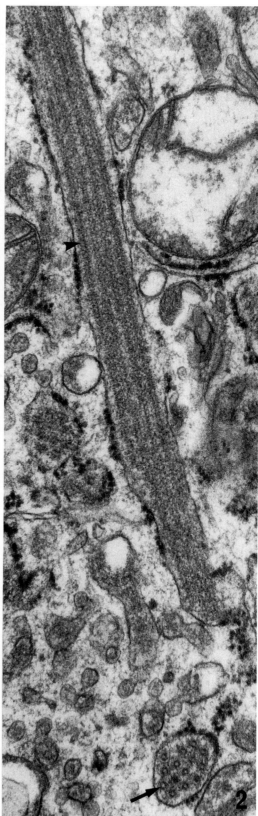

reflect the loss of variable amounts of proteinaceous material from the endoplasmic reticulum during tissue preparation. The presence of such material complicates accurate measurement of the diameter of these microtubules, but it seems to range from about 12–25 nm.

Straight rod-like microtubules in parallel arrays or crystalline formation have been seen in the rough endoplasmic reticulum of the cells of: (1) an adrenal cortical adenoma (Macadam, 1970); (2) a Mullerian adenosarcoma of the uterus (Damjanov et al., 1978); (3) metastatic malignant melanoma of man (Mackay and Ayala, 1980; Mazur and Katzenstein, 1980; Tillman, 1981); (4) an osteosarcoma (Marquart, 1981); (5) non-pigmented epithelial cells of the ciliary body of the Rhesus monkey (Martins-Green and Roth, 1982); (6) plasma cells in a renal biopsy from a patient with glomerulonephritis (Duyvené De Wit, 1986).

Randomly oriented, short and straight, or slightly wavy or curved microtubules, have been seen in the rough endoplasmic reticulum of the cells of: (1) myxoid chondrosarcoma (Dardick et al., 1983; Hinrichs et al., 1985; Wetzel and Reuhl, 1980; DeBlois et al., 1986) (Plate 216); (2) atypical benign fibrous histiocytoma (Battifora, 1983); (3) cartilage from a case of Morquio's syndrome (Sengel et al., 1971); (4) ochronotic articular cartilage (Plate 217); (5) pars intermedia of toad (Bufo paracnemis L) hypophysis (Valeri et al., 1971); (6) hepatocytes in the hyperplastic nodules or benign hepatomas of ageing mice (Hruban, 1979); and (7) hepatocytes of cirrhotic human liver containing a hepatocellular carcinoma (Ma and Blackburn, 1973).

By far the largest number of sightings of highly ordered (i.e. crystalline) parallel arrays of straight microtubules have been in cases of metastatic melanoma. These structures have been seen in secondary tumour deposits where melanosomes were present and also in tumours where no melanosomes were detectable. It is in the latter instance that (in the correct histopathological setting) these microtubules become of diagnostic value, for they suggest (but do not prove) the diagnosis of melanoma (for details, see Ghadially, 1985).

Plate 216
Myxoid chondrosarcoma (*From a block of tissue supplied by Dr B. Mackay*)
Fig. 1. The dilated cisternae of the rough endoplasmic reticulum are packed with microtubules. ×22 000
Fig. 2. Higher magnification showing microtubules which are randomly scattered in dilated cisternae of the rough endoplasmic reticulum. ×52 000

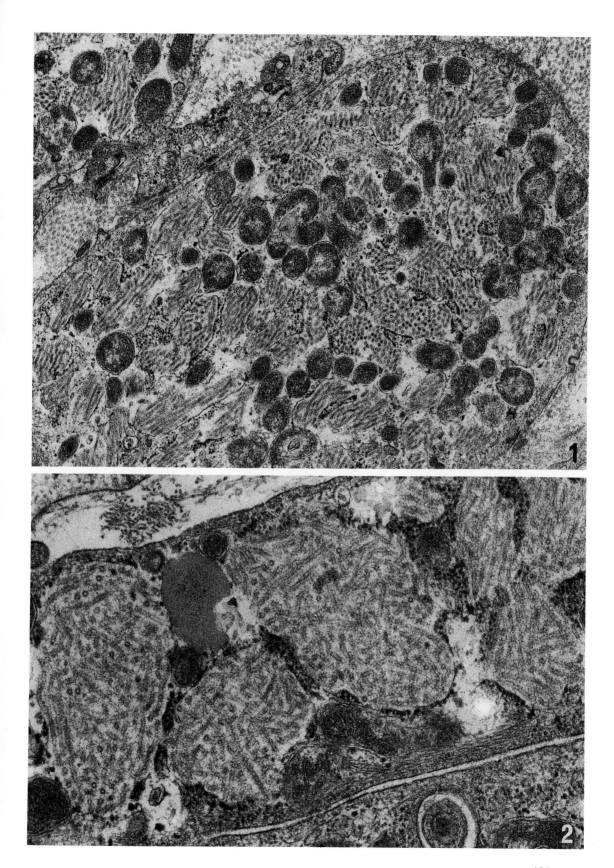

489

The chemical composition of these microtubules found in the rough endoplasmic reticulum is not known. Some of the reported diameters of the microtubules seem to be a bit too small (12 nm) for these to be the conventional tubulin microtubules (24 nm) yet this may be because it is difficult to see the walls (because of the proteinaceous coat) of these microtubules and measure them accurately. In a certain plane of sectioning, the microtubules in the rough endoplasmic reticulum show a striated appearance, so at times do the tubulin microtubules in flagella, but only when the microtubules run in a perfectly straight course. Thus, it is possible that the microtubules in the rough endoplasmic reticulum are the common microtubules composed of tubulin, but how they come to lie in the rough endoplasmic reticulum would need explaining, because normally tubulin is synthesized by polyribosomes lying free in the cytoplasm and not by those lying on the membranes of the rough endoplasmic reticulum.

Since these microtubules occur in the rough endoplasmic reticulum, virtually all authors have speculated that they comprise a secretory product which is presumably proteinaceous in nature. For example, microtubules were found in the rough endoplasmic reticulum most frequently in toads exposed to intense illumination and were rarely seen in animals kept in darkness. Therefore Valeri et al. (1971) suggest that these microtubules 'are secretory material'. In the case of the intracisternal microtubules in metastatic melanoma Mackay and Ayalla (1980) suggest that this might represent 'a distorted form of elaboration of the premelanosomal protein'. In the case of the intracisternal microtubules in plasma cells, one may point out that some cryoglobulin precipitates produced in vitro are composed of microtubules (Stoebner et al., 1979; Stoebner, 1986) so most likely the microtubules in the rough endoplasmic reticulum of plasma cells are derived from cryoglobulins. It seems to me that while some proteins in the rough endoplasmic reticulum precipitate as dense granules, filaments or crystals, others precipitate out as microtubules. Thus, it would appear that the straight and not so straight or well ordered microtubules in the rough endoplasmic reticulum seen in various sites and situations are a chemically heterogeneous group whose precise composition awaits elucidation by future studies. One thing, however, is certain; these rod-like microtubules are quite distinct and different from the undulating or reticulated microtubules (i.e. lupus type inclusions) and also the parallel microtubular arrays (natural killer lymphocyte inclusion). The frequent lumping together of all these structures as some authors do is quite unwarranted and confusing. The only thing they have in common is that they are all members of the microtubule group.

Plate 217

Chondrocytes from ochronotic articular cartilage.

Fig. 1. The dilated cisternae of the rough endoplasmic reticulum contain microtubules that are often not too well visualized because of their random orientation to the plane of sectioning. Profiles of transversely cut microtubules lying in dilated cisternae (arrows) are, however, well visualized. They lack the highly ordered crystalline arrangement of microtubules seen in the melanoma-type inclusion (*Plate 215*). ×50 000

Fig. 2. The microtubules lying in the rough endoplasmic reticulum are quite straight and hence they show a striated appearance. ×71 000

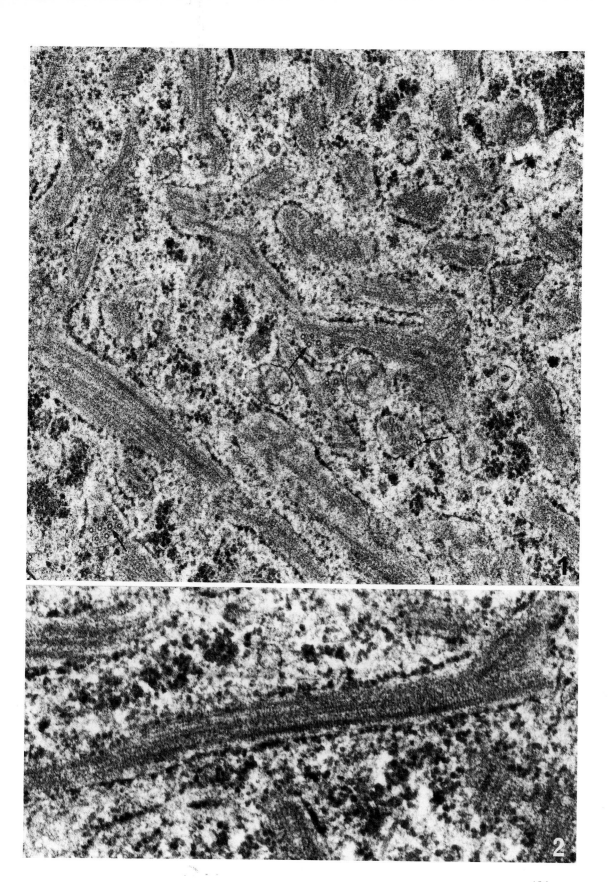

491

Microtubule group: parallel microtubular arrays

The structures or inclusions described here as 'parallel microtubular arrays'* are commonly referred to as 'parallel tubular arrays' (*Plates 218* and *219*). Curiously enough, even those who call these structures 'parallel tubular arrays' realize or suspect that these single-membrane-bound structures contain microtubules and not tubules, for when describing the morphology of these structures they speak about 'structures resembling microtubules' (White, 1972), 'microtubule-like structures comprising the inclusions' (Brunning and Parkin, 1975b), and 'typical microtubule-like structure' (Payne and Tennican, 1982).

Parallel microtubular arrays usually present as electron-dense inclusions in the cytoplasm of certain lymphocytes (*see below*). These round, oval or elongated, single-membrane-bound inclusions range in size from about 100 to 600 nm, but much larger inclusions (1–5 μm) of this type are at times seen. Basically, this inclusion is composed of bundles of parallel rather thick-walled microtubules (diameter of about 15–30 nm or more†) set in a sparse or abundant electron-dense matrix. In some profiles the bundles of microtubules run in one direction only, in others the bundles are oriented in various directions often at almost 90 degrees to each other. Yet other profiles show that some bundles of parallel microtubules follow a curvilinear course.

These parallel arrays of microtubules set in an electron-dense matrix usually lie in a single-membrane-bound vacuole, but at times they truly or apparently lie free in the cytoplasm. The membrane of the vacuole may be close-fitting and hence, at times, is difficult to visualize. On the other hand, at times complexes of microtubules and dense substance lie in large lucent vacuoles where the limiting membrane is easily visualized.

The nature of parallel microtubular arrays and their mode of genesis is not known. Acid phosphatase has on rare occasions been found in a few of these inclusions (White, 1972; McKenna *et al.*, 1977a), but this is probably because these structures at times fuse with primary or secondary lysosomes. No author has suggested that parallel microtubular arrays are lysosomal in nature. The idea that they develop by the laying down of microtubules within dilated rough endoplasmic reticulum has theoretical appeal (because a variety of microtubular inclusions do develop in the rough endoplasmic reticulum), but there is no clear evidence to support this idea. Another theoretically appealing suggestion would be that these structures develop by the laying down of microtubules in Golgi vacuoles (a precedent for this would be the rod-shaped microtubulated body). There is no firm evidence supporting this proposal but a

---

*At the moment this structure defies classification because we do not know its mode of genesis. Hence, I do not know which chapter to put it in. I include it in this chapter, not because I believe that it develops within the endoplasmic reticulum (it may or may not do so) but simply to put it in company with other structures, arrays or aggregates of microtubules and because it has been confused and at times is still confused with the lupus-type microtubuloreticular structure (described on pages 496–508).

†The electron-dense matrix in which the microtubules lie makes it extremely difficult to obtain reliable measurements of their external diameter. The diameter reported by a majority of authors (White, 1972; Belcher *et al.*, 1975; Brunning and Parkin, 1975; Imamura *et al.*, 1975; Schwendemann, 1976; Dryll *et al.* 1977; McKenna *et al.*, 1977a, b) lie in the 15–30 nm range (this is in keeping with what is seen in *Plate 218* and *Figs.* 1 and 2 in *Plate 219*). However, a few authors (Hovig *et al.*, 1968; Halie *et al.*, 1975; Payne *et al.*, 1977) have reported external diameters of up to 40 or 44 nm (this is in keeping with what is seen in *Plate 219, Fig. 3*). The internal diameters of these structures (which can be more confidently measured) are rather small (i.e. the microtubules are thick-walled) and show smaller variations in size (12–17 nm). Therefore, one may conclude that: (1) the marked variations of the external diameter reflect principally the amount of dense material deposited on the walls of these microtubules; and (2) the structures are basically less than 30 nm in diameter and hence qualify as microtubules.

Plate 218
Circulating lymphocyte in blood vessel in a lymph node from a case of AIDS. Several single membrane-bound bodies or inclusions which we call 'parallel microtubular arrays' are seen around the cell centre wherein lie the centriole (C) and Golgi complex (G). Such bodies were not present in the rest of the cell cytoplasm. Profiles of longitudinally cut parallel microtubules (arrowheads) and transversely cut microtubules (arrows) are seen in these inclusions. The microtubule indicated by the long arrow has an external diameter of about 30 nm and an internal diameter of about 15 nm. ×75 000

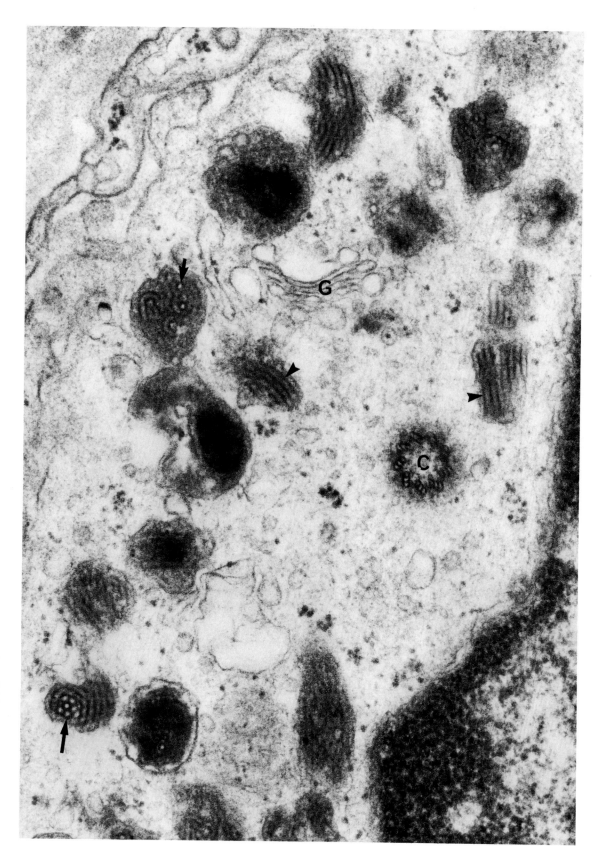

493

cluster of these inclusions are, at times, seen in the Golgi region. Yet another possibility is that the microtubules of this structure develop from the ends of the centriolar microtubules (the analogy here is microtubules of cilia), and indeed a fairly but not totally convincing illustration depicting this has been published (Fig. 3 in Brunning and Parkin, 1975b). The idea here is that microtubules are first assembled in the cytoplasm and then become enveloped by a membrane, but no suggestions as to how this happens or where the membrane comes from are forthcoming.

Parallel microtubular arrays have been found in lymphocytes from: (1) cases of rheumatoid arthritis (Hovig et al., 1968; Dryll et al., 1977); (2) late-onset amaurotic idiocy and Tay–Sachs disease (Witzleben, 1972; Noonan et al., 1976); (3) juvenile types of generalized ceroid-lipofuscinosis (Schwendemann, 1976); (4) Chediak–Higashi syndrome (White, 1972); (5) systemic and discoid lupus erythematosus (Goodman et al., 1973; Imamura et al., 1975); (6) Hodgkin's disease (Halie et al., 1975; Dryll et al., 1977); (7) sarcoidosis (Belcher et al., 1975); chronic lymphocytic leukaemia (Brunning and Parkin, 1975b; McKenna et al., 1977b); (9) severe combined immune deficiency disease (Payne et al., 1977); (10) infectious mononucleosis (Brunning and Parkin, 1975b; McKenna et al., 1977b; Payne and Tennican, 1982); (11) many normal or apparently normal individuals (Huhn, 1968; Imamura et al., 1975; Dryll et al. 1977; McKenna et al., 1977a; Payne et al., 1977, 1983; Payne and Glasser, 1978, 1981; Payne and Nagel, 1980; Payne and Tennican, 1982).

As noted above (item 11 above), lymphocytes containing parallel microtubular arrays have frequently been reported to occur in normal individuals. White (1972) suggested that they can be found in low numbers in any sample of normal lymphocytes. This view is now widely accepted. It would appear that in some pathological states there may be a relative or absolute increase in the number of lymphocytes bearing parallel microtubular arrays.

Payne and Glasser (1981) have shown that parallel microtubular array-containing cells constitute the major portion of the third population of lymphoid cells (non-T, non-B). These cells include K cells and NK cells. In a later study, Payne et al. (1983) state that 'It is probable that NK cells, K cells, and Tγ cells all belong to a distinct third mononuclear cell population which has properties of both T-lymphocytes and monocytes and are characterized morphologically at the light microscopic level as large granular lymphocytes (LGL), and at the ultrastructural level by the presence of parallel tubular arrays (PTA)'.

The function of parallel microtubular arrays is not known, but Payne et al. (1983) have hypothesized that these structures 'may represent accumulations of some metabolite necessary for the killing process'. This is in keeping with the studies of Henkart and Henkart (1982) who have shown that parallel microtubular arrays are released from killer cells in a cytotoxic assay system and that the size of the holes produced in cell membranes by effectors of antibody-dependent, cell-mediated cytotoxicity is similar to the size of the parallel microtubular arrays.

Plate 219

From circulating lymphocytes in normal peripheral blood donated by a technician in our department.

Figs. 1. 2 and 3. Examples of parallel microtubular arrays where the complexes of microtubules embedded in dense substance lie in large lucent vacuoles. Circular profiles of the rather thick-walled microtubules (arrows) are evident. The microtubules indicated by arrows in *Figs. 1 and 2* have an internal diameter of about 12nm and an external diameter of about 29nm, while that indicated by an arrow in *Fig. 3* has an internal diameter of about 16.6nm and an external diameter of about 40nm. The cells were well preserved and there was no evidence of mitochondrial swelling. Therefore the lucent vacuole is unlikely to be a swelling artefact. ×90 000, ×90 000, ×150 000

Fig. 4. This parallel microtubular array comprises a complex of microtubules and dense substance bounded by a loose fitting membrane. The microtubules are not too well visualized, hence reliable measurements are not possible. ×145 000

494

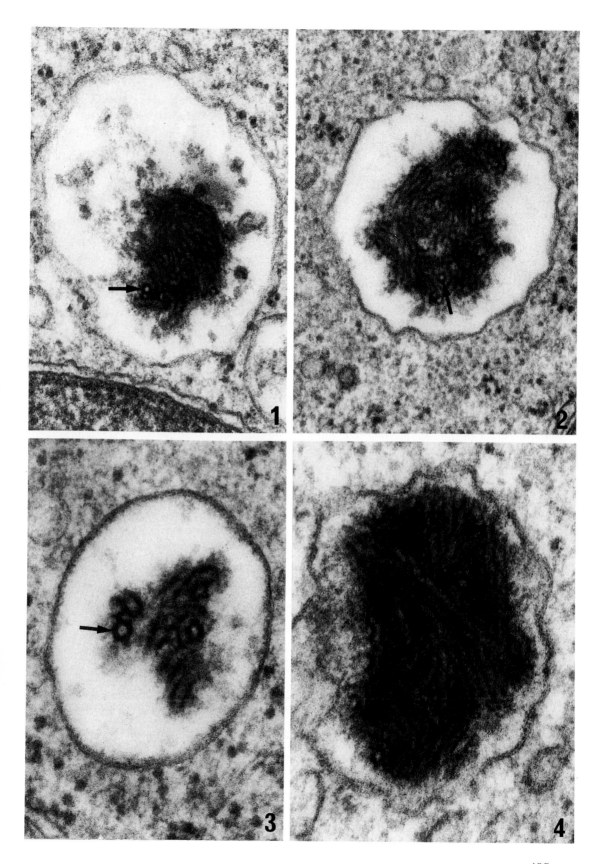

495

Microtuble group: microtubuloreticular structures (lupus type and others)

The term 'microtubuloreticular structures' is used to describe a group of structures composed of undulating or reticulated microtubules. Numerous names have been used in the past (particularly 'undulating tubules') to describe microtubuloreticular structures but they are now commonly referred to as 'tubuloreticular structures'. However, since the diameter of these 'tubules' is under 30 nm it is best to call them 'microtubuloreticular structures' and not 'tubuloreticular structures'*. Most examples of microtubuloreticular structures lie within the endoplasmic reticulum (e.g. lupus-type inclusion), some lie in the cytoplasmic matrix (e.g. chimpanzee hepatitis-type inclusion), and such an inclusion has also now been seen in the nucleus (*see below*).

The lupus type inclusion is the commonest and most studied inclusion, so we deal with it first. The overall size of these round, oval, elongated or irregular-shaped microtubuloreticular structures is usually about 100–400 nm, but some can be much larger (up to about 4 μm). The diameter of the microtubules in the inclusion ranges from 18–27 nm. The microtubules comprising a microtubuloreticular structure invariably or almost invariably lie within a dilated cisterna of the rough endoplasmic reticulum or the perinuclear cistern.

The three-dimensional morphology of the microtubules in microtubuloreticular structures is difficult to comprehend. In 1966 Bassot studied the luminous cells of the polynoid worm elytra (*Annelides polynoinae*) in which the photogenic grains are composed of a tightly packed system of undulating microtubules (20 nm diameter). Longitudinal sections through these microtubules would make one think that these were sections through paired membranous lamellae, but transverse sections clearly establish that these are microtubules while oblique sections at various angles reveal their undulating nature. Bassot (1966) found that these microtubules were continuous with the endoplasmic reticulum and he considered that this was a specialized form of endoplasmic reticulum.

In 1968 Chandra studied what he called 'undulating tubules' (in this text we call them microtubules) associated with the endoplasmic reticulum in cultured cell lines from normal and pathological tissues. He gave a detailed explanation as to how the various appearances seen in sectioned material can be correlated with different planes of sectioning through a system of undulating microtubules particularly when there is a superimposition of images of two parallel, overlaying, undulating microtubules where the crest of one lies opposite to the trough of another.

*For reasons given on page 478 and footnote on page 938, all hollow, cylindrical structures under 30 nm in diameter are referred to in this book as 'microtubules'; while structures above this size are called 'tubules'. Microtubuloreticular structures are members of the microtubule group. The distinction between tubule group, microtubule group and membrane group is explained on page 478. For various other members of the microtubule group *see* page 486.

Plate 220

Fig. 1. A microtubuloreticular structure in a cultured human embryonic kidney cell infected with HRV. Note the longitudinally sectioned undulating microtubules (arrowhead), and the thick-walled (small arrow) and double-walled (large arrow) circular profiles which are thought to be produced by overlaying of undulating microtubules within the section thickness. ×110 000 (*Chandra, unpublished electron micrograph*).

Fig. 2. A microtubuloreticular structure found in a lymphoblast in a leucocyte culture. Note the granular profiles (arrows) and the poorly defined thick-walled circular profiles (arrowheads) which seem to lie in an irregular ramifying dilated cistern the wall of which is continuous (arrows marked X) with the rough endoplasmic reticulum in several places. ×110 000 (*From Chandra, 1968*).

Figs. 3, 4 and 5. A diagrammatic demonstration of a few of the many theoretically possible ways in which two undulating microtubules (one hatched, the other filled with small circles so that their course can be easily traced) or even one undulating microtubule can produce thick-walled or double-walled circular profiles. *Fig. 3* demonstrates how circular profiles are produced when the crest of one microtubule overlays the trough of another. *Fig. 4* shows how abutting of crest and trough of neighbouring microtubules can produce circular profiles, while *Fig. 5* shows how longitudinal compression of a single undulating microtubule can produce circular profiles. Of the various possibilities, the concept illustrated in *Fig. 3* is the most plausible one.

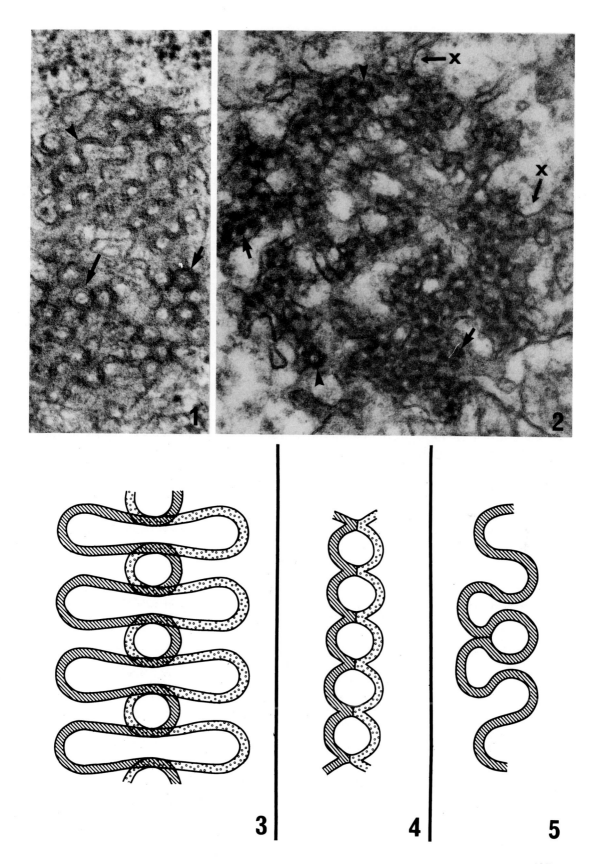

These important studies of Bassot (1966) and Chandra (1968) show that when the microtubules are not too closely packed, longitudinal sections through them clearly reveal long profiles of wavy or undulating microtubules. However, more often than not, what one sees are small granular profiles and double-walled or thick-walled circular profiles★. The small granular profiles probably represent transverse sections through microtubules with electron-dense contents and also perhaps points where the overlaying microtubules cross each other. Small circular profiles acceptable as transverse sections through microtubules are very rarely seen because of the electron-dense contents of the microtubules. The double-walled or thick-walled circular profiles can be produced in many ways, the most likely being the superimposition of the images of two microtubules where the crest of one overrides the trough of another (*Plate 220, Fig. 3*).

Other interpretations of the three-dimensional morphology of microtubules in microtubuloreticular structures include: (1) Hruban *et al.* (1976) who considered them to be a 'tangled skein of contorted microtubules'; (2) Gyorkey *et al.* (1972) who described them as 'curved and interwoven microtubular structures'†; and (3) my view that when there are relatively few randomly oriented wavy microtubules scattered in the rough endoplasmic reticulum they overlay each other to produce a reticular pattern. When the tubules are somewhat more numerous and more wavy or undulating, they present the granular and thick-walled circular profiles one expects to find in such a situation. When there is a close geometric packing of microtubules, a crystalline structure with a sieve-like appearance is produced. On close examination, each subunit of the 'sieve' is as a rule seen to be a thick-walled circular profile.

The microtubules in the microtubuloreticular structures are often quite electron-dense, and the lumen of these microtubules is difficult or impossible to visualize (*Plates 221–223*). It would appear that some electron-dense material is present in these microtubules. In places this material is absent or extracted or unstained and the walls of the microtubules are then more easily seen. It is thought that the microtubules are derived from the membranes of the rough endoplasmic reticulum because: (1) at times there appears to be continuity between the microtubules and the surrounding membrane of the dilated rough endoplasmic reticulum; (2) the microtubules at times seem to be bounded by a trilaminar membrane similar to the membranes of the rough endoplasmic reticulum; and (3) they do not contain RNA (i.e. not viral in nature) but they do contain phospholipids and proteins as do cytomembranes. Thus, the microtubules in these inclusions are not tubulin microtubules, but structures presumably derived from the membranes of the rough endoplasmic reticulum.

★The thick-walled circular profile is no more than a double-walled circular profile which cannot be recognized as such because of the electron-dense material between the walls (i.e. within the undulating microtubules).
†Note that both Hruban *et al.* (1976) and Gyorkey *et al.* (1972) recognized that they were microtubules, not tubules.

Plate 221
Microtubuloreticular structures found in vascular endothelial cells (glomerular capillaries) from the kidney of a case of systemic lupus erythematosus (*Ghadially and Larsen, unpublished electron micrographs*)
Fig. 1. Glomerular capillary showing microtubuloreticular structures (T). ×25 000
Figs. 2–6. Depicted here are microtubuloreticular structures at higher magnifications. Sometimes they appear to be within dilatations of the endoplasmic reticulum (e.g. *Figs. 5 and 6*) and in other instances where the surrounding membrane is absent or not well visualized, they appear to be in the cytoplasmic matrix (e.g. *Fig. 4*). ×62 000; ×115 000; ×62 000; ×62 000; ×62 000

498

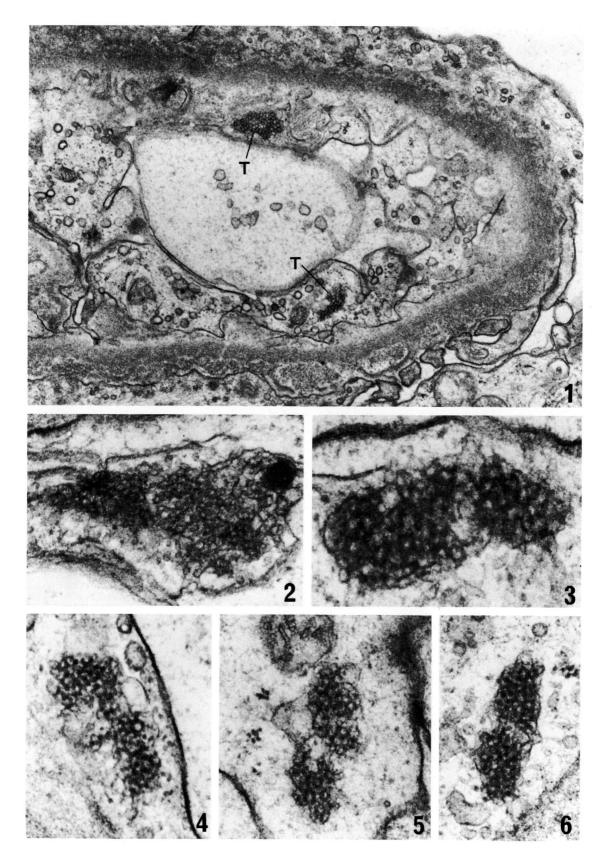

499

Microtubuloreticular structures have been seen in★: (1) photogenic grains in luminous cells of the elytra of polynoid worm (*Annelides polynoinae*) (Bassot, 1966); (2) vascular endothelial cells (in kidney and liver) of apparently normal Rhesus monkeys (Rosen and Tisher, 1968; De Martino *et al.*, 1969; Ruebner *et al.*, 1969); (3) endothelial cells of blood vessels (in prostate) and lymphatics (in hilum and capsule of kidney) of apparently normal dogs (Hruban *et al.*, 1976; Albertine *et al.*, 1980); (4) vascular endothelial cells (in kidney, skin, lung and synovium) and circulating lymphocytes in cases of systemic lupus erythematosus (Gyorkey *et al.*, 1969, 1972; Hurd *et al.*, 1969, 1971; Kawano *et al.*, 1969; Norton, 1969, 1970; Sinkovics *et al.*, 1969; Bloodworth and Shelp, 1970; Grausz *et al.*, 1970; Haas and Yunis, 1970a; Pincus *et al.*, 1970; Schumacher, 1970; Bariety *et al.*, 1971, 1973; Fraire *et al.*, 1971; Gyorkey and Sinkovics, 1971; Müller-Hermelink and Lennert, 1971; Müller-Hermelink *et al.*, 1971; Tannenbaum *et al.*, 1971; Tisher *et al.*, 1971; Andres *et al.*, 1972; Grimley *et al.*, 1972; Hashimoto and Chandler, 1972; Kobayasi and Asboe-Hansen, 1972; Kovacs *et al.*, 1972; Nieland *et al.*, 1972; Prunieras *et al.*, 1972; Goodman *et al.*, 1973; Klippel *et al.*, 1974a, b; Metz and Metz, 1974; Grimley and Schaff, 1976; Lyon *et al.*, 1984); (5) vascular endothelial cells (in skin) and circulating lymphocytes in discoid lupus erythematosus (Hashimoto and Thompson, 1970; Goodman *et al.*, 1973); (6) vascular endothelial cells (in synovium) from a case of palindromic rheumatism and cases of rheumatoid arthritis (Gyorkey *et al.*, 1972; Molnar *et al.*, 1972); (7) vascular endothelial cells (in synovium) from a case of pigmented villonodular synovitis (Molnar *et al.*, 1971); (8) vascular endothelial cells (in salivary glands and kidney) from cases of Sjögren's syndrome (Shearn *et al.*, 1970; Aübock and Albegger, 1972; Gyorkey *et al.*, 1972; Daniels *et al.*, 1974); (9) vascular endothelial cells (in skin, muscle and lymph node) and muscle cells from cases of dermatomyositis and polymyositis (Norton, 1970; Norton *et al.*, 1970; Hashimoto *et al.*, 1971; Gyorkey *et al.*, 1972; Chou and Miike, 1981); (10) vascular endothelial cells, histiocytes and lymphocytes in kidneys, small intestine, choroid and lymph nodes, and lymphocytes and monocytes from peripheral blood from cases of AIDS (acquired immune deficiency syndrome) and to a lesser extent in the prodrome of AIDS (persistent generalized lymphadenopathy) (Ewing *et al.*, 1983; Kostianovsky *et al.*, 1983; Orenstein, 1983; Rozman and Feliu, 1983; Sidhu, 1983; Allegra *et al.*, 1984; Anderson *et al.*, 1984; Onerheim *et al.*, 1984; Said *et al.*, 1984; Jensen, 1985; Liu *et al.*, 1985; Schenk and Konrad, 1985; Sidhu *et al.*, 1985; Rácz *et al.*, 1986; Schenk *et al.*, 1986); (11) neoplastic vascular endothelial cells, lymphocytes (peripheral blood) and hepatocytes of cases of Kaposi's sarcoma, particularly in homosexual men and patients with

★There is no review from which one can trace all or virtually all the papers on microtubuloreticular structures, principally because a major review on this topic has not been published recently. Since microtubuloreticular structures are currently the focus of much interest (because of AIDS), I have presented in this chapter about 95 per cent of the references I am aware of. The omissions are largely short abstracts and 'Letters to the Editor', which I am sure will not be missed.

Plate 222

Lymph node from a case of AIDS.

Fig. 1. A microtubuloreticular structure (arrow) is seen in a circulating lymphocyte lying adjacent to endothelial cells (E) of a blood vessel. ×17 000

Fig. 2. Microtubuloreticular structure in an endothelial cell. The profiles seen here are interpreted by some as reticulated (perhaps branching) microtubules, by others as undulating microtubules. It is difficult to choose between these alternatives. However, one does see here profiles expected from undulating microtubules deployed in various ways (*Plate 220*). Such profiles include: (1) small circular profiles (thin arrows) acceptable as transverse sections through microtubules; (2) electron-dense granules (thick arrows); and (3) thick-walled or double-walled circular profiles (between arrowheads). Clear demonstration of such details is impeded by the electron density of the contents of the microtubules, but they are just discernible in this electron micrograph. ×78 000

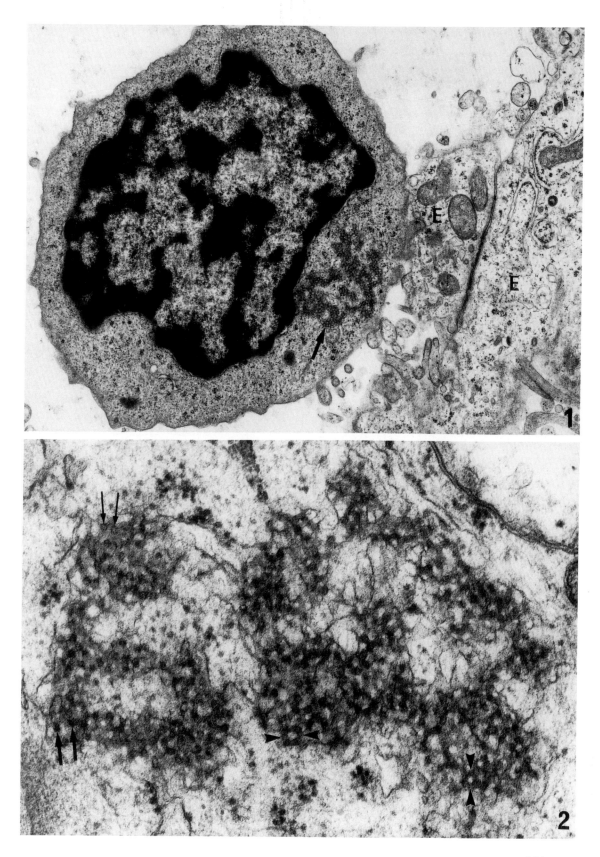

501

AIDS (Gyorkey et al., 1982; Schenk and Konrad, 1985; Rácz et al., 1986; Schenk et al., 1986); (12) circulating lymphocytes in a case of severe combined immune deficiency (Geha et al., 1974); (13) circulating lymphocytes from a child with an unidentified form of cerebroretinal degeneration (Anzil and Blinzinger, 1974); (14) vascular endothelial cells in a woman with Dego's disease (Nishida and Howard, 1968); (15) bursal lymphocytes of a 12-day-old male chicken afflicted by an undiagnosed disease (Alves de Matos and Camara e Sousa, 1978); (16) vascular endothelial cells, malignant osteoblasts and lymphocytes of a human osteosarcoma (patient had markedly elevated measles antibody titres) (Jenson et al., 1971); (17) vascular endothelial cells in a human insulinoma (Le Charpentier et al., 1973); (18) vascular endothelial cells in a human bronchial carcinoid (Alves de Matos, 1974); (19) vascular endothelial cells and lymphocytes in human pituitary tumours (Cure et al., 1972; Landolt et al., 1976); (20) presumably (cell type not clearly stated) the neoplastic cells of human rhabdomyosarcoma, liposarcoma and fibrosarcoma (Gyorkey et al., 1971); (21) neoplastic cells of human breast carcinoma (in biopsy specimens and/or cultures derived thereof. Report not too clear on this point) (Seman et al., 1971); (22) vascular endothelial cells and circulating lymphocytes in human melanoma and metastatic melanoma (questionably also in tumour cells) (Cesarini et al., 1973; Posalaky and McGinley, 1979; Moura Nunes et al., 1980); (23) vascular endothelial cells in human intracranial germinomas (Matsumura et al., 1984); (24) vascular endothelial cells (occasionally also in pericytes, lymphocytes and fibroblasts) in common warts, papillomas, Bowen's disease and basal cell carcinoma (Maciejewski et al., 1973); (25) neoplastic cells of American Burkitt's type lymphoma (Popoff and Malinin, 1976); (26) lymphocytes in lymph nodes from cases of lymphosarcoma, malignant IgM-lymphoma without macroglobulinaemia, and in a lymph node containing metastasis of breast carcinoma (Kaiserling, 1972); (27) neoplastic cells of Japanese adult T-cell leukaemia (Shamoto et al., 1981); (28) leukaemic cells (leukaemia following whole-body proton irradiation) in a Rhesus monkey (Macaca mulatta) (Siegal et al., 1968); (29) neoplastic cells of canine lymphomas and breast carcinoma (Seman et al., 1968); (30) vaginal epithelial cells and connective tissue cells from a case of Sticker sarcoma (transmissible venereal tumour of the dog) (Lombard et al., 1967); (31) neoplastic cells of gliomas and meningiomas produced in dogs by Rous sarcoma virus (Bucciarelli et al., 1967; Haguenau et al., 1972); (32) neoplastic cells and vascular endothelial cells of tumours (no diagnosis given, said to be composed of spindle cells) induced in Rhesus monkey by a variant of Rous sarcoma virus (Munro et al., 1964); (33) human cultured cells from normal blood leucocytes and normal lymph nodes, Chediak–Higashi syndrome, lymphomas and leukaemias, Hodgkin's disease, fibrosarcoma, rhabdomyosarcoma, chondrosarcoma, osteosarcoma, melanoma, recurrent paraganglioma and also in tumours produced by injecting some of these cells into laboratory animals (Chandra, 1968; Chandra et al., 1968, 1969; Moore and Chandra, 1968; Douglas et al., 1969; Recher et al., 1969; Gyorkey et al., 1971; Sinkovics et al., 1971; Uzman et al., 1971; Dalton et al., 1973; Sinkovics and Gyorkey, 1973); (34) vascular endothelial cells in the heart of a human case of Coxsackie myocarditis (Haas and Yunis, 1970b); (35) perivascular cells, endothelial cells and fibroblasts in the skin of an infant with the rubella

---

Plate 223

From an ovarian carcinoma.

Fig. 1. A long (3.6 μm approximately) microtubuloreticular structure in a vascular endothelial cell. ×39 000

Fig. 2. Two microtubuloreticular structures are present in an endothelial cell. The lumen of the microtubules is difficult to discern because of electron-dense contents. Hence, they have the 'solid' look of filaments and fibrils rather than the 'hollow' look expected of microtubules and tubules. These loosely packed microtubules are clearly not undulating microtubules and hence thick-walled circular profiles are nowhere evident. These randomly oriented straight and slightly curved microtubules form a reticulum. Appearances suggesting branching (arrows) could be real but they are more likely an illusion produced by overlaying of two or three microtubules within the section thickness. ×60 000

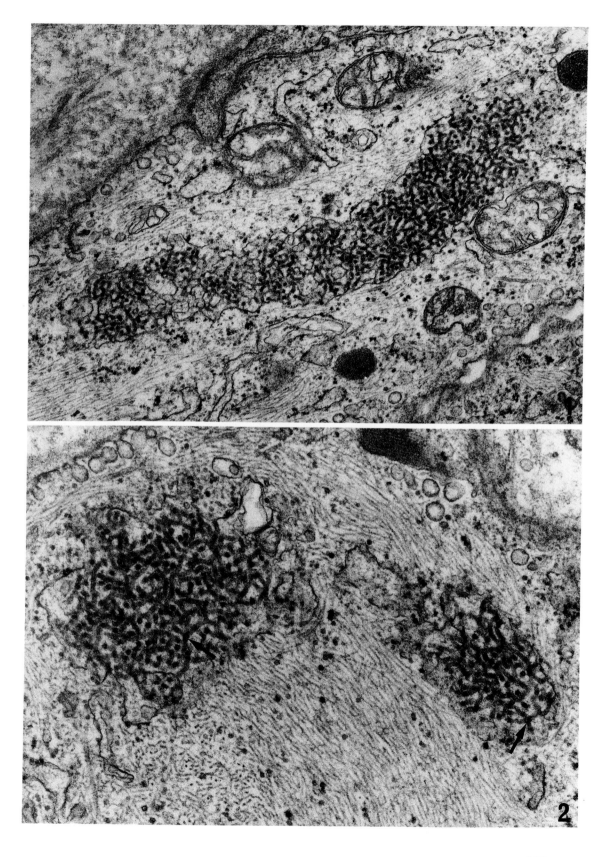

syndrome (Hanissian and Hashimoto, 1972); (36) vascular endothelial cells, fibroblasts, glioblasts and cytotrophoblasts in fetuses and placenta of 85 per cent of women with serologically confirmed rubella infection (Kistler, 1975); (37) sinusoidal endothelial cells of the liver in human cases of viral hepatitis (Schaff et al., 1982); (38) vascular endothelial cells in lungs of patients with viral pneumonia (Hammar et al., 1983); (39) vascular endothelial cells and macrophages in human brain from a patient with herpes simplex encephalitis (Baringer and Griffith, 1969; Baringer and Swoveland, 1972; Blinzinger et al., 1972; McGinley and Posalaky, 1984); (40) vascular endothelial cells and macrophages in the brain of rabbits with experimentally produced herpes virus encephalitis (Baringer and Griffith, 1969); (41) cultured human lymphoma cells infected with herpes simplex virus (Bedoya et al., 1968); (42) vascular endothelial cells of kidney of mink with Aleutian disease (Tsai et al., 1968); (43) littoral cells in liver of dogs infected with canine hepatitis virus (Givan and Jezequel, 1969); (44) vascular endothelial adventitial cells, macrophages, microglial cells and ependymal cells in the brain of the central nervous system of dogs with distemper (Blinzinger et al., 1972); (45) vascular endothelial cells and mononuclear cells in the spinal cord of cynomolgus monkeys infected with poliovirus (Blinzinger et al., 1969); (46) vascular endothelial cells in spinal cord of pigs injected with porcine polioencephalitis virus (Koestner et al., 1966); and (47) vascular endothelial cells in horses with equine viral arteritis (Estes and Cheville, 1970).

An analysis of the large literature on microtubuloreticular structures shows that: (1) although these structures occasionally occur in normal or apparently normal mammalian cells, most examples come from tissues of diseased individuals; particularly from cases of autoimmune diseases and viral infections; (2) these structures have been found in human tissues and tissues of monkey, pig, dog, horse, rabbit, squirrel and mink, but they do not appear to have been reported to occur in tissues of mouse, rat, hamster and guinea pig; (3) a singularly large number of reports have dealt with the occurrence of microtubuloreticular structures in cultured cells, particularly tumour cells, cells from the spleen and thymus, and white blood cells obtained from patients with a variety of disorders, including tumours such as lymphoma and leukaemia, melanoma, carcinoma of the pancreas, carcinoma of the colon and multiple myeloma; (4) microtubuloreticular structures have been seen in various tissues and organs such as kidney, skin, muscle, myocardium, synovium, brain, lymph nodes, liver, jejunum and blood. The cells (in tissue or in culture) in which they have been seen include endothelium, fibroblasts, glial cells, lymphoid cells, mononuclear cells, macrophages and tumour cells.

The diagnostic value of microtubuloreticular structures will now be considered. The fact that these structures are seen in many different disease states shows that they are neither pathognomonic nor diagnostic of any particular disease. However, their high incidence in lupus erythematosus and AIDS★ may be of some diagnostic value when taken in conjunction with other clinicopathological findings.

In renal biopsies, microtubuloreticular structures have been seen not only from cases of systemic lupus erythematosus but also from other nephropathies and apparently normal kidneys. Nevertheless, these structures do occur much more frequently in lupus nephritis. Norton (1969) found that such inclusions were 'present in 100 per cent of active lesions of SLE', while an incidence of '62 per cent was noted in lupus biopsies as opposed to 2.4 per cent from non-lupus biopsies' by Bloodworth and Shelp (1970).

★Rácz et al. (1986) found microtubuloreticular structures in the lymph nodes of 100 per cent of cases of AIDS and in 85 per cent of patients with persistent generalized lymphadenopathy. This contrasts with tubular confronting cisternae, which are seen in only about 27 per cent of cases of AIDS and 14 per cent of cases with persistent generalized lymphadenopathy (page 474).

Plate 224
Microtubuloreticular structure in the hepatocyte of a chimpanzee inoculated with serum from a case of non-A, non-B hepatitis. In contrast to the lupus-type inclusion, this inclusion is not membrane-bound. The microtubules (diameter about 23 nm) forming the reticulum lie free in the cytoplasmic matrix. The circular profiles (arrowheads) of transversely cut microtubules are clearly evident. ×62 000 (*From a block of tissue supplied by Dr H.P. Dienes*)

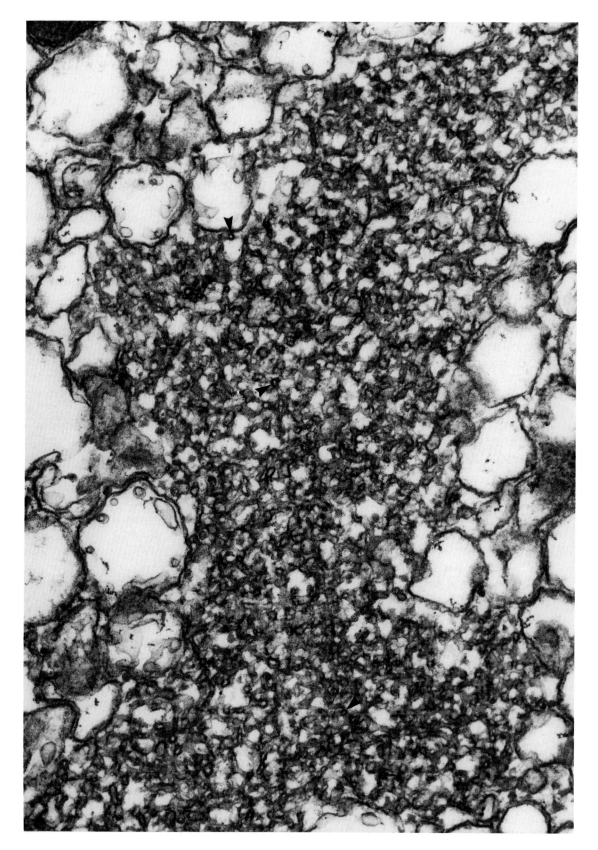

505

The pathogenesis and nature of microtubuloreticular structures in diseased humans have not been fully clarified, but many interesting observations have been made. Their occurrence in autoimmune diseases and viral infections and the morphology of the microtubules which bear some resemblance to viral microtubules (i.e. nucleocapsids of myxoviruses (influenza or parainfluenza virus) or paramyxoviruses) led some workers (Gyorkey *et al.*, 1969; De Sousa and Pritchard, 1974) to speculate that these were virions or derivatives thereof.

The possibility that microtubuloreticular structures are viral in nature has not been completely abandoned, but the current view is that these structures are of cellular derivation (Grimley and Henson, 1983). Against the viral hypothesis is: (1) the failure to isolate virus from inclusion-bearing tissues (Norton, 1969; Feorino *et al.*, 1970); (2) immunofluorescence, tissue culture and ultrastructural studies by Pincus *et al.* (1970) who point out that the strands of paramyxoviruses are somewhat smaller in diameter and occur in the cytoplasm and not in the endoplasmic reticulum; and (3) histochemical studies which show that microtubuloreticular structures do not contain RNA (Grimley and Schaff, 1976).

The occurrence of microtubuloreticular structures in a variety of virus infections led Kistler (1973) to hypothesize that interferon might be the agent which induces the formation of microtubuloreticular structures. Later workers (Rich, 1981; Carrette *et al.*, 1982; Grimley *et al.*, 1983, 1985; Rich *et al.*, 1983; Kuyama *et al.*, 1986) have amply vindicated this thesis by showing that tubuloreticular structures are produced when: (1) lymphoid cell line (Dandi) is treated with sera from lupus cases; (2) cancer patients are treated with alpha-interferon; and (3) lymphocytes from healthy donors are treated (*in vitro*) with interferon. Thus interferon appears to be a factor in provoking cells to produce microtubuloreticular structures but the relationship between the level of interferon and production of microtubuloreticular structures is not a simple one. For example: (1) Grimley *et al.* (1984) found that serum interferon levels were elevated in all cases of AIDS which they studied but microtubuloreticular structures could not be detected in peripheral blood lymphocytes in every case. They also did not find microtubuloreticular structures in two asymptomatic homosexual males with raised levels of interferon; and (2) Carrette *et al.* (1982) studied 33 cases of systemic lupus erythematosus, 11 of whom had raised

---

Plate 225

Microtubuloreticular inclusion in the hepatocyte of a chimpanzee inoculated with serum from a case of non-A, non-B hepatitis. Besides microtubules (transversely cut ones indicated by arrowheads) the inclusion contains electron–dense material (D) of an unknown nature. There appears to be a continuity (arrows) between the microtubules and the surrounding endoplasmic reticulum. ×63 000 (*From a block of tissue supplied by Dr H.P. Dienes*)

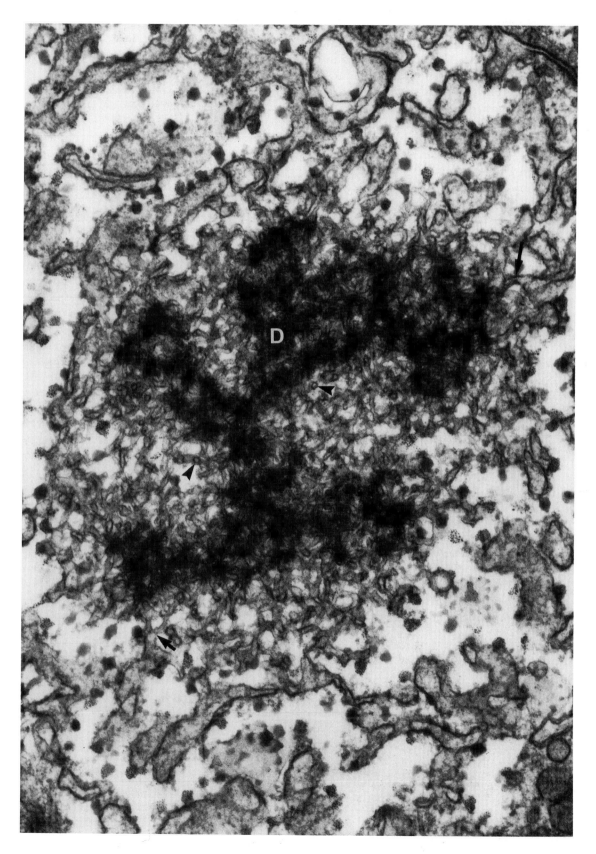

507

interferon levels while 22 of them did not. Not only did the 11 cases with raised interferon levels show microtubuloreticular structures, but so also did 14 of the cases without elevated serum interferon. These studies show that it would be an oversimplification to say that raised interferon levels produce microtubuloreticular structures.

Some observations suggest that the type of lymphoid cells bearing microtubuloreticular structures may vary according to the disease process. Thus according to Grimley et al. (1984) and Rácz et al. (1986) in AIDS, microtubuloreticular structures occur in T-cells, while Müller-Hermelink and Lennert (1971) and Müller-Hermelink et al. (1971) find that in systemic lupus erythematosus, microtubuloreticular structures occur not only in lymphocytes but also in immunoblasts, immature plasma cells and plasma cells. It remains for future studies to determine whether there is a preferential location of microtubuloreticular structures which is related to specific diseases.

Until now we have discussed microtubuloreticular structures of the type seen principally in lupus and AIDS. These develop within the rough endoplasmic reticulum and hence, invariably or almost invariably present as membrane-bound inclusions. In contrast to this, the microtubuloreticular inclusion found in the hepatocytes of chimpanzees inoculated with serum from patients with non-A, non-B hepatitis, invariably lies in the cytoplasmic matrix and is not bounded by a membrane (Plates 224 and 225). The small or early lesion consists of a reticulum of microtubules (diameter about 23 nm) lying free in the cytoplasmic matrix. At the periphery of the inclusion continuity between the microtubules and the endoplasmic reticulum is often demonstrable. The larger or more mature inclusion has a similar appearance except that some dense material of an unknown nature is trapped in the reticulum of microtubules.

To the best of my knowledge, microtubuloreticular structures have not been seen in the nucleus (as true non-membrane-bound inclusions), except in a case of epilepsy (cause unknown) where the neurons contained intranuclear microtubuloreticular structures (Plate 226). The diameter of the microtubules was about 19–23 nm. Virtually any and every cytoplasmic organelle and inclusion has at one time or other been seen to lie in a double-membrane-bound pseudoinclusion in the nucleus. Therefore, one would not be too surprised to see a microtubuloreticular structure in an intranuclear pseudoinclusion. However, what we are looking at in Plate 226 are true intranuclear inclusions which presumably developed within the nucleus.

At a casual glance and at low magnifications some of the inclusions appear membrane-bound, but closer examination at higher magnifications show that they are not. Myelin figures of the type one associates with glutaraldehyde fixation are seen adjacent to some of these inclusions. This suggests that the microtubular inclusions contain phospholipids, which when liberated and hydrated, form myelinoid membranes and myelin figures. This leads one to suspect that these microtubules were probably derived from the inner membrane of the nuclear envelope, even though no connections between the two were detected.

Plate 226
Inclusions found in neurons from a patient with epilepsy (*Electron micrographs supplied by Dr T. Stanley*)
Fig. 1. Several intranuclear microtubuloreticular structures are seen here. They are not membrane-bound, but at times microtubules (arrowheads) lying at the periphery of the inclusions create such an impression. Note also the myelinoid membranes (arrows) closely associated with these structures. ×25 000
Fig. 2. Higher-power view showing a small portion of a large intranuclear microtubuloreticular inclusion (M). Note also the solitary microtubules (arrows) lying free in the nuclear matrix. ×85 000

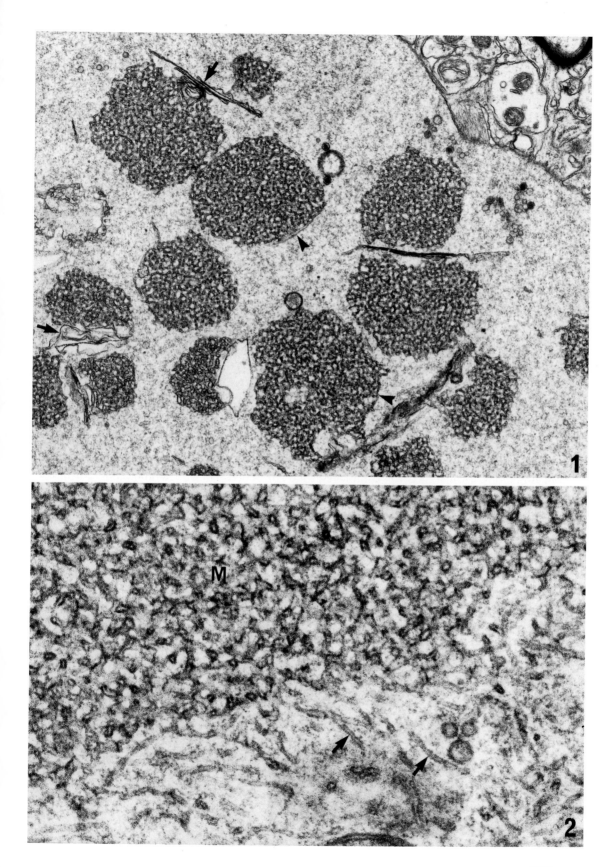

Membrane group: reticulated, knotted, undulating, pouched, radiate and cross-banded membranous formations or complexes

As its name implies the membrane group★ comprises structures composed mainly or entirely of membranes (usually as paired membranous lamellae) deployed in unusual or abnormal patterns and where circular profiles acceptable as transverse sections through tubules or microtubules are very rare or absent. There has been no formal attempt in the literature to classify these structures and the term 'membrane complex' has been used to describe several membranous formations of quite different patterns. In view of this, the best use one can make of this term now is to use it as a generic term for all members of the membrane group, and then wherever possible label each variety with a specific name. The terms used to describe various membrane complexes include: 'folded membrane complex', 'undulating membranes' or 'undulating membrane complex', 'pouched membranes' or 'pouched membrane complex', 'crystalloid configuration of membranes', 'unusual form of endoplasmic reticulum', 'radiate cisternae', 'convoluted membranes', 'tortuous membranes', 'knotted membranes' or 'knotted membrane complex', 'concentric membranous bodies' and several others.

Unless tilting stage and serial section studies are executed, it is difficult or impossible to say whether a given membranous formation is composed of undulating paired membranous lamellae or pouched paired membranous lamellae†. Before classifying the membranous structures described in the literature, it is worth noting that while some are composed 'purely' of membranes, others have electron-dense material associated with them.

The members of this group include: (1) concentric membranous formations, arrays, complexes or bodies of the endoplasmic reticulum (dealt with on pages 516–523). Three main subtypes are recognized: (a) the Nebenkern which is composed of whorls of rough endoplasmic reticulum; (b) concentric smooth membrane arrays; and (c) the glycogen body which is composed of smooth membranes and glycogen particles; (2) knotted membranous formations or complexes which are usually associated with radiating cisternae; (3) undulating membranous formations or complexes; (4) pouched membranous formations or complexes; (5) folded membranous formations or complexes; and (6) cross-banded membranous formations (ladder-like appearance).

We will now consider the knotted membranous formations which are usually associated with radiating cisternae of the rough endoplasmic reticulum. The 'knot' comprises a focal accumulation of reticulated or irregularly deployed undulating membranes (usually paired membranous lamellae). Electron-dense material may or may not be entrapped in the reticulated interstices of the knot. Cisternae of the rough endoplasmic reticulum at times radiate from the knot. Such structures have been called 'radiate cisternae' (for illustrations *see* Filshie and

---

★The general system of classification employed and the differences between the tubule group, microtubule group and membrane group are explained on page 478.
†The differences between undulating and pouched membranes is explained in a large footnote on page 94. Briefly, an undulating membrane is like a corrugated sheet, a pouched membrane is like an egg-tray. Closely apposed pairs of such sheets (corrugated or pouched) deployed in certain ways can on section yield double-walled circular profiles and double-walled wavy or undulating profiles.

Plate 227

Fig. 1. A cultured Burkitt's lymphoma cell showing two knots (K) composed of reticulated or undulating membranes (actually paired membranous lamellae, but this is difficult to discern at this low magnification) which are continuous with stacks of confronting cisternae (C). ×21 000 (*Chandra, unpublished electron micrograph*)

Fig. 2. Radiating cisternae in a macrophage from the olfactory bulb of a squirrel (*Citellus lateralis*) seven days after a subcutaneous injection of Coxsackie virus. The cisternae radiate from focal dilatations of the endoplasmic reticulum containing some vesicles (arrows). ×90 000 (*Grodums, unpublished electron micrograph*)

510

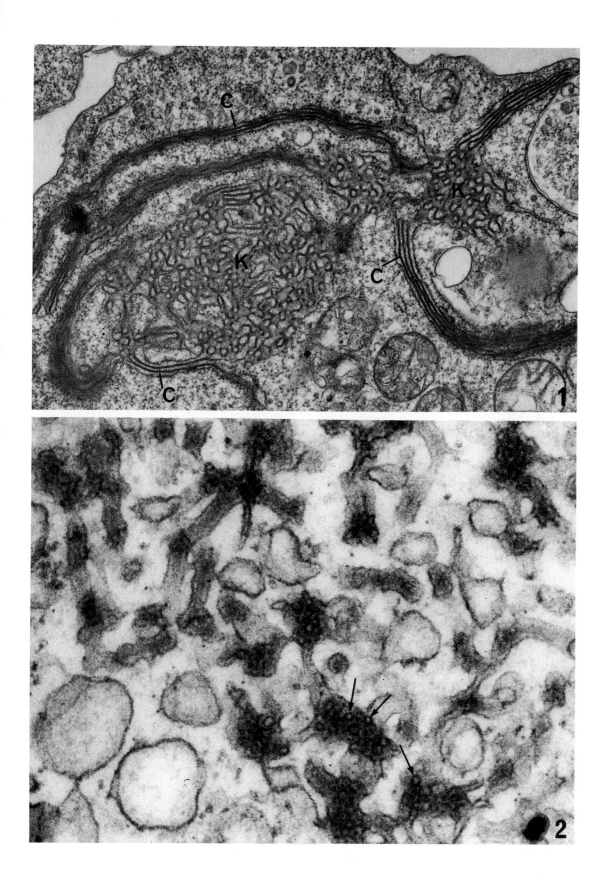

Rehacek, 1968; Tandler *et al.*, 1973). At other times, however, parallel arrays (at times coming together to form confronting cisternae) of meandering cisternae may be seen emerging from the 'knot' (*Plate 227, Fig. 1*). Not all radiating cisternae, however, radiate from a knot, in some instances the centre of radiation is expanded endoplasmic reticulum containing some vesicles (*Plate 227, Fig. 2*).

We will now consider together, the structures composed of undulating or pouched paired membranous lamellae (items 3 and 4) because as mentioned earlier it is difficult to distinguish between the two. The simplest variety of this structure presents in sectioned material as discrete C-shaped, U-shaped or S-shaped profiles (at times called 'comma-shaped' or 'worm-like' profiles) of paired membranous lamellae (some electron-dense or medium density material is usually seen between the paired membranes) scattered in the cell cytoplasm. These structures which are best referred to as 'curvilinear membranous formations' have been seen in: (1) Langerhans cells from cases of histiocytosis X (Turiaf *et al.*, 1969; Gianotti and Caputo, 1971; Basset *et al.*, 1972; Mierau *et al.*, 1982); (2) malignant lymphoma of the skin (Pruniéras *et al.*, 1971); (3) histiocyte from a Kaposi's sarcoma (Sterry *et al.*, 1979); (4) pleural mesothelioma (Wang, 1974); and (5) mononuclear cells in a giant cell tumour of bone (Marquart, 1984). In a couple of early reports and in a recent one (Marquart, 1984)★ these structures have been misinterpreted as tubules when in fact they are paired membranous lamellae.

In the better developed form of this structure (i.e. curvilinear membranous formations), instead of the small, discrete comma-shaped or worm-like profiles, we have long runs of undulating profiles composed of paired membranous lamellae (with or without electron-dense material between the paired membranes). Double-walled circular profiles are also quite commonly seen. These profiles clearly lie in the cell cytoplasm but occasionally a solitary circular profile is seen lying in dilated endoplasmic reticulum. This, almost certainly, is an illusion created by a transverse section through a 'pouch' protruding into neighbouring dilated endoplasmic reticulum.

Undulating or pouched membranous formations (at times so well ordered and packed as to produce a crystalloid or crystalline appearance) have been seen in: (1) liver of a hamster treated with barbiturates (*Plate 228*); (2) a novel or new organelle of a trypanosomatid flagellate (*Leptomonas collosoma*). (Freeze fracture images in their Figs. 3 and 4 have an egg-tray-like (i.e. pouched membrane) appearance (Linder and Staehelin, 1980); (3) Rous sarcoma virus-induced

---

★In *Fig. 5* of Marquart (1984) some 25 profiles of scattered comma-shaped structures (unbranched) are present but not a single solitary circular profile acceptable as a transverse section through the alleged 'tubular comma-shaped structures' is seen in the cell cytoplasm. The dense material between the paired membranous lamellae forming the comma-shaped structures appears extracted and striated. In a couple of instances, a circular profile is seen lying within the comma-shaped profile, probably reflecting a lucent area created by loss of substance in the region. Whatever the explanation of the circular profiles may be, they certainly cannot be accepted as evidence supporting the idea that the comma-shaped structures are tubules.

Plate 228

A membrane complex (composed of paired membranous lamellae) found within an area of hypertrophied smooth endoplasmic reticulum in the hepatocyte of a phenobarbitone-treated hamster. Note the undulating profiles (arrows) and the double-walled circular profiles (between arrowheads). This seems to be an undulating membrane complex rather than a pouched membrane complex. ×71 000

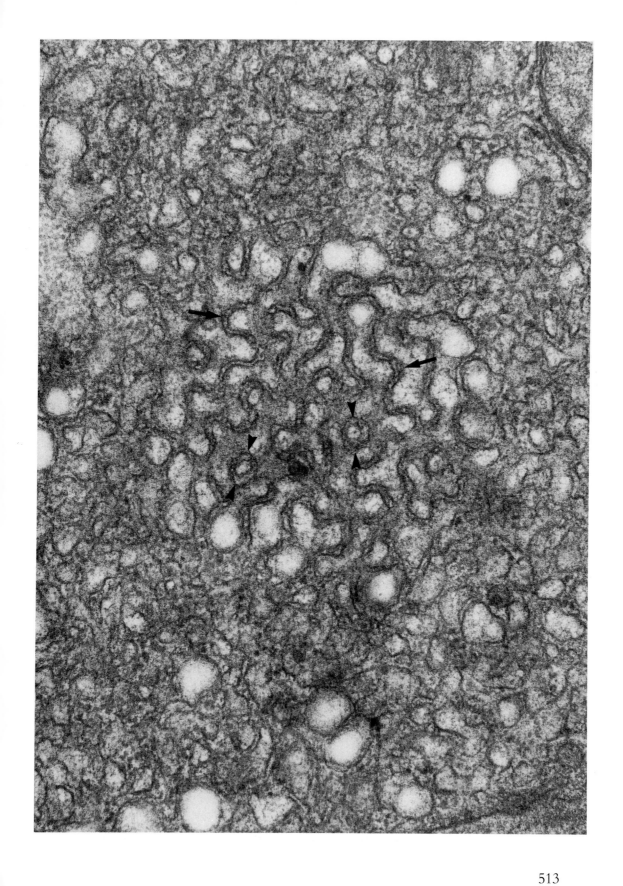

513

intracerebral and subcutaneous tumours in the marmoset (*Saquinus* sp.) (Smith and Deinhardt, 1968); (excellent electron micrographs and diagrams of pouched membranes are provided in this paper); (4) hepatocytes of chimpanzees inoculated with serum from patients with non-A, non-B hepatitis (*Plate 229*) (Jackson *et al.*, 1979; Shimizu *et al.*, 1979; Pfeifer *et al.*, 1980, Schaff, 1984); and (5) hepatocytes of chimpanzees infected with HBsAg-associated delta agent (Canese *et al.*, 1984).

Yet another type of membrane complex is the so-called 'folded membrane complex'. There is, however, no evidence whatsoever that this structure evolves by a process of membrane folding, in fact the appearances suggest that it is composed of aggregations of short slightly dilated cisternae forming small rosettes or parallel stacks.

Folded membrane complexes have been seen in: (1) cells of human corpus luteum (Van Lennep and Madden, 1965; Adams and Hertig, 1969); (2) interstitial cells (steroidogenic cells) of the antebrachial organ of the ring-tailed lemur (*Lemur catta*) (Sisson and Fahrenbach, 1967); (3) cultured mouse liver cells infected with a mouse hepatitis virus (David-Ferreira and Manaker, 1965); (4) HEp-2 cells (human epidermoid carcinoma cell line) infected with Ilheus virus (Tandler *et al.*, 1973); (5) spermatids of the American chameleon (*Anolis carolinensis*) and rat (Clark, 1967; Posalaki *et al.*, 1968); and (6) endodermal cells of the yolk sac of the bat (*Tadarida brasiliensis cynocephala*).

The final variety of membrane complex we deal with is the cross-banded membranous formation or aggregate. Here, a ladder-like pattern is seen between the apposed walls of dilated cisternae of the rough endoplasmic reticulum. This modification of the rough endoplasmic reticulum has been seen in hepatocytes of mice infected with Rift Valley fever virus (McGavran and Easterday, 1963).

The significance of the various membrane complexes described in this section of the text is not clear. Some of them have been seen in normal cells, but most of them have been seen in pathological cells, including several types of tumour cells and many virus infected cells. The best interpretation one can put forward at the moment is that these are specialized forms of endoplasmic reticulum which occur in some normal cells and that they increase in frequency and variety as a reaction to various stimuli such as viral, hormonal and neoplasmic transformation.

Plate 229

From the liver of a chimpanzee inoculated with serum from a patient with non-A, non-B hepatitis (*From a block of tissue supplied by Dr H.P. Dienes*)

Fig. 1. Part of large membrane complex found in the cytoplasm of a hepatocyte. ×41 000

Fig. 2. Higher-power view of a similar complex found in another hepatocyte. The appearances seen here suggest that this is a pouched membrane complex. One may interpret the double-membrane-bound circular profiles (arrowheads) as transverse sections through projections or pouches arising from tangentially cut membranes which present as grey areas (arrows) in this electron micrograph. The inset shows a double-walled circular profile lying in a dilated cisterna. Such a profile can be explained as a transverse section through a finger-like pouch protruding into a dilated cisterna of endoplasmic reticulum. ×75 000, inset ×88 000

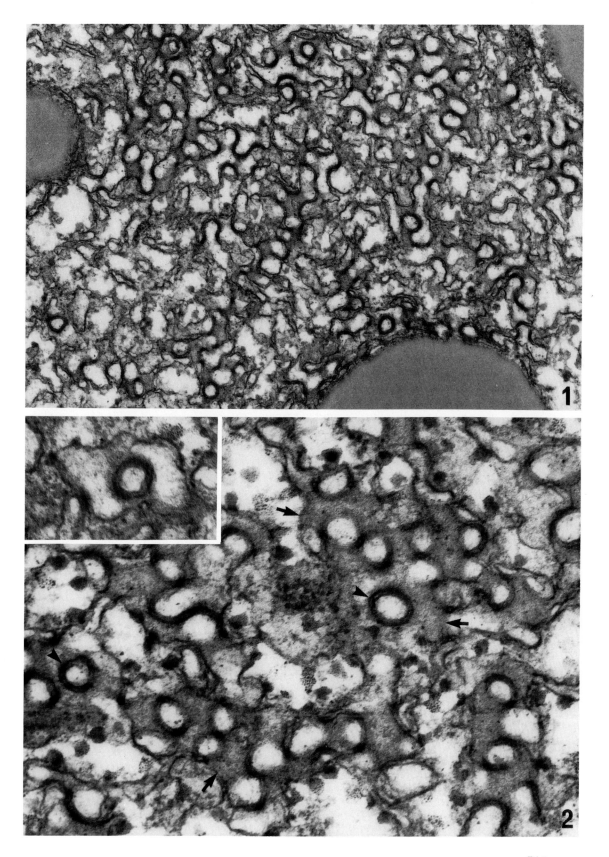

Membrane group: concentric membranous bodies of the endoplasmic reticulum

Some of the members of this group have been dealt with earlier (pages 510–515). Here we will deal with those members of the group which are characterized by a concentric arrangement of membranes. Such structures called 'concentric membranous bodies' (*Plates 230–233*) are derived from the endoplasmic reticulum* and they are usually composed of paired membrane arrays. Sequestrated at the centre of the concentric profiles of such bodies there lies a portion of the cell cytoplasm often containing some organelles and inclusions, particularly common being lipid droplets and mitochondria.

On a morphological basis, one might divide these concentric membranous bodies into three varieties: (1) those composed of rough endoplasmic reticulum; (2) those composed of smooth membranes; and (3) those composed of membranes in association with glycogen. However, intermediate forms occur which are difficult to classify in this fashion.

Terms such as 'ergastoplasmic Nebenkern' (Haguenau, 1958) or 'Nebenkern' may aptly be applied to those concentric membranous bodies composed of ribosome-studded membranes, for they are likely to present as juxtanuclear basophilic bodies at light microscopy. Terms such as 'myelin figures', 'myelinoid figures', and 'finger-prints' have been used to describe concentric membranous structures devoid of particles (i.e. ribosomes or glycogen). These are likely to present as eosinophilic bodies at light microscopy. The term 'glycogen body' was coined by Steiner *et al.* (1964) to describe bodies which contain both membrane and glycogen.

Most of the above-mentioned terms are acceptable, but terms such as 'myelin figures' and 'myelinoid figures' or 'bodies' should be avoided, for they relate to other structures such as the myelin figures produced at times by glutaraldehyde fixation (page 616) and the highly electron-dense membranous whorls found in certain lysosomes (pages 614–626). However, the situation is complicated somewhat by the fact that the membranous bodies may suffer degenerative changes and be converted into cytolysosomes (autolysosomes) and myelinosomes (i.e. lysosomes containing myelin figures), or myelin figures (*Plate 231, Fig. 2*).

It is said that concentric membranous bodies do not occur in normal liver (Steiner *et al.*, 1964) but they have often been observed in hepatocytes altered by disease or experimental procedure. Thus they have been seen in: (1) viral infections and viral hepatitis of man and mouse (Albot and Jézéquel, 1962; Leduc and Bernhard, 1962; Miyai *et al.*, 1963; McGavran and Easterday, 1963); (2) guinea-pig hepatocytes after the administration of diphtheria toxin (Caesar and Rapaport, 1963); (3) liver from a case of systemic lupus erythematosus (Shapiro *et al.*, 1985); (4) hepatomas, hepatocellular carcinomas and cholangiocarcinomas of man, rat and mouse (Fawcett and Wilson, 1955; Rouiller, 1957; Driessens *et al.*, 1959; Ghadially and Parry, 1966; Flaks, 1968; Moyer *et al.*, 1970; Ordóñez and Mackay, 1983) (*Plate 233*). Such bodies have also been seen in rat hepatocytes after the administration of: (5) DL-ethionine (Herman *et al.*, 1962; Steiner *et al.*, 1964; Shinozuka *et al.*, 1970); (6) thioacetamide (Salomon, 1962a, b; Rouiller and Simon, 1962; Thoenes, 1962; Thoenes and Bannasch, 1962); (7) α-naphthylisothiocyanate (Steiner and Baglio, 1963); (8) dimethylnitrosamine (Benedetti and Emmelot, 1960; Emmelot and Benedetti, 1960, 1961); (9) thiohydantoin compound (Bax 4222) (Herdson *et al.*, 1964a;

---

*Cup-shaped mitochondria, particularly when they form chondriospheres can produce another variety of concentric membranous body (page 282). However, such bodies are usually distinguishable on the basis of their morphology and alterations in adjoining mitochondria. In this section we deal only with concentric membranous bodies derived from the endoplasmic reticulum.

Plate 230

From a hepatocyte of a rat treated with yellow phosphorus. The membranes of the rough endoplasmic reticulum have formed a whorl in the cytoplasm enclosing mitochondria and lipid droplets. ×21 000 (*Ganote and Otis, unpublished electron micrograph*)

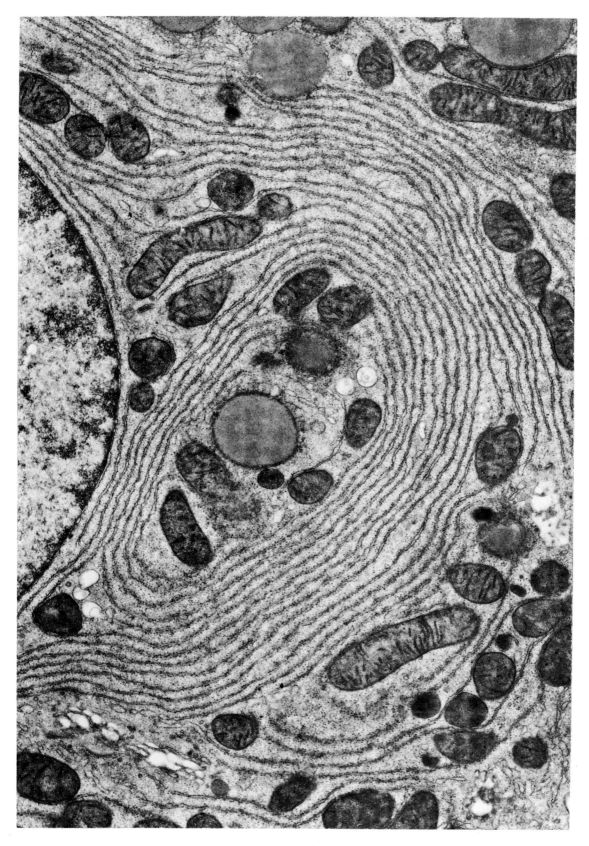

Herdson and Kaltenbach, 1965); (10) N-2-fluorenyldiacetamide (Mikata and Luse, 1964); (11) aflatoxin B1 (Svoboda *et al.*, 1966); (12) carbon tetrachloride (Stenger, 1964, 1966); (13) yellow phosphorus (Ganote and Otis, 1969) (*Plate 230*); (14) dichlorodiphenyltrichloroethane (DDT) (Ortega *et al.*, 1956); (15) phenobarbitone (Herdson *et al.*, 1964b; Burger and Herdson, 1966) (*Plate 232, Fig. 1*); (16) toxic fat (Norback and Allen, 1969); and (17) fructose (Phillips *et al.*, 1970).

Besides altered hepatocytes, a variety of other normal and pathologically altered cells have shown concentric membranous bodies in their cytoplasm. These include: (1) germinal epithelial cells of the testes of guinea-pigs (Fawcett and Ito, 1958); (2) testicular interstitial cells of 28-day-old mice (Ichihara, 1970); (3) lutein cells of rabbit ovary (Blanchette, 1966); (4) spermatocytes of *Ascaris megalocephala* (Favard, 1958); (5) oocyte of *Spisula solidissima* (Rebhun, 1961); (6) parietal endoderm cells of guinea-pig yolk sac (King, 1971); (7) acinar cells of salivary gland in *Chironomus* larvae (Haguenau, 1958); (8) transitional epithelium of urinary bladder of mouse (Walker, 1960); (9) sympathetic ganglion cells of the rat (Palay and Palade, 1955); (10) sensory nerve fibres of cat muscle spindles (Corvaja *et al.*, 1971); (11) ciliated epithelium of rabbit fallopian tube (Le Beux, 1969); (12) adrenal cortical cells of cat, guinea-pig and hamster (Cotte, 1959); (13) oxyphil cells of parathyroid in monkey (Trier, 1958); (14) pancreatic acinar cells of the rat after DL-ethionine (Herman and Fitzgerald, 1962; Herman *et al.*, 1962), and of the mouse after fasting and re-feeding (Weiss, 1953); (15) argyrophil cells of gastric mucosa of mouse after fasting and water deprivation (Helander, 1961); (16) Rous sarcoma cells (Epstein, 1957b); (17) oestrogen-induced pituitary adenoma (Haguenau, 1958); (18) Ehrlich ascites tumour cells infected with Newcastle virus (Adams and Prince, 1959); (19) 7,12 dimethyl-benz-α-anthracine-induced subcutaneous sarcoma (*Plate 232, Fig. 2*); (20) parathyroid adenomas of man (Elliott and Arhelger★, 1966) (*Plate 231, Fig. 1*); and (21) secondary deposit of an adenocarcinoma in the lung (*Plate 231, Fig. 2*).

A study of the above mentioned literature shows that probably the most common type of concentric membranous body is that composed of smooth membranes but concentric membranous bodies composed of ribosome-studded membranes are also quite common and both varieties may be found in the same situations. Much rarer by comparison is the glycogen body. However, it is difficult to classify all concentric membranous bodies in this fashion for often the membranes are sparsely populated with ribosomes or some of the concentric whorls

---

★Besides concentric membranous bodies derived from the rough endoplasmic reticulum, Elliott and Arhelger (1966) illustrate a concentric membranous body derived from annulate lamellae.

Plate 231

Fig. 1. Parathyroid adenoma. A tumour cell showing a concentric membranous body composed of ribosome studded membranes. ×36 000

Fig. 2. Secondary deposit of adenocarcinoma in the lung. A tumour cell showing a large myelin figure which is presumed to have developed from whorled endoplasmic reticulum. The peripheral paired membranes of this structure appears to be continuous with the endoplasmic reticulum in the cell. ×16 000

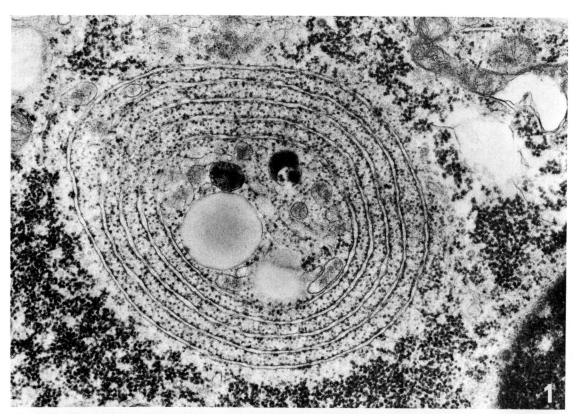

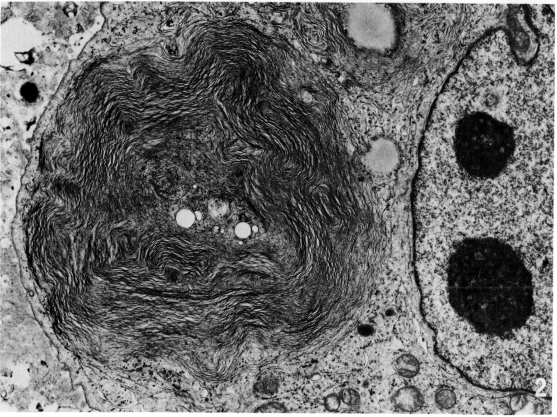

are devoid of ribosomes while others bear ribosomes. It is difficulties of this type and difficulties in interpreting some not too clear electron micrographs or statements about what was actually observed which have led to the presentation of the amorphous list above. However, the glycogen body has attracted much attention and these bodies with their picturesque morphology are more readily identified; hence a list of the situations in which they have been seen is now presented.

The glycogen body★ has been found in: (1) hepatocytes under various experimental and pathological conditions (Steiner *et al.*, 1964; Biava and Mukhlova-Montiel, 1965; Porta *et al.*, 1965); (2) human and rat hepatoma cells (Ghadially and Parry, 1966; Flaks, 1968) (*Plate 233*); (3) striated muscle cells of rat, mouse and rabbit (Heuson-Stiennon and Drochmans, 1967; Schiaffino and Hanlíková, 1972; Davidowitz *et al.*, 1983); (4) endodermal cells of fetal yolk sac of man and guinea-pig (Hoyes, 1969; King, 1971); (5) ciliated epithelial cells of the fallopian tube of rabbit (Le Beux, 1968, 1969); (6) glial cells of rat spinal cord in culture (Bunge *et al.*, 1965); (7) neurons from spinal ganglia of rat, guinea-pig, rabbit and hamster (Pannese, 1969; Hirano, 1978); (8) sympathetic neurons of cat (Seïte, 1969); (9) sensory nerve fibres of cat muscle spindle (Corvaja *et al.*, 1971); (10) photoreceptor cells of various vertebrates (here the glycogen body has been called a 'paraboloid') (Carasso, 1960; Yamada, 1960; Cohen, 1963; Petit, 1968); and (11) maternal elements (glandular and decidual cells) of placenta of the cat (Malassine, 1974).

A variety of structures such as lipid droplets, mitochondria and microbodies have been found at the centre of concentric membranous bodies. A reasonable assumption would be that this is fortuitous and not meaningful.

★Other terms used to describe the glycogen body include 'glycogen-membrane complexes' and 'glycogen membrane arrays'. The term 'glycogen body' has also been used to describe a certain type of intranuclear glycogen inclusions (*see* page 102).

Plate 232

Fig. 1. From a hepatocyte of a hamster treated with phenobarbitone. A smooth-membraned concentric body is seen enclosing a portion of cytoplasm containing numerous mitochondria and two microbodies, one of which contains glycogen. The significance of this unusual finding (glycogen in a microbody) is obscure. (*See* page 778 for further details.) ×18 000

Fig. 2. A membranous body in a tumour cell. From a fibrosarcoma produced in the flank of a rat by injection of 7,12 dimethyl-benz-α-anthracene. ×12 000 (*Ghadially and Parry, unpublished electron micrograph*)

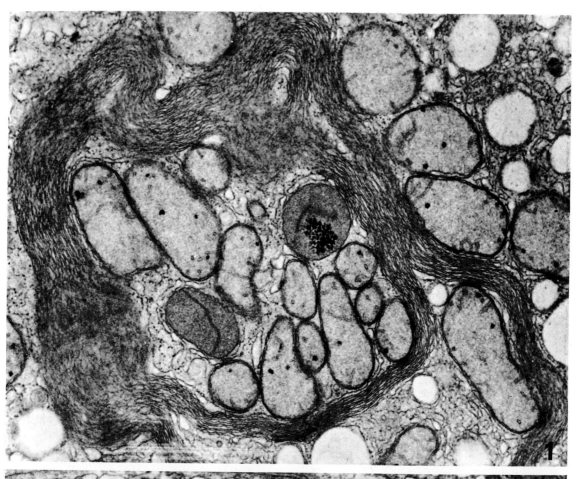

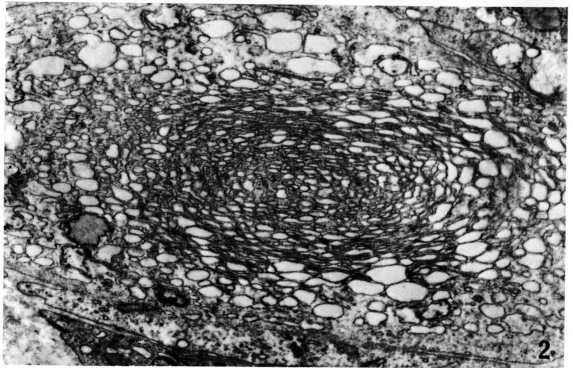

Since continuities between the peripheral membranes of smooth-membraned bodies and adjacent rough endoplasmic reticulum in the cell have been observed, it has been proposed that these membranous bodies represent either (1) a new formation of smooth endoplasmic reticulum, or that (2) they are produced by a degranulation of pre-existing rough endoplasmic reticulum. Both mechanisms are probably operative but often the amount of membranous material is so abundant that it is difficult to reconcile this as being derived solely by degranulation of pre-existing rough endoplasmic reticulum. There is now much evidence indicating that the biogenesis of the membranes of the smooth endoplasmic reticulum occurs in the rough endoplasmic reticulum where the necessary protein synthesis and the incorporation of lipid involved is achieved (Dallner et al., 1966; Jones and Fawcett, 1966). Thus, the concentric membranes in these bodies could be regarded as modified smooth endoplasmic reticulum arising from the rough endoplasmic reticulum, as does the normal smooth endoplasmic reticulum in the hepatocyte.

Broadly speaking, two views have been expressed regarding the nature of concentric membranous bodies: (1) that they represent a degenerative change or an elaborate autophagic vacuole; and (2) that this is a regenerative change leading to a specialized type of hypertrophy of the endoplasmic reticulum which may have a functional significance. Since cytomembranes clearly in excess of normal occur at least in the larger concentric membranous bodies, and since no limiting membrane is apparent, the second hypothesis seems more attractive.

There is little doubt, however, that these concentric membranous bodies found in various sites and situations, may suffer degenerative changes and that they can ultimately transform into large myelin figures (*Plate 231, Fig. 2*). For example, such a sequence of events is well depicted by Cassier (1979) in the *Corpora allata* of the adult female migratory locust (*Locusta migratoria migratorioides*) where large concentric whorls of smooth endoplasmic reticulum are transformed into myelin figures during oviposition and the following two days.

The concentric smooth membrane arrays produced as a result of drugs may be looked upon as a specialized type of smooth endoplasmic reticulum hypertrophy and one may speculate that this probably helps in the detoxication of drugs, as does the smooth endoplasmic reticulum in the hepatocyte (pages 458–461). The association of glycogen with some of these membrane systems is reminiscent of its close association with the smooth endoplasmic reticulum in the hepatocyte (page 422).

Since the rough endoplasmic reticulum is involved in the production of secretory proteins, one may speculate that the ribosome-studded membranous bodies may indicate enhanced protein secretory activity. This seems to be so at least in the spermatocytes of *Ascaris megalocephala* (Favard, 1958).

The significance of the occurrence of concentric membranous bodies in hepatomas and other neoplasms is obscure, but one may speculate that it represents yet another example of atypical or exaggerated growth associated with the neoplastic state.

Plate 233
A glycogen body found in a human hepatoma. ×23 000 (*Ghadially and Parry, unpublished electron micrograph*)

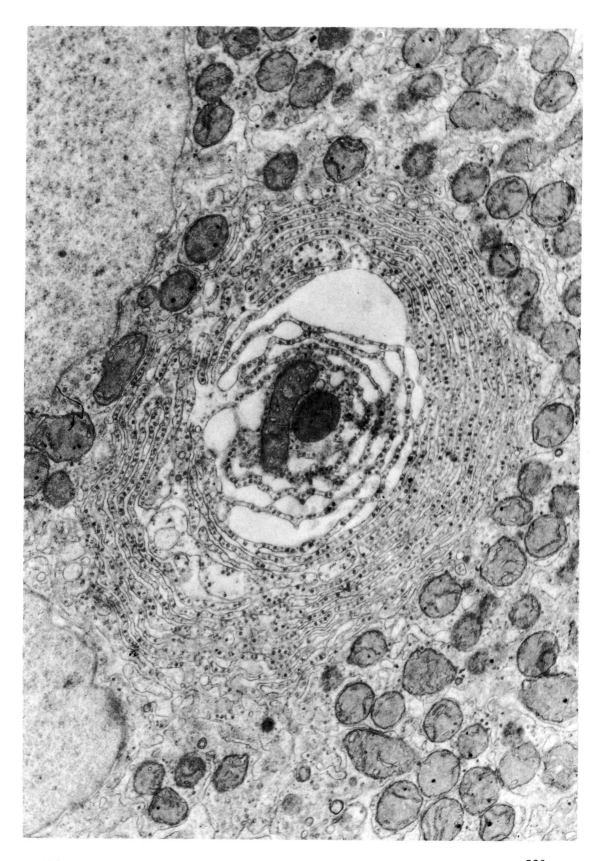

Glycogen in rough endoplasmic reticulum

Although typically glycogen occurs in the cytoplasmic matrix (page 962) in certain physiological and pathological states glycogen has also been found in other cell compartments such as the nucleus (page 100), mitochondrion (page 288), microbody (*Plate 232*) and the lysosome (page 720). In a few instances, glycogen has been seen within dilated and vesiculated cisternae of the rough endoplasmic reticulum. Such examples include: (1) hypobranchial gland of certain molluscs (Fain-Maurel, 1966); (2) epididymal epithelial cells of golden hamsters (Fouquet, 1970); (3) murine pulmonary adenomas (Flaks and Flaks, 1969); (4) a canine plasmacytoma (Ghadially *et al.*, 1977) (*Plate 234*); and (5) a malignant small cell chest wall tumour (Askin tumour?) from an 18-year-old male (Gaffney and Cottell, 1986)★.

Histochemical studies show that the plasma cells in the canine tumour had a pyroninophilic cytoplasm and contained numerous PAS-positive diastase sensitive particles. Electron microscopy revealed monoparticulate and rosette forms of glycogen in the rough endoplasmic reticulum and also monoparticulate glycogen (rare rosettes were also present) in mitochondria. However, no glycogen could be detected in the cytoplasmic matrix.

As we have already noted (page 422) cell fractionation studies have shown that the main enzymes of glycogen metabolism lie in the cytoplasmic matrix (i.e. the soluble fraction) and not the endoplasmic reticulum (microsomal fraction), the only exception being glucose-6-phosphatase which is associated with the endoplasmic reticulum.

The occurrence of glycogen in various other cell compartments besides the cytoplasmic matrix raises grave doubts as to whether glycogen-synthesizing enzymes are really so restricted in their distribution and whether the situation varies from cell type to cell type and in pathological states. In each instance at least two main possibilities have to be considered: (1) that glycogen from the cytoplasmic matrix was transported into another cellular compartment; or (2) that some or all the stages of glycogen synthesis occurred in the atypical site.

In the case of intranuclear glycogen in hepatoma cells, Karasaki (1971) has provided experimental evidence supporting the idea that synthesis of glycogen occurs in the nucleus, while in the case of intramitochondrial glycogen Tandler *et al.* (1970) concluded that 'at a minimum oncocytoma mitochondria possess the enzymes necessary to convert β-glycogen to α-glycogen'; because while only monoparticulate glycogen (β-form) was present in the cytoplasm, glycogen rosettes (α-form) were found in mitochondria.

In our (Ghadially *et al.*, 1977) plasmacytoma monoparticulate glycogen was found in mitochondria while both monoparticulate and rosette forms were found in the endoplasmic reticulum. Since no glycogen could be detected in the cytoplasm it would appear that synthesis of glycogen was occurring both in the mitochondria and in the rough endoplasmic reticulum of the neoplastic plasma cells.

★These authors presented this tumour as a case for discussion by the panel in *Ultrastructural Pathology*. There is no doubt whatsoever that their illustrations show glycogen in endoplasmic reticulum (partially degranulated rough endoplasmic reticulum), yet they erroneously imagine that they are glycogen-ER complexes or glycogen bodies (page 520), and so does one of the panel members (Rosai) who adds 'I have seen them in several human tumours'. Other members of the panel (Erlandson, Ghadially and Mierau) correctly distinguish these structures from glycogen bodies and point out that they have not seen glycogen in the endoplasmic reticulum in human material that they have examined. It is difficult to understand how one can confuse glycogen in the endoplasmic reticulum for glycogen bodies.

Plate 234

This plasmacytoma was collected by a veterinarian in neutral buffered formalin. Upon receipt three days later small pieces of the tumour were fixed in 1 per cent osmium tetroxide in phosphate buffer and processed in the usual way for electron microscopy. Despite this treatment the preservation of ultrastructural morphology is not too bad. (*From Ghadially, Lowes and Mesfin, 1977*)

Fig. 1. Dilated cisternae of the rough endoplasmic reticulum containing glycogen. ×28 000

Fig. 2. Vesiculated rough endoplasmic reticulum containing glycogen. ×18 000

Fig. 3. High-power view showing monoparticulate and rosette forms of glycogen in the rough endoplasmic reticulum. ×44 000

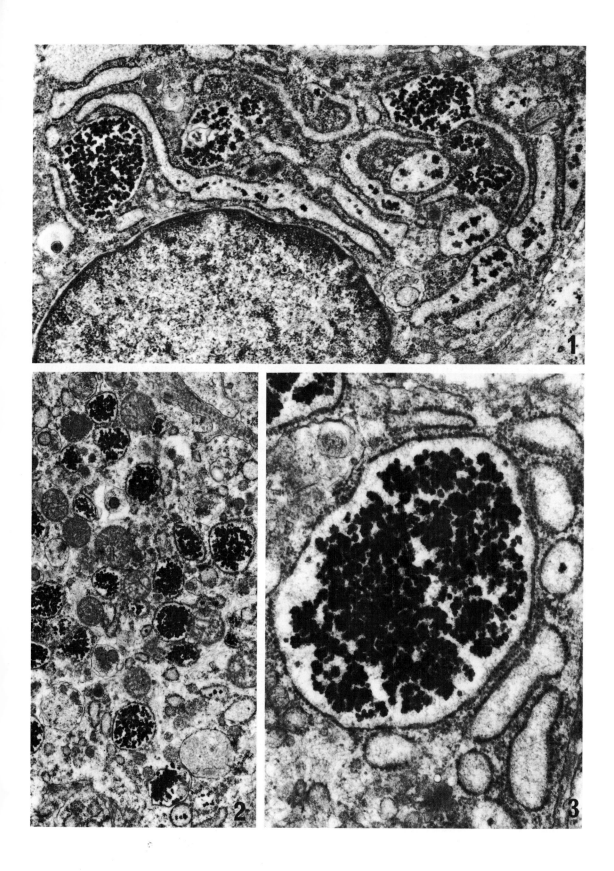

Lipid in endoplasmic reticulum (liposomes)

Lipids (triglycerides) generally occur as non-membrane-bound droplets lying free within the cytoplasm of various cell types. Occasionally, however, lipid droplets may be found in the endoplasmic reticulum (*Plate 235*), and also in the Golgi complex★. Such deposits may present in various ways, such as lipid droplets lying within: (1) dilated cisternae of the rough endoplasmic reticulum; (2) ribosome-studded vesicles clearly derived from the rough endoplasmic reticulum; or (3) smooth membrane-bound vesicles and tubules representing or derived from the Golgi complex, smooth endoplasmic reticulum or degranulated rough endoplasmic reticulum.

Such membrane-bound lipidic bodies, particularly those encountered in the liver, are often called liposomes†—a term first introduced by Baglio and Farber (1965b) to describe these bodies in rat hepatocytes.

A few liposomes may be found in the livers of fasted but otherwise normal rats (Baglio and Farber, 1965b; Stein and Stein, 1965). Liposomes in great number, however, are characteristic of fatty livers where an abnormal accumulation of triglycerides is occurring. Since a large number of drugs, dietary regimens and experimental procedures can produce fatty livers, liposomes have frequently been observed and studied (for details and references, *see* Schlunk and Lombardi, 1967; Stenger, 1970).

Thus, shortly after the administration of agents such as carbon tetrachloride, ethionine, orotic acid or yellow phosphorus, membrane-bound lipidic material collects in the hepatocytes (*Plate 235*). Later much larger non-membrane-bound lipidic droplets appear in the cytoplasm of the hepatocyte but it is not clear how these evolve from the membrane-bound liposomes. One can only speculate that a dissolution of membranes and fusion of smaller droplets to form larger ones probably occurs.

The lipidic nature of liposomes was indicated by the histochemical studies of Novikoff *et al.* (1964), and this has now been amply confirmed by isolation and chemical characterization studies such as those of Schlunk and Lombardi (1967), which show that isolated liposomes contain mainly neutral fat.

Many theories have been advanced to explain the occurrence of liposomes and fatty livers, and it is clear that not all drugs produce this change in precisely the same fashion. However, one

★The occurrence of lipid and lipoprotein in the Golgi complex has already been discussed on page 344. This topic is so closely linked with the subject dealt with in this section that it is recommended that both sections are read conjointly.
†The term 'liposomes' is now also used to describe micelles of enzymes or drugs sequestrated in lipidic particles (Gregoriadis, 1976), but these 'liposomes' do not concern us here. However, in passing one may note that the liposomes in such therapeutic preparations can 'home' selectively into lysosomes. Thus it is possible that with this method one may be able to make good the deficiency of certain lysosomal enzymes in lysosomal diseases. However, the most dramatic result to date is in the treatment of experimental leishmaniasis (Black *et al.*, 1977; Alving *et al.*, 1978; New *et al.*, 1978) where there is a parasitic infestation of the reticuloendothelial cells. Treatment with liposome-encapsulated antimony salts has been found to be more than 300 times as effective as the antimonal drug alone.

Plate 235

Liver of a rat given yellow phosphorus, showing numerous liposomes (L) which have collected mainly near the vascular pole of the hepatocytes. There was a marked hypertrophy of the smooth endoplasmic reticulum in this liver. This, combined with the fact that the liposomes are covered with a smooth membrane, and many show a tubular profile, suggests that the lipid accumulated in the smooth endoplasmic reticulum. In hepatocytes the Golgi complex is often located adjacent to the cell membrane in the same position as some of the liposomes. Hence one may speculate that some of the liposomes could also have been derived from the Golgi complex. Some of the liposomes (arrows) appear to have lost lipid during processing. This permits a good demonstration of the membrane covering liposomes. ×27 000

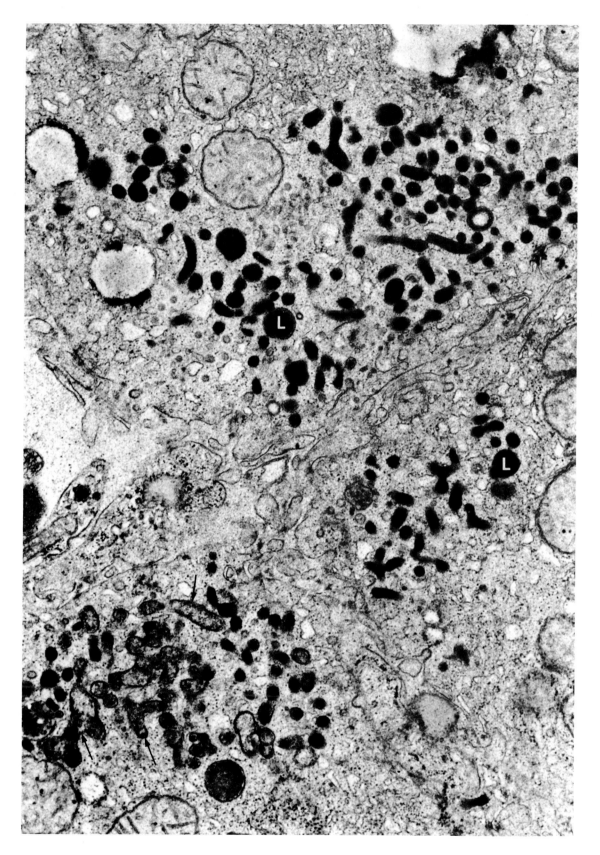

concept that seems applicable in many instances and has gained wide acceptance is that lipid accumulation is secondary to depressed protein synthesis, a point supported by the disorganization of rough endoplasmic reticulum which is so commonly seen in such livers (page 436). It is believed that in the normal situation a lipid acceptor protein is produced by the rough endoplasmic reticulum and this combines with triglycerides to form very low-density lipoproteins which are then released in the blood. It has hence been argued by many workers that any toxic agent which damages the rough endoplasmic reticulum and depresses the synthesis of this protein but not the synthesis of triglyceride will lead to a pathological accumulation of fat in the liver (for references, *see* Stenger, 1970). Other mechanisms that have been evoked to explain fat accumulation in the liver include: (1) ineffective coupling of lipid and acceptor protein; (2) impaired release of lipoproteins from liver to blood; (3) hypermobilization of free fatty acids from fat stores; and (4) enhanced lipogenesis.

However, as already indicated, liposome formation is not necessarily a pathological phenomenon. It may be no more than a morphological expression of fatty acid esterification in the endoplasmic reticulum. Membrane-enclosed lipids acceptable as liposomes have been described and isolated by Sheldon (1964) and by Angel and Sheldon (1965) for adipose tissue cells engaged in active triglyceride synthesis, and it is now well known that the endoplasmic reticulum of intestinal epithelial cells comes to contain lipid droplets during fat absorption (Palay and Karlin, 1959; Onoe and Ohno, 1963; Fawcett, 1981) (*Plate 236*).

Since, in the latter example, lipid can be demonstrated in pinocytotic vesicles, argument has raged as to whether this is how the bulk of the lipid is picked up and the endoplasmic reticulum merely transports the lipid or whether most of the lipid is first hydrolysed and the fatty acids are picked up and resynthesized into triglycerides within the endoplasmic reticulum. There is now much evidence to support the latter concept.

The role of the microsomal fraction (derived from endoplasmic reticulum) in fatty acid esterification is now well-established (Stein and Shapiro, 1959; Hultin, 1961; Tzur and Shapiro, 1964) and considerable evidence has also accumulated which shows that, although some cells (e.g. neutrophils and Kupffer cells) can pick up lipid by a process of pinocytosis or phagocytosis generally in the majority of instances, the lipid is first hydrolysed and the fatty acids are picked up and the lipid is resynthesized in the endoplasmic reticulum. Such a concept has been evoked to explain lipid uptake in many tissues, such as adipose, mammary, hepatic, cartilage, cardiac and skeletal muscle (Stein and Stein, 1967; Scow, 1970; Ghadially *et al.*, 1970; Mehta and Ghadially, 1973; Sprinz and Stockwell, 1976).

Plate 236

Intestinal epithelial cells during fat absorbtion. From a rat that had been given 1 ml of corn oil by stomach tube. Sample of gut (one inch from the pylorus) was collected 1 hour later.

Fig. 1. Longitudinal section through an intestinal epithelial cell showing osmiophilic lipid droplets (L) within membrane-bound vacuoles. ×17 000

Fig. 2. Transverse section through a deeper part (as compared with *Fig.1*) of intestinal epithelial cells showing lipid in; Golgi-associated vacuoles (G), several other membrane-bound vacuoles (V), and in the intercellular space (S). ×19 500

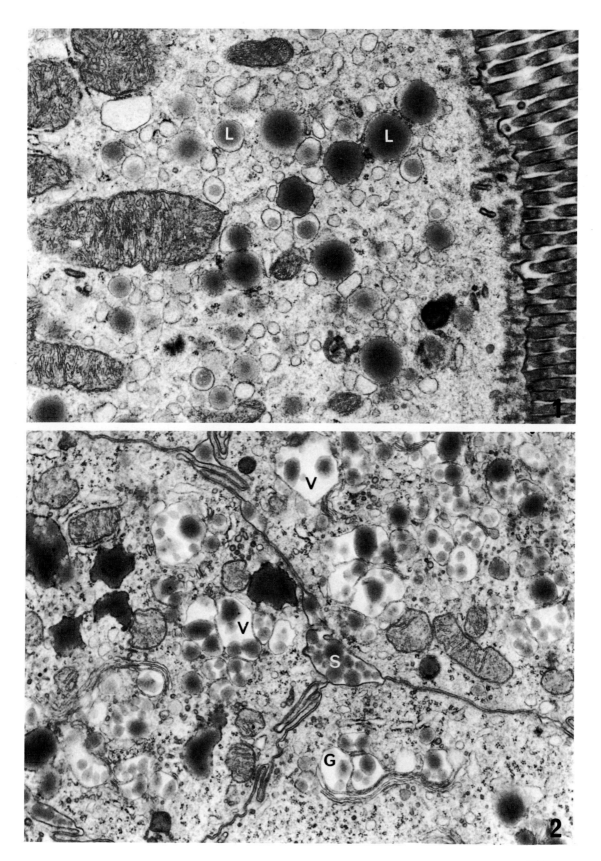

Proteinaceous granules and crystalline inclusions in rough endoplasmic reticulum

As a rule, the contents of the rough endoplasmic reticulum are fairly homogeneous and usually of medium or low electron density. One therefore gets the impression that the proteinaceous secretion in the rough endoplasmic reticulum exists in a fairly dilute state. The power to concentrate this material into the more electron-dense secretory granules is thought to lie in the Golgi complex and not in the rough endoplasmic reticulum itself.

However, exceptions to these generalizations exist and it is clear that in some circumstances the secretory products can become concentrated in the rough endoplasmic reticulum and the proteinaceous material then presents as medium- or high-density granules or bodies within the dilated cisternae (*Plate 237–240, Fig. 1*). In some instances the proteinaceous material separates out not as amorphous granules but as crystals (*Plate 240, Fig. 2* and *Plates 241* and *242*). In most instances the composition of these granules is a matter of conjecture. Since they occur in the rough endoplasmic reticulum there is strong presumptive evidence that they contain protein. In some situations, however, they could represent glycoprotein (e.g. Russell bodies in plasma cells, *see below*). Hence the term 'proteinaceous granules' is used here.

An interesting example of this phenomenon is seen in the pancreatic acinar cells. Here, normally, the protein-rich secretion produced in the rough endoplasmic reticulum is transported to the Golgi complex and condensed to form zymogen granules. However, in some animals, such as the guinea-pig, dog and cat, small electron-dense granules resembling zymogen granules are also found in occasional dilated cisternae of the rough endoplasmic reticulum (Palade, 1956; Ichikawa, 1965; Fawcett, 1966; Brown and Still, 1970). Intracisternal dense granules have also been noted in the pancreas of rats kept on a protein-free diet or following the administration of various agents such as ethionine, puromycine or colchicine (Herman *et al.*, 1964; Longnecker *et al.*, 1975; Seybold *et al.*, 1975). The situation in the normal human pancreas is not known but intracisternal granules have been seen in a human pancreas in the Zollinger-Ellison syndrome (Brown and Schatzki, 1971) and in the neoplastic cells of a giant cell tumour* of the pancreas (Rosai, 1968). The proteinaceous nature of the granules in the pancreatic tumour was confirmed by their sensitivity to pepsin.

*Somewhat larger medium density granules were also present in the stromal cells of this tumour.

Plate 237

Figs. 1 and 2. Tumour cells from a well differentiated osteogenic sarcoma of man, showing dilated and vesiculated rough endoplasmic reticulum containing numerous electron-dense granules (G) thought to be proteinaceous in nature. ×32 000; ×27 000 (*Fig. 1, Ghadially and Mehta, unpublished electron micrograph; Fig. 2, from Ghadially and Mehta, 1970*)

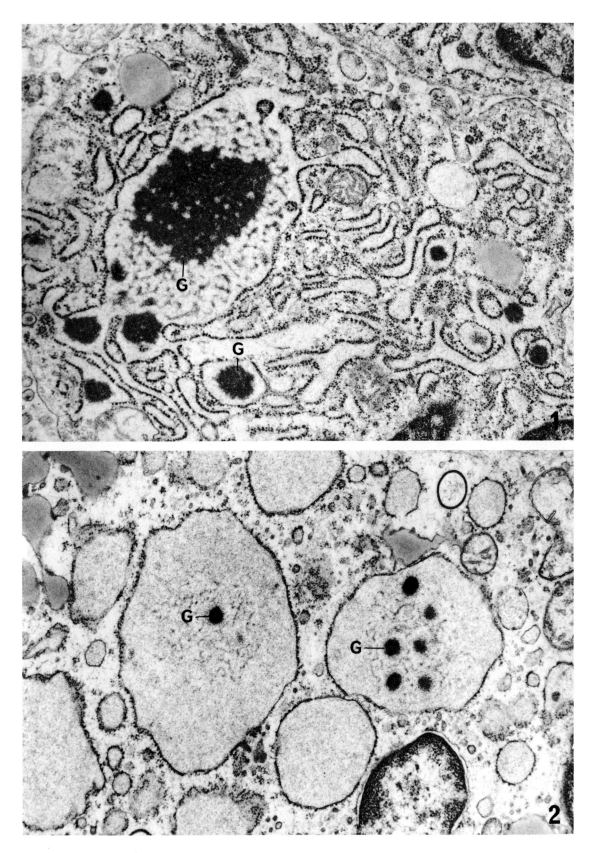

531

The true significance of these pancreatic intracisternal granules is not clear. At one time it was thought (Siekevitz and Palade, 1958) that this might be an intermediate step in zymogen granule formation in some species where a condensation of proteinaceous material occurred not only in the Golgi complex but also in the rough endoplasmic reticulum. However, autoradiographic studies have cast doubt on this thesis because no significant labelling of these intracisternal granules was found during zymogen granule production (Caro and Palade, 1964). This, taken in conjunction with the fact that intracisternal granules are seen in ethionine-treated but not normal rats*, has led to the idea that they could be the result of blockage of transport within the rough endoplasmic reticulum and subsequent concentration of products therein.

Such a concept is also supported by the fact that intracisternal dense granules have been seen in pathological tissues, particularly tumours, where one can with some justification also speculate that the rough endoplasmic reticulum may be malformed and the passage of substances impeded.

Besides the above mentioned examples, intracisternal granules (i.e. dense granules, reticulated granules and medium density granules) have been seen in: (1) Paneth cells of the rat (Behnke and Moe, 1964); (2) crayfish oocytes (Beams and Kessel, 1962, 1963); (3) endosperm of barley grain (Buttrose et al., 1960); (4) glomerular endothelial cells in a case of Alport's syndrome (Sengel and Stoebner, 1971); (5) podocytes in a case of Imerslund-Najman-Gräsbeck syndrome (intrinsic factor independent vitamin B_{12} malabsorption with a benign nephropathy) (Rumpelt and Michl, 1979); (6) human giant cell tumour of bone (Boquist et al., 1976); (7) human carcinoma of the breast (Hollman, 1959); (8) osteogenic sarcoma of man (Plate 237) (Ghadially and Mehta, 1970); (9) type B synovial cells from cases of rheumatoid arthritis (Plate 240, Fig. 1) (Ghadially and Roy, 1969); (10) hepatomas of man and mouse (Norkin and Campagna-Pinto, 1968; Keeley et al., 1972; Smetana et al., 1972; Dekker and Krause, 1973; Palmer and Wolfe, 1976; Helyer and Petrelli, 1978) (Plate 238); (11) human liver in cases of α_1-antitrysin deficiency (Eriksson and Larsson, 1975; Yunis et al., 1976); and (12) secretory cells of the venom gland of the South American rattlesnake (Warshawsky et al., 1973).

*Strangely enough the converse appears to be true in the case of the dog. Intracisternal granules occur in the normal dog pancreatic cells but they disappear when pancreatitis is induced by the administration of staphylococcal α-toxin (Schoning et al., 1972). This is probably explainable by the disaggregation of polyribosomes that also occurs, for this would inhibit protein synthesis and hence intracisternal granule production.

Plate 238

Fig. 1. Reticulated intracisternal dense granules found in spontaneous hepatomas of mice. ×18 000 (*From Helyer and Petrelli, 1978*)

Fig. 2. High-power view of intracisternal granules showing reticular structure. ×24 000 (*Petrelli, unpublished electron micrograph*)

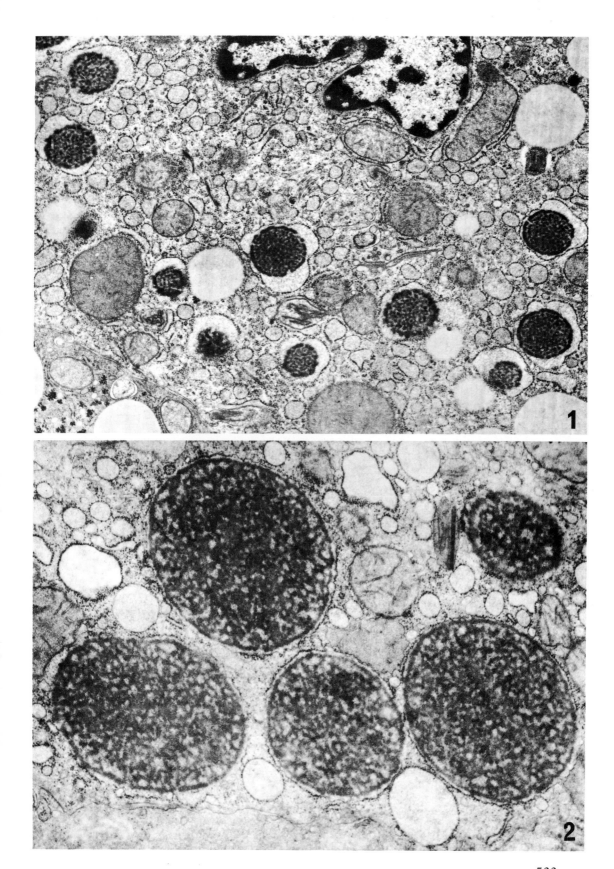

Autoradiographic studies on venom production have led Warshawsky *et al.* (1973) to conclude that 'the interstitial granules are not a part of the main sequence in the secretion of venom protein' and that 'they may represent a storage form of immature protein which condenses out of the otherwise flocculent content of the distended rough endoplasmic reticulum cisternae'.

However, the best-known intracisternal dense granule is the one that occurs in plasma cells (*Plate 239*) and has long been known to light microscopists as the Russell body* (Russell, 1890; Stich *et al.*, 1955; Welsh, 1960; Sorenson, 1964; Zucker-Franklin, 1964). Although Russell thought that this body† was a fungus and an aetiological agent of cancer, it is now well known that this glycoprotein-rich body may be found in both reactive and neoplastic plasma cells and that its formation can be induced by immunization (White, 1954; Ortega and Mellors, 1957). Here, too, the idea that excessive production of secretory material and/or a disordered secretory mechanism is responsible appears tenable.

Much confusion exists in the literature regarding the ultrastructural equivalents of the many morphological (light microscopic) variations of the plasma cells, variously referred to as thesaurocytes, flame cells, Mott cells, morula cells and grape cells. An extended discussion on this point and the ultrastructural differences between these varieties of plasma cells is beyond the scope of this text (*see* instead Thiery, 1960). It would appear, however, that the above-mentioned variants reflect no more than the highly pleomorphic character of the rough endoplasmic reticulum and its contents in plasma cells. Illustrations in this chapter (*Plates 180, 199* and *239*) demonstrate this point; the cisternae can be collapsed, dilated or vesiculated and their contents can vary from electron-lucent to quite dense. At the end of this scale is the

*For Russell bodies in the nucleus *see* page 78.
†It would appear that Russell must have seen the bodies which now bear his name in reactive plasma cells found in or adjacent to tumours.

Plate 239

Figs. 1 and 2. Plasma cells showing dilated and vesiculated rough endoplasmic reticulum, containing numerous Russell-type bodies (R). The bodies shown here are somewhat small and would be difficult to discern with the light microscope, but larger bodies of the type shown would present as classic Russell bodies. From bronchial mucosa adjacent to a bronchial carcinoma. ×18 000; ×45 000

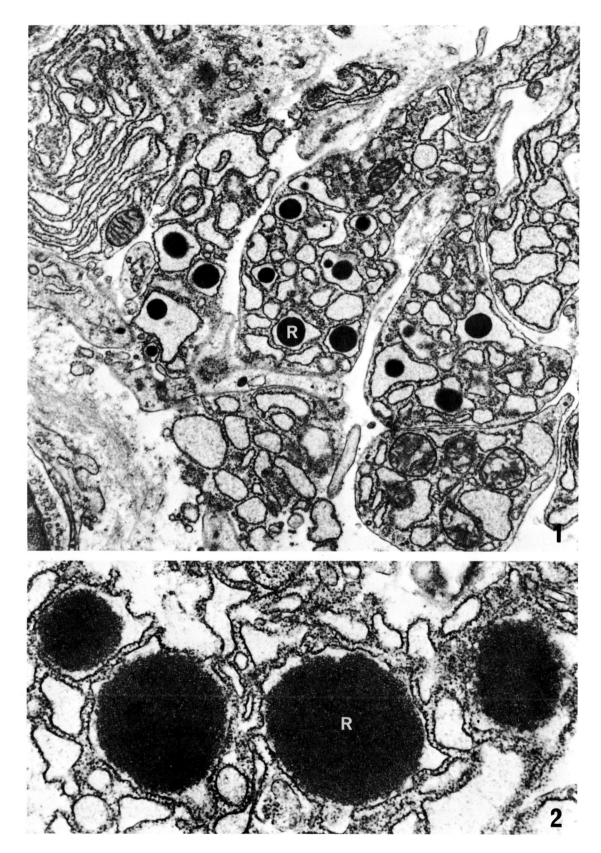

compact, rounded, electron-dense Russell body. In rare instances the proteins separate out to form crystals which are at times detectable by the light microscope and are clearly seen by electron microscopy to lie within the rough endoplasmic reticulum (*Plate 240, Fig. 2*) (for references, *see* Sanel and Lepore, 1968).

Crystals are not found in normal plasma cells, but they may be found in any state where there is increased immunoglobulin (or fraction thereof) production. Such conditions include: cryoglobulinaemia, macroglobulinaemia, of Waldenstrom's disease, or the hyperglobulinaemia of multiple myeloma, plasmacytoma or hyperimmune states. Crystals have also been found in reactive plasma cells of an equine granuloma (Wilkie, unpublished observation) (*Plate 241*). Plasmacytoid cells and immunoblasts (*Plate 240, Fig. 2* and *Plate 416*) also at times contain crystals. The crystals mentioned above generally lie in the rough endoplasmic reticulum, but they may be translocated into the cytoplasm, and when such cells disintegrate a collection of crystals is seen lying in the intercellular matrix (Schvartz *et al.*, 1985).

Besides the examples mentioned above, crystalline or paracrystalline inclusions in the endoplasmic reticulum have been seen in: (1) Paneth cells of the rat (Behnke and Moe, 1964); (2) dog hepatocytes (Gueft and Kikkawa, 1962); (3) liver of slender salamander (Hamilton *et al.*, 1966; Fawcett, 1981); (4) submucosal gland cells of the fowl proventriculus (Toner, 1963);

Plate 240

Fig. 1. A type B synovial cell from a case of rheumatoid arthritis, showing medium-density proteinaceous granules (G) in dilated rough endoplasmic reticulum. ×50 000 (*Ghadially and Roy, unpublished electron micrograph*)

Fig. 2. Part of the cytoplasm of a plasmacytoid cell from a case of Hodgkin's disease, showing crystalline inclusions (C) lying within the cisternae (between arrows) of the rough endoplasmic reticulum. ×110 000 (*From Sanel and Lepore, 1968*)

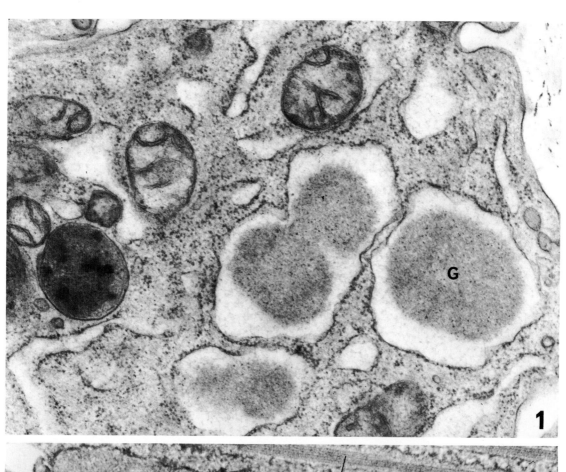

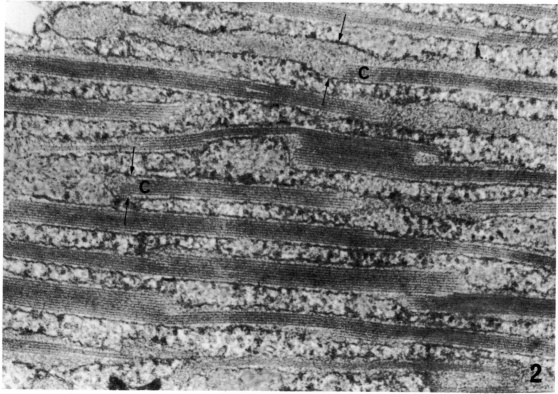

(5) root cells of radish (Bonnett and Newcomb, 1965); (6) spinal cord of the lung fish (*Polypterus enlicheri*) and the aquarium guppy (*Poecila reticulata*) (Marquet and Sobel, 1969); (7) malpighian tubules of the mosquito (*Celex tarsalis*) (Houk, 1977); (8) fat body of *Coccygomimus dispar*, a hymenopterous parasite of gipsy moth pupae (*Plate 242*); (9) parathyroid glands removed from patients with tertiary hyperparathyroidism (Cinti *et al.*, 1982; Krause and Hedinger, 1985) (*Plate 242*); and (10) human meningioma (Hammar *et al.*, 1983b).

Crystals in the rough endoplasmic reticulum resemble crystals in other sites such as those found in the nucleus and mitochondria. In sectioned material they can present long rod-like profiles or square, rectangular or polygonal profiles★. Their substructure is often difficult to establish but they may be composed of spherical units, short cylindrical units or filaments or microtubules. In sectioned material (depending upon the plane of sectioning) the most common profiles seen are a series of 'dots' and/or 'parallel lines'.

Regarding the mode of formation, the view repeatedly expressed in the literature is that crystals result from an excess of protein production and/or an 'obstruction' (mechanical or biochemical) to the flow of secretory products from the rough endoplasmic reticulum. Thus for example, Marquet and Sobel (1969) (item 6 above) noted that the frequency of crystalline inclusions was greater in lordotic than normal guppies, and it was postulated that 'the volume

---

★Those not familiar with the terms crystalline, paracrystalline and filamentous inclusions and profiles produced by these inclusions should consult pages 108 and 298.

Plate 241

Plasma cells from a granuloma on the face of a 3-year-old horse. (*From a block of tissue supplied by Dr I. Wilkie*)

Fig. 1. Pleomorphic profiles of intracisternal crystals are seen here. Note the crystal with a triangular profile (T), and another with a hexagonal profile (H). Two unusual hexagonal crystals (U) appear to have a hollow centre in which lies reticulated electron-dense material set in a flocculent or lucent matrix. It would appear that some of the central portion of the material in the rough endoplasmic reticulum precipitated out as electron-dense granules and strands, while the peripheral portion crystallized around it. ×14 000

Fig. 2. Portion of an intracisternal rectangular crystal (2 × 1.2 μm) showing striations with a periodicity of 17 nm. ×83 000

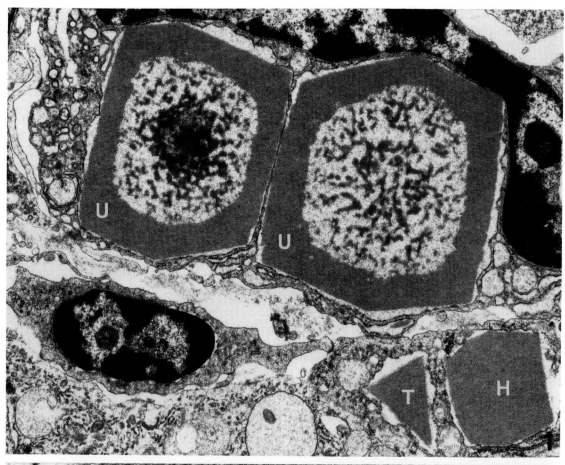

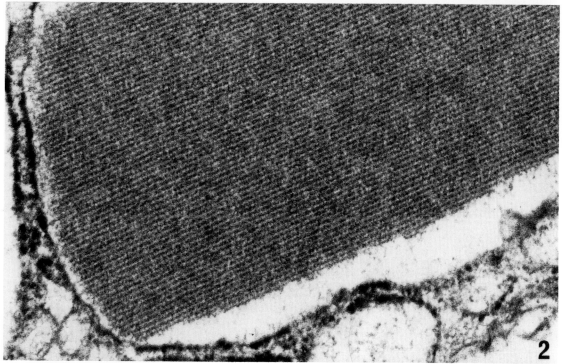

of protein produced exceeds the volume which the Golgi complex can package and which the cell can utilize*, and that subsequent accumulation and crystallization of this material occur in the nuclear envelope and dilated sacs of endoplasmic reticulum'. In some instances, however, intracisternal crystals may have a physiological role in the economy of the organism. Such a view is expressed by Fawcett (1966) regarding the protein crystals in the liver of the slender salamander; he states that 'they are presumed to be the storage form of a protein synthesized by the cell'.

The crystalline or paracrystalline inclusion which presents as rows of 'dots' (Plate 242, Fig. 2) in dilated rough endoplasmic reticulum was first described by Cinti et al. (1982). Since it was found in parathyroid cells from cases of tertiary parathyroidism Cinti et al. (1982) suggested that the globular particles in the dilated rough endoplasmic reticulum may represent proparathyroid hormone or some other protein unrelated to parathyroid hormone production. The discovery of identical inclusions in a meningioma by Hammar et al. (1983b) shows that this quite rare inclusion is not specific for parathyroids or for parathyroid hormone production.

It is generally assumed (and for good reasons) that virtually all crystals are composed of proteins but the proteins in crystals have rarely been characterized. Electron-probe x-ray analysis has shown that the crystals in the rough endoplasmic reticulum in the gipsy moth contain iron (Adams, personal communication and my own analysis of these crystals). The particles in these crystals are too large to be ferritin molecules but they could be aggregates of such molecules. However this would leave unexplained how the ferritin got into the rough endoplasmic reticulum, for ferritin is synthesized by polyribosomes lying free in the cytoplasm. If we consider them to be haemosiderin crystals then once more we are faced with the same dilemma, because haemosiderin is a substance derived from the breakdown of haemoglobin in lysosomes (see pages 636–645).

*This statement is correct but a bit off the mark because the rough endoplasmic reticulum usually produces export proteins and not proteins which the cell utilizes.

Plate 242

Fig. 1. A lipocyte from the fat body of a hymenopterous parasite of gipsy moth pupae. The high electron density of the intracisternal crystals reflects the presence of iron in them. The crystals are probably composed of spherical subunits, which depending upon the plane of sectioning present as a series of dots or dotted lines. ×118 000 *(From a block of tissue supplied by Dr J.R. Adams)*

Fig. 2. Parathyroid cell from a case of tertiary hyperparathyroidism. This inclusion presents as two rows of 'dots' adjacent to membranes of a dilated segment of the rough endoplasmic reticulum. Because of the ordered arrangement this inclusion deserves to be called a crystalline inclusion. The true three-dimensional morphology of this inclusion is not known, but it is probably composed of sheets of spherical particles covering the inner surfaces of dilated rough endoplasmic reticulum cisternae. ×102 000 *(From Cinti, Osculati and Parravicini, 1982)*

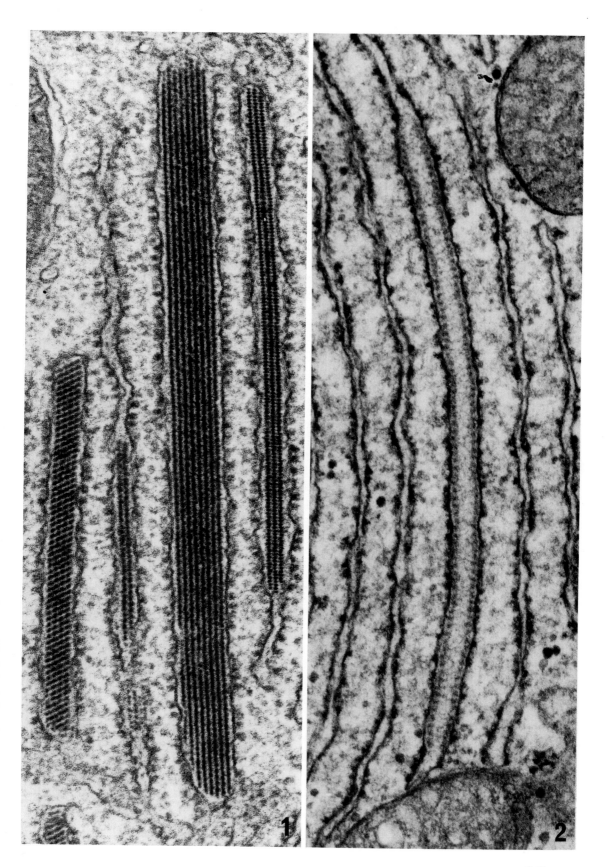

541

Laminated inclusions in rough endoplasmic reticulum

It would appear that large laminated inclusions* (*Plate 243*) in the rough endoplasmic reticulum have so far been found only in the chondrocytes of pseudochondroplastic dwarfs. Such affected chondrocytes have been seen in biopsies from the costochondral junction, iliac crest and epiphysis of long bones (Lindseth *et al.*, 1967; Phillips, 1970; Maynard *et al.*, 1972; Cooper *et al.*, 1973a, b).

In the report by Lindseth *et al.* (1967) only one small electron micrograph is presented and the inclusion is described as 'bodies of an unidentified nature within the chondrocytes'. The report by Phillips (1970) is a brief abstract which describes succinctly the inclusions as containing alternating dense and lucent lamellae repeating at a periodicity of 100–150 nm. These lamellae are said to have formed 'a distinct moiré pattern of the kind seen in watered silk'.

The detailed and elegant studies of Maynard *et al.* (1972) and Cooper *et al.* (1973a, b) show numerous such inclusions indubitably situated in dilated and vesiculated rough endoplasmic reticulum. They refer to them as 'curvilamellar bodies' and state that they were PAS-negative† and that they had no affinity for phosphotungstic acid. The chemical composition of these inclusions is obscure but these authors suggest that the material might be 'abnormal protein, perhaps lipoprotein or glycoprotein'. Electron-dense granules are also at times seen trapped within these inclusions; they could be lipid or proteinaceous dense granules.

Since chondrocytes normally secrete the precursors of matrical collagen‡ and proteoglycans one may speculate that the laminated inclusions contain such precursors or an abnormal product which is not too easily transported in the rough endoplasmic reticulum probably as a result of a genetic defect.

Reticulated and laminated patterns have been seen in the secretory granules of the salivary glands of Drosophila (Rizki, 1967) and mouse (Kumegawa *et al.*, 1967) so it would appear that glycoproteins can at times form laminated structures. Such an idea is also supported by our studies (Ghadially and Lalonde, 1980) which show that intranuclear laminated inclusions can develop from zymogen granules (page 80–85), and the fact that mucous granules (human material) can at times have quite a prominent reticulated pattern (*Plate 153*). Thus the idea that the laminated inclusions in the rough endoplasmic reticulum comprise mainly glycoprotein or proteoglycans is attractive.

---

*These inclusions are quite large and totally fill the dilated cisternae in chondrocytes. They may occupy up to about 75 per cent or more of the profile of a sectioned chondrocyte. This contrasts them from small round or oval laminated inclusions composed of two or three dense lamellae which are on rare occasions seen in the rough endoplasmic reticulum. I have seen such an inclusion in a rhabdomyosarcoma. These small laminated bodies are more akin to the dense granules and reticulated granules shown in *Plates 237* and *238*, than the inclusions shown in *Plate 243*.
†It is worth recalling that chondroitin sulphate and keratan sulphate are PAS-negative.
‡It is perhaps worth stating that collagen is now considered to be a glycoprotein.

Plate 243

From Maynard, Cooper and Ponseti (1972)
Figs. 1 and 2. Chondrocytes from pseudochondroplastic dwarfs showing reticulated (*Fig. 1*) and laminated inclusions in dilated rough endoplasmic reticulum. ×15 000; ×43 000

542

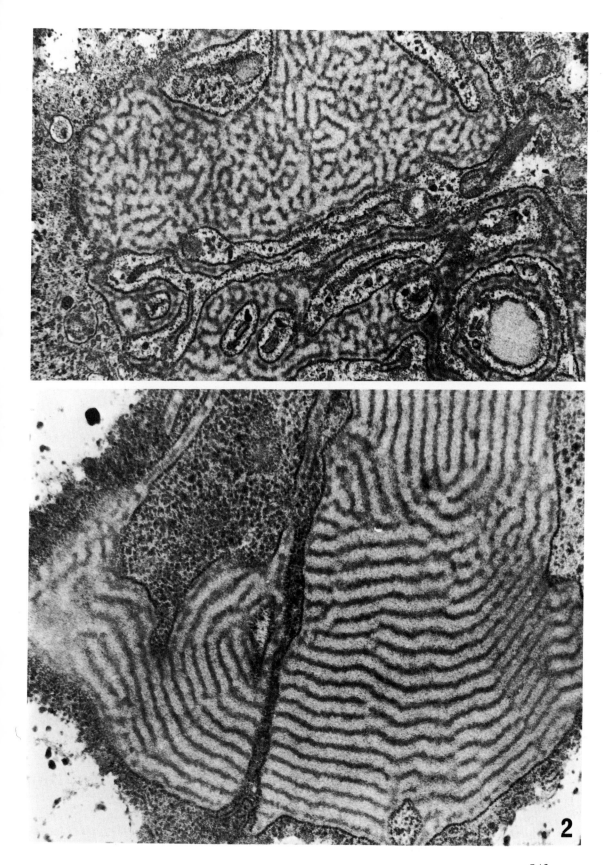

2

Intracisternal sequestration

'Intracisternal sequestration' or 'microsequestration' are terms used to describe a pattern of organization of the rough endoplasmic reticulum where vesicular profiles of rough endoplasmic reticulum are seen lying within dilated cisternae. It is thought that the primary stage of this process is the formation of papillary processes from the walls of dilated cisternae. Later such processes may be pinched off to form vesicular structures which come to lie free within the cisternae (*Plate 244*). When such a change is extensive, so that numerous vesicular profiles of rough endoplasmic reticulum are seen lying in a few grossly dilated but perhaps not too well visualized cisternae, one may at a casual glance confuse this change with vesiculation of the rough endoplasmic reticulum—quite a different phenomenon, which has already been described (page 428). This point is well illustrated and discussed by Blackburn and Vinijchaikul (1969), who point out that in vesiculation of the rough endoplasmic reticulum the ribosomes line the outside of the vesicles, but, since intracisternal sequestration represents an invagination of the rough endoplasmic reticulum into the cisternae, the ribosomes line the inner surface of the vesicles in this condition. Such vesicles may contain only the cytoplasmic matrix, but at times they also contain other structures such as lipid droplets, mitochondria and microbodies (*Plate 244*).

The vesicular profiles seen within the dilated cisternae may in some instances represent transverse sections through papillary processes, but there is often quite a preponderance of vesicular profiles over papillary forms, suggesting that these are portions of the invaginated rough endoplasmic reticulum which have indeed become detached from the walls of the cisternae and are now lying free within them. Such a concept is further supported by evidence of regressive or degenerative changes in the sequestrated material.

The formation of papillary projections from ductal and surface epithelia has long been linked in the minds of histopathologists with proliferative processes, and it could be argued that here, also, one is witnessing a similar process and that intracisternal sequestration could be a type of hypertrophy of the rough endoplasmic reticulum. However, the situations in which this phenomenon occurs militate against this view. Thus one of the most marked examples of intracisternal sequestration has been noted in the pancreatic acinar cells in kwashiorkor (Blackburn and Vinijchaikul, 1969) where there is a marked diminution in the quantity of rough

---

Plate 244

Fig. 1. Papilliferous (P) and vesicular (V) profiles of rough endoplasmic reticulum containing cytoplasmic matrix are seen within the dilated cisternae (arrow) of a human hepatocyte. From non-neoplastic liver adjacent to a hepatoma. ×51 000 (*From Ghadially and Parry, 1966*)

Fig. 2. Within the dilated cisternae of the rough endoplasmic reticulum of a hepatocyte are seen papillary (P) and vesicular structures (arrows) containing cytoplasmic matrix and microbodies (M). Note that the ribosomes line the inner surface of these vesicles. From an ill canary which had refused food for many days. ×28 000

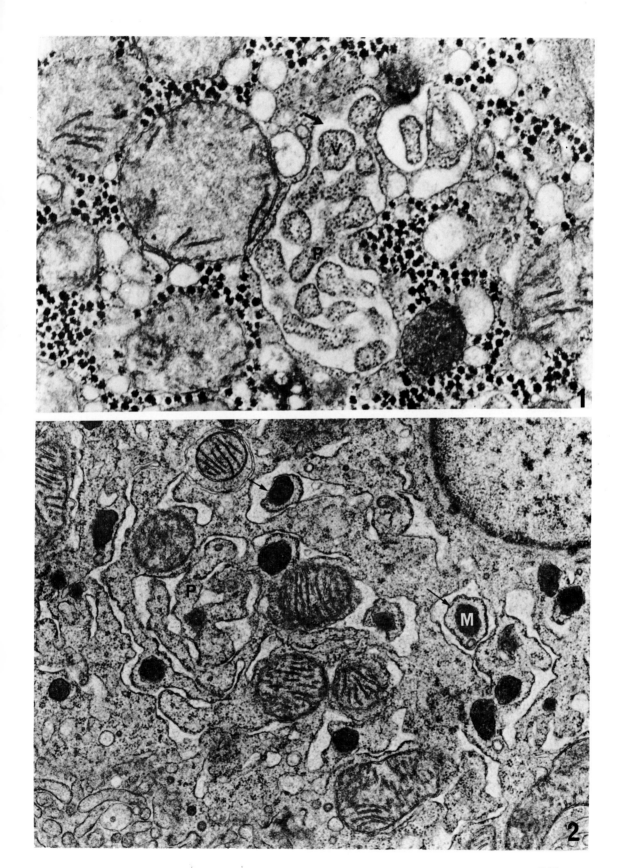

endoplasmic reticulum and much of what remains shows intracisternal sequestration. These authors have therefore suggested that intracisternal sequestration is a mechanism by which cytoplasmic atrophy may occur in cells with abundant rough endoplasmic reticulum. In other words, this is a process by which 'excess' rough endoplasmic reticulum is disposed of by the cell. It is postulated that such disposal may be achieved by degradation of the sequestrated rough endoplasmic reticulum and transport of this material to the Golgi and then into lysosomes. Svoboda and Higginson (1964) noted intracisternal sequestration (which they called microsequestration) in protein-deficient rats and considered this arrangement of the rough endoplasmic reticulum as a non-specific reaction of the cell to injury, leading to the formation of autolysosomes.

Besides the above mentioned examples intracisternal sequestration has been seen during: (1) holocrine cell lysis in the rat sebaceous preputial gland (Mesquita-Guimarães and Coimbra, 1976; Mesquita-Guimarães et al., 1979); (2) prolonged treatment with 4-acetylaminofluorene in the rat pancreas (Flaks and Lucas, 1972); and (3) cytoplasmic reduction phase in the spermiogenesis of *Eisenia foetida* (Stang-Vos, 1972).

We (Ghadially and Parry, unpublished observations) have observed occasional cells showing intracisternal sequestration in a wide variety of situations and, since such cells have shown other regressive changes also, we are inclined to agree with these hypotheses. For example, we have found cells showing intracisternal sequestration in the atrophic liver of a starving canary and in the liver tissue surrounding a hepatoma (*Plate 244*). It is our experience that senescent cells in culture and regressing or dying tumour cells adjacent to an area of necrosis also show this change.

We (Ghadially and Larsen, unpublished observations) have observed a somewhat different pattern of intracisternal sequestration in the pancreas of a child who had an islet cell adenoma. Here occasional pancreatic acinar cells showed quite sizeable masses of rough endoplasmic reticulum and mitochondria sequestrated within focal vacuolar dilatations of rough endoplasmic reticulum. Support for the idea that such sequestrated material suffers disintegration was also seen (*Plate 245*).

The manner in which autolysosomes (also called autophagic vacuoles) form and how the acid hydrolases arrive in these structures is not too clearly established, but various ideas have been put forward (*see* discussion on pages 596–598). Intracisternal sequestration is thought to be one of the ways in which an autolysosome forms, the necessary enzymes being synthesized by the ensheathing rough endoplasmic reticulum.

Plate 245

From a case of islet cell adenoma of the pancreas. (*Ghadially and Larsen, unpublished electron micrographs*)

Fig. 1. Pancreatic acinar cell showing a rounded mass of rough endoplasmic reticulum (R) and a mitochondrion (M) lying within a vacuole clearly lined by ribosome-studded rough endoplasmic reticulum (arrow). ×25 000

Fig. 2. Appearances seen in this illustration are thought to represent a further stage of evolution of the type of lesion shown in *Fig. 1*. Here the sequestrated material (presumably rough endoplasmic reticulum) appears disorganized, clumped and electron-dense. ×38 000

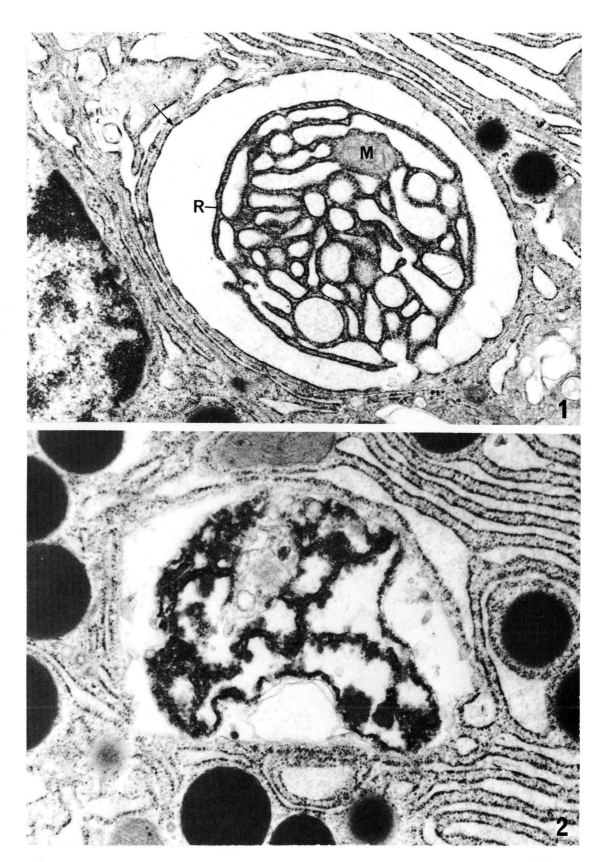

Virus in endoplasmic reticulum

Several types of viruses have been observed lying in or budding from walls of cytoplasmic vacuoles. Such vacuoles may represent sections through invaginations of the cell membrane (plasma membrane), or they could be derived from the endoplasmic reticulum or Golgi complex (intracytoplasmic membranes). Both phenomena are known to occur, and in some instances the virus particles have also been clearly demonstrated to lie in relatively unaltered cisternae of the rough endoplasmic reticulum or elements of the Golgi complex. Only a brief review of some of the instances where virus particles have been seen in such circumstances can be dealt with in the space available.

It has already been noted (page 42) that herpesvirus nucleocapsids assembled in the nucleus acquire one or two membranous coats from the nuclear envelope. In their subsequent passage through the cell they may acquire another coat by budding into vacuoles probably derived from intracytoplasmic membranes. The same phenomenon may also occur at the cell membrane as the virus leaves the cell.

Several RNA viruses have been found in the endoplasmic reticulum and Golgi complex, or in vacuoles derived from them. For example, the cores of rubella virus and some arboviruses assembled in the cytoplasm or close to intracytoplasmic membranes acquire their membranous coat by budding into these structures (Murphy *et al.*, 1968, 1970; Holmes *et al.*, 1969; Grimley and Friedman, 1970; Zlotnik and Harris, 1970; Boulton and Webb, 1971; Whitfield *et al.*, 1971).

Murine leukaemia viruses and avian tumour viruses are usually formed at the plasma membrane of the tumour cells by a process of budding; however, in some instances, they have been seen within vacuoles derived from intracytoplasmic membranes. A different situation, however, prevails in the megakaryocytes of such leukaemic mice. These cells do not become neoplastic but harbour many virus particles. Here the virus particles do not form and bud from the plasma membrane but into the endoplasmic reticulum, Golgi complex and numerous interconnecting channels and vacuoles clearly derived from these structures.

Viruses are now known to be associated with many transplantable mouse carcinomas and sarcomas. A well-known example of this is the Ehrlich ascites tumour, which shows many virus particles within smooth-membraned tubules and vesicles derived from the rough endoplasmic reticulum and at times also in the region of the Golgi complex (*Plate 246*). This virus, however, is not the causative agent of this particular tumour, for cell-free extracts of this tumour injected into newborn mice produces a high incidence of leukaemias but not Ehrlich ascites tumour. It is therefore thought that this and other transplantable mouse tumours harbour a latent leukaemogenic virus. (The extensive literature on oncogenic viruses cannot be adequately quoted here. For references supporting the statements made, the reader is referred to Dalton and Haguenau, 1962, and Gross, 1970.)

Plate 246
Ehrlich ascites tumour showing many virus particles budding into the endoplasmic reticulum and vesicles derived therefrom. The probable sequence of events is indicated by letters A to D. ×92 000

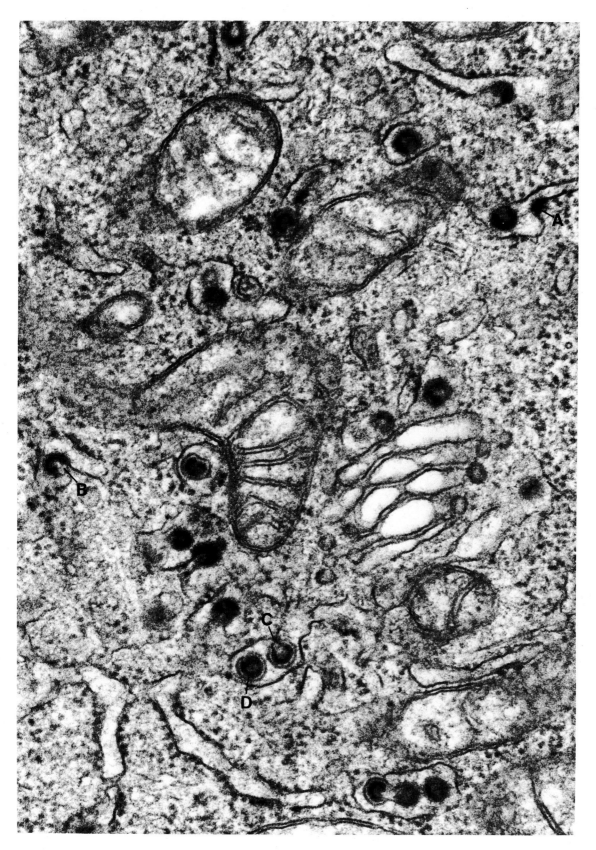

References

Adams, E.C. and Hertig, A.T. (1969). Studies on the human corpus luteum. *J. Cell Biol.* **41**, 696

Adams, W.R. and Prince, A.M. (1959). Cellular changes associated with infection of the Ehrlich ascites tumor with Newcastle disease virus. *Ann. N.Y. Acad. Sci.* **81**, 89

Albertine, K.H., Fox, L.M. and O'Morchoe, C.C.C. (1980). Lymphatic endothelial cell inclusion bodies. *J. Ultrastruct. Res.* **73**, 199

Albot, P.M.G. and Jezequel, A.M. (1962). Ultrastructure du foie et pathogenie de l'ictere au cours des hepatites virales. *Archs. Mal. Appar. dig.* **51**, 38

Alexander, R.W. (1984). Honeycomb structures in tumor cells. *Ultrastructural Pathol.* **6**, 99

Allegra, S.R., Chao, T. and Pella, J.A. (1984). Acquired immune deficiency syndrome (AIDS). Light microscopic, ultrastructural and immunocytochemical studies of one case. *J. Submicrosc. Cytol.* **16**, 561

Alves de Matos, A.P. (1974). Tubuloreticular structures in a case of bronchialadenom (carcinoid type). *Experientia* **30**, 1465

Alves de Matos, A.P. and Camara e Sousa, R. (1978). Tubuloreticular structures in chicken bursa Fabricii lymphocytes. *Experientia* **34**, 1218

Alving, C.R., Steck, E.A., Hanson, W.L., Loizeaux, P.S., Chapman, W.L., Jr. and Waits, V.B. (1978). Improved therapy of experimental Leishmaniasis by use of a liposome-encapsulated antimonial drug. *Life Sci.* **22**, 1021

Amagase, H. (1975). An ultrastructural-cytochemical study on the proliferation of smooth endoplasmic reticulum induced by chlorobiphenyls (PCB) in the guinea pig liver cells. *Arch. Histol. Jap.* **38**, 285

Anday, G.J., Goodman, J.R. and Tishkoff, G.H. (1973). An unusual cytoplasmic ribosomal structure in pathologic lymphocytes. *Blood* **41**, 439

Anderson, M.G., Dixey, J., Key, P., Ellis, D.S., Tovey, G., McCaul, T.F., Murray-Lyon, I.M., Gazzard, B., Lawrence, A., Evans, B., Byrom, N. and Zuckerman, A.J. (1984). Persistent lymphadenopathy in homosexual men: A clinical and ultrastructural study. *Lancet* **i**, 880

Andres, G.A., Spiele, H. and McCluskey, R.T. (1972). Viruslike structures in systemic lupus erythematosus. In *Progress in Clinical Immunology*, Vol 1. Ed. R.S. Schwartz. New York: Grune and Stratton

Angel, A. and Sheldon, H. (1965). Adipose cell organelles: isolation, morphology and possible relation to intracellular lipid transport. *Ann. N.Y. Acad. Sci.* **131**, 157

Anitschkow, N. (1914). Zur Frage der tropfigen Entmischung. *Verh. deutsch. Ges. Path.* **17**, 103

Anzil, A.P. and Blinzinger, K. (1974). Cytoplasmic tubule-containing vacuoles and endoplasmic tubuloreticular inclusions in the lymphocytes of a child with an unidentified form of cerebroretinal degeneration. *Biomedicine* **21**, 210

Arai, T., Kino, I., Nakamura, S-i. and Koda, K. (1986). Solid and cystic acinar cell tumors of the pancreas. *Acta Pathol. Jpn* **36**, 1887

Arcasoy, M., Smuckler, E.A. and Benditt, E.P. (1968). Acute effects of 3-methyl-4-dimethyl aminoazobenzene intoxication on rat liver. Structural and functional changes in the endoplasmic reticulum and NADPH-related electron transport. *Am. J. Path.* **52**, 841

Arhelger, R.B., Broom, S. and Boler, R.K. (1965). Ultrastructural hepatic alterations following tannic acid administration to rabbits. *Am. J. Path.* **46**, 409

Armstrong, D.T., O'Brien, J. and Greep, R.O. (1964). Effects of luteinizing hormone on progestin biosynthesis in the luteinized rat ovary. *Endocrinology* **75**, 488

Ashworth, C.T., Werner, D.J., Glass, M.D. and Arnold, N.J. (1965). Spectrum of fine structural changes in hepatocellular injury due to thioacetamide. *Am. J. Path.* **47**, 917

Aübock, L. and Albegger, K.W. (1972). Virusahnliche Strukturen bei Sjogrens Syndrom. *Archiv klin. exp. Ohren-, Nasen- und Kehlkopfheilk.* **202**, 427

Baglio, C.M. and Farber, E. (1965a). Correspondence between ribosome aggregation patterns in rat liver homogenates and in electron micrographs following administration of ethionine. *J. molec. Biol.* **12**, 466

Baglio, C.M. and Farber, E. (1965b). Reversal by adenine of the ethionine-induced lipid accumulation in the endoplasmic reticulum of the rat liver. *J. Cell. Biol.* **27**, 591

Banfield, W.G., Dawe, C.J., Lee. C.E. and Sonstegard, R. (1976). Cylindroid lamella-particle complexes in lymphoma cells of northern pike (*Esox lucius*). *J. Natl. Cancer Inst. US.* **57**, 415

Banfield, W.G., Lee, C.W., Tralka, T.S. and Rabson, A.S. (1977). Lamella-particle complexes in nuclei of owl monkey kidney cells infected with *Herpesvirus saimiri*. *J. Natl. Cancer Inst. US* **58**, 1421

Barbieri, M., Simonelli, L., Simoni, P. and Maraldi, N.M. (1970). Ribosome crystallization, II. Ultrastructural study on nuclear and cytoplasmic ribosome crystallization in hypothermic cell cultures. *J. Submicr. Cytol.* **2**, 33

Barer, R., Joseph, S. and Meek, G.A. (1961). Membrane interrelationships during meiosis. In *Electron Microscopy in Anatomy*, pp. 160–175, Ed. by J.D. Boyd *et al.* London: Edward Arnold

Bariety, J., Amor, B., Kahan, A., Balafrej, J.L. and Delbarre, F. (1971). Ultrastructural anomalies in mononuclear cells of peripheral blood in SLE: Presence of virus-like inclusions. *Rev. Europ. Etudes Clin. et Biol.* **16**, 715

Bariety, J., Richer, D., Appay, M.D., Grosseetete, J. and Callard, P. (1973). Frequency of intraendothelial 'virus-like' particles: An electron microscopy study of 376 human renal biopsies. *J. clin. Path.* **26**, 21

Baringer, J.R. and Griffith, J.F. (1969). Experimental herpes encephalitis: Crystalline arrays in endoplasmic reticulum. *Science* **165**, 1381

Baringer, J.R., and Swoveland, P. (1972). Tubular aggregates in endoplasmic reticulum: Evidence against their viral nature. *J. Ultrastruct. Res.* **41**, 270

Barka, T. and Popper, H. (1967). Liver enlargement and drug toxicity. *Medicine, Baltimore* **46**, 103

Bartels, P.G. and Weier, T.E. (1967). Particle arrangements in proplastids of *Triticum vulgare L*, seedlings, *J. Cell Biol.* **33**, 243

Basset, F., Escraig, J. and Le Crom, M. (1972). A cytoplasmic membranous complex in histiocytosis X. *Cancer* **29**, 1380

Bassi, M. (1960). Electron microscopy of rat liver after carbon tetrachloride poisoning. *Exp. Cell. Res.* **20**, 313

Bassot, J.M. (1966). Une forme microtubulaire et paracristalline de reticulum endoplasmique dans les photocytes des annelides polynoinae. *J. Cell Biol.* **31**, 135

Battifora, H. (1983). Case 7. *Ultrastructural Pathol.* **5**, 315

Beams, H.W. and Kessel, R. (1962). Intracisternal granules of the endoplasmic reticulum in the crayfish oocyte. *J. Cell Biol.* **13**, 158

Beams, H.W. and Kessel, R. (1963). Electron microscope studies on developing crayfish oocytes with special reference to the origin of yolk. *J. Cell Biol.* **18**, 621

Bedoya, V., Rabson, A.S. and Grimley, P.M. (1968). Growth *in vitro* of herpes simplex virus in human lymphoma cell lines. *J. Nat. Cancer Inst.* **41**, 635

Begin, L.R., Osborne, B.M. and Mackay, B. (1981). Monocytic leukaemia with cutaneous involvement: Ultrastructural observations on unusual cytoplasmic complexes. *Ultrastructural Pathol.* **2**, 11

Behnke, O. (1963). Helical arrangement of ribosomes in the cytoplasm of differentiating cells of the small intestine of rat foetuses. *Exp. Cell Res.* **30**, 597

Behnke, O. and Moe, H. (1964). An electron microscope study of mature and differentiating Paneth cells in the rat, especially of their endoplasmic reticulum and lysosomes. *J. Cell Biol.* **22**, 633

Belcher, R.W., Czarnetzki, B.M. and Campbell, P.B. (1975). Ultrastructure of inclusions in peripheral blood mononuclear cells in sarcoidosis. *Am. J. Path.* **78**, 461

Benedetti, E.L. and Emmelot, P. (1960). Changes in the fine structure of rat liver cells brought about by dimethylnitrosamine. In *Proceedings of the European Regional Conference on Electron Microscopy, Delft*, Vol. 2, p. 875. Ed. by A.L. Henwick and B.J. Spit. Uppsala: Almqvist and Wiksell

Benedetti, E.L., Bont, W.S. and Bloemendal, H. (1966). Electron microscopic observations on polyribosomes and endoplasmic reticulum fragments isolated from rat liver. *Lab. Invest.* **15**, 196

Bernhard, W. (1969). Ultrastructure of the cancer cell. In *Handbook of Molecular Cytology*. Ed. by A. Lima-De-Faria. Amsterdam and London: North Holland Publ.

Biava, C. and Mukhlova-Montiel, M. (1965). Electron microscopic observations on councilman-like acidophilic bodies and other forms of acidophilic changes in human liver cells. *Am. J. Path.* **46**, 775

Biempica, L., Kosower, N.S. and Roheim, P.S. (1971). Cytochemical and ultrastructural changes in rat liver in experimental porphyria. II. Effects of repeated injections of allylisopropylacetamide. *Lab. Invest.* **24**, 110

Bini, A., Botti, B., Calligaro, A., Congiu, L., Tomasi, A. and Vannini, V. (1978). Morphological changes and free radical rate in early hepatic injury from carbon tetrachloride and monobromotrichloromethane. *J. Submicr. Cytol.* **10**, 215

Black, C.D.V., Watson, G.J. and Ward, R.J. (1977). The use of Pentostam liposomes in the chemotherapy of experimental Leishmaniasis. *Roy. Soc. trop. Med. Hyg. Trans.* **71**, 550

Blackburn, W.R. and Vinijchaikul, K. (1969). The pancreas in kwashiorkor. An electron microscopic study. *Lab. Invest.* **20**, 305

Blanchette, E.J. (1966). Ovarian steroid cells. II. The lutein cell. *J. Cell Biol.* **31**, 517

Blinzinger, K., Simon, J., Magrath, D. and Boulger, L. (1969). Poliovirus crystals within the endoplasmic reticulum of endothelial and mononuclear cells in the monkey spinal cord. *Science* **163**, 1336

Blinzinger, K., Anzil, A.P. and Deutschlander, N. (1972). Nature of tubular aggregates. *New Engl. J. Med.* **286**, 157

Bloodworth, J.M.B. and Shelp, W.D. (1970). Endothelial cytoplasmic inclusions. *Arch. Path.* **90**, 252

Bloom, W. and Fawcett, D.W. (1975). *A Textbook of Histology*, 10th edn. Philadelphia and London: Saunders

Bockus, D., Remington, F., Friedman, S. and Hammar, S. (1985). Electron microscopy what izzits. *Ultrastructural Pathol.* **9**, 1

Bonnett, H.T. and Newcomb, E.H. (1965). Polyribosomes and cisternal accumulations in root cells of radish. *J. Cell Biol.* **27**, 423

Boquist, L., Larsson, S.-E. and Lorentzon, R. (1976). Genuine giant-cell tumour of bone; a combined cytological, histopathological and ultrastructural study. *Path. Europ.* **11**, 117

Boulton, P.S. and Webb, H.E. (1971). An electron microscopic study of Langat virus encephalitis in mice. *Brain* **94**, 411

Brenner, R.M. (1966). Fine structure of adrenocortical cells in adult male rhesus monkeys. *Am. J. Anat.* **119**, 429

Brinkley, B.R., Stubblefield, E. and Hsu, T.C. (1967). The effects of Colcemid inhibition and reversal on the fine structure of the mitotic apparatus of Chinese hamster cells *in vitro*. *J. Ultrastruct. Res.* **19**, 1

Brown, R.E. and Schatzki, P.F. (1971). Intracisternal granules in the human pancreas. *Archs Path.* **91**, 351

Brown, R.E. and Still, W.J.S. (1970). Acinar-islet cells in the exocrine pancreas of the adult cat. *Am. J. dig. Dis.* **15**, 327

Brunelli, M.A., Marini, M., Pettazzoni, P. and Bubola, G. (1977). Ribosomal crystallization in hypothermized chicken bone marrow. *J. Ultrastruct. Res.* **60**, 140

Brunning, R.D. and Parkin, J. (1975a). Ribosome-lamella complexes in neoplastic hematopoietic cells. *Am. J. Path.* **79**, 565

Brunning, R.D. and Parkin, J. (1975b). Ultrastructural studies of parallel tubular arrays in human lymphocytes. *Am. J. Pathol.* **78**, 59

Bucciarelli, E., Rabotti, G.F. and Dalton, A.J. (1967). Ultrastructure of meningeal tumors induced in dogs with Rous sarcoma virus. *J. Nat. Cancer Inst.* **38**, 359

Buck, R.C. (1961). Lamellae in the spindle of mitotic cells of Walker 256 carcinoma. *J. biophys. biochem. Cytol.* **2**, 227

Bulger, R.E. (1968). Granule-lamella complex in monkey renal proximal tubular cells. *J. Ultrastruct. Res.* **24**, 150

Bull, T.B. and McCartney, A.C.E. (1986). The ribosome–lamellar complex: Is it a normal structure? *Ultrastructural Pathol.* **10**, 363

Bunge, R.P., Bunge, M.B. and Peterson, E.R. (1965). An electron microscope study of cultured rat spinal cord. *J. Cell Biol.* **24**, 163

Burger, P.C. and Herdson, P.B. (1966). Phenobarbital-induced fine structural changes in rat liver. *Am. J. Path.* **48**, 793

Buttrose, M.S., Frey-Wyssling, A. and Muhlethaler, K. (1960). Intracisternal granules in the endosperm cell of the barley grain. *J. Ultrastruct. Res.* **4**, 258

Byers, B. (1967). Structure and formation of ribosome crystals in hypothermic chick embryo cells. *J. molec. Biol.* **26**, 155

Byers, B. (1971). Chick embryo ribosome crystals: analysis of bonding and functional activity *in vitro*. *Proc. Natn Acad. Sci., USA* **68**, 440

Caesar, R. and Rapaport, M. (1963). Elektronenmikroskopische Untersuchung des Leberzellschadens bei der Diphtherietoxinvergiftung. *Frankfurt. Ztschr. Path.* **72**, 517

Cameron, A.M. and Conroy, J.D. (1974). Rabies-like neuronal inclusions associated with a neoplastic reticulosis in a dog. *Vet. Path.* **11**, 29

Canese, M.G., Rizzetto, M., Novara, R., London, W.T. and Purcell, R.H. (1984). Experimental infection of chimpanzees with the HBsAg-Associated delta (δ) Agent: An ultrastructural study. *J. Med. Virol.* **13**, 63

Cappelli-Gotzos, B., Gotzos, V. and Conti, G. (1983). Peculiar ultrastructural features in the cytoplasm of cells from human effusions associated with malignant disease. *Ultrastructural Pathol.* **5**, 243

Carasso, N. (1960). Role de l'érgastoplasme dans l'elaboration du glycogène au cours de la formation du 'paraboloide' des cellules visuelles. *C.R. Acad. Sci. (Paris)* **250**, 600

Carette, S., Klippel, J.H., Preble, O.T., Grimley, P.M., Decker, J.L. and Friedman, R.M. (1982). Association of human leukocyte interferon and lymphocyte tubuloreticular inclusions in systemic lupus erythematosus. *Arthritis Rheum.* **25**(Suppl), S57

Caro, L.G. and Palade, G.E. (1964). Protein synthesis, storage, and discharge in the pancreatic exocrine cell – an autoradiographic study. *J. Cell Biol.* **20**, 473

Carstens, P.H.B. (1984). Honeycomb structures in tumor cells. *Ultrastructural Pathol.* **6**, 99

Cassier, P. (1979). The Corpora Allata of Insects. *Int. Rev. Cytol.* **57**, 1

Catovsky, D. (1977). Hairy-cell leukaemia and pro-lymphocytic leukaemia. *Clin. Haematol.* **6**, 245

Cawley, J.C., Emmines, J., Goldstone, A.H., Hamblin, T., Hough, D. and Smith, J.L. (1975). Distinctive cytoplasmic inclusions in chronic lymphocytic leukaemia. *Europ. J. Cancer* **11**, 91

552

Cedergren, B. and Harary, I. (1964). *In vitro* studies on single beating rat heart cells. VI. Electron microscopic studies of single cells. *J. Ultrastruct. Res.* **11**, 428

Cesarini, J.-P., Pruniéras, M. and Clark, W.H. (1973). Branched tubular structures in human malignant melanoma. *Yale J. Biol Med.* **46**, 482

Chandra, S. (1968). Undulating tubules associated with endoplasmic reticulum in pathologic tissues. *Lab. Invest.* **18**, 422

Chandra, S. and Stefani, S.S. (1976). A possible mode of formation of tubuloreticular structures. *J. Ultrastruct. Res.* **56**, 304

Chandra, S. and Stefani, S.S. (1978). Ultrastructure of granulofilamentous bodies in pathologic spleen and lymph node. *J. Ultrastruct. Res.* **64**, 148

Chandra, S., Moore, G.E. and Brandt, P.M. (1968). Similarity between leukocyte cultures from cancerous and noncancerous human subjects: An electron microscopic study. *Cancer Res.* **28**, 1982

Chandra, S., Brown, D.E., Aldenderfer, P., Garon, C., Buscheck, F.T. and Manaker, R.A. (1969). Morphologic and serologic studies of transplanted human leukocyte culture (M-1) cells in laboratory animals. *Cancer Res.* **29**, 1829

Chang, J.P. and Gibley, C.W. Jr. (1968). Ultrastructure of tumor cells during mitosis. *Cancer Res.* **28**, 521

Chapman, J.A. (1962). Fibroblasts and collagen. *Br. med. Bull.* **18**, 233

Cheville, N.F. (1972). Ultrastructure of canine carotid body and aortic body tumors. Comparison of tissues of thyroid and parathyroid origin. *Vet. Path.* **9**, 166

Chiesara, E., Clementi, F., Conti, F. and Meldolesi, J. (1967). The induction of drug-metabolizing enzymes in rat liver during growth and regeneration. *Lab. Invest.* **16**, 254

Chou, S.M. and Miike, T. (1981). Ultrastructural abnormalities and perifascicular atrophy in childhood dermatomyositis. *Arch. Path. Lab. Med.* **105**, 76

Christensen, A.K. (1965). The fine structure of testicular interstitial cells in guinea pigs. *J. Cell Biol.* **26**, 911

Christensen, A.K. and Fawcett, D.W. (1961). The normal fine structure of opossum testicular interstitial cells. *J. biophys. biochem. Cytol.* **9**, 653

Cinti, S. and Osculati, F. (1982). Ribosome-lamellae complex in the adenoma cells of the human parathyroid gland. *J. Submicrosc. Cytol.* **14**, 521

Cinti, S., Osculati, F. and Parravicini, C. (1982). RER-associated structure in parathyroid glands removed because of tertiary hyperparathyroidism. *Ultrastructural Pathol.* **3**, 263

Clark, A.W. (1967). Some aspects of spermiogenesis in a lizard. *Am. J. Anat.* **121**, 369

Cockrell, B.Y., Hall, B.V. and Simon, J. (1972). Morphometric analysis of anthelmintic- and prednisolone-induced alterations in the ultrastructure of beagle liver parenchymal cells. *Am. J. vet. Res.* **33**, 687

Cohen, A.I. (1963). The fine structure of the visual receptors of the pigeon. *Exp. Eye Res.* **2**, 88

Conney, A.H. (1965). Enzyme induction and drug toxicity. In *Proceedings of the Second International Pharmacological Meeting*, Vol. 4, *Drugs and Enzymes*. p. 277, Ed. by B.B. Brodie. Oxford: Pergamon Press.

Cooper, R.R., Ponseti, I.V. and Maynard, J.A. (1973a). Pseudochondroplastic dwarfism. A rough-surfaced endoplasmic reticulum storage disorder. *J. Bone Jt Surg.* **55A**, 475

Cooper, R.R., Pedrini-Mille, A. and Ponseti, I.V. (1973b). Metaphyseal dystosis. A rough-surfaced endoplasmic reticulum storage defect. *Lab. Invest.* **28**, 119

Corvaja, N., Magherini, P.C. and Pompeiano, O. (1971). Ultrastructure of glycogen-membrane complexes in sensory nerve fibres of cat muscle spindles. *Z. Zellforsch. mikrosk. Anat.* **121**, 199

Cotte, G. (1959). Quelques problèmes posés par l'ultrastructure des lipides de la cortico-surrenale. *J. Ultrastruct. Res.* **3**, 186

Crisp, T.M., Dessouky, D.A. and Denys, F.R. (1970). The fine structure of the human corpus luteum of early pregnancy and during the progestational phase of the menstrual cycle. *Am. J. Anat.* **127**, 37

Cure, M., Trouillas, J., Lheritier, M., Girod, C. and Rollet, J. (1972). Inclusions tubulaires dans une tumeur hypophysaire. *Nouv. Presse med.* **1**, 2309

Dallner, G., Siekevitz, P. and Palade, G.E. (1966). Biogenesis of endoplasmic reticulum membranes. I. Structural and chemical differentiation in developing rat hepatocyte. *J. Cell Biol.* **30**, 73

Dalton, A.J., Heine, U., Kondratick, J.M., Ablashi, D.V. and Blackham, E.A. (1973). Ultrastructural and complement-fixation studies on suspension cultures derived from human solid tumors. *J. Natl. Cancer Inst.* **50**, 879

Dalton, J.A. (1964). An electron microscopical study of a series of chemically induced hepatomas. In *Cellular Control, Mechanisms and Cancer*, p. 211. Ed. by P. Emmelot and O. Muhlbock. New York: American Elsevier

Dalton, J.A. and Haguenau, F. (1962). *Tumors Induced by Viruses: Ultrastructural Studies.* New York and London: Academic Press

Damjanov, I., Casey, M.J., Maenza, R.M. and Kennedy, A.W. (1978). Müllerian adenosarcoma of the uterus. *Am. J. Clin. Path.* **70**, 96

Daniel, M. Th, and Flandrin, G. (1974). Fine structure of abnormal cells in hairy cell (Tricholeukocytic) leukaemia, with special reference to their *in vitro* phagocytic capacity. *Lab. Invest.* **30**, 1

Daniels, T.E., Sylvester, R.A., Silverman, S., Polando, V. and Talal, N. (1974). Tubuloreticular structures within labial salivary glands in Sjogren's syndrome. *Arthritis Rheum.* **17**, 593

Dardick, I., Lagace, R., Carlier, M.T. and Jung, R.C. (1983). Chordoid sarcoma (extraskeletal myxoid chondrosarcoma). *Virchows Arch. A Path. Anat.* **399**, 61

David-Ferreira, J.F. and Manaker, R.A. (1965). An electron microscope study of the development of a mouse hepatitis virus in tissue culture cells. *J. Cell Biol.* **24**, 57

Davidowitz, J., Philips, G. and Breinin, G.M. (1983). Membrane-glycogen complexes in rabbit extraocular muscle. *J. Ultrastruct. Res.* **82**, 64

David, H. (1964). *Submicroscopic Ortho- and Pathomorphology of the Liver.* Oxford: Pergamon Press

Dawe, C.J., Banfield, W.G., Sonstegard, R., Lee, C.W. and Michelitch, H.J. (1976). Cylindroid lamella-particle complexes and nucleoid intracytoplasmic bodies in lymphoma cells of northern pike (*Esox lucius*). *Prog. Exp. Tumor Res.* **20**, 166

DeBlois, G., Wang, S. and Kay, S. (1986). Microtubular aggregates within rough endoplasmic reticulum: An unusual ultrastructural feature of extraskeletal myxoid chondrosarcoma. *Human Pathol.* **17**, 469

Dekker, A. and Krause, J.R. (1973). Hyaline globules in human neoplasms. *Arch. Pathol.* **95**, 178

De Martino, C., Accini, L., Andres, G.A. and Archetti, I. (1969). Tubular structures associated with the endothelial endoplasmic reticulum in glomerular capillaries of Rhesus monkey and Nephritic man. *Z. Zellforsch.* **97**, 502

De Sousa, M. and Pritchard, H. (1974). The cellular basis of immunological recovery in nude mice after thymus grafting. *Immunology* **26**, 769

Djaczenko, W., Benedetto, A. and Pezzi, R. (1970). Formation of helical polyribosomes in poliovirus-infected cells of the 37 RC line. *J. Cell Biol.* **45**, 173

Djaldetti, M. (1976). 'Hairy Cell' Leukaemia. *Case Histories in Human Medicine No. 9.* Philips Monographs

Djaldetti, M., Landau, M., Mandel, E.M., Har-Zaav, L. and Lewinski, U. (1974). Electron microscopic study of lymphosarcoma cell leukemia. *Blut* **29**, 210

Douglas, S.D., Blume, R.S., Glade, P.R., Chessin, L.N. and Wolff, S.M. (1969). Fine structure of continuous long term lymphoid cell cultures from a Chediak-Higashi patient and heterozygote. *Lab. Invest.* **21**, 225

Driessens, J., Dupont, A. and Demaille, A. (1959). L'hepatome experimental azoique du rat examine au microscope electronique. *C.R. Soc. Biol.* **153**, 788

Dryll, A., Cazalis, P. and Ryckewaert, A. (1977). Lymphocyte tubular structures in rheumatoid arthritis. *J. clin. Path.* **30**, 822

Duyvené De Wit, L.J. (1986). Microtubules in plasma cells. *Ultrastructural Pathol.* **10**, 275

Echlin, P. (1965). An apparent helical arrangement of ribosomes in developing pollen mother cells of *Ipomoea purpurea (L.)* Roth. *J. Cell Biol.* **24**, 150

Elliott, R.L. and Arhelger, R.B. (1966). Fine structure of parathyroid adenomas with special reference to annulate lamellae and septate desmosomes. *Arch. Path.* **81**, 200

Emmelot, P. and Benedetti, E.L. (1960). Changes in the fine structure of rat liver cells brought about by dimethylnitrosamine. *J. biophys. biochem. Cytol.* **7**, 393

Emmelot, P. and Benedetti, E.L. (1961). Some observations on the effect of liver carcinogens on the fine structure and function of the endoplasmic reticulum of rat liver cells. In *Protein Biosynthesis*, p. 99. Ed. by R.J.C. Harris. London and New York: Academic Press

Enders, A.C. (1962). Observations on the fine structure of lutein cells. *J. Cell Biol.* **12**, 101

Enders, A.C. and Lyons, W.R. (1964). Observations on the fine structure of lutein cells. II. The effects of hypophysectomy and mammotrophic hormones in the rat. *J. Cell Biol.* **22**, 127

Epstein, M.A. (1957a). The fine structure of the cells in mouse sarcoma 37 ascitic fluids. *J. biophys. biochem. Cytol.* **3**, 567

Epstein, M.A. (1957b). The fine structural organization of Rous tumor cells. *J. biophys. biochem. Cytol.* **3**, 851

Epstein, M.A. (1961). Some unusual features of fine structure observed in HeLa cells. *J. biophys. biochem. Cytol.* **10**, 153

Eriksson, S. and Larsson, C. (1975). Purification and partial characterization of PAS-positive inclusion bodies from the liver in Alpha$_1$-antitrypsin deficiency. *New Engl. J. Med.* **292**, 176

Ernst, P. (1914). *Verh. deutsch. Ges. Path.* **17**, 43, (Quoted by Cameron, G.R. (1952). *Pathology of the Cell.* Edinburgh: Oliver and Boyd

Ernster, L., Siekevitz, P. and Palade, G.E. (1962). Enzyme-structure relationships in the endoplasmic reticulum of rat liver. A morphological and biochemical study. *J. Cell Biol.* **15**, 541

Estes, P.C. and Cheville, N.F. (1970). The ultrastructure of vascular lesions in equine viral arteritis. *Am. J. Pathol.* **58**, 235

Ewing, E.P., Spira, T.J., Chandler, F.W., Callaway, C., Brynes, R.K. and Chan, W.C. (1983a). Ultrastructural markers in AIDS. *Lancet* **ii**, 285

Ewing, E.P., Spira, T.J., Chandler, F.W., Callaway, C.S., Brynes, R.K. and Chan, W.C. (1983b). Unusual cytoplasmic body in lymphoid cells of homosexual men with unexplained lymphadenopathy. *New Engl. J. Med.* **308**, 819

Fahr, R. (1914). Zur Frade der sogenannten hyalintropfigen Zelldegeneration. *Verh. deutsch. Ges. Path.* **17**, 119

Fain-Maurel, M.A. (1966). Localisations intramitochondriale et intracisternale de glycogène monoparticulaire. *C.R. hebdomadaires des Séances de l'académie des Sciences Paris, Series D* **263**, 1107

Favard, P. (1958). L'origine ergastoplasmique des granules proteiques dan les spermatocytes d'Ascaris. *C.R. Acad. Sci.* **247**, 531

Fawcett, D.W. (1964). Morphological considerations of lipid transport in the liver. *Proceedings of the International Symposium on Lipid Transport,* p. 1. Springfield, Illinois: Charles C. Thomas

Fawcett, D.W. (1966). *The Cell. An Atlas of Fine Structure.* Philadelphia and London: W.B. Saunders.

Fawcett, D.W. (1981). *The Cell.* Philadelphia and London: W.B. Saunders

Fawcett, D.W. and Ito, S. (1958). Observations on the cytoplasmic membranes of testicular cells examined by phase contrast and electron microscopy. *J. biophys. biochem. Cytol.* **4**, 135

Fawcett, D.W. and Revel, J.P. (1961). The sarcoplasmic reticulum of a fast-acting fish muscle. *J. biophys. biochem. Cytol.* **10**, Suppl. 89

Fawcett, D.W. and Selby, C.C. (1958). Observations on the fine structure of the turtle atrium. *J. biophys. biochem. Cytol.* **4**, 63

Fawcett, D.W. and Wilson, J.W. (1955). A note on the occurrence of virus-like particles in the spontaneous hepatomas of C3H mice. *J. natn. Cancer Inst.* **15**, 1505

Feorino, P.M., Hierholzer, J.C. and Norton, W.L. (1970). Viral isolation studies of inclusion positive biopsy from human connective tissue diseases. *Arthritis Rheum.* **13**, 378

Feremans, W.W., Menu, R., Hupin, J., Bieva, C.J. and Caudron, M. (1980). Acute promonocytic leukaemia with ribosome-lamella complexes and elevated muramidase activity in serum and urine. A clinical, morphological, cytochemical and immunochemical study. *Acta Clinica Belg.* **35**, 212

Filshie, B.K. and Rehacek, J. (1968). Studies of the morphology of Murray Valley encephalitis and Japanese encephalitis viruses growing in cultured mosquito cells. *Virology* **34**, 435

Flaks, B. (1968). Formation of membrane-glycogen arrays in rat hepatoma cells. *J. Cell Biol.* **36**, 410

Flaks, B. (1971). Fine structure of rat hepatocytes during the late phase of chronic 2-acetylaminofluorene intoxication. *Chem-Biol. Interactions* **3**, 157

Flaks, B. and Flaks, A. (1969). Fine structure of murine pulmonary adenomata induced by carcinogen treatment in organ culture. *Cancer Res.* **29**, 1781

Flaks, B. and Lucas, J. (1972). Fine structural changes in rat pancreatic cells during prolonged treatment with 4-acetylaminofluorene. *Chem.-Biol. Interactions* **5**, 217

Flickinger, C.J. (1969). Fine structure of the Wolffian duct and cytodifferentiation of the epididymis in fetal rats. *Z. Zellforsch.* **96**, 344

Fouquet, J.-P. (1970). Glycogène et activité glycogène—synthetastique dans les cisterns ergastoplasmiques de l'épididyme du Hamster doré *Mesocricetus auratus* W. *C.R. hebdomadaires des Séances de l'Académie des Sciences, Paris, Series D* **270**, 2821

Fraire, A.E., Smith, M.N., Greenberg, S.D., Weg, J.G. and Sharp, J.T. (1971). Tubular structures in pulmonary endothelial cells in systemic lupus erythematosus. *Am. J. Clin. Pathol.* **56**, 244

Fritzler, M.J., Church, R.B. and Wagenaar, E.B. (1973). Ultrastructure of Taper hepatoma ascites cells. *J. electron Micr.* **22**, 73

Gaffney, E.F. and Cottell, D.C. (1986). Random glycogen-ER complexes in small cell chest wall tumor. *Ultrastructural Pathol.* **10**, 203

Ganote, C.E. and Otis, J.B. (1969). Characteristic lesions of yellow phosphorus-induced liver damage. *Lab. Invest.* **21**, 207

Geha, R.S., Schneeberger, E., Gatien, J., Rosen, F.S. and Merler, E. (1974). Synthesis of an M component by circulating B lymphocytes in severe combined immunodeficiency. *New Engl. J. Med.* **290**, 726

Gessaga, E.C. (1982). Intracellular structures in an astrocytoma. *Ultrastructural Pathol.* **3**, 199

Ghadially, F.N. (1985). *Diagnostic Electron Microscopy of Tumours.* 2nd Edition. London: Butterworths

Ghadially, F.N. (1984). *Diagnostic Ultrastructural Pathology.* London: Butterworths

Ghadially, F.N. (1983). *Fine Structure of Synovial Joints.* London: Butterworths

Ghadially, F.N. (1982). *Ultrastructural Pathology of the Cell and Matrix* London: Butterworths

Ghadially, F.N. (1980a). *Diagnostic Electron Microscopy of Tumours.* 1st Edition, London: Butterworths

Ghadially, F.N. (1980b). Overview article. The articular territory of the reticuloendothelial system. *Ultrastruct. Path.* **1**, 249

Ghadially, F.N. (1975). *Ultrastructural Pathology of the Cell,* London: Butterworths

Ghadially, F.N. and Lalonde, J-M.A. (1980). Genesis of concentric laminated inclusions in the nucleus. *Experientia* **36**, 59

Ghadially, F.N. and Mehta, P.N. (1970). Ultrastructure of osteogenic sarcoma. *Cancer* **25**, 1457

Ghadially, F.N. and Parry, E.W. (1966). Ultrastructure of a human hepatocellular carcinoma and surrounding non-neoplastic liver. *Cancer* **19**, 1989

Ghadially, F.N. and Roy, S. (1969). *Ultrastructure of Synovial Joints in Health and Disease.* London: Butterworths

Ghadially, F.N., Lowes, N.R. and Mesfin, G.M. (1977). Atypical glycogen deposits in a plasmacytoma. An ultrastructural study. *J. Path.* **122**, 157

Ghadially, F.N., Mehta, P.N. and Kirkaldy-Willis, W.H. (1970). Ultrastructure of articular cartilage in experimentally produced lipoarthrosis. *J. Bone Jt Surg.* **52A**, 1147

Ghadially, F.N., Senoo, A., Fuse, Y. and Chan, K.W. (1987). A serial section study of the so-called 'test-tube and ring-shaped forms' in AIDS. *J. Submicrosc. Cytol.* **19**, 175

Ghiara, G. and Taddei, C. (1966). Dati citologici e ultrastrutturali su di un particolare tipo di constituenti basofili del citoplasma di cellule follicolari e di ovociti ovarisi di rettili. *Boll. Soc. ital. Biol. sper.* **42**, 784

Gianotti, F. and Caputo, R. (1971). Skin ultrastructure in Letterer-Siwe disease treated with vinblastine. *Br. J. Derm.* **84**, 335

Givan, K.F. and Jezequel, A-M. (1969). Infectious canine hepatitis. *Lab. Invest.* **20**, 36

Godman, G. and Porter, K.R. (1960). Chondrogenesis, studied with the electron microscope. *J. biophys. biochem. Cytol.* **8**, 719

Goldblatt, P.J. (1969). The endoplasmic reticulum. In *Handbook of Molecular Cytology,* p. 1101. Ed. by A. Lima-de-Faria. Amsterdam and London: North Holland Publ.

Gompel, C. (1971). Ultrastructure of endometrial carcinoma. *Cancer* **28**, 745

Goodman, H.M. and Rich, A. (1963). Mechanism of polyribosome action during protein synthesis. *Nature, Lond.* **199**, 318

Goodman, J.R., Sylvester, R.A., Talal, N. and Tuffanelli, D.L. (1973). Virus-like structures in lymphocytes of patients with systemic and discoid lupus erythematosus. *Ann. Intern. Med.* **79**, 396

Graf, R. and Heitz, Ph.U. (1980). Tubuloampullar structures associated with the endoplasmic reticulum in pancreatic B-cells. *Cell Tissue Res.* **208**, 507

Grausz, H., Earley, L.E., Stephens, B.G., Lee, J.C. and Hopper, J. (1970). Diagnostic import of virus-like particles in the glomerular endothelium of patients with systemic lupus erythematosus. *New Engl. J. Med.* **283** 506

Gray, E.G. (1959). Axo-somatic and axo-dendritic synapses of the cerebral cortex: An electron microscope study. *J. Anat.* **93**, 420

Gregoriadis, G. (1976). Medical applications of liposome-entrapped enzymes. *Methods in Enzymology* **44**, 698

Grimley, P.M. and Friedman, R.M. (1970). Developments of Semliki Forest virus in mouse brain: an electron microscopic study. *Expl Molec. Path.* **12**, 1

Grimley, P.M. and Schaff, Z. (1976). Significance of tubuloreticular inclusions in the pathobiology of human diseases. *Pathobiology Annual* **6**, 221

Grimley, P.M. and Henson, D.E. (1983). Electron microscopy in virus infections. In *Diagnostic Electron Microscopy* **4**, 1. New York: Wiley

Grimley, P.M., Frantz, M.M., Michelitch, H.J. and Decker, J.L. (1972). Tubuloreticular structures of circulating lymphocytes in systemic lupus erythematosus (SLE). *Arthritis Rheum.* **15**, 112

Grimley, P.M., Kang, Y.-H., Silverman, R.H., Davis, G. and Hoofnagle, J.H. (1983). Blood lymphocyte inclusions associated with α-interferon. *Lab. Invest.* **48**, 30A

Grimley, P.M., Kang, Y-H., Frederick, W., Rook, A.H., Kostianovsky, M., Sonnabend, J.A., Macher, A.M., Quinnan, G.V., Friedman, R.M. and Masur, H. (1984). Interferon-related leukocyte inclusions in acquired immune deficiency syndrome: Localization in T cells. *Am. J. Clin Pathol.* **81**, 147

Grimley, P.M., Davis, G.L., Kang, Y-S., Dooley, J.S., Strohmaier, J. and Hoofnagle, J.H. (1985). Tubuloreticular inclusions in peripheral blood mononuclear cells related to systemic therapy with α-interferon. *Lab. Invest.* **52**, 638

Gross, L. (1970). *Oncogenic Viruses.* 2nd Ed. Oxford: Pergamon Press

Gueft, B. and Kikkawa, Y. (1962). The periodic structure of nuclear and cytoplasmic crystals of dog liver cells. In *Electron Microscopy,* Fifth International Congress on Electron Microscopy, Vol. 2, p. T-5. Ed. by S. Breese. Jr. New York: Academic Press

556

Gyorkey, F. and Sinkovics. J.G. (1971). Microtubules of systemic lupus erythematosus. *Lancet* **i**, 131

Gyorkey, F., Sinkovics, J.G. and Gyorkey, P. (1971). Electron microscopic observations on structures resembling myxovirus in human sarcomas. *Cancer* **27**, 1449

Gyorkey, F., Sinkovics, J.G. and Gyorkey, P. (1982). Tubuloreticular structures in Kaposi's sarcoma. *Lancet* **ii**, 984

Gyorkey, F., Min, K-W., Sinkovics, J.G. and Gyorkey, P. (1969). Systemic lupus erythematosus and myxovirus. *New Engl. J. Med.* **280**, 333

Gyorkey, F., Sinkovics, J.G., Min, K.W. and Gyorkey, P. (1972). A morphologic study on the occurrence and distribution of structures resembling viral nucleocapsids in collagen diseases. *Am. J. Med.* **53**, 148

Haas, J.E. and Yunis, E.J. (1970a). Tubular inclusions of systemic lupus erythematosus. *Exp. Molec. Pathol.* **12**, 257

Haas, J.E. and Yunis, E.J. (1970b). Viral crystalline arrays in human Coxsackie myocarditis. *Lab. Invest.* **23**, 442

Hadjiolov, D. and Markov, D. (1973). Effect of aminoacetonitrile on the fine structure and cytochemistry of hepatic cells in rats fed two carcinogenic N-nitrosodialkylamines. *J. Natl. Cancer Inst.* **50**, 979

Haguenau, F. (1958). The ergastoplasm. Its history, ultrastructure and biochemistry. *Int. Rev. Cytol.* **7**, 425

Haguenau, Fr., Rabotti. G.-F., Lyon, G. and Moraillon, A. (1972). Tumeurs cerebrales experimentales d'etiologie virale chez le chien. *Rev. Neurologique (Paris)* **126**, 347

Halie, M.R., Splett-Romascano, M., Molenaar, I. and Nieweg, H.O. (1975). Parallel tubular structures in lymphocytes. *Acta Haemat.* **54**, 18

Hamdy, F., Holt, S.C. and Sevoian, M. (1974). Ultrastructure of hamster kidney cell culture infected with herpesvirus. *Infection & Immunity* **10**, 270

Hamilton, D.W., Fawcett, D.W. and Christensen, A.K. (1966). The liver of the slender salamander *Batrachoseps attenuatus*. I. The structure of its crystalline inclusions. *Z. Zellforsch. mikrosk. Anat.* **70**, 347

Hammar, S.P., Bockus, D. and Remington, F. (1983b). RER-associated structure in parathyroid glands removed because of tertiary hyperparathyroidism. *Ultrastructural Pathol.* **4**, 283

Hammar, S.P., Bockus, D., Remington, F. and Friedman, S. (1984). More on ultrastructure of AIDS lymph nodes. *New Engl. J. Med.* **310, 924**

Hammar, S.P., Winterbauer, R.H., Bockus, D., Remington, F., Sale, G.E. and Meyers, J.D. (1983a). Endothelial cell damage and tubuloreticular structures in interstitial lung disease associated with collagen vascular disease and viral pneumonia. *Am. Rev. Resp. Dis.* **127**, 77

Hammar, S.P., Winterbauer, R.H., Bockus, D., Remington, F. and Friedman, S. (1985). Idiopathic fibrosing alveolitis: A review with emphasis on ultrastructural and immunohistochemical features. *Ultrastructural Pathol.* **9**, 345

Hanaoka, H. and Friedman, B. (1970). Paired cisternae in human tumor cells. *J. Ultrastruct. Res.* **32**, 323

Hanaoka, H., Friedman, B. and Mack, R.P. (1970). Ultrastructure and histogenesis of giant-cell tumor of bone. *Cancer* **25**, 1408

Hanissian, A.S. and Hashimoto, K. (1972). Paramyxovirus-like inclusions in rubella syndrome. *Pediatrics* **81**, 231

Hardesty, B., Miller, R. and Schweet, R. (1963). Polyribosome breakdown and hemoglobin synthesis. *Proc. natn. Acad. Sci.* **50**, 924

Hashimoto, K. and Chandler, R.W. (1972). Paramyxovirus-like inclusions in systemic lupus erythematosus. *Acta Dermatovener. (Stockholm)* **52**, 263

Hashimoto, K. and Thompson, D.F. (1970). Discoid lupus erythematosus. *Arch. Derm.* **101**, 565

Hashimoto, K., Robison, L.., Velayos, E. and Niizuma, K. (1971). Dermatomyositis. *Arch. Derm.* **103**, 120

Helander, H.F. (1961). A preliminary note on the ultrastructure of the argyrophile cells of the mouse gastric mucosa. *J. Ultrastruct. Res.* **5**, 257

Helyer, B.J. and Petrelli, M. (1978). Cytoplasmic inclusions in spontaneous hepatomas of CBA/H-T6T6 mice. Histochemistry and electron microscopy. *J. Natl. Cancer Inst.* **60**, 861

Henkart, M.P. and Henkart, P.A. (1982). Lymphocyte mediated cytolysis as a secretory phenomenon. *Adv. Exp. Med.* **146**, 227

Henry, K. (1975). Electron microscopy in the non-Hodgkin's lymphomata. *Br. J. Cancer* **31**, Suppl. II, 73

Herdson, P.B. and Kaltenbach, J.P. (1965). Electron microscope studies on enzyme activity and the isolation of thiohydantoin induced myelin figures in rat liver. *J. Cell Biol.* **25**, 485

Herdson, P.B., Garvin, P.J. and Jennings, R.B. (1964a). Reversible biological and fine structural changes produced in rat liver by a thiohydantoin compound. *Lab. Invest.* **13**, 1014

Herdson, P.B., Garvin, P.J. and Jennings, R.B. (1964b). Fine structural changes in rat liver induced by phenobarbital. *Lab. Invest.* **13**, 1032

557

Herman, L. and Fitzgerald, P.J. (1962). Restitution of pancreatic acinar cells following ethionine *J. Cell Biol.* **12**, 297

Herman, L., Eber, L. and Fitzgerald, P.J. (1962). Liver cell degeneration with ethionine administration. In *Proceedings of the Fifth International Congress for Electron Microscopy*, Vol. 2, p. vv-6. Ed. by S.S. Breese, Jr. New York: Academic Press

Herman, L., Sato, T. and Fitzgerald, P.J. (1964). The pancreas. In *Electron Microscopic Anatomy*, p. 72, Ed. by S.M. Kurtz. New York: Academic Press

Herndon, R.M. (1964). Lamellar bodies, an unusual arrangement of the granular endoplasmic reticulum. *J. Cell Biol.* **20**, 338

Heuson-Stiennon, J-A. and Drochmans, P. (1967). Morphogenèse de la cellule musculaire striée étudiée au microscope électronique II. Localisation et structure de glycogène. *J. Microscopie* **6**, 639

Hinrichs, S.H., Jaramillo, M.A., Gumerlock, P.H., Gardner, M.B., Lewis, J.P. and Freeman, A.E. (1985). Myxoid chondrosarcoma with a translocation involving chromosomes 9 and 22. *Cancer Genet. Cytogenet.* **14**, 219

Hinton, D.E., Glaumann, H. and Trump, B.F. (1978). Studies on the cellular toxicity of polychlorinated biphenyls (PCBs). *Virchows Arch. B Cell Path.* **27**, 279

Hirano, A. (1978). Changes of the neuronal endoplasmic reticulum in the peripheral nervous system in mutant hamsters with hind leg paralysis and normal controls. *J. Neuropath. exp. Neurol.* **37**, 75

Hollmann, K.H. (1959). L'ultrastructure de la glande mammaire normale de la souris en lactation étude au microscope electronique. *J. Ultrastruct. Res.* **2**, 423

Holmes, I.H., Wark, M.C. and Warburton, M.F., (1969). Is rubella an arbovirus? II. Ultrastructural morphology and development. *Virology* **37**, 15

Hope, J. (1970). Stereological analysis of the ultrastructure of liver parenchymal cells during pregnancy and lactation. *J. Ultrastruct. Res.* **33**, 292

Hoshino, M. (1969). 'Polysome-lamellae complex' in the adenoma cells of the human adrenal cortex. *J. Ultrastruct. Res.* **27**, 205

Houk, E.J. (1977). Endoplasmic reticular inclusions in the Malpighian tubules of the Mosquito, *Culex tarsalis. J. Ultrastruct. Res.* **60**, 63

Hovig, T., Jeremic, M. and Stavem, P. (1968). A new type of inclusion bodies in lymphocytes. *Scand. J. Haemat.* **5**, 81

Hoyes, A.D. (1969). The human foetal yolk sac. An ultrastructural study of four specimens. *Z. Zellforsch.* **99**, 469

Hruban, Z. (1979). Ultrastructure of hepatocellular tumors. *J. Toxicol.envir. Hlth* **5**, 403

Hruban, Z., Swift, H. and Wissler, R.W. (1963). Alterations in the fine structure of hepatocytes produced by β-3-thienylalanine. *J. Ultrastruct. Res.* **8**, 236

Hruban, Z., Swift, H. and Rechcigl. M. Jr. (1965a). Fine structure of transplantable hepatomas of the rat. *J. natn. Cancer Inst.* **35**, 459

Hruban, Z., Swift, H., Dunn, F.W. and Lewis, D.E. (1965b). Effects of β-3-furylalanine on the ultrastructure of the hepatocytes and pancreatic acinar cells. *Lab. Invest.* **14**, 70

Hruban, Z., Wong, T.-W., Itabashi, M. and Lyon, E.S. (1976). Glomiform and fibrillar cytoplasmic inclusions. *Virchows Arch. B Cell Path.* **20**, 91

Huhn, D. (1968). Neue Organelle im peripheren Lymphozyten? *Deutsch Med. Wschr.* **93**, 2099

Hultin, T. (1961). On the functions of the endoplasmic reticulum. *Biochem. Pharmac.* **5**, 359

Hurd, E.R., Eigenbrodt, E., Ziff, M. and Strunk, S.W. (1969). Cytoplasmic tubular structures in kidney biopsies in systemic lupus erythematosus. *Arthritis Rheum.* **12**, 541

Hurd, E.R., Eigenbrodt, E., Worthen, H., Strunk, S.S. and Ziff, M. (1971). Glomerular cytoplasmic tubular structures in renal biopsies of patients with systemic lupus erythematosus and other diseases. *Arthritis Rheum.* **14**, 539

Hutterer, F., Schaffner, F., Klion, F.M. and Popper, H. (1968). Hypertrophic hypoactive smooth endoplasmic reticulum: a sensitive indicator of hepatotoxicity exemplified by dieldrin. *Science* **161**, 1017

Hutterer, F., Klion, F., Wengraf, A., Schaffner, F. and Popper, H. (1969). Hepatocellular adaptation and injury—structural and biochemical changes following dieldrin and methyl butter yellow. *Lab. Invest.* **20**, 455

Ichihara, I. (1970). The fine structure of testicular interstitial cells in mice during postnatal development. *Z. Zellforsch. mikrosk. Anat.* **108**, 475

Ichikawa, A. (1965). Fine structural changes in response to hormonal stimulation of the perfused canine pancreas. *J. Cell Biol.* **24**, 369

Imamura, M., Block, S.R. and Mellors, R.C. (1975). Electron microscopic study of distinctive structures in peripheral blood lymphocytes obtained from twins with systemic lupus erythematosus. *Am. J. Path.* **81**, 561

Ito, S. (1961). The endoplasmic reticulum of gastric parietal cells. *J. biophys. biochem. Cytol.* **11**, 333

Ito, S. and Winchester, R.J. (1963). The fine structure of the gastric mucosa in the bat. *J. Cell Biol.* **16**, 541

Jackson, D., Tabor, E. and Gerety, R.J. (1979). Acute non-A, non-B hepatitis: specific ultrastructural alterations in endoplasmic reticulum of infected hepatocytes. *Lancet* (June 9) 1249

Jacob, F. and Monod, J. (1961). Genetic regulatory mechanisms in the synthesis of proteins. *J. molec. Biol.* **3**, 318

Jenson, A.B., Spjut, H.J., Smith, M.N. and Rapp, F. (1971). Intracellular branched tubular structures in osteosarcoma. *Cancer* **27** 1440

Jensen, O.A. (1985). Cytoplasmic structures in endothelial cells of the choroid. *Ultrastructural Pathol.* **8**, 375

Jensen, W.A. (1968). Cotton embryogenesis. *J. Cell. Biol.* **36**, 403

Jones, A.L. and Armstrong, D.T. (1965). Increased cholesterol biosynthesis following phenobarbital induced hypertrophy of agranular endoplasmic reticulum in liver. *Proc. Soc. exp. Biol. Med.* **119**, 1136

Jones, A.L. and Fawcett, D.W. (1966). Hypertrophy of the agranular endoplasmic reticulum in hamster liver induced by phenobarbital (with a review of the functions of the organelle in the liver). *J. Histochem. Cytochem.* **14**, 215

Kaiserling, E. (1972). Verzweigte tubulare cytoplasmaeinschlusse im menschlichen Lymphknoten. *Beitr. Path. Bd.* **147**, 237

Kamimura, T., Ponzetto, A., Bonino, F., Feinstone, S.M., Gerin, J.L. and Purcell, R.H. (1983). Cytoplasmic tubular structures in liver of HBsAg carrier chimpanzees infected with delta agent and comparison with cytoplasmic structures in non-A, non-B hepatitis. *Hepatology* **3**, 631

Kamiyama, R., Nozawa, Y., Hara, M., Kimoto, M., Yamaguchi, H., Asai, I. and Tsukada, T. (1979). Ribosome-lamella complex and annulate lamellae in acute lymphatic leukaemia. *Acta Haematol. Jpn* **42**, 626

Karasaki, S. (1971). Cytoplasmic and nuclear glycogen synthesis in Novikoff Ascites hepatoma cells. *J. Ultrastruct. Res.* **35**, 181

Katayama, I. and Finkel, H.E. (1974). Leukemic reticuloendotheliosis. A clinicopathologic study with review of the literature. *Am. J. Med.* **57**, 115

Katayama, I. and Schneider, G.B. (1977). Further ultrastructural characterization of hairy cells of leukemic reticuloendotheliosis. *Am. J. Path.* **86**, 163

Katayama, I., Li, C.Y. and Yam, L.T. (1972). Ultrastructural characteristics of the 'Hairy Cells' of leukemic reticuloendotheliosis. *Am. J. Path.* **67**, 361

Katayama, I., Nagy, G.K. and Balogh, K. (1973). Light microscopic identification of the ribosome-lamellae complex in 'hairy cells' of leukemic reticuloendotheliosis. *Cancer* **32**, 843

Kawano, K., Miller, L. and Kimmelstiel, P. (1969). Virus-like structures in lupus erythematosus. *New Engl. J. Med.* **281**, 1228

Keeley, A.F., Iseri, O.A. and Gottlieb, L.S. (1972). Ultrastructure of hyaline cytoplasmic inclusions in a human hepatoma: relationship to Mallory's alcoholic hyalin. *Gastroenterology* **62**, 280

Kelley, R.O. (1971). Ultrastructural comparisons of paired cisternae in leukemic and mesenchymal cells during mitosis. *Anat. Rec.* **171**, 559

Kendrey, G. (1968). Fine structural changes in rat liver cells in response to prolonged thioacetamide. *Path. europ.* **3**, 96

Kimbrough, R.D., Linder, R.E. and Gaines, T.B. (1972). Morphological changes in livers of rats fed polychlorinated biphenyls. Light microscopy and ultrastructure. *Arch. environ. Hlth* **25**, 354

King, B.F. (1971). Differentiation of parietal endoderm cells of the guinea pig yolk sac, with particular reference to the development of endoplasmic reticulum. *Dev. Biol.* **26**, 547

King, N.W., Daniel, M.D., Barahona, H.H. and Meléndez, L.V. (1972). Viruses from South American monkeys: ultrastructural studies. *J. Natl Cancer Inst.* **49**, 273

Kingsbury, E.W. and Voelz, H. (1969). Induction of helical arrays of ribosomes by vinblastine sulfate in *Escherichia coli*. *Science* **166**, 768

Kistler, G. (1973). Discussion in *Intrauterine Infections*. Ciba Foundation Symposium 10 (new series) p. 95. Amsterdam-London-New York: Elsevier-Excerpta Medica-North Holland

Kistler, G.S. (1975). Zytoplasmatische tuburoretikulare Komplexe und Kernspharidien in Zellen rotelninfizierter menschlicher Embryonen und Feten. *Beitr. Path. Bd.* **155**, 101

Klippel, J.H., Grimley, P.M. and Decker, J.L. (1974a). Lymphocyte inclusions in newborns of Mothers with systemic lupus erythematosus. *New Engl. J. Med.* **290**, 96

Klippel, J.H., Grimley, P.M., Decker, J.L. and Michelitch, H.J. (1974b). Lymphocyte tuboreticular structures in lupus erythromatosus. *Ann. Intern. Med.* **81**, 355

Kobayasi, T. and Asboe-Hansen, G. (1972). Virus particles in lupus erythematosus. *Acta Dermatovener. (Stockholm)* **52**, 425

Koestner, A., Kasza, L. and Holman, J.E. (1966). Electron microscopic evaluation of the pathogenesis of porcine polioencephalomyelitis. *Am. J. Path.* **49**, 325

Komiyama, A., Ogawa, M., Eurenius, K. and Spicer, S.S. (1976). Unusual cytoplasmic inclusions in blast cells in acute leukemia. *Arch. Path. Lab. Med.* **100**, 590

Kostianovsky, M. and Ghadially, F.N. (1987). Intracisternal tubules in a case of chronic lymphocytic leukaemia. *J. Submicroscopic Cytol.* **19**, 509

Kostianovsky, M. and Grimley, P.M. (1985). Ultrastructural findings in the acquired immunodeficiency syndrome (AIDS). *Ultrastructural Pathol.* **8**, 123

Kostianovsky, M., Kang, Y.H. and Grimley, P.M. (1983). Disseminated tubuloreticular inclusions in acquired immunodeficiency syndrome (AIDS). *Ultrastructural Pathol.* **4**, 331

Kovacs, E., Horvath, E., and Warren, R.E. (1972). Hepatic lesion in systemic lupus erythematosus: Cytoplasmic tubules in sinusoidal endothelium. *J. Am. Med. Ass.* **219**, 510

Krause, M.W. and Hedinger, C.E. (1985). Pathologic study of parathyroid glands in tertiary hyperparathyroidism. *Human Pathol.* **16**, 772

Krishan, A. (1970). Ribosome-granular material complexes in human leukaemic lymphoblasts exposed to vinblastine sulfate. *J. Ultrastruct. Res.* **31**, 272

Krishan, A. and Hsu, D. (1969). Observations on the association of helical polyribosomes and filaments with vincristine-induced crystals in Earle's L-cell fibroblasts. *J. Cell Biol.* **43**, 553

Krishan, A. and Stenger, R.J. (1966). Effects of starvation on the hepatotoxicity of carbon tetrachloride. A light and electron microscopic study. *Am. J. Path.* **49**, 239

Kumegawa, M., Cattoni, M. and Rose, G.G. (1967). An unusual droplet in submandibular gland of newborn mice. *J. Cell Biol.* **33**, 720

Kumegawa, M., Cattoni, M. and Rose, G.G. (1968). Electron microscopy of oral cells *in vitro* II. Subsurface and intracytoplasmic confronting cisternae in strain KB cells. *J. Cell Biol.* **36**, 443

Kuntzman, R. and Jacobson, M. (1965). Effect of drugs on the metabolism of progesterone by liver microsomal enzymes from various animal species. *Fedn. Proc.* **24**, 152

Kuyama, J., Kanayama, Y., Katagiri, S., Tamaki, T., Yonezawa, T. and Tarui, S. (1985). Tubuloreticular inclusions and paired cisternae induced in human lymphocytes cultured with *Staphylococcus aureus* Cowan 1. *Ultrastructural Pathol.* **8**, 155

Kuyama, J., Kanayama, Y., Mizutani, H., Katagiri, S., Tamaki, T., Yonezawa, T. and Tarui, S. (1986). Formation of tubuloreticular inclusions in mitogen-stimulated human lymphocyte cultures by endogenous or exogenous alpha-interferon. *Ultrastructural Pathol.* **10**, 77

Lafontaine, J.G. and Allard, C. (1964). A light and electron microscope study of the morphological changes induced in rat liver cells by the azo dye 2-Me-DAB. *J. Cell Biol.* **22**, 143

Landolt, A.M., Ryffel, U., Hosbach, H.U. and Wyler, R. (1976). Ultrastructure of tubular inclusions in endothelial cells of pituitary tumors associated with acromegaly. *Virchows Arch. A Path. Anat. Histol* **370**, 129

Lane, B.P. and Lieber, C.S. (1967). Effects of butylated hydroxytoluene on the ultrastructure of rat hepatocytes. *Lab. Invest.* **16**, 342

Leak, L.V., Caulfield, J.B., Burke, J.F. and McKhann, C.F. (1967). Electron microscopic studies on a human fibromyxosarcoma. *Cancer Res.* **27**, 261

Le Beux, Y. (1968). Présence de corpuscules glycogéniques dans le cellule ciliée de l'épithélium tubaire de la lapine. *J. Microscopie* **7**, 445

Le Beux, Y.J. (1969). An unusual ultrastructural association of smooth membranes and glycogen particles: the glycogen body. *Z. Zellforsch. mikrosk. Anat.* **101**, 433

Le Charpentier, Y., Louvel, A., De Saint-Maur, P.P., Daudet-Monsac, M., Leger, L. and Abei Anet, R. (1973). Inclusions tubuleuses endotheliales dans un insulome a stroma amyloide. *Nouv. Presse med.* **2**, 2125

Leduc, E.H. and Bernhard, W. (1962). Electron microscope study of mouse liver infected by ectromelia virus. *J. Ultrastruct. Res.* **6**, 466

Lewis, J.H., Sundeen, J.T., Simon, G.L., Schulof, R.S., Wand, G.S., Gelfand, R.L., Miller, H., Garrett, C.T., Jannotta, F.S. and Orenstein, J.M. (1985). Disseminated talc granulomatosis. *Arch. Path. Lab. Med.* **109**, 147

Linder, J.C. and Staehelin, L.A. (1980). The membrane lattice: A novel organelle of the trypanosomatid flagellate *Leptomonas collosoma*. *J. Ultrastruct. Res.* **72**, 200

Lindseth, R.E., Danigelis, J.A., Murray, D.G. and Wray, J.B. (1967). Spondylo-epiphyseal dysplasia (Pseudochondroplastic type). *Am. J. Dis. Child.* **113**, 721

Lipetz, J. (1970). The fine structure of plant tumours. I. Comparison of crown gall and hyperplastic cells. *Protoplasma* **70**, 207

Lipetz, J. and Galston, A.W. (1959). Indole acetic acid oxidase and peroxidase activities in normal and crown gall tissues of *Parthenocissus tricuspidata*. *Am. J. Bot.* **46**, 193

Liu, P.I., Britton, J.C., Lim, J. and Jennings, D. (1985). Morphological alterations in the lymphoreticular system in acquired immunodeficiency syndrome. *Ann. Clin. Lab. Sci.* **15**, 212

Lombard, C., Cabanie, P. and Izared, J. (1967). Images evoquant l'aspect de virus dans les cellules du sarcome de Sticker. *J. Microscop.* **6**, 81

Long, J.A. and Jones, A.L. (1967a). Observations on the fine structure of the adrenal cortex of man. *Lab. Invest.* **17**, 355

Long, J.A. and Jones, A.L. (1967b). The fine structure of the zona glomerulosa and the zona fasciculata of the adrenal cortex of the opossum. *Am. J. Anat.* **120**, 463

Longnecker, D.S., Crawford, B.G. and Nadler, D.J. (1975). Recovery of pancreas from mild puromycin-induced injury. *Arch. Path.* **99**, 5

Lucky, A.W., Mahoney, M.J., Barrnett, R.J. and Rosenberg, L.E. (1975). Electron microscopy of human skin fibroblasts *in situ* during growth in culture. *Exp. Cell Res.* **92**, 383

Lyon, M.G., Bewtra, C., Kenik, J.G. and Hurley, J.A. (1984). Tubuloreticular inclusions in systemic lupus pneumonitis. *Arch. Path. Lab. Med.* **108**, 599

Ma, M.H. and Blackburn, C.R.B. (1973). Fine structure of primary liver tumors and tumor-bearing livers in man. *Cancer Res.* **33**, 1766

Ma, M.H. and Webber, A.J. (1966). Fine structure of liver tumours induced in the rat by 3'-methyl-4-dimethylaminoazobenzene. *Cancer Res.* **26**, 935

Macadam, R.F. (1970). Fine structure of a functional adrenal cortical adenoma. *Cancer* **26**, 1300

Machín-Santamaría, C. (1978). Ultrastructure of the hypothalamic neurosecretory nuclei of the dormouse (*Eliomys quercinus* L.) in the awakening and hibernating states. *J. Anat.* **127**, 239

Maciejewski, W., Dabrowski, J., Jablonska, S. and Jakubowicz, K. (1973). Virus-like tubular cytoplasmic inclusions in epithelial tumors. *Dermatologica* **146**, 141

McGavran, M.H. and Easterday, B.C. (1963). Rift valley fever virus hepatitis. Light and electron microscopic studies in the mouse. *Am. J. Path.* **42**, 587

McGinley, D.M. and Posalaky, Z. (1984). Microtubuloreticular structures in the cerebral vasculature of a patient with herpes simplex encephalitis. *Ultrastructural Pathol.* **7**, 177

Mackay, B. and Ayala, A.G. (1980). Intracisternal tubules in human melanoma cells. *Ultrastruct. Path.* **1**, 1

McKenna, R.W., Parkin, J., Gajl-Peczalska, K.J., Kersey, J.H. and Brunning, R.D. (1977a). Ultrastructural, cytochemical, and membrane surface marker characteristics of the atypical lymphocytes in infectious mononucleosis. *Blood* **50**, 505

McKenna, R.W., Parkin, J., Kersey, J.H., Gajl-Peczalska, K.J., Peterson, L, and Brunning, R.D. (1977b). Chronic lymphoproliferative disorder with unusual clinical, morphologic, ultrastructural and membrane surface marker characteristics. *Am. J. Med.* **62**, 588

McLean, N. (1978). Unusual aggregations of tubules associated with endoplasmic reticulum in digestive cells of *Alderia modesta* (Mollusca: gastropoda: sacoglossa). *Cell Tiss. Res.* **194**, 179

McNutt, N.S. and Jones, A.L. (1970). Observations on the ultrastructure of cytodifferentiation in the human fetal adrenal cortex. *Lab. Invest.* **22**, 513

Mair, W.G.P. and Tomé, F.M.S. (1972). *Atlas of the Ultrastructure of Diseased Human Muscle.* Edinburgh and London: Churchill Livingstone

Malassine, A. (1974). Localisation ultrastructurale et cytochimique de glycogéne dans le placenta de Chatte: présence de "corps glycogénique". *C.R. Acad. Sc. Paris (Series (D)).* **278**, 629

Maraldi, N.M. and Barbieri, M. (1969). Ribosome crystallization. I. Study on electron microscope of ribosome crystallization during chick embryo development. *J. Submicr. Cytol.* **1**, 159

Maraldi, N.M., Simonelli, L., Pettazzoni, P. and Barbieri, M. (1970). Ribosome crystallization. III. Ribosome and protein crystallization in hypothermic cell cultures treated with vinblastine sulfate. *J. Submicr. Cytol.* **2**, 51

Marks, B.H., Alpert, M. and Kruger, F.A. (1958). Effect of amphenone upon steroidogenesis in adrenal cortex of the golden hamster. *Endocrinology* **63**, 75

Marks, P.A., Rifkind, R.A. and Danon, D. (1963). Polyribosomes and protein synthesis during reticulocyte maturation *in vitro*. *Proc. natn. Acad. Sci.* **50**, 336

Maron, B.J. and Ferrans, V.J. (1974). Aggregates of tubules in human cardiac muscle cells. *J. Mol. Cell. Cardiol.* **6**, 249

Marquart, K-H. (1984). An unusual form of endoplasmic reticulum in mononuclear cells of a giant cell tumor of bone. *Ultrastructural Pathol.* **7**, 161

Marquart, K-H. (1981). Intracisternal crystalline arrays of coated parallel tubules in cells of a human osteosarcoma. *Virchows Arch. A Pathol. Anat.* **391**, 309

Marquet, E. and Sobel, H.J. (1969). Crystalline inclusions in the nuclear envelope and granular endoplasmic reticulum of the fish spinal cord. *J. Cell Biol.* **41**, 774

Martins-Green, M. and Roth, A.M. (1982). Tubular aggregates in the nonpigmented epithelial cells of the ciliary body of the Rhesus monkey. *J. Ultrastruct. Res.* **80**, 206

Matsumura, H., Setoguti, T., Mori, K., Ross, E.R., and Koto, A. (1984). Endothelial tubuloreticular structures in intracranial germinomas. *Acta Path. Jpn* **34**, 1

Maynard, J.A., Cooper, R.R. and Ponseti, I.V. (1972). A unique rough surfaced endoplasmic reticulum inclusion in pseudoachondroplasia. *Lab. Invest.* **26**, 40

Mazur, M.T. and Katzenstein, A-L.A. (1980). Metastatic melanoma: The spectrum of ultrastructural morphology. *Ultrastruct. Path.* **1**, 337

Mehta, P.N. and Ghadially, F.N. (1973). Articular cartilage in corn oil induced lipoarthrosis. *Ann. Rheum. Dis.* **32**, 75

Meldolesi, J., Clementi, F., Chiesara, E., Conti, F. and Fanti, A. (1967). Cytoplasmic changes in rat liver after prolonged treatment with low doses of ethionine and adenine. An ultrastructural and biochemical study. *Lab. Invest.* **17**, 265

Mesquita-Guimarães, J. and Coimbra, A. (1976). Holocrine cell lysis in the rat preputial sebaceous gland. Evidence of autophagocytosis during cell involution. *Anat. Rec.* **186**, 49

Mesquita-Guimarães, J., Pignatelli, D. and Coimbra, A. (1979). Autophagy during holocrine cell lysis in skin sebaceous glands. *J. Submicr. Cytol.* **11**, 435

Metz, G. and Metz, J. (1974). Ultrastrukturelle Cytoplasmastrukturen in peripheren Blutzellen bei Erythematodes. *Arch. Derm. Forsch.* **249**, 35

Mierau, G.W., Favara, B.E. and Brenman, J.M. (1982). Electron microscopy in histiocytosis X. *Ultrastructural Pathol.* **3**, 137

Mikata, A. and Luse, S.A. (1964). Ultrastructural changes in the rat liver produced by N-2-fluorenyldiacetamide. *Am. J. Path.* **44**, 455

Mikata, A., Suzuki, S., Suzuki, H., Higo, O. and Shimoyama, M. (1984). Ribosome-lamella complex of the lymphocytes in a case of plasmacytic lymphadenopathy with polyclonal hypergammaglobulinemia. *Ultrastructural Pathol.* **6**, 161

Min, K-W. (1982). Intracellular structures in an astrocytoma. *Ultrastructural Pathol.* **3**, 199

Mirra, S.S., Miles, M.L. and Jacobs, J. (1981). The coexistence of ribosome-lamella complex and annulate lamellae in chronic lymphocytic leukaemia. *Ultrastructural Pathol.* **2**, 249

Miyai, K., Slusser, R.J. and Ruebner, B.H. (1963). Viral hepatitis in mice: electron microscopic study. *Exp. Molec. Path.* **2**, 464

Mizuhira, V., Amakawa, T., Yamashina, S., Shirai, N. and Utida, S. (1970). Electron microscopic studies on the localization of sodium ions and sodium-potassium activated adenosinetriphosphatase in chloride cells of eel gills. *Exp. Cell Res.* **59**, 346

Möbius, W., Hennekeuser, H.H., Westerhausen, M., Stang-Voss, C. and Lesch, R. (1975). Haarzell-leukämie. *Acta haemat.* **53**, 1

Molnar, Z., Stern, W.H. and Stoltzner, G.H. (1971). Cytoplasmic tubular structures in pigmented villonodular synovitis. *Arthritis Rheum.* **14**, 784

Molnar, Z., Metzger, A.L. and McCarty, D.J. (1972). Tubular structures in endothelium in palindromic rheumatism. *Arthritis Rheum.* **15**, 553

Monneron, A. (1969). Experimental induction of helical polysomes in adult rat liver. *Lab. Invest.* **20**, 178

Moore, G.E. and Chandra, S. (1968). Is Degos' disease of viral origin? *Lancet* **ii**, 406

Morales, R. and Duncan, D. (1966). Multilaminated bodies and other unusual configurations of endoplasmic reticulum in the cerebellum of the cat. An electron microscopic study. *J. Ultrastruct. Res.* **15**, 480

Morris, M.D. and Chaikoff, I.L. (1959). The origin of cholesterol in liver, small intestine, adrenal gland, and testis of the rat: dietary versus endogenous contributions. *J. Biochem.* **234**, 1095

Moses, H.L., Stein, J.A. and Tschudy, D.P. (1970). Hepatocellular changes associated with allylisopropylacetamide-induced hepatic porphyria in rats. *Lab. Invest.* **22**, 432

Moura Nunes, J.F., Soares, J.O., Alves de Matos, A.P. and Aguas, A.P. (1980). Tubuloreticular structures in human malignant melanoma. *Arch. Path. Lab. Med.* **104**, 610

Moyer, G.H., Murray, R.K., Khairallah, L.H., Suss, R. and Pitot, H.C. (1970). Ultrastructural and biochemical characteristics of endoplasmic reticulum fractions of the Morris 7800 and Reuber H-35 hepatomas. *Lab. Invest.* **23**, 108

Müller-Hermelink, H.K. and Lennert, K. (1971). Virusahnliche Strukturen in einem Lymphknoten bei Lupus erythematosus visceralis. *Virchows Arch. B Cell Path.* **7**, 367

Müller-Hermelinck, H.K., Lennert, K. and Schlaack, M. (1971). Virusahnliche Strukturen in Leukocyten des peripheren Blutes bei Lupus erythematosus visceralis. *Klin. Wschr.* **49**, 661

Munroe, J.S., Shipkey, F., Erlandson, R.A. and Windle, W.F. (1964). Tumors induced in juvenile and adult primates by chicken sarcoma virus. *Nat. Cancer Inst. Monograph* **17**, 365

Murphy, F.A., Halonen, P.E. and Harrison, A.K. (1968). Electron microscopy of the development of rubella virus in BHK-21 cells. *J. Virol.* **2**, 1223

Murphy, F.A., Harrison, A.K. and Collin, W.K. (1970). The role of extraneural arbovirus infection in the pathogenesis of encephalitis. *Lab. Invest.* **22**, 318

Nabarra, B., Sonsino, E. and Andrianarison, I. (1977). Ultrastructure of a polysome-lamellae complex in a human paraganglioma. *Am. J. Path.* **86**, 523

562

Nakanishi, I., Katsuda, S., Okada, Y., Oda, Y. and Matsubara, F. (1986). The presence of intracytoplasmic confronting cisternae of the endoplasmic reticulum in osteosarcoma cells in interphase. *Acta Pathol., Jpn* **36**, 261

Napolitano, L. and Gagne, H.T. (1963). Lipid-depleted white adipose cells: an electron microscope study. *Anat. Res.* **147**, 273

New, R.R.C., Chance, M.L., Thomas, S.C. and Peters, W. (1978). Antileishmanial activity of antimonials entrapped in liposomes. *Nature* **272**, 55

Newstead, J.D. (1971). Observations on the relationship between 'Chloride-Type' and 'Pseudobranch Type' cells in the gills of a fish, *Oligocottus maculosus*. *Z. Zellforsch.* **116**, 1

Nieland, N.W., Hashimoto, K. and Masi, A.T. (1972). Microtubular inclusions in normal skin of systemic lupus erythematosus patients. *Arthritis Rheum.* **15**, 193

Nii, S., Morgan, C. and Rose, H.M. (1968). Electron microscopy of Herpes Simplex Virus. II. Sequence of development. *J. Virol.* **2**, 517

Nimmo Wilkie, J.S. and Ghadially, F.N. (1987). Confronting cisternae complexes in Purkinje cells of a dog. *J. Submicroscopic Cytol.* **19**, 433

Nishida, S. and Howard, R.O. (1968). Is Dego's disease of viral origin? *Lancet* **i**, 1200

Nishizumi, M. (1970). Light and electron microscope study of chlorobiphenyl poisoning in mouse and monkey liver. *Arch. environ. Hlth* **21**, 620

Noonan, S.M., Weiss, L. and Riddle, J.M. (1976). Ultrastructural observations of cytoplasmic inclusions in Tay-Sachs lymphocytes. *Arch. Pathol. Lab. Med.* **100**, 595

Norback, D.H. and Allen, J.R. (1969). Morphogenesis of toxic fat-induced concentric membrane arrays in rat hepatocytes. *Lab. Invest.* **20**, 338

Norkin, S.A. and Campagna-Pinto, D. (1968). Cytoplasmic hyaline inclusions in hepatoma. *Arch. Path.* **86**, 25

Norton, W.L. (1969). Endothelial inclusions in active lesions of systemic lupus erythematosus. *J. lab. clin. Med.* **74**, 369

Norton, W.L. (1970). Comparison of the microangiopathy of systemic lupus erythematosus, dermatomyositis, scleroderma, and diabetes mellitus. *Lab. Invest.* **22**, 301

Norton, W.L., Velayos, E. and Robison, L. (1970). Endothelial inclusions in dermatomyositis. *Ann rheum. Dis.* **29**, 67

Novi, A.M. (1977). Liver carcinogenesis in rats after aflatoxin B_1 administration. In *Current topics in Pathology* **65**, 115. Ed. by E. Grundmann and W.H. Kirsten, Berlin: Springer-Verlag.

Novikoff, A.B., Roheim, P.S. and Quintana, N. (1964). Lipid in the liver cells of rats fed orotic acid and adenine. *Fedn Proc.* **23**, 126

Oberling, Ch. and Bernhard, W. (1961). The morphology of the cancer cells. In *The Cell,* Vol. 5, p. 405. Ed. by J. Brachet and A.E. Mirsky. New York and London: Academic Press

O'Connell, K.M. (1977). Kaposi's sarcoma in lymph nodes: histological study of lesions from 16 cases in Malawi. *J. clin. Path.* **30**, 696

Ohtsuki, Y., Dmochowski, L., Seman, G., Bowen, J.M. and Johnson, D.E. (1978). Particle-lamella complexes in a case of human benign prostate hyperplasia: Brief communication. *J. Natl. Cancer Inst.* **60**, 299

Oikawa, K. (1975). Electron microscopic observation of inclusion bodies in plasma cells of multiple myeloma and Waldenström's macroglobulinemia. *Tohoku J. exp. Med.* **117**, 257

Onerheim, R.M., Wang, N-S., Gilmore, N. and Jothy, S. (1984). Ultrastructural markers of lymph nodes in patients with acquired immune deficiency syndrome and in homosexual males with unexplained persistent lymphadenopathy. *Am. J. Clin. Pathol.* **82**, 280

Onoe, T. and Ohno, K. (1963). Role of endoplasmic reticulum in fat absorption. In *Intracellular Membranous Structure*, Vol. 14. Ed. by S. Seno and E.V. Cowdry. Okayama, Japan: Japan Society for Cell Biology

Ordóñez, N.G. and Mackay, B. (1983). Ultrastructure of liver cell and bile duct carcinomas. *Ultrastructural Pathol.* **5**, 201

Orenstein, J.M. (1983). Ultrastructural markers in AIDS. *Lancet* **ii**, 284

Orenstein, J.M., Schulof, R.S., and Simon, G.L. (1984). Ultrastructural markers in acquired immune deficiency syndrome. *Arch. Pathol. Lab. Med.* **108**, 857

Orenstein, J.M., Simon, G.L., Kessler, C.M. and Schulof, R.S. (1985). Ultrastructural markers in circulating lymphocytes of subjects at risk for AIDS. *Am. J. Clin. Pathol.* **84**, 603

Orrenius, S. and Ericsson, J.L.E. (1966a). Enzyme-membrane relationship in phenobarbital induction of synthesis of drug-metabolizing enzyme system and proliferation of endoplasmic membranes. *J. Cell Biol.* **28**, 181

Orrenius, S. and Ericsson, J.L.E. (1966b). On the relationship of liver glucose-6-phosphatase to the proliferation of endoplasmic reticulum in phenobarbital induction. *J. Cell Biol.* **31**, 243

Orrenius, S., Ericsson, J.L.E. and Ernster, L. (1965). Phenobarbital induced synthesis of microsomal drug-metabolizing enzyme system and its relationship to the proliferation of endoplasmic membranes. A morphological and biochemical study. *J. Cell Biol.* **25**, 627

Ortega, L.G. and Mellors, R.C. (1957). Cellular sites of formation of gamma globulin. *J. exp. Med.* **106**, 627

Ortega, P. (1966). Light and electron microscopy of dichlorodiphenyltrichlorothane (DDT) poisoning in the rat liver. *Lab. Invest.* **15**, 657

Ortega, P., Hayes, W.J.Jr., Durham, W.F. and Mattson, A. (1956). *DDT in the diet of the Rat; its effect on DDT storage, liver function and cell morphology.* Public Health Monograph, No. 43. Washington DC: US Government Printing Office

Palade, G.E. (1955). Studies on the endoplasmic reticulum. II. Simple dispositions in cells *in situ. J. biophys. biochem. Cytol.* **1**, 567

Palade, G.E. (1956). Intracisternal granules in the exocrine cells of the pancreas. *J. biophys. biochem. Cytol.* **2**, 417

Palay, S. (1958). The morphology of secretion. In *Frontiers of Cytology*, p. 305. New Haven, Conn: Yale University Press

Palay, S. and Karlin, L.J. (1959). An electron microscopic study of the intestinal villus. II. The pathways of fat absorption. *J. biophys. biochem. Cytol.* **5**, 373

Palay, S. and Palade, G.E. (1955). The fine structure of neurons. *J. biophys. biochem. Cytol.* **1**, 69

Palmer, P.E. and Wolfe, H.J. (1976). α_1 antitrypsin deposition in primary hepatic carcinomas. *Arch. Path. Lab. Med.* **100**, 232

Pannese, E. (1969). Unusual membrane-particle complexes within nerve cells of the spinal ganglia. *J. Ultrastruct. Res.* **29**, 334

Papadimitriou, J.M. and Mastaglia, F.L. (1982). Ultrastructural changes in human muscle fibres in disease. *J. Submicrosc. Cytol.* **14**, 525

Pathak, R.K., Luskey, K.L. and Anderson, R.G.W. (1986). Biogenesis of the crystalloid endoplasmic reticulum in UT-1 cells: Evidence that newly formed endoplasmic reticulum emerges from the nuclear envelope. *J. Cell Biol.* **102**, 2158

Payne, C.M. and Glasser, L. (1978). The effect of steroids on peripheral blood lymphocytes containing parallel tubular arrays. *Am. J. Pathol.* **92**, 611

Payne, C.M. and Glasser, L. (1981). Evaluation of surface markers on normal human lymphocytes containing parallel tubular arrays: A quantitative ultrastructural study. *Blood* **57**, 567

Payne, C.M. and Nagle, R.B. (1980). Complement receptors on normal human lymphocytes containing parallel tubular arrays. *Am. J. Pathol.* **99**, 645

Payne, C.M. and Tennican, P.M. (1982). A quantitative ultrastructural study of peripheral blood lymphocytes containing parallel tubular arrays in Epstein-Barr virus and cytomegalovirus mononucleosis. *Am. J. Pathol.* **106**, 71

Payne, C.M., Jones, J.F., Sieber, O.F., Fulginiti, V.A. (1977). Parallel tubular arrays in severe combined immunodeficiency disease: An ultrastructural study of peripheral blood lymphocytes. *Blood* **50**, 55

Payne, C.M., Glasser, L., Fiederlein, R. and Lindberg, R. (1983). New ultrastructural observations: Parallel tubular arrays in human T_γ lymphoid cells. *J. Immun. Meth.* **65**, 307

Perez-Atayde, A.R. (1982). Intracellular structures in an astrocytoma. *Ultrastructural Path.* **3**, 199

Perez-Atayde, A.R., Chang, Y.C. and Seiler, M.W. (1982a). Retroperitoneal lymphoma with ribosome-lamellae complexes, cytoplasmic projections, and desmosome-like junctions: An ultrastructural study. *Ultrastructural Pathol.* **3**, 43

Perez-Atayde, A.R., Hartman, A.S. and Seiler, M.W. (1982b). Ribosome-lamellae complexes in a symptomatic insulinoma. *Arch. Pathol. Lab. Med.* **106**, 221

Perk, K., Hod, I. and Nobel, T.A. (1971). Pulmonary adenomatosis of sheep (Jaagsiekte). 1. Ultrastructure of the tumor. *J. Nat. Cancer Inst.* **46**, 525

Petit, A. (1968). Ultrastructure de la rétine de l'oeil pariétal d'un Lacertilien *Anguis fragilis. Z. Zellforsch.* **92**, 70

Petrik, P. (1968). The demonstration of chloride ions in the 'chloride cells' of the gills of eels (*Anguilla anguilla* L.) adapted to sea water. *Z. Zellforsch. mikrosk. Anat.* **92**, 422

Pfeifer, U., Thomssen, R., Legler, K., Böttcher, U., Gerlich, W., Weinmann, E. and Klinge, O. (1980). Experimental Non-A, Non-B hepatitis: Four types of cytoplasmic alteration in hepatocytes of infected chimpanzees. *Virchows Arch. B. Cell Path.* **33**, 233

Pfeiffer, C.J., Weibel, J., Bair, J.W., Jr. and Roth, J.L.A. (1971). Aspirin-induced damage to the gastric mucosa. *29th Ann. Proc. Electron Microscopy Soc. Am.*, Boston, Mass. Ed. by C.J. Arceneaux

Phillips, M.J., Hetenyi, G. and Adachi, F. (1970). Ultrastructural hepatocellular alterations induced by *in vitro* fructose infusion. *Lab. Invest.* **22**, 370

Phillips, S.J. (1970). A rough endoplasmic reticulum storage disease in chondrocytes. *Anat. Rec.* **166**, 363

Pilotti, S., Carbone, A., Lombardi, L., Tavolato, C. and Rilke, F. (1978). Hairy cell leukemia: Enzyme-histochemical and ultrastructural investigation of one case. *Tumori* **64**, 535

Pincus, T., Blacklow, N.R., Grimley, P.M. and Bellanti, J.A. (1970). Glomerular microtubules of systemic lupus erythematosus. *Lancet* **2**, 1058

Popoff, N.A. and Malinin, T.I. (1976). Cytoplasmic tubular arrays in cells of American Burkitt's type lymphoma. *Cancer* **37**, 275

Porta, E.A., Bergman, B.J. and Stein, A.A. (1965). Acute alcoholic hepatitis. *Am. J. Path.* **46**, 657

Porter, E.R. (1955). Changes in cell fine structure accompanying mitosis. In *Fine Structure of Cells*. VIIIth Congress of Cell biology Symposium held in Leiden 1954. New York: Interscience Publishers

Porter, K.R. (1961). The ground substance; observations from electron microscopy. In *The Cell*, Vol. 2, p. 621. Ed. by J. Brachet and A.E. Mirsky. New York and London: Academic Press

Porter, K.R. (1964). Cell fine structure and biosynthesis of intercellular macromolecules. In *Connective Tissue: Intercellular Macromolecules*, New York Heart Ass. Symp., p. 167. Edinburgh and London: Churchill Livingstone

Porter, K.R. and Bruni, C. (1959). An electron microscope study of the early effects of 3'-Me-DAB on rat liver cells. *Cancer Res.* **19**, 997

Porter, K.R. and Kallman, F.L. (1952). Significance of cell particulates as seen by electron microscopy. *Ann. N.Y. Acad. Sci.* **54**, 882

Porter, K.R. and Pappas, G.D. (1959). Collagen formation by fibroblasts of the chick embryo dermis. *J. biophys. biochem. Cytol.* **5**, 153

Porter, K.R. and Thompson, H.P. (1948). A particulate body associated with epithelial cells cultured from mammary carcinomas of mice of a milk-factor strain. *J. exp. Med.* **88**, 15

Porter, K.R. and Yamada, E. (1960). Studies on the endoplasmic reticulum. V. Its form and differentiation in pigment epithelium cells of the frog retina. *J. biphys. biochem. Cytol.* **8**, 181

Porter, K.R., Claude, A. and Fullam, E.F. (1945). A study of tissue culture cells by electron microscopy. Methods and preliminary observations. *J. exp. Med.* **81**, 233

Posalaki, Z. and Barka, T. (1968). Alterations of hepatic endoplasmic reticulum in porphyric rats. *J. Histochem. Cytochem.* **16**, 337

Posalaki, Z., Szabo, D., Bacsi, E. and Okros, I. (1968). Hydrolytic enzymes during spermatogenesis in rat. An electron microscopic and histochemical study. *J. Histochem. Cytochem.* **16**, 249

Posalaky, Z. and McGinley, D. (1979). Cytoplasmic microtubular structures in metastatic melanoma. *Arch. Pathol. Lab. Med.* **103**, 543

Prineas, J.W. and Wright, R.G. (1978). Macrophages, lymphocytes and plasma cells in the perivascular compartment in chronic multiple sclerosis. *Lab. Invest.* **38**, 409

Procicchiani, G., Miggiano, V. and Arancia, G. (1968). A peculiar structure of membranes in PHA-stimulated lymphocytes. *J. Ultrastruct. Res.* **22**, 195

Pruniéras, M., Cachard-Berger, D. Durepaire, R.M. and Grupper, C. (1971). Étude sur les hématodermies. I. Microscopie électronique. *Acta Dermatol. Syphiligr. (Paris)* **98**, 316

Pruniéras, M., Grupper, C., Durepaire, R., Eisenmann, D. and Regnier, M. (1972). Les inclusions type lupus dans la peau. *Nouv. Presse Med.* **1**, 1133

Prutkin, L. (1967). An ultrastructure study of the experimental keratoacanthoma. *J. Invest. Derm.* **48**, 326

Prutkin, L. and Bogart, B. (1970). The uptake of labelled vitamin A acid in keratoacanthoma. *J. Invest. Derm.* **55**, 249

Quan, S.G., Poolsawat, S.S. and Golde, D.W. (1980). Ultrastructure and tartrate-resistant acid phosphatase localization in a T-cell hairy-cell leukemia cell line. *J. Histochem. Cytochem.* **28**, 434

Rácz, P., Tenner-Rácz, K., Kahl, C., Feller, A.C., Kern, P. and Dietrich, M. (1986). Spectrum of morphologic changes of lymph nodes from patients with AIDS or AIDS-related complexes. *Prog. Allergy* **37**, 81

Rebhun, L.I. (1961). Some electron microscopic observations on membranous basophilic elements of invertebrate eggs. *J. Ultrastruct. Res.* **5**, 208

Recher, L., Sinkovics, J.G., Sykes, J.A. and Whitescarver, J. (1969). Electron microscopic studies of suspension cultures derived from human leukemic and nonleukemic sources. *Cancer Res.* **29**, 271

Reger, J.F. (1961). The fine structure of neuromuscular junctions and the sarcoplasmic reticulum of extrinsic eye muscles of *Fundulus heteroclitus. J. biophys. biochem. Cytol.* **10**, No. 4 Suppl., 111

Reid, I.M., Shinozuka, H. and Sidransky, H. (1970). Polyribosomal disaggregation induced by puromycin and its reversal with time. An ultrastructural study of mouse liver. *Lab. Invest.* **23**, 119

Remmer, H. and Merker, H.J. (1963). Enzyminduktion und Vermehrung von endoplasmatischen Reticulum in der Leberzelle wahrend der Behandlung mit phenobarbital (Luminal). *Klin. Wschr.* **41**, 276

Revel, J.P. (1961). Electron microscopic study of the bat cricothyroid muscle. *Anat. Rec.* **139**, 267 (abstract)

Revel, J.P., Napolitano, L. and Fawcett, D.W. (1960). Identification of glycogen in electron micrographs of thin tissue sections. *J. biophys. biochem. Cytol.* **8**, 575

Reynolds, E.S. (1963). Liver parenchymal cell injury. I. Initial alterations of the cell following poisoning with carbon tetrachloride. *J. Cell Biol.* **19**, 139

Reynolds, E.S. and Yee, A.G. (1967). Liver parenchymal cell injury. V. Relationships between patterns of chloromethane-C incorporation into constituents of liver *in vitro* and cellular injury. *Lab. Invest.* **16**, 591

Rich, A., Penman, S., Becker, Y., Darnell, J. and Hall, C. (1963). Polyribosomes: size in normal and polio-infected HeLa cells. *Science* **142**, 1658

Rich, S.A. (1981). Human lupus inclusions and interferon. *Science* **213**, 772

Rich, S.A., Owens, T.R., Bartholomew, L.E. and Gutterman, J.U. (1983). Immune interferon does not stimulate formation of alpha and beta interferon induced human lupus-type inclusions. *Lancet* **i**, 127

Rifkind, R.A., Danon, D. and Marks, P.A. (1964). Alterations in polyribosomes during erythroid cell maturation. *J. Cell Biol.* **22**, 599

Rizki, T.M. (1967). Ultrastructure of the secretory inclusions of the salivary gland cell in drosophila. *J. Cell Biol.* **32**, 531

Robbins, S.L. (1974). *Pathologic Basis of Disease*, p. 8, Philadelphia: W.B. Saunders Co.

Rosai, J. (1968). Carcinoma of pancreas simulating giant cell tumor of bone. Electron-microscopic evidence of its acinar cell origin. *Cancer* **22**, 333

Rosen, S. and Tisher, C.C. (1968). Observations on the Rhesus monkey glomerulus and juxtaglomerular apparatus. *Lab. Invest.* **18**, 240

Rosenbaum, R.M. and Wittner, M. (1970). Ultrastructure of bacterized and axenic trophozoites of *Entamoeba histolytica* with particular reference to helical bodies. *J. Cell Biol.* **45**, 367

Rosenbluth, J. (1969). Sarcoplasmic reticulum of an unusual fast-acting crustacean muscle. *J. Cell Biol.* **42**, 534

Rosner, M.C. and Golomb, H.M. (1980). Ribosome-lamella complex in hairy cell leukemia. *Lab. Invest.* **42**, 236

Ross, R. and Benditt, E.P. (1964). Wound healing and collagen formation. IV. Distortion of ribosomal patterns of fibroblasts in scurvy. *J. Cell Biol.* **22**, 365

Ross, R. and Benditt, E.P. (1965). Wound healing and collagen formation. V. Quantitative electron microscope radioautographic observations of proline H^3 utilisation by fibroblasts. *J. Cell Biol.* **27**, 83

Ross, W.T. and Cardell, R.R. (1972). Effects of halothane on the ultrastructure of rat liver cells. *Am. J. Anat.* **135**, 5

Rothschild, J. (1963). The isolation of microsomal membranes. *Biochem. Soc. Symp.* **22**, 4

Rouiller, Ch. (1957). Contribution de la microscopie electronique a l'etude du foie normal et pathologique. *Annls. Anat. path.* **2**, 548

Rouiller, Ch. and Simon, G. (1962). Contribution de la microscopie electronique au progres de nos connaissances en cytologie et en histo-pathologie hepatique. *Revue int. Hépat.* **12**, 167

Rozman, C. and Feliu, E. (1983). Ultrastructural markers in AIDS. *Lancet* **ii**, 285

Rozman, C. and Woessner, S. (1978). Caracterización de la tricoleucemia por medio de la microscopia electrónica cuantitativa. *SNGRA* **23**, 303

Rubin, E., Hutterer, F. and Lieber, C.S. (1968). Ethanol increases hepatic smooth endoplasmic reticulum and drug metabolizing enzymes. *Science* **159**, 1469

Ruebner, B.H., Moore, J., Rutherford, R.B., Seligman, A.M. and Zuidema, G.D. (1969). Nutritional cirrhosis in Rhesus monkeys: Electron microscopy and histochemistry. *Exp. Mol. Pathol.* **11**, 53

Rumpelt, H.J. and Michl. W. (1979). Selective vitamin B_{12} malabsorption with proteinuria (Imerslund-Najman-Gräsbeck-syndrome): ultrastructural examinations on renal glomeruli. *Clin. Nephol.* **11**, 213

Russell, W. (1890). An address on a characteristic organism of cancer. *Br. med. J.* **2**, 1356

Said, J.W., Shintaku, I.P., Teitelbaum, A., Chien, K. and Sassoon, A.F. (1984). Distribution of T-cell phenotypic subsets and surface immunoglobulin-bearing lymphocytes in lymph nodes from male homosexuals with persistent generalized adenopathy. *Hum. Pathol.* **15**, 785

Salomon, J.C. (1962a). Modifications ultrastructurales des hepatocytes au cours de l'intoxication chronique par la thioacetamide. In *Electron Microscopy*, Vol. 7, Fifth Int. Congress for Electron Microscopy. Ed. by S.S. Breese, Jr. New York: Academic Press

Salomon, J.C. (1962b). Modifications des cellules du parenchyme hepatique du rat sous l'effet de la thioacetamide. Etude au microscope électronique des lesions observées a la phase tardive d'une intoxication chronique. *J. Ultrastruct. Res.* **7**, 293

Sanel, F.T. and Lepore, M.J. (1968). Granular and crystalline deposits in perinuclear and ergastoplasmic cisternae of human lamina propria cells. *Exp. Molec. Path.* **9**, 110

Schaff, Z., Tabor, E., Jackson, D.R. and Gerety, R.J. (1983). AIDS-associated ultrastructural changes. *Lancet* **i**, 1336

Schaff, Z., Tabor, E., Jackson, D.R. and Gerety, R.J. (1984). Ultrastructural alterations in serial liver biopsy specimens from chimpanzees experimentally infected with a human non-A, non-B hepatitis agent. *Virchows Arch B Cell Pathol.* **45**, 301

566

Schaff, Z., Lapis, K., Keresztury, S., Kollath, Z., Herics, M. and Hollos, I. (1982). Occurrence of tubuloreticular inclusions in acute viral hepatitis. *Ultrastructural Pathol.* **3**, 169

Schaffner, F. (1966). Intralobular changes in hepatocytes and the electron microscopic mesenchymal response in acute viral hepatitis. *Medicine, Baltimore* **45**, 547

Scharff, M.D. and Robbins, E. (1966). Polyribosome disaggregation during metaphase. *Science* **151**, 992

Schenk, P. and Konrad, K. (1985). Ultrastructure of Kaposi's sarcoma in acquired immune deficiency syndrome (AIDS). *Arch. Otorhinolarygol.* **242**, 305

Schenk, P., Konrad, K. and Rappersberger, K. (1986). Tubuloreticular structures in peripheral blood cells from patients with AIDS-associated Kaposi's sarcoma. *Arch. Dermatol. Res.* **278**, 249

Schiaffino, S. and Hanzlíková, V. (1972). Autophagic degradation of glycogen in skeletal muscles of the newborn rat. *J. Cell Biol.* **52**, 41

Schindler, W.J. and Knigge, K.M. (1959). Adrenal cortical secretion by the golden hamster. *Endocrinology* **65**, 739

Schlunk, F.F. and Lombardi, B. (1967). Liver liposomes. I. Isolation and chemical characterization. *Lab. Invest.* **17**, 30

Schnitzer, B. and Kass, L. (1974). Hairy-cell leukemia. A clinicopathologic and ultrastructural study. *Am. J. clin. Path.* **61**, 176

Schoning, P., Anderson, N.V. and Westfall, J.A. (1972). Effect of staphylococcal α-toxin on the fine structure of pancreatic acinar cells of dogs. *Am. J. Path.* **66**, 497

Schubert, M. and Hamerman, D. (1968). *A Primer on Connective Tissue Biochemistry.* Philadelphia, Pa: Lea & Febiger

Schumacher, H.R. (1970). Tubular paramyxovirus-like structures in synovial vascular endothelium. *Ann. rheum. Dis.* **29**, 445

Schuurmans Stekhoven, J.H. and van Haelst, U.J.G.M. (1975). Intracytoplasmic granule-lamella structures in visceral epithelial cells of human glomeruli. *Virchows Arch. B Cell Path.* **18**, 61

Schvartz, H., Bonhomme, P., Caulet, S., Beorchia, A., Patey, M. and Caulet, T. (1985). Bone marrow lambda-type light chain crystalline structures associated with multiple myeloma. *Virchows Arch A Pathol. Anat.* **407**, 449

Schwendemann, G. (1976). Lymphocyte inclusions in the juvenile type of generalized ceroid-lipofuscinosis. *Acta neuropath. (Berlin).* **36**, 327

Scow, R.O. (1970). Transport of tryglyceride. Its removal from blood circulation and uptake by tissues. In *Parenteral Nutrition*, p. 294. Ed. by H.C. Meng and D.H. Law. Springfield, Illinois: Charles C. Thomas.

Sebahoun, G., Bayle, J., Muratore, R. and Carcassonne, Y. (1979). Ribosome lamella complex in neoplastic cells of a Sezary's syndrome. *J. Clin. Pathol.* **32**, 1041

Seïte, R. (1969). Recherches sur l'ultrastructure, la nature et la signification des inclusions microfibrillaires paracristallines des neurones sympathiques. *Z. Zellforsch,* **101**, 621

Seman, G., Gallager, H.S., Lukeman, J.M., Dmochowski, L. (1971). Studies on the presence of particles resembling RNA virus particles in human breast tumors, pleural effusions, their tissue cultures, and milk. *Cancer* **28**, 1431

Seman, G., Guillon, J.C., Proenca, M. and Mery, A-M. (1968). Enterovirus observes au microscope electronique dans des biopsies de tumeurs malignes chez le chien. *Rev. Franc. Etudes Clin. et Biol.* **13**, 1006

Sengel, A. and Stoebner, P. (1971). Intracisternal granules in endothelial cells of human pathologic glomeruli. *Virchows Arch. Abt. B. Zellpath.* **7**, 157

Sengel, A., Stoebner, P. and Juif, J. (1971). Les chondrocytes de la maladie de morguio. Vacuoles ergastoplasmiques a inclusions specifiques. *J. Microscop.* **10**, 33

Seybold, J., Bieger, W. and Kern, H.F. (1975). Studies on intracellular transport of secretory proteins in the rat exocrine pancreas. II. Inhibition by antimicrotubular agents. *Virchows Arch. A Path. Anat. Histol.* **368**, 309

Shamoto, M., Murakami, S. and Zenke, T. (1981). Adult T-cell leukemia in Japan: An ultrastructural study. *Cancer* **47**, 1804

Shapiro, S.H., Wessely, Z. and Lipper, S. (1985). Concentric membranous bodies in hepatocytes from a patient with systemic lupus erythematosus. *Ultrastructural Pathol.* **8**, 241

Shearn, M.A., Tu, W.H., Stephens, B.G. and Lee, J.C. (1970). Virus-like structures in Sjogren's syndrome. *Lancet* **i**, 568

Sheldon, H. (1964). The fine structure of the fat cell. In *Fat as a Tissue*, p. 41. Ed. by K. Rodahl and B. Issekutz. New York: McGraw-Hill

Shimizu, Y.K., Feinstone, S.M., Purcell, R.H., Alter, H.J., and London, W.T. (1979). Non-A, non-B hepatitis: ultrastructural evidence for two agents in experimentally infected chimpanzees. *Science* **205**, 197

Shinozuka, H., Reid, I.M., Shull, K.H., Liang, H. and Farber, E. (1970). Dynamics of liver cell injury and repair. I. Spontaneous reformation of the nucleolus and polyribosomes in the presence of extensive cytoplasmic damage induced by ethionine. *Lab. Invest.* **23**, 253

Siddiqui, W.A. and Rudzinska, M.A. (1963). A helical structure in ribonucleoprotein-bodies of *Entamoeba invadens. Nature, Lond.* **200**, 74

Siddiqui, W.A. and Rudzinska, M.A. (1965). The fine structure of axenically-grown trophozoites of *Entamoeba invadens* with special reference to the nucleus and helical ribonucleoprotein bodies. *J. Protozool.* **12**, 448

Sidhu, G.S. (1983). Ultrastructure of AIDS lymph nodes. *New Engl. J. Med.* **309**, 1188

Sidhu, G.S., Stahl, R.E., El-Sadr, W., Cassai, N.D., Forrester, E.M. and Zolla-Pazner, S. (1985). The acquired immunodeficiency syndrome: An ultrastructural study. *Hum. Pathol.* **16**, 377

Siegal, A.M., Casey, H.W., Bowman, R.W. and Traynor, J.E. (1968). Leukemia in a Rhesus monkey (*Macaca mulatta*) following exposure to whole-body proton irradiation. *Blood* **32**, 989

Siekevitz, P. and Palade, G.E. (1958). A cytochemical study on the pancreas of the guinea pig. II. Functional variations in the enzymatic activity of microsomes. *J. biophys. biochem. Cytol.* **4**, 309

Sinkovics, J.G. and Gyorkey, F. (1973). Hodgkin's disease: Involvement of viral agents in the etiology. *J. Med.* **4**, 282

Sinkovics, J.G., Gyorkey, F. and Thoma, G.W. (1969). A rapidly fatal case of systemic lupus erythematosus: Structures resembling viral nucleoprotein strands in the kidney and activities of lymphocytes in culture. *Texas Rep. Biol. Med.* **27**, 3

Sinkovics, J.G., Shirato, E., Martin, R.G., Cabiness, J.R. and White, E.C. (1971). Chondrosarcoma, immune reactions of a patient to autologous tumor. *Cancer* **27**, 782

Sisson, J.K. and Fahrenbach, W.H. (1967). Fine structure of steroidogenic cells of a primate cutaneous organ. *Am. J. Anat.* **121**, 337

Sjostrand, F.S. (1964). The endoplasmic reticulum. In *Cytology and Cell Physiology*, 3rd edn., p. 311. Ed. by G.H. Bourne. New York: Academic Press

Skinnider, L.F. and Ghadially, F.N. (1975). Ultrastructure of acute myeloid leukemia arising in multiple myeloma. *Human Path.* **6**, 379

Slater, T.F. and Sawyer, B.C. (1969). The effects of carbon tetrachloride on rat liver microsomes during the first hour of poisoning *in vitro*, and the modifying actions of promethazine. *Biochem. J.* **111**, 317

Smetana, K., Gyorkey, F., Gyorkey, P. and Busch, H. (1972). Studies on nucleoli and cytoplasmic fibrillar bodies of human hepatocellular carcinomas. *Cancer Res.* **32**, 925

Smith, D.S. (1961). The organization of the flight muscle in a dragonfly, *Aeshna sp. (Odonata). J. biophys. biochem. Cytol.* **11**, 119

Smith, D.S. (1966). The organization and function of the sarcoplasmic reticulum and T-system of muscle cells. *Prog. Biophys. mol. Biol.* **16**, 109

Smith, R.D. and Deinhardt, F. (1968). Unique cytoplasmic membranes in Rous sarcoma virus-induced tumors of a subhuman primate. *J. Cell Biol.* **37**, 819

Smuckler, E.A. and Benditt, E.P. (1963). Carbon tetrachloride poisoning in rats: alteration in ribosomes of the liver. *Science* **140**, 308

Smuckler, E.A., Iseri, O.A. and Benditt, E.P. (1962). An intracellular defect in protein synthesis induced by carbon tetrachloride. *J. exp. Med.* **116**, 55

Sobel, H.J., Marquet, E. and Seely, J.C. (1983). Viruslike particles in hamster liver. *Ultrastructural Pathol.* **5**, 257

Sorenson, G.D. (1964). Electron microscopic observations of bone marrow from patients with multiple myeloma. *Lab. Invest.* **13**, 196

Sprinz, R. and Stockwell, R.A. (1976). Changes in articular cartilage following intraarticular injection of triated glyceryl trioleate. *J. Anat.* **122**, 91

Srere, P.A., Chaikoff, I.L. and Dauben, W.B. (1968). The *in vitro* synthesis of cholesterol from acetate by surviving adrenal cortical tissue. *J. biol. Chem.* **176**, 829

Staehelin, W. and Noll, H. (1963). Breakdown of rat-liver ergosomes *in vivo* after actinomycin inhibition of messenger RNA synthesis. *Science* **140**, 180

Stang-Voss, C. (1972). Ultrastrukturen der zellulären Autophagie. *Z. Zellforsch.* **127**, 580

Stefani, S., Chandra, S., Schrek, R., Tonaki, H. and Knospe, W.H. (1977). Endoplasmic reticulum-associated structures in lymphocytes from patients with chronic lymphocytic leukemia. *Blood* **50**, 125

Stein, Y. and Shapiro, B. (1959). Assimilation and dissimilation of fatty acids by the rat liver. *Am. J. Physiol.* **196**, 1238

Stein, Y. and Stein, Y. (1965). Fine structure of ethanol induced by fatty liver in the rat. *Israel J. Med. Sci.* **1**, 378

568

Stein, Y. and Stein, Y. (1967). The role of the liver in the metabolism of chylomicrons, studied by electron microscopic autoradiography. *Lab. Invest.* **17**, 436

Steiner, J.W. and Baglio, C.M. (1963). Electron microscopy of the cytoplasm of parenchymal liver cells in α-napthylisothiocyanate-induced cirrhosis. *Lab. Invest.* **12**, 765

Steiner, J.W., Carruthers, J.S. and Kalifat, R.S. (1962). Observations on the fine structure of rat liver cells in extrahepatic cholestasis. *Z. Zellforsch, mikrosk. Anat.* **58**, 141

Steiner, J.W., Miyai, K. and Phillips, M.J. (1964). Electron microscopy of membrane-particle arrays in liver cells of ethionine-intoxicated rats. *Am. J. Path.* **44**, 169

Stenger, R.J. (1964). Regenerative nodules in carbon tetrachloride induced cirrhosis. A light and electron microscopic study of lamellar structures encountered therein. *Am. J. Path.* **44**, 31A

Stenger, R.J. (1966). Concentric lamellar formations in hepatic parenchymal cells of carbon tetrachloride-treated rats. *J. Ultrastruct. Res.* **14**, 240

Stenger, R.J. (1970). Progress in gastroenterology. Organelle pathology of the liver. The endoplasmic reticulum. *Gastroenterology* **58**, 554

Sterry, W., Steigleder, G.K., and Bodeux, E. (1979). Kaposi's sarcoma: Venous capillary haemangioblastoma. A histochemical and ultrastructural study. *Arch. Dermatol. Res.* **266**, 253

Stich, M.H., Swiller, A.I. and Morrison, M. (1955). The grape cell of multiple myeloma. *Am. J. clin. Path.* **25**, 601

Stinson, J.C. (1981). Unidentified intracellular structures in an astrocytoma. *Ultrastruct. Pathol.* **2**, 397

Stoebner, P. (1986). Microtubules in plasma cells. *Ultrastruct. Pathol.* **10**, 277

Stoebner, P., Renversez, J.C., Groulade, J., Vialtel, P. and Cordonnier, D. (1979). Ultrastructural study of human IgG and IgG-IgM crystalcryoglobulins. *Am. J. Clin. Pathol.* **71**, 404

Sutherland, J.C., Middleton, E.B., Banfield, W.G. and Lee, C.W. (1980). Lamella-particle complexes in the human placenta. *Path. Res. Pract.* **169**, 323

Suzuki, I., Kamei, H. and Takahashi, M. (1969). Ultrastructural study on the ribosome helix and its change after antigenic stimulation in P3-J cells. *Exp. mol. Path.* **11**, 28

Svoboda, D.J. and Higginson, J. (1963). Ultrastructural changes in liver cells during carcinogenesis. *Am. Ass. Cancer Res. Proc.* **4**, 70

Svoboda, D. and Higginson, J. (1964). Ultrastructural changes produced by protein and related deficiencies in rat liver. *Am. J. Path.* **45**, 353

Svoboda, D., Grady, H.J. and Higginson, J. (1966). Aflatoxin B_1 injury in rat and monkey liver. *Am. J. Path.* **49**, 1023

Tamarin, A. (1971a). Submaxillary gland recovery from obstruction. I. Overall changes and electron microscopic alterations of granular duct cells. *J. Ultrastruct. Res.* **34**, 276

Tamarin, A. (1971b). Submaxillary gland recovery from obstruction. II. Electron microscopic alterations of acinar cells. *J. Ultrastruct. Res.* **34**, 288

Tandler, B. (1984). Honeycomb structures in tumor cells. *Ultrastruct. Path.* **6**, 99

Tandler, B., Erlandson, R.A. and Southam, C.M. (1973). Unusual membrane formations in HEp-2 cells infected with Ilheus virus. *Lab. Invest.* **28**, 217

Tandler, B., Hutter, R.V.P. and Erlandson, R.A. (1970). Ultrastructure of oncocytoma of the parotid gland. *Lab. Invest.* **23**, 567

Tani, E. and Higashi, N. (1972). Particle-lamella complex and lamellar crystalloid in human meningioma. *J. Ultrastruct. Res.* **41**, 334

Tannenbaum, M., Hsu, K.C., Buda, J., Grant, J.P., Lattes, C. and Lattimer, J.K. (1971). Electron microscopic virus-like material in systemic lupus erythematosus: With preliminary immunologic observations on presence of measles antigen. *J. Urol.* **105**, 615

Taura, M. (1978). Origin and fate of paired cisternae in mitotic aortic cells of swine. *J. electron Micros.* **27**, 283

Thiery, J.P. (1960). Microcinematographic contributions to the study of plasma cells. In *Cellular Aspects of Immunity*, p. 59. Ed. by G.E.W. Wolstenholme and M. O'Connor. Ciba Foundation Symposium. Boston, Mass: Little, Brown.

Thoenes, W. (1962). Zur kenntnis des glatten endoplasmatischen retikulums der leberzelle. *Verhand. deutsch. Ges. Path.* **46**, 202

Thoenes, W. and Bannasch, P. (1962). Elektronen- und lichtmikroskopische untersuchungen am cytoplasma der Leberzellen nach akuter und chronischer thioacetamid-vergiftung. *Virchows Arch. path. Anat. Physiol.* **335**, 556

Tillman, L.J. (1981). Metastatic malignant melanoma. A case study with unusual ultrastructure. *Dermatologica* **163**, 343

Tisher, C.C., Kelso, H.B., Robinson, R.R., Gunnells, J.C. and Burkholder, P.M. (1971). Intraendothelial inclusions in kidneys of patients with systemic lupus erythematosus. *Ann. Intern. Med.* **75**, 537

Tokue, A., Yonese, Y., Mato, M. and Ookawara, S. (1985). Unusual intracytoplasmic lamellar bodies in a malignant gonadal stromal tumor. *Virchows Arch. B Cell Path.* **49**, 261

Toner, P.G. (1984). Honeycomb structures in tumor cells. *Ultrastruct. Pathol.* **6**, 99

Toner, P.G. (1963). The fine structure of resting and active cells in the submucosal glands of the fowl proventriculus *J. Anat.* **97**, 575

Trier, J.S. (1958). The fine structure of the parathyroid gland. *J. biophys. biochem. Cytol.* **4**, 13

Tsai, K.S., Grinyer, I., Pan, I.C. and Karstad, L. (1969). Electron microscopic observation of crystalline arrays of virus-like particles in tissues of mink with Aleutian disease. *Can. J. Microbiol.* **15**, 138

Turiaf, J., Basset, F., Nezelof, Ch., Basset, G. and Georges, R. (1969). Histiocytose X pulmonaire. Données de l'exploration fonctionnelle pulmonaire, de l'analyse histopathologique et ultrastructurale des lésions. *Gazz. Sanit. (Milano)* **40**, 1

Turner, A. and Kjeldsberg, C.R. (1978). Hairy cell leukemia: A review. *Medicine* **57**, 477

Tzur, R. and Shapiro, B. (1964). Dependence of microsomal lipid synthesis on added protein. *J. Lipid Res.* **5**, 542

Uzman, B.G., Saito, H. and Kasac, M. (1971). Tubular arrays in the endoplasmic reticulum in human tumor cells. *Lab. Invest.* **24**, 492

Valeri, V., Goncalves, R.P., Cruz, A.R. and Laicine, E.M. (1971). Tubular structure within the granular endoplasmic reticulum of the Pars intermedia of toad hypophysis. *J. Ultrastruct. Res.* **35**, 197

Van Lennep, E.W. and Madden, L.M. (1965). Electron microscopic observations on the involution of the human corpus luteum of menstruation. *Z. Zellforsch.* **66**, 365

Villa-Trevino, S., Farber, R., Staehelin, T., Wettstein, F.O. and Noll, H. (1964). Breakdown and reassembly of rat liver ergosomes after administration of ethionine or puromycin. *J. biol. Chem.* **239**, 3826

Virchow, R. (1858). *Die Cellularpathologie*. Berlin

Vuillaume, M. and de-Thé, G. (1973). Nasopharyngeal carcinoma. III. Ultrastructure of different growths leading to lymphoblastoid transformation *in vitro*. *J. Natl Cancer Inst.* **51**, 67

Waddington, C.H. and Perry, M.M. (1963). Helical arrangement of ribosomes in differentiating muscle cells. *Exp. Cell Res.* **30**, 599

Walker, B.E. (1960). Electron microscopic observations on transitional epithelium of the mouse urinary bladder. *J. Ultrastruct. Res.* **3**, 345

Wang, N-S. (1974). Fine structural alterations in mesothelial cells associated with cardiac anomaly. *Virchows Arch. B Cell Path.* **15**, 217

Ward, A.M., Shortland, J.R. and Darke, C.S. (1971). Lymphosarcoma of the lung with monoclonal (IgM) gammapathy. *Cancer* **27**, 1009

Warner, J.R., Knopf, P.M. and Rich A. (1963). A multiple ribosomal structure in protein synthesis. *Proc. natn. Acad. Sci., USA* **49**, 122

Warren, B.A., Greenblatt, M. and Kommineni, V.R.C. (1972). Tumour angiogenesis: ultrastructure of endothelial cells in mitosis. *Br. J. exp. Path.* **53**, 216

Warshawsky, H., Haddad, A., Goncalves, R.P., Valeri, V. and de Lucca, F.L. (1973). Fine structure of venom gland epithelium of the South American rattlesnake and radioautographic studies of protein formation by the secretory cells. *Am. J. Anat.* **138**, 79

Wassef, M., Leclerc, J.P., Lavergne, A. and Ferrand-Lougnon, J. (1979). Inclusions cylindriques grillagees dans un hemangioblastome cerebelleux. *Arch. Anat. Cytol. Path.* **27**, 171

Weiss, J.M. (1953). The ergastoplasm. Its fine structure and relation to protein synthesis as studied with the electron microscope in the pancreas of the Swiss albino mouse. *J. exp. Med.* **98**, 607

Weiss, P. and Grover, N.B. (1968). Helical array of polyribosomes. *Nat. acad. Sci. USA Proc.* **59**, 763

Welsh, R.A. (1960). Electron microscopic localization of Russell bodies in the human plasma cell. *Blood* **16**, 1307

Werbin, H. and Chaikoff, I.L. (1961). Utilization of adrenal gland cholesterol for synthesis of cortisol by the intact normal and ACTH-treated guinea pig. *Archs Biochem.* **93**, 476

Wetzel, W.J. and Reuhl, K.R. (1980). Microtubular aggregates in the rough endoplasmic reticulum of a myxoid chondrosarcoma. *Ultrastructural Pathol.* **1**, 519

White, J.G. (1972). Giant organelles containing tubules in Chediak-Higashi lymphocytes. *Am. J. Pathol.* **69**, 225

White, R.G. (1954). Observations on the formation and nature of Russell bodies. *Br. J. exp. Path.* **35**, 365

Whitfield, S.G., Murphy, F.A. and Sudia, W.D. (1971). Eastern equine encephalomyelitis virus: an electron microscopic study of *Aedes triseriatus (Say)* salivary gland infection. *Virology* **43**, 110

Winborn, W.B. and Seelig, L.L. (1970). Cytologic effects of reserpine on hepatocytes. An ultrastructural study of drug toxicity. *Lab. Invest.* **23**, 216

Witzleben, C.L. (1972). Lymphocyte inclusions in late-onset amaurotic idiocy. *Neurology* **22**, 1075

Woessner, S. and Rozman, C. (1976). Ribosome-lamellae complex in chronic lymphatic leukaemia. *Blut* **33**, 23

Wood, R.L. (1964). Morphological changes in hepatic cells during recovery from ethionine poisoning. *Anat. Rec.* **148**, 352

Wood, R.L. (1965). The fine structure of hepatic cells in chronic ethionine poisoning and during recovery. *Am. J. Path.* **46**, 307

Wooding, F.B.P. (1968). Ribosome helices in mature cells. *J. Ultrastruct. Res.* **24**, 157

Yamada, E. (1960). The fine structure of the paraboloid in the turtle retina as revealed by electron microscopy. *Anat. Rec.* **137**, 172(abst.)

Yamada, E. and Ishikawa, T.M. (1960). The fine structure of the corpus luteum in the mouse ovary as revealed by electron microscopy. *Kyushu J. med. Sci.* **11**, 235

Yunis, E.J., Agostini, R.M. and Glew, R.H. (1976). Fine structural observations of the liver in α-I-antitrypsin deficiency. *Am. J. Path.* **82**, 265

Zimmerman, K.G., Payne, C.M. and Nagle, R.B. (1984). Ribosome-lamellae complexes in benign plasma cells accompanying neoplastic infiltrates. *Am. J. Clin. Pathol.* **81**, 364

Zlotnik, I. and Harris, W.J. (1970). The changes in cell organelles of neurons in the brains of adult mice and hamsters during Semliki forest virus and Louping ill encephalitis. *Br. J. exp. Path.* **51**, 37

Zucker-Franklin, D. (1963). Virus-like particles in the lymphocytes of a patient with chronic lymphocytic leukaemia. *Blood* **21**, 509

Zucker-Franklin, D. (1964). Structural features of cells associated with the paraproteinemias. *Semin. Hemat.* **1**, 165

6
_____

Annulate lamellae

Introduction

The term 'annulate lamellae' is used to describe an intracytoplasmic membrane system composed of parallel arrays of cisternae bearing at regular intervals small annuli or fenestrae. On rare occasions annulate lamellae have also been found in the nucleus.

Probably the first observations on annulate lamellae were made by McCulloch (1952) and Lansing *et al.* (1952) in oocytes of marine animals. Palade (1955) described this organelle as fenestrated cisternae in the rat spermatocyte and considered it to be a differentiation of the endoplasmic reticulum. The term 'annulate lamellae' was coined by Swift (1956) to describe this organelle in the pancreatic acinar cells of the larval salamander, oocytes of snail and clam, and rat spermatids. Various other terms that have been used to describe this organelle include; 'coarse fibrous component' (McCulloch, 1952), 'periodic lamellae' (Rebhun, 1956), 'secondary membranes' (Merriam, 1959), 'pitted membranes' (Balinsky and Devis, 1963), and 'porous cytomembranes' (Kessel, 1968).

The occurrence of this organelle in vertebrate and invertebrate germ cells, embryonic cells and some tumour cells has frequently been documented. However, this organelle is also found occasionally in some adult somatic cells. The structure and distribution of this organelle in various cell types is dealt with in great detail in an excellent review by Kessel (1968). The functional significance of this organelle is still unknown but, since it is better developed and found more frequently in embryonic and tumour cells than in adult somatic cells, it is speculated that it has a role in cell growth and differentiation.

Intracytoplasmic and intranuclear annulate lamellae

This membrane system, which is now regarded as an organelle in its own right is usually found in the cytoplasm but it is sometimes also seen in the nucleus (*Plates 247–251*). Cytoplasmic annulate lamellae usually present as stacks of cisternae, the edges of which tend to be slightly or markedly dilated. In some cases the cisternae of the annulate lamellae have been reported to be continuous with the cisternae of the rough endoplasmic reticulum. Regular periodic fusion of the paired membranes of the cisternae produces structures reminiscent of nuclear pores.

Indeed, annulate lamellae bear a close resemblance to the structure of the nuclear envelope. The appearance created is that of segments of nuclear envelope stacked in parallel arrays in the cytoplasm. Such stacks may be scattered in the cytoplasm or lie in the juxtanuclear position. In the latter instance such stacks are usually orientated parallel to the nuclear envelope, but examples of annulate lamellae lying at right angles to the nuclear envelope are also known to occur (*Plate 247, Fig. 2*). The number of stacks and the number of lamellae per stack seen in various cells studied to date are also very variable. Kessell (1968) has stated that 'In general, cytoplasmic annulate lamellae in somatic cells are much less extensively developed than in germ cells, especially oocytes'.

Intranuclear annulate lamellae (*Plates 249–251*) have not as yet been observed to occur in stacked parallel arrays. They usually present as solitary lamellae showing straight, branched, curved or circular profiles.

Most reports deal with the occurrence of annulate lamellae in the cytoplasm, a few with their occurrence in the nucleus and fewer still relate to situations where annulate lamellae have been seen both in the cytoplasm and nucleus. Examples where annulate lamellae have been seen both in the cytoplasm and nucleus include: (1) sand dollar eggs (*Dendraster excentricus*) (Merriam, 1959) (*Plate 249*); (2) oocyte of the Ascidian, *Boltenia villosa* Stimpson (Hsu, 1963, 1967); (3) certain plant cells (Franke *et al.*, 1972); (4) trophoblast giant cells of rat placenta (Jollie, 1969); (5) rat hepatoma★ (Merkow *et al.*, 1972); and (6) HeLa cells subjected to periods of hypothermia during cultivation (Newstead, personal communication).

Intracytoplasmic annulate lamellae have been seen in a large number of vertebrate and invertebrate oocytes, spermatocytes, embryonic cells and cells of juveniles, such as: (1) oocytes of (a) echinoderms (Afzelius, 1955; Gross *et al.*, 1960; Kane, 1960; Kessel, 1964a); (b) snail and clam (Rebhun, 1956, 1961; Swift, 1956), (c) sand dollar (Merriam, 1959), (d) tunicates (Hsu, 1963; Kessel, 1964b, 1965) (*Plate 249, Figs. 2 and 3*) (e) necturus (Kessel, 1963a, b), (f) *Drosophila* (Okada and Waddington, 1959), (g) dragon fly (Kessel and Beams, 1969; Kessel, 1983), (h) teleosts (Yamamoto and Onozato, 1965; Kessel 1968; Kessel *et al.*, 1984, 1985), (i) amphibia (Wischnitzer, 1960; Balinsky and Devis, 1963; Kessel, 1969; Scheer and Franke, 1969), (j) several other lower forms such as the planktic foraminifer (*Hastigerin pelagica*), jelly fish (*Hydrozoa* sp.), various worms (Platyhelminths, Acanthocephala, Annelida) (for references *see*

★Numerous cytoplasmic annulate lamellae were present and what appeared to be the early stages of development of intranuclear annulate lamellae, but indubitable intranuclear annulate lamellae were not found.

Plate 247

The annulate lamellae shown in these electron micrographs were found in ciliated columnar cells of bronchial mucosa of patients with pulmonary tuberculosis or bronchial carcinoma. However, the specimens were collected some distance from the lesions in the lung where the mucosa appeared normal. (*From Frasca, Auerbach, Parks and Stoeckenius, 1967*)

Fig. 1. A large stack of annulate lamellae (arrow) is seen in the cytoplasm of a ciliated columnar cell. ×7000

Fig. 2. Orientated perpendicular to the nuclear envelope lie some 50 cisternae of annulate lamellae. Many of the 'pores' in the stack are in register and an ill-defined, filamentous, material is seen extending through them. ×26 000

Fig. 3. Apparent continuity of the cisternae of rough endoplasmic reticulum and annulate lamellae is seen here. Note also the filamentous material extending across the 'pores' in the cisternae and nuclear pore (between arrows). ×52 000

Fig. 4. The cisternae of the rough endoplasmic reticulum are well aligned with the cisternae of the annulate lamellae. The images seen here indicate a continuity between the two cisternal systems. ×72 000

574

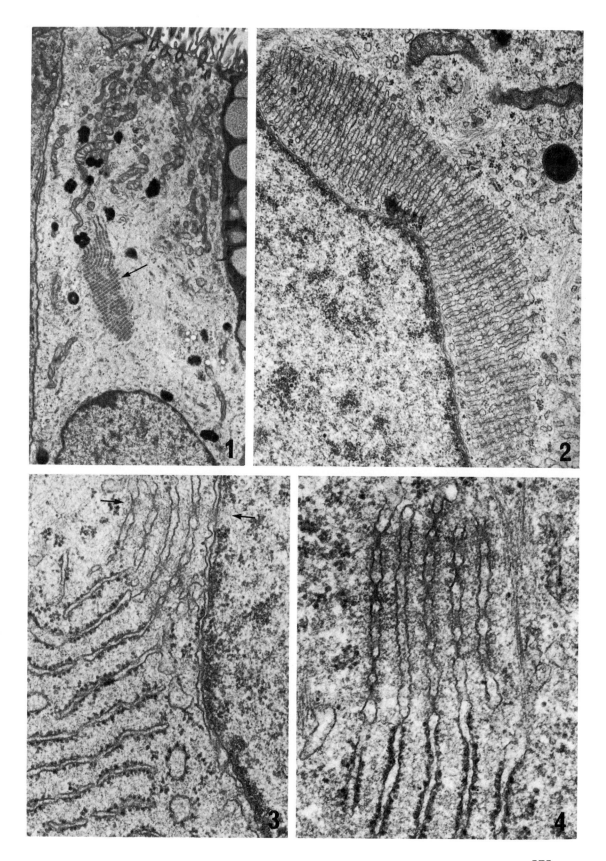

Kessel 1985a), and (k) mammals (rabbit, hamster, chimpanzee, human) (Wartenberg and Stegner, 1960; Hertig and Adams, 1967; Zamboni et al., 1972; Weakley 1969; Longo and Anderson, 1969; Merchant, 1970); (2) spermatocytes or spermatids of: (a) crayfish (Ruthmann, 1958; Kaye et al., 1961), (b) locust (Barer et al., 1960), Drosophila (Kessel, 1981, 1985b), and (c) rat (Swift, 1956); (3) rabbit zygote (Gulyas, 1971); (4) blastoderm of Drosophila (Mahowald, 1962); (5) epithelial cells of rete ovarii of juvenile rabbits (Mori and Fukunishi, 1977); (6) hepatic and pancreatic beta cells of chick embryo (Benzo, 1974); (7) adrenal cortical cells of embryo rat (Ross, 1962); and (8) pancreatic acinar cells of Amblystoma larva (Swift, 1956).

Intracytoplasmic annulate lamellae have been seen in normal and pathological (non-neoplastic) adult somatic cells such as: (9) human axillary apocrine gland cells (Gross, 1966); (10) human parathyroid cells (Boquist, 1980); (11) human pancreatic cells (Lechène-de la Porte, 1973); (12) ciliated columnar cells of human bronchial mucosa (Frasca et al., 1967) (Plate 247); (13) Sertoli cells from normal and azoospermic human testis (Bawa, 1963; Livni et al., 1977); (14) human erythroblasts of dyserythropoietic anaemia (Verwilghen et al., 1975); (15) salivary gland cells of Drosophila (Gay, 1955); (16) islet organ and associated tissues of the cyclostome (Myxine glutinosa) (Boquist and Östberg, 1975); (17) lateral geniculate body neurons in the adult cat (Doolin et al., 1967); (18) adrenal cortical cells of alligator and seagull (Harrison, 1966); (19) epithelium of the ductuli efferentes testis in the common starling (Sturnus vulgaris) (Bellamy and Kendall, 1985); (20) intestinal epithelial cells of rat bearing a subcutaneous sarcoma (Plate 249, Fig. 1); (21) hepatocytes of rats injured by azaserine or 2-fluorenylacetamide or β-3-furylalanine (Hruban et al., 1965a, b; Merkow et al., 1967); and (22) phloem cells of virus infected plants (Steinkamp and Hoefert, 1977).

Intracytoplasmic annulate lamellae have been seen in various cultured cells (normal, neoplastic, virus infected and treated in various ways). These include: (23) chick embryo cells in culture (Benzo, 1972); (24) myocardial cells of chick embryo incubated at abnormal temperatures (Merkow and Leighton, 1966); (25) cultured cells (normal and neoplastic) exposed to antitubulin agents (colchicine or vinblastine) (Krishan et al., 1968; Chemnitz et al., 1977; Kessel and Katow, 1984); (26) cultured cells infected with rubella virus and porcine polioencephalitis virus (Koestner et al., 1966; Merkow et al., 1970; Patrizi and Middelkamp, 1970); (27) HeLa cells (Epstein, 1961); (28) KB cells (human epidermoid carcinoma) (Kumegawa et al., 1967); and (29) cultured neoplastic phaeochromocytes (Kadin and Bensch, 1971).

Intracytoplasmic annulate laminae have been seen in several tumours of experimental animals. These include: (30) mouse sarcoma (Chambers and Weiser, 1964); (31) rat hepatomas (Hruban et al., 1965c; Hoshino, 1963; Locker et al., 1969; Ma and Webber, 1966; Svoboda, 1964); (32) transplantable ascitic plasmacytoma of mice (Grieshaber et al., 1969); (33) Ehrlich ascites tumour and Yoshida ascites tumour (Wessel and Bernhard, 1957); (34) breast carcinoma of rat (Schulz, 1957); and (35) simian adenovirus induced tumours (Merkow et al., 1968).

Intracytoplasmic annulate lamellae have been seen in a few benign human tumours such as: (36) apocrine hidrocystoma (Gross, 1965); (37) adenolymphoma (Tandler, 1966); (38) parathyroid adenomas of man (Elliott and Arhelger, 1966; Boquist, 1970; Ghadially unpublished observations); (39) pituitary adenoma (Kuromatsu, 1968; Horvath and Kovacs, 1974; Kovacs et al., 1975); (40) leiomyoma (Nakayama et al., 1977); and (41) clear cell odontogenic tumour (Eversole et al., 1985).

Plate 248
Rhabdomyosarcoma of prostate. Intracytoplasmic annulate lamellae found in a tumour cell. ×50 000

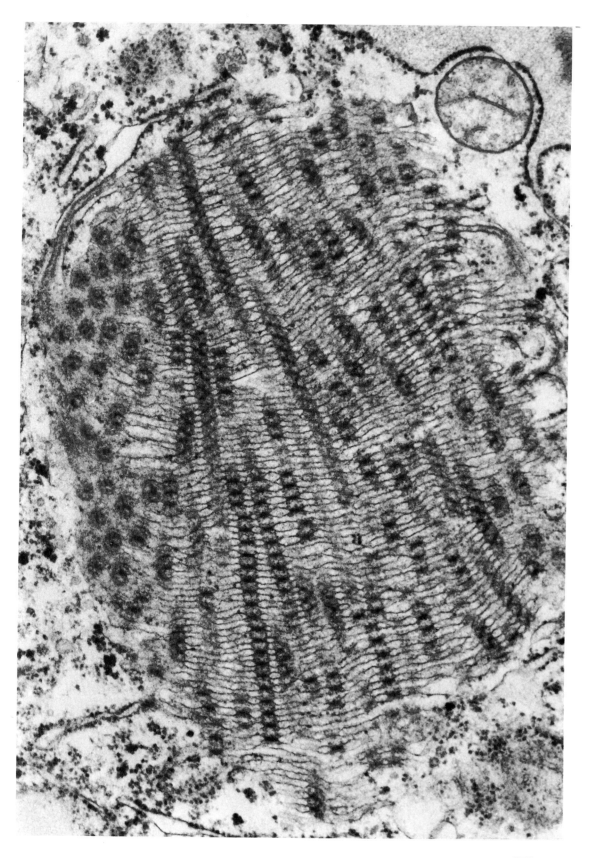

577

The list of human malignant tumours in which intracytoplasmic annulate lamellae have been seen is somewhat more substantial. These include: (42) malignant melanoma (Ainsworth *et al.*, 1976; Nakayama *et al.*, 1977; Tschang *et al.*, 1978; Sun and White, 1979; Hammar *et al.*, 1982); (43) papillary serous cystadenocarcinoma (Roberts *et al.*, 1970); (44) metastatic adenocarcinoma in lymph node (Sobel and Marquet, 1981); (45) metastatic ovarian carcinoma in lymph node (Rennison, 1983); (46) adenocarcinoma and adenosquamous carcinoma of lung (Dingemans, 1982; Schurch, 1982); (47) renal cell carcinoma (Ghadially, unpublished observation) (*Plate 250*); (48) testicular seminoma (Sun and White, 1979); (49) retinoblastoma (Sun and White, 1979); (50) primitive neuroectodermal tumour (Boesel *et al.*, 1978; Sun and White, 1979); (51) metastatic cerebellar tumour (Sun and White, 1979); (52) lymphomas and leukaemias (Hagon and Gunz, 1973; Watanabe *et al.*, 1977; Tschang *et al.*, 1978); (53) fibrous mesothelioma (Tschang *et al.*, 1978); (54) malignant mesenchymal tumour (Bhawan *et al.*, 1978); (55) fibromyxosarcoma (Leak *et al.*, 1967); (56) fibroxanthosarcoma (Merkow *et al.*, 1971); (57) leiomyosarcoma (Nakayama *et al.*, 1977); and (58) rhabdomyosarcoma (Nakayama *et al.*, 1977; Ghadially, 1985) (*Plate 248*).

Intranuclear annulate lamellae have been found in: (1) the oocytes of a variety of vertebrates and invertebrates (Hsu, 1963, 1967; Kessel, 1964b, 1965, 1968; Everingham, 1968a, b); (2) spermatocytes of crayfish (Kessel, 1968); (3) trophoblastic cells of rat and mouse chorioallantoic placenta (Jollie, 1969; Ollerich and Carlson, 1970; Pope and Ollerich, 1973); (4) mouse embryonic cells (Calarco and Brown, 1969; Hillman and Tasca, 1969); (5) certain plant cells (Franke *et al.*, 1972); (6) human melanoma cell in culture (Maul, 1970); (7) Ehrlich ascites cells (Ghadially and Parry, 1974) (*Plate 251*); (8) primitive neuroectodermal tumour (Sun and White, 1979); and (9) a metastatic squamous cell carcinoma in the brain (*Plate 250, Fig. 2*).

The morphological similarity between annulate lamellae and the nuclear envelope has led most workers to conclude that this organelle is in some way derived from the nuclear envelope. It has been suggested that cytoplasmic annulate lamellae may be formed: (1) from fragments of nuclear envelope left behind after mitosis; (2) by delamination from nuclear envelope with the nuclear envelope serving as a mould or template; or (3) from a large evagination of the outer membrane of the nuclear envelope which later becomes infolded to form the cisternae of the annulate lamellae.

Kessel (1968), however, has found that in tunicate oocytes cytoplasmic annulate lamellae are derived from the nuclear envelope by a process of blebbing. He presents convincing morphological evidence that the vesicles derived by this process subsequently fuse and flatten out to form the cisternae of the annulate lamellae. At each 'point' of fusion between two vesicles a 'pore' develops. Harrison (1966) found a similar mechanism operating in alligator adrenal cortical tissue, but in the seagull, annulate lamellae appeared to originate as sheets delaminated from the nuclear envelope, as suggested by Swift (1956).

Plate 249

Fig. 1. Annulate lamellae found in the small intestinal epithelial cell of a rat bearing a carcinogen-induced (7,12-dimethylbenz-α-anthracine) subcutaneous sarcoma in its flank. ×32 000

Fig. 2. Tangential section through the annulate lamellae of a tunicate oocyte showing numerous annulae with a dense central granule. ×25 000 (*From a block of tissue supplied by Dr L.W. Oliphant*)

Fig. 3. Both stacked cytoplasmic annulate lamellae (C) and solitary intranuclear annulate lamellae (N) are seen in this electron micrograph from a tunicate oocyte. ×17 000 (*From a block of tissue supplied by Dr L.W. Oliphant*)

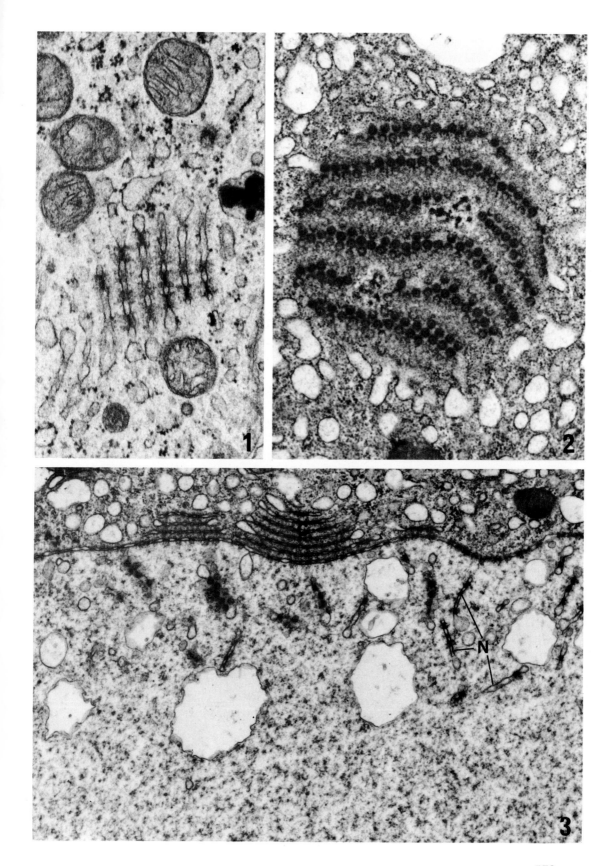

However, the idea that the nuclear envelope serves as a template for the production of annulate lamellae is not too attractive, for studies on the newt oocyte show that, although there are remarkable morphological similarities between the pores on both these structures, there are about twice as many pores on the cytoplasmic annulate lamellae as on the corresponding nuclear envelope (Scheer and Franke, 1969).

It is generally conceded that intranuclear annulate lamellae arise from the inner membrane of the nuclear envelope, but the manner in which these structures arise has been the subject of controversy. According to Kessel (1968) (who studied the oocytes of various invertebrates) intranuclear annulate lamellae arise by a process of blebbing of the inner membrane of the nuclear envelope. It is thought that the vesicles so produced fuse and flatten out to form the lamellae, the points of such fusion presenting as pores. However, other studies have now shown that annulate lamellae can arise in continuity with the inner membrane of the nuclear envelope where no evidence of blebbing is seen (Everingham, 1968b; Jollie, 1969; Ollerich and Carlson, 1970; Ghadially and Parry, 1974). It therefore seems likely that these structures can also arise by a process of growth and elongation of the inner membrane of the nuclear envelope.

The origin of annulate lamellae from pseudoinclusions or invaginations of the nuclear envelope appears to be a rare phenomenon. In the rat placenta Jollie (1969) and Ollerich and Carlson (1970) saw a few examples of annulate lamellae arising from the invaginated nuclear envelope, but most of the intranuclear annulate lamellae were found to originate from the peripheral nuclear envelope. In the Ehrlich ascites tumour cells (*Plate 251*) and in the metastatic squamous cell carcinoma (*Plate 250, Fig. 2*), these structures sprang from the inner membrane of the nuclear envelope only in regions where the envelope was invaginated and formed pseudoinclusions. It would appear that, in these examples at least, the folding and distortion of the nuclear envelope involved in pseudoinclusion formation was probably a factor responsible for the proliferation of the inner membrane of the nuclear envelope leading to the formation of intranuclear annulate lamellae.

Experimental studies where alterations have been noted in the number and size of annulate lamellae (cytoplasmic) are few. They include the work of: (1) Van de Velde and Van de Velde (1968) who found that annulate lamellae present in the epithelial cells of ductus epididymis of castrated rats break down and disappear when androgen therapy is provided; (2) Vandré *et al.* (1979), who found that when certain cultured cells (e.g. KB cells) are exposed to macromomycin (antibiotic and antitumour agent) one of the effects is a proliferation of annulate lamellae; (3) Merkow and Leighton (1966), which shows that enhanced numbers of annulate lamellae are seen when chick embryos are reared at 90°F instead of the normal 100°F; (4) Procicchiani *et al.* (1968) which shows that lymphocytes treated with phytohaemagglutinin develop annulate lamellae; (5) Kessel and Subtelny (1981) which shows that a breakdown of stacks of annulate lamellae occurs in frog (*Rana pipiens*) oocytes after prolonged treatment with progesterone; and (6) Krishan *et al.* (1968) and Kessel and Katow (1984) which shows that

Plate 250

Fig. 1. Renal cell carcinoma. Seen here are profiles of normally sectioned (i.e. perpendicular to the surface of the cisternae) and tangentially sectioned annulate lamellae found in a tumour cell. The former show periodically fused cisternal membranes producing pores (arrows). The latter show an *en face* view of the pores which present as annuli (arrowheads). Note the continuity of annulate lamellae with the rough endoplasmic reticulum. ×31 000

Fig. 2. Metastatic (primary site now known) squamous cell carcinoma in the brain. An annulate lamella with a well demonstrated pore (arrow) is seen in the nucleus of a tumour cell. It arises from an invagination of the nuclear envelope containing cytoplasmic material (C). ×42 000

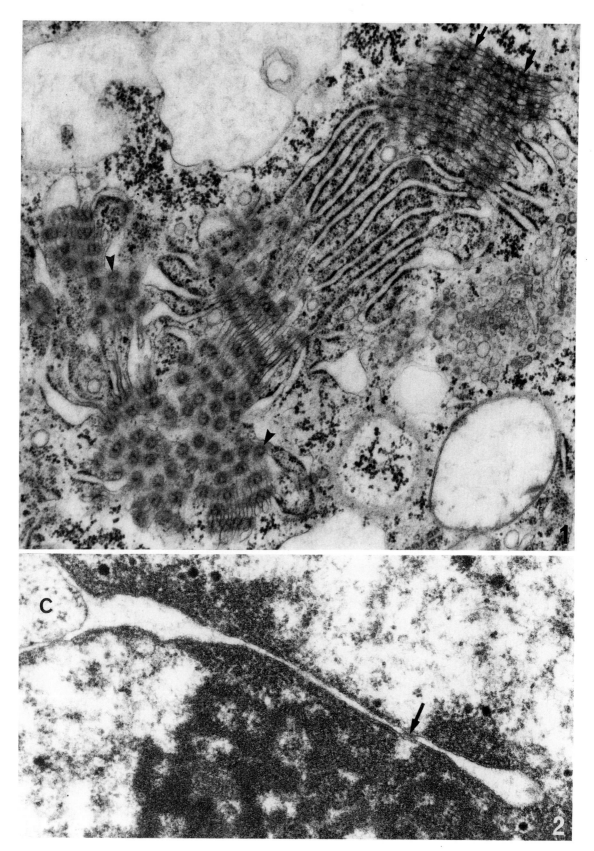

several, but not all cell types (*see* review by Kessel, 1985b) when exposed to various antitubulins (e.g. colchicine, vinblastine sulphate and others) develop an increased amount and number of annulate lamellae as compared to untreated controls.

These studies show that alterations can be produced in the number and size of cytoplasmic annulate lamellae by physical, chemical and hormonal agents, but they shed little light on the function of this organelle.

Despite these experimental studies and observations on annulate lamellae in various cells, the significance and function of this organelle remains unknown.

The difficulty of isolating annulate lamellae precludes biochemical analysis and this hampers our ability to probe the function of this organelle. Under the circumstances its association with other cell constituents (besides the well known association with rough endoplasmic reticulum) is worth studying for it may provide clues as to its function. Kessel (1981, 1985a) has drawn attention to an interesting association between certain dense cytoplasmic masses (also called 'nucleolus-like bodies', *see* pages 1020–1025 for more details) and cytoplasmic annulate lamellae which occur in certain situations such as the spermatocyte stage of spermatogenesis in *Drosphila melanogaster* (and also in some other cell types, especially oocytes and spermatocytes). Dense cytoplasmic masses appear to arise from fragmentation of the nucleolus and the passage of the fragments through the nuclear pores into the cytoplasm. In the very early spermatid stage, annulate lamellae appear within or in close proximity to these dense masses and the appearances seen suggest that the differentiation of annulate lamellae results in utilization or dispersal of the components of the dense cytoplasmic masses and the concomitant development of extensive rough endoplasmic reticulum and many polyribosomes.

Based on this and other studies and observations, Kessel (1985a) has hypothesized that 'annulate lamellae are somehow involved with the mobilization of stored gene products or with the processing of long-lived developmental information' and he considers that pores in annulate lamellae are 'important in the release of stored informational material and consequently involved in gene expression'.

The nature, significance and function of intranuclear annulate lamellae are also obscure. One may look upon such structures found in Ehrlich ascites tumour cells as yet another aberration of nuclear morphology associated with neoplasia or one can argue that since such structures occur also in germ cells and embryonic cells they are a sign of heightened metabolic activity and have some role in cell growth or differentiation.

The close association of intranuclear annulate lamellae and the nucleolus which often occurs also tends to support such a view. This association between annulate lamellae and the nucleolus was frequently noted by us in the Ehrlich ascites tumours and also by Pope and Ollerich (1973) in the rat placenta. These authors suggest that intranuclear annulate lamellae may be involved in the transfer of RNA from the nucleolus to the cytoplasm, or that 'intranuclear annulate lamellae function in the transfer of basic raw materials required for nuclear synthesizing activity'.

Plate 251

From Ehrlich ascites cells.

Fig. 1. An annulate lamella with a well demonstrated pore (arrow) is seen arising from the outer membrane (i.e. an extension of the inner membrane of the nuclear envelope) of a pseudoinclusion (P). ×70 000 (*From Ghadially and Parry, 1974*)

Fig. 2. Two annulate lamellae arising from the outer membrane of a pseudoinclusion (P). ×41 000 (*From Ghadially and Parry, 1974*)

Fig. 3. An annulate lamella is seen arising from the apex of a deep invagination of the nuclear envelope (i.e. a longitudinally cut pseudoinclusion) containing cytoplasmic material (C). ×58 000· (*Ghadially and Parry, unpublished electron micrograph*)

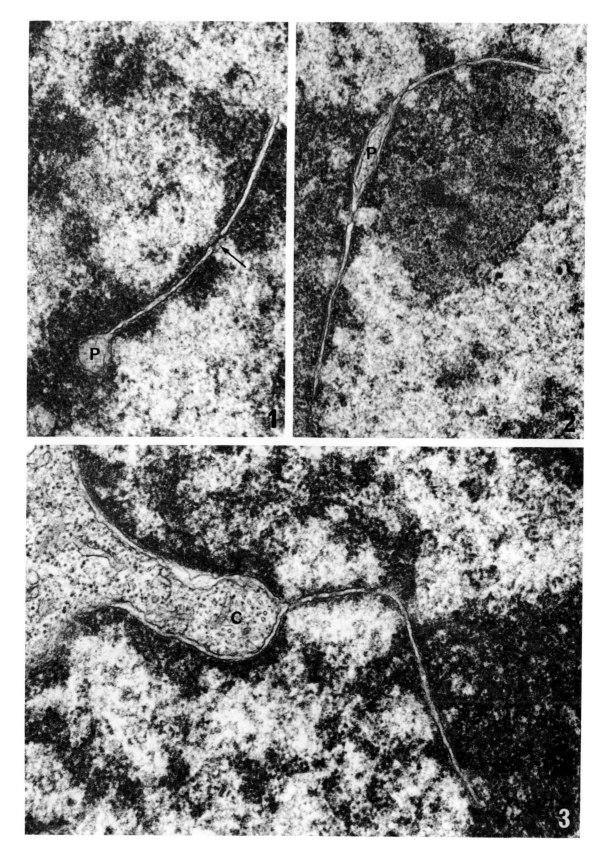

583

References

Afzelius, B.A. (1955). The ultrastructure of the nuclear membrane of the sea urchin oocyte as studied with the electron microscope. *Exp. Cell Res.* **8**, 147

Ainsworth, A.M., Clark, W.H., Mastrangelo, M. and Conger, K.B. (1976). Primary malignant melanoma of the urinary bladder. *Cancer* **37**, 1928

Balinsky, B.I. and Devis, R.J. (1963). Origin and differentiation of cytoplasmic structures in the oocytes of *Xenopus laevis. Acta embryol. morphol. Exp. Palermo* **6**, 55

Barer, R., Joseph, S. and Meek, G.A. (1960). The origin and fate of the nuclear membrane in meiosis. *Proc. R. Soc. B.* **152**, 353

Bawa, S.R. (1963). Fine structure of the Sertoli cell of the human testis. *J. Ultrastruct. Res.* **9**, 459

Bellamy, S.J. and Kendall, M.D. (1985). The ultrastructure of the epithelium of the ductuli efferentes testis in the common starling (*Sternus vulgaris*). *J. Anat.* **140**, 189

Benzo, C.A. (1972). The annulate lamellae of chick embryo liver cells in organ culture. *Anat. Rec.* **174**, 399

Benzo, C.A. (1974). Annulate lamellae in hepatic and pancreatic beta cells of the chick embryo (1). *Am. J. Anat.* **140**, 139

Bhawan, J., Ceccacci, L. and Cranford, J. (1978). Annulate lamellae in a malignant mesenchymal tumor. *Virchows Arch. B Cell Path.* **26**, 261

Boesel, C.P., Suhan, J.P. and Bradel, E.J. (1978). Ultrastructure of primitive neuroectodermal neoplasms of the central nervous system. *Cancer* **42**, 194

Boquist, L. (1980). On the relationship between annulate lamellae and mitochondria in human parathyroid adenomas. *Z. Zellforsch. Anat. Forsch. (Leipzig)* **94**, 241

Boquist, L. (1970). Annulate lamellae in human parathyroid adenoma. *Virchows Arch. B Zellpath.* **6**, 234

Boquist, L. and Östberg, Y. (1975). Annulate lamellae and crystalline inclusions in granular endoplasmic reticulum of the islet organ and associated tissues of a cyclostome, *Myxine glutinosa. Cell Tiss. Res.* **158**, 75

Calarco, P.G. and Brown, E.H. (1969). An ultrastructural and cytological study of preimplantation development of the mouse. *J. Exp. Zool.* **171**, 253

Chambers, V.C. and Weiser, R.S. (1964). Annulate lamellae in sarcoma I cells. *J. Cell Biol.* **21**, 133

Chemnitz, J., Salmberg, K. and Bierring, F. (1977). Observations on the association of annulate lamellae with vinblastine-induced paracrystals in tumour cells *in vitro. Virchows Arch. B Cell Path.* **24**, 147

Dingemans, K.P. (1982). Lymph node adenocarcinoma. *Ultrastructural Path.* **3**, 201

Doolin, P.F., Barron, K.D. and Seber, A. (1967). Annulate lamellae in cat lateral geniculate neurons. *Anat. Rec.* **159**, 219

Elliott, R.L. and Arhelger, R.B. (1966). Fine structure of parathyroid adenomas with special reference to annulate lamellae and septate desmosomes. *Archs Path.* **81**, 200

Epstein, M.A. (1957). The fine structure of the cells in mouse sarcoma 37 ascitic fluids. *J. biophys. biochem. Cytol.* **3**, 567

Epstein, M.A. (1961). Some unusual features of fine structure observed in HeLa cells. *J. biophys. biochem. Cytol.* **10**, 153

Everingham, J.W. (1968a). Intranuclear annulate lamellae in ascidian embryos. *J. Cell Biol.* **37**, 551

Everingham, J.W. (1968b). Attachment of intranuclear annulate lamellae to the nuclear envelope. *J. Cell Biol.* **37**, 540

Eversole, L.R., Belton, C.M. and Hansen, L.S. (1985). Clear cell odontogenic tumor: histochemical and ultrastructural features. *J. Oral Path.* **14**, 603

Franke, W.W., Scheer, U. and Fritsch, H. (1972). Intranuclear and cytoplasmic annulate lamellae in plant cells. *J. Cell Biol.* **53**, 823

Frasca, J.M., Auerbach, O., Parks, V.R. and Stoeckenius, W. (1967). Electron microscopic observations of bronchial epithelium. I. Annulate lamellae. *Exp. molec. Path.* **6**, 261

Gay, H. (1955). Nucleo-cytoplasmic relations in salivary-gland cells of Drosophila. *Proc. natn. Acad. Sci., USA* **41**, 370

Ghadially, F.N. (1985). *Diagnostic Electron Microscopy of Tumours.* 2nd Edition. London: Butterworths

Ghadially, F.N. and Parry. E.W. (1974). Intranuclear annulate lamellae in Ehrlich ascites tumour cells. *Virchows Archs.* **15**, 131

Grieshaber, E., Pedio, G. and Rüttner, J.R. (1969). On plasmacytoma oncogenesis of mice. III. Annulate lamellae with unusual morphology in a plasmacytoid neoplasia of mice (HIPA tumor). *Path. Microbiol. (Basle)* **33**, 1

Gross, B.G. (1965). The apocrine hidrocystoma. An electron microscope study. *Fedn Proc.* **24**, 432

Gross, B.G. (1966). Annulate lamellae in the axillary apocrine glands of adult man. *J. Ultrastruct. Res.* **14**, 64

Gross, P.R., Philpott, D.E. and Nass, S. (1960). 'Electron microscopy of the centrifuged sea urchin egg, with a note on the structure of the ground cytoplasm. *J. biophys. biochem. Cytol.* **7**, 135

Gulyas, B.J. (1971). The rabbit zygote: formation of annulate lamellae. *J. Ultrastruct. Res.* **35**, 112

Hagon, E.E. and Gunz, F.W. (1973). Annulate lamellae in human lymphosarcoma and chronic lymphocytic leukaemia. *Cytobios* **7**, 7

Hammar, S.P., Bockus, D. and Remington, F. (1982). Lymph node adenocarcinoma. *Ultrastructural Path.* **3**, 204

Harrison, G.A. (1966). Some observations on the presence of annulate lamellae in alligator and sea gull adrenal cortical cells. *J. Ultrastruct. Res.* **14**, 158

Hertig, A.T. and Adams, E.C. (1967). Studies on the human oocyte and its follicle. I. Ultrastructural and histochemical observations on the primordial follicle stage. *J. Cell Biol.* **34**, 647

Hillman, N. and Tasca, R.J. (1969). Ultrastructural and autoradiographic studies of mouse cleavage stages. *Am. J. Anat.* **126**, 151

Horvath, E. and Kovacs, K. (1974). Misplaced exocytosis. Distinct ultrastructural feature in some pituitary adenomas. *Arch. Path.* **97**, 221

Hoshino, M. (1963). Submicroscopic characteristics of four strains of Yoshida ascites hepatoma of rats: a comparative study. *Cancer Res.* **23**, 209

Hruban, Z., Swift, H. and Slesers, A. (1965a). Effect of azaserine on the fine structure of the liver and pancreatic acinar cells. *Cancer Res.* **25**, 708

Hruban, Z., Swift, H., Dunn, F.W. and Lewis, D.E. (1965b). Effects of β-3-furylalanine on the ultrastructure of the hepatocytes and pancreatic acinar cells. *Lab. Invest.* **14**, 70

Hruban, Z., Swift, H. and Rechcigl, M. (1965c). Fine structure of transplantable hepatomas of the rat. *Natn. Cancer Inst. J. (US)* **35**, 459

Hsu, W.S. (1963). The nuclear envelope in the developing oocytes of the tunicate *Boltenia villosa*. *Z. Zellforsch. mikrosk. Anat.* **58**, 660

Hsu, W.S. (1967). The origin of annulate lamellae in the Oocyte of the Ascidian, *Boltenia villosa* Stimpson. *Zeitschrift fur Zellforschung* **82**, 376

Jollie, W.P. (1969). Nuclear and cytoplasmic annulate lamellae in trophoblast giant cells of rat placenta. *Anat. Record* **165**, 1

Kadin, M.E. and Bensch, K.G. (1971). Comparison of pheochromocytes with ganglion cells and neuroblasts grown *in vitro*. *Cancer* **27**, 1148

Kane, R.E. (1960). The effect of partial protein extraction on the structure of the eggs of the sea urchin. *Arbacia punctulata*. *J. biophys. biochem. Cytol.* **7**, 21

Kaye, G.I., Pappas, G.D., Yasuzumi, G. and Yamamoto, H. (1961) The distribution of the endoplasmic reticulum during spermatogenesis in the crayfish *Cambaroides japonicus*. *Z. Zellforsch. mikrosk. Anat.* **53**, 159

Kessel, R.G. (1963a). The formation and subsequent differentiation of cytoplasmic vesicles in oocytes of Necturus. *Anat. Res.* **145**, 363

Kessel, R.G. (1963b). Electron microscope studies on the origin of annulate lamellae in oocytes of Necturus. *J. Cell Biol.* **19**, 391

Kessel, R.G. (1964a). Electron microscopic studies on oocytes of an echinoderm. *Thyone briareus*, with special reference to the origin and structure of the annulate lamellae. *J. Ultrastruct. Res.* **10**, 498

Kessel, R.G. (1964b). Intranuclear annulate lamellae in oocytes of the tunicate, *Styela partita*. *Z. Zellforsch. mikrosk. Anat.* **63**, 37

Kessel, R.G. (1965). Intranuclear and cytoplasmic annulate lamellae in tunicate oocytes. *J. Cell Biol.* **24**, 471

Kessel, R.G. (1968). Annulate lamellae. *J. Ultrastruct Res.* Supp. 10

Kessel, R.G. (1969). The effect of glutaraldehyde fixation on the elucidation of the morphogenesis of annulate lamellae in oocytes of *Rana pipiens*. *Z. Zellforsch.* **94**, 454

Kessel, R.G. (1985a). Annulate lamellae (porous cytomembranes): With particular emphasis on their possible role in differentiation of the female gamete. *Develop. Biol.* **1**, 179

Kessel, R.G. (1985b). The relationships of annulate lamellae, fibrogranular bodies, nucleolus, and polyribosomes during spermatogenesis in *Drosophila melanogaster*. *J. Ultrastruct. Res.* **91**, 183

Kessel, R.G. (1983). Fibrogranular bodies, annulate lamellae, and polyribosomes in the dragonfly oocyte. *J. Morphol.* **176**, 171

Kessel, R.G. (1981). Origin, differentiation, distribution and possible functional role of annulate lamellae during spermatogenesis in *Drosophila melanogaster*. *J. Ultrastruct. Res.* **75**, 72

Kessel, R.G. and Beams, H.W. (1969). Annulate lamellae and 'Yolk Nuclei' in oocytes of the dragonfly *Libellula pulchella*. *J. Cell Biol.* **42**, 185

Kessel, R.G. and Katow, H. (1984). Effects of prolonged antitubulin culture on the ultrastructure of anterior limb bud cells of the chick embryo. *J. Morphol.* **179**, 263

Kessel, R.G. and Subtelny, S. (1981). Alteration of annulate lamellae in the *in vitro*, progesterone-treated, full grown *Rana pipiens* oocyte. *J. Exp. Zool.* **217**, 119

Kessel, R.G., Beams, H.W. and Tung, H.N. (1984). Relationships between annulate lamellae and filament bundles in oocytes of the zebrafish, *Brachydanio rerio. Cell Tissue Res.* **236**, 725

Kessel, R.G., Tung, H.N., Beams, H.W. and Roberts, R. (1985). Freeze-fracture studies of annulate lamellae in zebrafish oocytes. *Cell Tissue Res.* **240**, 293

Koestner, A., Kasza, L. and Kindig, O. (1966). Electron microscopy of tissue cultures infected with porcine polioencephalomyelitis virus. *Am. J. Path.* **48**, 129

Kovacs, K., Horvath, E. and Bilbao, J.M. (1975). Annulate lamellae in adenomas of human pituitary glands. *Acta Anat.* **93**, 249

Krishan, A., Hsu, D. and Hutchins, P. (1968). Hypertrophy of granular endoplasmic reticulum and annulate lamellae in Earle's L Cells exposed to vinblastine sulphate. *J. Cell Biol.* **39**, 211

Kumegawa, M., Cattoni, M. and Rose, G.G. (1967). Electron microscopy of oral cells *in vitro*. 1. Annulate lamellae observed in strain KB cells. *J. Cell Biol.* **34**, 897

Kuromatsu, C. (1968). The fine structure of the human pituitary chromophobe adenoma with special reference to the classification of this tumour. *Arch. Histol. Jpn* **29**, 41

Lansing, A.I., Hillier, J. and Rosenthal, T.B. (1952). Electron microscopy of some marine egg inclusions. *Biol. Bull.* **103**, 294 (Abstract)

Leak, L.V., Caulfield, J.B., Burke, J.F. and McKhann, C.F. (1967). Electron microscopic studies on a human fibromyxosarcoma. *Cancer Res.* **27**, 261

Lechène-de la Porte, P. (1973). Description de structures analogues aux annulate lamellae dans les cellules du pancreas exocrine de l'homme et du rat, normaux ou pathologiques. *C.R. Acad. Sci. (D) (Paris)* **276**, 2549

Livni, N., Palti, Z., Segal, S. and Laufer, A. (1977). Fine structure of Sertoli and Leydig cells in Azoospermic human testis. *Arch. Path. Lab. Med.* **101**, 442

Locker, J., Goldblatt, P.J. and Leighton, J. (1969). Hematogenous metastasis of Yoshida ascites hepatoma in the chick embryo liver: ultrastructural changes in tumour cells. *Cancer Res.* **29**, 1244

Longo, F.J. and Anderson, E. (1969). Cytological events leading to the formation of the two-cell stage in the rabbit: Association of the maternally and paternally derived genomes. *J. Ultrastruct. Res.* **29**, 86

Ma, M.H. and Webber, A.J. (1966). Fine structure of liver tumors induced in the rat by 3'-methyl-4-dimethylaminoazobenzene. *Cancer Res.* **26**, 935

McCulloch, D. (1952). Fibrous structures in the ground cytoplasm of the Arbacia egg. *J. expl. Zool.* **119**, 47

Mahowald, A.P. (1962). Fine structure of pole cells and polar granules in *Drosophila melanogaster. J. exp. Zool.* **151**, 201

Mahowald, A.P. (1963). Ultrastructural differentiation during formation of the blastoderm in the *Drosophila melanogaster* embryo. *Dev. Biol.* **8**, 186

Maul, G.G. (1970). The presence of intranuclear annulate lamellae shortly after mitosis in human melanoma cells *in vitro. J. Ultrastruct. Res.* **31**, 375

Merchant, H. (1970). Ultrastructural changes in preimplantation rabbit embryos. *Cytologia* **35**, 319

Merkow, L. and Leighton, J. (1966). Increased numbers of annulate lamellae in myocardium of chick embryos incubated at abnormal temperatures. *J. Cell Biol.* **28**, 127

Merkow, L., Epstein, S.M., Caito, B.J. and Bartus, B. (1967). The cellular analysis of liver carcinogenesis: ultrastructural alterations within hyperplastic liver nodules induced by 2-fluorenylacetamide. *Cancer Res.* **27**, 1712

Merkow, L., Slifkin, M., Pardo, M. and Rapoza, N.P. (1968). Studies on the pathogenesis of Simian adenovirus-induced tumors. III. The histopathology and ultrastructure of intracranial neoplasms induced by SV 20. *J. Natn. Cancer Inst.* **41**, 1051

Merkow, L.P., Slifkin, M., Pardo, M. and Rapoza, N.P. (1970). Pathologenesis of oncogenic Simian adenoviruses VII. The origin of annulate lamellae in LLC-MK 2 cells infected with SV 30. *J. Ultrastruct. Res.* **30**, 344

Merkow, L.P., Frich, J.C., Slifkin, M., Kyreages, C.G. and Pardo, M. (1971). Ultrastructure of a fibroxanthosarcoma (malignant fibroxanthoma). *Cancer* **28**, 372

Merkow, L.P., Epstein, S.M., Slifkin, M., Farber, E. and Pardo, M. (1972). The cellular analysis of liver carcinogenesis. V. Ultrastructural alterations within hepatocellular carcinoma induced by ethionine. *Lab. Invest.* **26**, 300

Merriam, R.W. (1959). The origin and fate of annulate lamellae in maturing sand dollar eggs. *J. biophys. biochem. Cytol.* **5**, 117

Mori, H. and Fukunishi, R. (1977). Annulate lamellae in rete ovarii of juvenile rabbits. *Virchows Arch. B Cell Path.* **23**, 29

Nakayama, I., Moriuchi, A., Taira, Y., Takahara, O., Itoga, T. and Tsuda, N. (1977). Fine structure study of annulate lamellae complexes in human tumors. *Acta Path. Jap.* **27**, 25

Okada, E. and Waddington, C.H. (1959). The submicroscopic structure of the Drosophila egg. *J. embryol. expl Morphol.* **7**, 583

Ollerich, D.A. and Carlson, E.C. (1970). Ultrastructure of intranuclear annulate lamellae in giant cells of rat placenta. *J. Ultrastruct. Res.* **30**, 411

Palade, G.E. (1955). Studies on the endoplasmic reticulum. II. Simple dispositions in cells *in situ*. *J. biophys. biochem. Cytol.* **1**, 567

Patrizi, G. and Middlekamp, J.N. (1970). Development and changes of annulate lamellae complexes in rubella virus-infected RK-13 cells. *J. Ultrastruct. Res.* **31**, 407

Pope, R.S. and Ollerich, D.A. (1973). Intranuclear annulate lamellae in giant cells of the mouse chorioallantoic placenta. *Anat. Record* **176**, 101

Procicchiani, G., Miggliano, V. and Arancia, G. (1968). A peculiar structure of membranes in PHA-stimulated lymphocytes. *J. Ultrastruct. Res.* **22**, 195

Rebhun, L.I. (1956). Electron microscopy of basophilic structures of some invertebrate oocytes. I. Periodic lamellae and the nuclear envelope. *J. biophys. biochem. Cytol.* **2**, 93

Rebhun, L.I. (1961). Some electron microscope observations on membranous basophilic elements of invertebrate eggs. *J. Ultrastruct. Res.* **5**, 208

Rennison, A. (1983). Annulate lamellae. *Ultrastructural Pathol.* **4**, 281

Roberts, D.K., Marshall, R.B. and Wharton, J.T. (1970). Ultrastructure of ovarian tumors. I. Papillary serous cystadenocarcinomas. *Cancer* **25**, 947

Ross, M.H. (1962). Annulate lamellae in the adrenal cortex of the fetal rat. *J. Ultrastruct. Res.* **7**, 373

Ruthmann, A. (1958). Basophilic lamellar systems in the crayfish spermatocyte. *J. biophys. biochem. Cytol.* **4**, 267

Scheer, U. and Franke, W.W. (1969). Negative staining and adenosine triphosphatase activity of annulate lamellae of newt oocytes. *J. Cell Biol.* **42**, 519

Schulz, H. (1957). Elektronenmikroscopische untersuchungen eines Mammakarzinoms der Ratte. *Oncologia* **10**, 307

Schurch, W. (1982). Lymph node adenocarcinoma. *Ultrastructural Path.* **3**, 201

Sobel, H.J. and Marquet, E. (1981). Lymph node adenocarcinoma. *Ultrastructural Path.* **2**, 395

Steinkamp, M.P. and Hoefert, L.L. (1977). Annulate lamellae in phloem cells of virus-infected *Sonchus* plants. *J. Cell Biol.* **74**, 111

Sun, C.N. and White, H.J. (1979). Annulate lamellae in human tumor cells. *Tissue & Cell* **11**, 139

Svoboda, D.J. (1964). Fine structure of hepatomas induced in rats with *p*-dimethylaminoazobenzene. *J. Natl Cancer Inst.* **33**, 315

Swift, H. (1956). The fine structure of annulate lamellae. *J. biophys. biochem. Cytol.* **2**, 415

Tandler, B. (1966). Warthin's tumour, electron microscopic studies. *Archs Otolar.* **84**, 90

Tschang, T-P., Kasin, J.V., Parnell, D. and Kraus, F.T. (1978). Annulate lamellae in human malignant tumors. *Arch. Path. Lab.* **102**, 426

Van De Velde, R.L. and Van De Velde, S.C. (1968). Annulated lamellae in the ductus epididymidis of fetal and castrated adult rats. *Anat. Rec.* **161**, 427

Vandré, D.D., Shepherd, V.L. and Montgomery, R. (1979). Effects of macromomycin on the ultrastructure and biological properties of cultured mammalian cells. *Cancer Res.* **39**, 4091

Verwilghen, R.L., Broeckaert-van Orshoven, A. and Heynen, M.J. (1975). Dyserythropoiesis and annulate lamellae. *Br. J. Haematol.* **30**, 307

Wartenberg, H. and Stegner, H.E. (1960). Uber die Electronenmikroskopische Feinstruktur des Menschlichen ovarialeies. *Z. Zellforsch. mikrosk. Anat.* **52**, 450

Watanabe, S., Berard, C.W. and Triche, T. (1977). Brief Communication: Annulate lamellae in four cases of diffuse lymphocytic lymphoma. *J. Natl. Cancer Inst.* **58**, 777

Weakley, B.S. (1969). Annulate lamellae in the oocyte of the golden hamster. *Z. Zellforsch Mikrosk. Anat.* **96**, 229

Wessel, W. and Bernhard, W. (1957). Vergleichende elektronenmikroskopische Untersuchung von Ehrlichund Yoshida-Ascitestumorzellen. *J. Krebsforsch,* **62**, 140

Wischnitzer, S.J. (1960). Observations on the annulate lamellae of immature amphibian oocytes. *J. biophys. biochem. Cytol.* **8**, 558

Yamamoto, K. and Onozato, H. (1965). Electron microscope study on the growing oocyte of the goldfish during the first growth phase. *Mem. Fac. Fisheries, Hokkaido Univ.* **13**, 69. (Quoted by Kessel, R.G. (1968). *J. Ultrastruct. Res.* Supp. 10)

Zamboni, L., Thompson, R.S. and Smith D.M. (1972). Fine morphology of human oocyte maturation *in vitro*. *Biol. Reprod.* **7**, 425